DECODING AND ENCODING ENGLISH WORDS

A HANDBOOK FOR LANGUAGE TUTORS

THOMAS BALDWIN JONES, Ph.D.

Second Edition

YORK
PRESS

Baltimore, Maryland

This book was manufactured in the United States of America.

Copyright page by Type Shoppe II Productions, Ltd.
Printing and Binding by Data Reproductions Corporation.

Library of Congress Cataloging-in-Publication Data
Jones, Thomas Baldwin.
    Decoding and encoding English words : a handbook for language tutors / Thomas
Baldwin Jones.--2nd ed.
        p. cm.
    Includes bibliographical references ( ).
    ISBN 0-912752-58-0
    1. Dyslexic children--Education--Handbooks, manuals, etc. 2. Reading--Phonetic
    method--Handbooks, manuals, etc. 3. Language arts--Handbooks, manuals, etc. 4. Tutors
    and tutoring--Handbooks, manuals, etc. I. Title: Handbooks for language tutors. II. Title.

LC4708.5 J66 2000
371.91'44--dc21   00-043409

DECODING AND ENCODING ENGLISH WORDS
TABLE OF CONTENTS

Phonics At a Glance . . . . (Inside of Front Cover.)

Specific Table of Contents for Chapters 1, 2, & 3 . . . . (On Back of this Page.)

Preface i

Introduction ii

Abbreviations used in this book iv

Ch. 1. Basic Phonics & Level 1 Rules *(Getting the Show on the Road.)* . . . 1

Ch. 2. Intermediate Phonics & Level 2 Rules *(And, a Bit More Subtlety.)* 18

Ch. 3. Advanced Phonics & Level 3 Rules *(Onward and Ever Upwards.)* 28

Ch. 4. Rules of "R" Pronunciation *(R's Are Easy.)* 47

Ch. 5. Plurals *(Just How Many Are There?)* 50

Ch. 6. Verbs *(Let's Do or Be Something.)* 53

Ch. 7. Gender *(Masculine, Feminine, or Neuter?)* 57

Appendix i Common Phonics *(Bits and Pieces.)*

Appendix ii Syllabication *(The Cutting Edge.)*

Appendix iii Prefixes *(A Good Beginning.)*

Appendix iv Suffixes *(All's Well That Ends Well.)*

Appendix v Old & Middle English, Old Norse, and other Germanic Languages *(Anglos We Have Heard On High.)*

Appendix vi Old, Middle, & Anglo-French *(The French Connection.)*

Appendix vii Latin Roots *(For Latin Lovers.)*

Appendix viii Modern French, Italian, Spanish and Portuguese *(The Romantic Romance Languages.)*

Appendix ix Greek Combining Forms *(It's All Greek To Me!)*

Appendix x Borrowings from Other Languages *(Yes, There's More!)*

Appendix xi Odds and Ends (Abbreviations, Acronyms, Akin To, Alterations, Apheresis, Aphesis, Back Formations, Coined Words, Contractions, Doublets, Homophones, Imitations, Initials, Interjections, Reduplications, Short For, Trade Names, Variants, Word Blends.)

Appendix xii Words from Names and Places *(Who? Where?)*

Appendix xiii Americanisms, Informal American, Notes on the Term MIND, American Slang *(Only in America!)*

Appendix xiv Black English Vernacular *(Ebonics Bees Fine!)*

Appendix xv A Brief History of the English Language *(Very Brief.)*

The Long Vowel Song; Mini-Flash Card Deck, Bibliography (At end of book.)

Vowel & Consonant Mouth Positions . . . . (Inside back cover.)

> *To* **Barbara A. Bliss**, *a loving and caring teacher,*
> *And to* **Janet**, *my loving and caring wife.*

> Special thanks to my numerous teachers and students who each in his or her own way provided some new insight for me into the nature of the English language.

SPECIFIC TABLE OF CONTENTS FOR CHAPTERS 1, 2, & 3

CHAPTER 1:

1. ă, t, n, c /k/, p, r, f, m, b, v, s, h, d, j, l, g /g/; <u>the</u>, <u>as</u>, <u>has</u>.
2. a /uh/, ĭ, w, k; <u>is</u>, <u>his</u>, <u>was</u>. 3. -ck, qu-, x, y, z, ŏ; <u>said</u>, <u>are</u>, <u>you</u>, <u>your</u>, <u>do</u>, <u>to</u>.
4. *Closed Syllable;* ĕ; egg. 5. *Fizzle Rule;* -ing, -ang, -ink, -ank, th-, sh-, ch-, wh-,
4. *Open syllable;* <u>one</u>, <u>of</u>, <u>off</u>, <u>Mr.</u> <u>Mrs.</u> <u>Ms.</u> <u>there</u>, <u>their</u>, <u>what</u>, <u>where</u>.
6. *Silent E;* bl-, cl-, fl-, gl-, pl-, sl-, br-, cr-, dr-, fr-, gr-, pr-, shr-, thr-, tr-, wr-;
6. <u>does</u>, <u>goes</u>, <u>blood</u>, <u>flood</u>, <u>once</u>, <u>only</u>, <u>done</u>, <u>gone</u>, <u>any</u>, <u>many</u>.
7. dw-, sw-, tw-, ŭ, -tch, g /j/, -dge; <u>who</u>, <u>whom</u>, <u>whose</u>, <u>put</u>, <u>two</u>.
8. sc-, sk-, sm-, sn-, sp-, squ-, st-; -ct, -ft, -ld, -lk, -lp, -lt, -mp, -nch, -nd, -nt, -pt, -sk, -sp,
8. -st, spl-, scr-, spr, str-; <u>some</u>, <u>come</u>, <u>could</u>, <u>should</u>, <u>would</u>, <u>bull</u>, <u>pull</u>, <u>bush</u>, <u>push</u>, <u>odd</u>.
9. c /s/; -all, ar, or, ai-, -ay, ee, er, ir, ur; <u>false</u>, <u>always</u>, <u>door</u>, <u>floor</u>, <u>says</u>, <u>four</u>, <u>sure</u>.
10. oi-, -oy, au-, -aw, ou-, -ow, -ve; <u>our</u>, <u>hour</u>, <u>owe</u>, <u>love</u>, <u>both</u>, <u>whole</u>.
11. o͞o, o͝o, oa-, ea, -igh; <u>move</u>, <u>prove</u>, <u>been</u>, <u>busy</u>.
12. eigh, ie, ear, -ild, -ind, -old, -ost; ū; <u>often</u>, <u>listen</u>, <u>build</u>, <u>buy</u>.
13. oe, o /ô/; *VC/CV;* ei, ey, ui, <u>shoe</u>, <u>toward</u>.
14. war, wor, -alt, -alk; gn, kn, -mb, eu, ue, ew, augh; <u>aunt</u>, <u>sign</u>, <u>sew</u>.
15. a /ä/; qua-, wa-, -ough, gh; <u>though</u>, <u>through</u>, <u>thorough</u>, <u>enough</u>, <u>rough</u>, <u>tough</u>, <u>cough</u>, <u>laugh</u>.
16. *Adjective, Adverb;* -ly, -tion, quar-, -sion, -y; <u>woman</u>, <u>women</u>, <u>bye</u>, <u>eye</u>.
17. sc, -ar, -or; *Adding vowel ending to Silent-E Word. Spelling the Alphabet.*

CHAPTER 2:

18. -ture, -age; *Accent;* <u>sugar</u>, <u>minute</u>, <u>ocean</u>, <u>view</u>, <u>lose</u>, <u>straight</u>.
19. *Schwa;* -ion; *1-1-1-V Rule.* 20. *Voiced & Unvoiced Consonant Pairs;* -mn.
21. *Plurals with -s & -es;* -ed; *More silent letters; Deliberate mispronunciations;*
21. *Plurals of words ending in -y;* <u>usual</u>, <u>beauty</u>.
22. du, tu, -ble, -dle, -fle, -gle, -kle, -ple, -tle, -zle; <u>again</u>, <u>against</u>, <u>cloth</u>, <u>clothes</u>, <u>people</u>.
23. -stle; *Adding suffixes to words ending in -y.*
24. *From Greek:* -y-, ph, rh, th, ch; ch (French); <u>iron</u>, <u>bury</u>.
25. *Blends in syllabication;* -que, -ique, -gue, -igue, gu-, ou,
25. -ation, -etion, -ition, -otion, -ution.
26. *Syllable types; V/CV or VC/V? Ways of protecting the short vowel.*
27. -cial, -tial, -cian, -tian, -cient, -tient, -cious, -tious, -ciate, -tiate, -ial, -ian, -ient, -ious, iate; *V/V.*

CHAPTER 3:

28. -oll; *Adjective degrees; The 2-1-1 V Rule.*
29. *The principal parts of a verb;* ar-r, er-r, ar-V, er-V, -less, -let, -ness.
30. *Parts of speech & pronunciation:* -ate, -ace;
30. *Parts of speech & spelling:* -ous, -us; -ism, -ist
31. *Old English;* -y /ī/ *at end of multi-syllable words; Words ending in -u; Old Norse.*
32. *Silent letters come to life;* More *ough* words; *Case of nouns and pronouns.*
33. -cle, -able, -ible. 34. *Old English prefixes; Latin prefixes, Greek prefixes.*
35. *Old English prefix + root; Latin prefix + root; Greek prefix + root.* 36-37. *Suffixes.*
38. *Latin word indicators.* 39. *Greek word indicators.* 40. *Greek Medical Terms.*
40. *French word indicators.* 41. *Spanish word indicators; Italian word indicators;*
41. *Borrowings from other Sources.* 42-44. *Chameleon prefixes.* 44. *British spellings.*
45-46. *When "i" sounds /ē/.* 46. *Words from names & places; Contractions.*

> Cover: Third grader Carlos Tejeda /tā-h̲ā-thə/; Photographer: Mary Tejeda.

Preface

Although this book may be used as a college text for introducing new reading teachers to the phonetic-rule basis of English, as an introduction for the young linguist, as supplementary material for the speech therapist, as a reference in the whole-language classroom, as a vocabulary enhancement for ACT or SAT test takers, as a parental reference for aiding a child's linguistic development (especially the home schoolers), as a resource for the ambitious adult who just wants to learn more about the nature and structure of the English language, as a guide for the adult and senior classroom reading help volunteers, it is also of special use to the tutors and teachers of students with special language problems, e.g., dyslexic students, who need a multi-sensory approach in learning to read and to spell.

"This d*ay* in v*ai*n th*ey* g*au*ged the *eig*ht gr*ea*t v*a*n*e*s on the g*ao*l , while l*a*zy v*ei*ns danced the ball*et* in the caf*é*." Not a very meaningful sentence, but it does demonstrate twelve ways to spell *long a, /ā/* and three words, *vain, vane,* and *vein,* that sound alike, but have different spellings and meanings! What is this English language? How in the world do we teach it? One can see the temptation to learn individual words in context, to despair of any phonetic help, and to stop a search for sure rule guidance. Yet, as this book will demonstrate, there are good reasons for what goes on in this sentence. These will be considered one by one and as logic dictates, we will go from the common and general to the more unusual and exceptional in our linguistic considerations.

Since *phonics* is absolutely essential for those needing special help with English, three chapters concern its ordered presentation and Appendix i is included as a compendium of all English sounds and their spellings with near exhaustive example listings. Rules of spelling and pronunciation are included. Other chapters explore pronunciation of "R" combinations, plurals, verbs, and gender. Since *Syllabication* aids greatly in "breaking the code" of reading and spelling, it will be a concern in Appendix ii. Appendix iii, *Prefixes,* and Appendix iv, *Suffixes,* show the multifarious beginnings and endings that may be added to root words to aid in our vocabulary expansion. Appendices v through x show the many contributors to English: *Anglo-Saxon, Old French, Latin, Greek, modern French, Spanish, Italian, American Indian,* and a few words here and there from countries and cultures all over the world. Since unusual spellings and pronunciations often accompany the words that English has borrowed, it is most helpful to know the derivation or source of a word. An interesting conglomeration of topics can be found in Appendix xi, *Odds and Ends.* See the Table of Contents for the listing of topics here: Acronyms, Coined Words, Contractions, Homophones, Imitations, Interjections, *etc.* Appendix xii contains a surprising twelve pages of English words that come from people's *Names* and geographical *Places. Only In America,* Appendix xiii, gives attention to Americanisms, Informal American, Notes on the Term "Mind," and American Slang. Appendix xiv concerns *Black English Vernacular* and how its acceptance may well be the first step for many in developing a proficiency in Standard English. Appendix xv, the last, is *A Brief History of the English Language.* The book concludes with appropriate *Flash Card* material that may be enlarged and printed on heavier stock at one's local print shop. A multi-sensory overlay predominates for those not reading and spelling up to their grade level. Suggestions on method of instruction are included in the Introduction.

INTRODUCTION

If you are using this book, you probably do not have to be convinced that about 20% of students need a *MULTI-SENSORY, PHONETIC* orientation in their learning to read and to spell. This has been well documented. So we'll get right to the task at hand. In addition to this book you will need a set of phonics flash cards and reading material appropriate to the expertise and interests of your student. You may use the material at the end of this book for your *card deck*, buy a commercial set, or make your own.

The success of this method can be established early, if the teacher insists that when a student is writing, he or she is also speaking. Thus when asked to represent /s/ on paper, the student will be sounding /s/ while writing *s*. This adds the sense of *hearing* to the sense of *seeing* to the *kinesthetic* (muscular) sense (hand, mouth position and movement of these). A teacher on occasion may also add the *tactile* (touch) sense by having a student trace a letter or letters with his finger on the table or in a sand tray. For writing words, the student will be saying the word aloud, coordinating individual sounds with individual letters (saying /kat/ while writing *cat*) or individual sounds with appropriate symbols and letters (saying /fō-tō/ while writing *photo)*. On a few occasions the student will spell a word instead of sounding while writing. This procedure is reserved for *Spell-Words*. In the text these are listed in bold print in the right hand margin. The teacher should underline these special, non-phonetic words in the **Decode and Encode** lists and identify them as "Spell-Words" when asking the student to write them. Thus the teacher will say, "spell-word /sed/," and the student will write *said* while saying each individual letter, "s-a-i-d."

As a reminder to both teacher and student, the following box will occur occasionally:

☞ **Remember: Whenever you write, you are sounding or spelling!** ✍

(Saying sounds for *phonetic words*, saying letters for *Spell-words*.)

After second or third grade it is worth the effort to convert the *printers* into *cursive* writers gradually. The slight lifting of the pencil between each letter in printed manuscript is counterproductive to a smooth kinesthetic, mental impression:

$$d\text{-}e\text{-}m\text{-}o\text{-}c\text{-}r\text{-}a\text{-}c\text{-}y \quad vs. \quad democracy.$$

To get started, you will have to proceed in a manner similar to that presented in Chapter 1. It is well, even for readers and spellers who are beyond a beginning stage, but are new to a multi-sensory phonetic approach, to start with *short a*. They may proceed rapidly, but it will be obvious where the "gaps" in their abilities occur.

Once a routine has been established, a typical multi-sensory, phonetic language lesson (30 to 60 minutes depending on student) might proceed like this:

1. Teacher shows various flash cards with which the student has had some experience; student says sounds. (Any unwanted symbol may be covered with a thumb.)

2. Teacher turns flash cards around and says same sounds; student writes. (There may be more than one possibility, but only the most common should be used first.)

3. Student reads a teacher-generated word list, *Decode and Encode*, containing only *phonetic* material or *Spell-Words* with which the student is already familiar.

4. The same or similar words are dictated to the student to write. Spell-Words are so identified.

5. A new sound and its representation and/or a new rule may be added as the student shows proficiency with present material.

6. Student reads appropriate material.

Aspects of punctuation and grammar can be introduced from the very start. Even in the first *Decode and Encode/Reading* section (Page 1), the notion of a *capital letter, period, sentence, question mark, rhyming* and *two uses for a word* (the girl, *Pat,* and the motion, *pat)* can be introduced. In the second *Decode and Encode/Reading* section (Page 2), the idea of a *comma* to separate items and putting things into a *category*, (e.g., names or things to put on the head), can be considered. With *is, was* and *has, had*, present and past tense can be contrasted; *said* (Page 3) can introduce the notion of quotation, *etc.*

As the lessons progress, circle back and mix up examples so that the student is not relying on repeated patterns to decode. With all the material it is important to make a distinction between <u>phonetic</u> and <u>non-phonetic</u> *Spell-word* material. Not making this distinction causes serious and unnecessary confusion in the student. If the Spell-Words become cumbersome or too time consuming, do only a few and return to those missed later.

The symbol / / will be used to indicate pronunciation. Thus /ā/ *mate,* /ē/ *Pete,* /ī/ *side,* /ō/ *pole,* /ū/ *cube,* indicate long vowels sounds, "letters saying their own name." Although /ă/ *at,* /ĕ/ *Ed,* /ĭ/ *it,* /ŏ/ *ox,* /ŭ/ *up,* can indicate short vowels, since these sounds are used so often in English, they will be simplified eventually to merely /a/, /e/, /i/, /o/, /u/. The consonant sounds of /b/, /d/, /f/, /g/, /h/, /j/, /k/, /l/, /m/, /n/, /p/, /s/, /t/, /v/, /w/, /y/, and /z/ should give no trouble, providing they are 'cleansed' of any vowel sound: /t/, not /tuh/, /v/, not /vuh/. Careful attention should be paid to /qu/ and /x/ since each is a combining symbol for two sounds: /qu/ = /kw/ and /x/ = /ks/. And /r/, often mispronounced /er/, is like *r* in *rat* without the *-at*---much like a little dog barking. Other pronunciation aids are: /aw/ *saw,* /ow/ *cow,* /oi/ *oil,* /o͞o/ *moon,* /o͝o/ *good,* /ä/ *ma* (same as /ŏ/, but spelled *a*), /ô/ *dog* (same as /aw/, but spelled *o*). *Vowel-R* combinations are simplified: /er/ *her,* /or/ *for,* /are/ *car,* /air/ *care,* /ear/ *hero.* And, of course, there is everyone's favorite, the *schwa,* /ə/, which will get its due in the text.

As the teacher, you are welcome to follow the lesson order as suggested in the following chapters; however, although there has been an attempt to go from the less to the more complicated, there is nothing sacred about this arrangement. As you improvise, make generous use of the appendices which are there to aid you. You may find the student covers some material quickly and with assurance and has unexpected difficulties elsewhere. This will affect your timing and how many extra examples for drill you might want to get from the appendices. Do not assume that what a student has learned today, he or she will continue to know tomorrow. There will be many memory lapses and only continual review will ensure that the student finally internalizes the material and makes it his or her own.

The appendices can be used to augment word listings demonstrating certain sounds or spellings, to practice syllabication, to build vocabulary (an occasional Latin or Greek prefix, root, or suffix has never been known to hurt anyone), to learn how our language has evolved from earlier forms, to begin a journey into Black English Vernacular, and in general, to become more *language-wise*. Most of the appendices are not intended for sequential reading, but as references as needed.

This book is admittedly designed for the student who has already fallen behind his or her grade level in reading and spelling and because of this, comprehension also. Although this *multi-sensory* program would be tedious for the majority of students who seem to learn well, or at least get by, with any method of instruction, nevertheless to deprive these "OK" students of some of the more useful phonic and rule material, is to ensure them some linguistic irritations, often lasting into their adult lives.

Abbreviations Used in This Book:

abbr. abbreviation	Eng. English	masc. masculine	rel. related to
adj. adjective	fem. feminine	M.Du. Middle Dutch	Rus. Russian
adv. adverb	F French	ME Middle English	Scot. Scottish
AF Anglo-French	Ger. German	MF Middle French	sing. singular
alter. alteration	Gk. Greek	n. noun	Skt. Sanskrit
Am. American	Gmc. Germanic	neut. neuter	sl. slang
Ar. Arabic	Heb. Hebrew	Nor. Norwegian	Sp. Spanish
Br. British	Hin. Hindi	OE Old English	suf. suffix
Cel. Celtic	inf. informal	OF Old French	super. superlative
Chin. Chinese	inter. interjection	ON Old Norse	Sw. Swedish
comp. comparative	Ir. Irish	Per. Persian	TN Trade Name
conj. conjunction	It. Italian	pl. plural	Turk. Turkish
dial. dialect	Jap. Japanese	Pg. Portuguese	var. variation of
Du. Dutch	L Latin	pref. prefix	v. verb
Egy. Egyptian	LL Late Latin	prep. preposition	< derives from

If needed, a tab index can be fashioned with the labels at the right edge of the Table of Contents page. Without cutting, merely place a folded, adhesive colored dot at the beginning of each appendix at the level of the appropriate label. Or, the labels can be cut and each placed in a transparent tab.

Bon voyage!

GETTING THE SHOW ON THE ROAD

Basic Phonics and Level 1 Rules

◆	**a**	[Short /ǎ/ as in the word *at.*]

t	/ǎ/	/t/	at		
n	/ǎ/	/n/	an		*"SPELL-WORDS"*
c /k/	at	an	cat	can	
p	at	an	pat	pan	
r	at	an	rat	ran	**the**
f	at	an	fat	fan	[Say the letters: "t-h-e."]
m	at	an	mat	man	
b	at	an	bat	ban	
v	at	an	vat	van	

> ☞ **Remember: whenever you write, you are sounding or spelling!** ✍
>
> (Saying sounds for *phonetic words*, saying letters for *Spell-words*.)

Decode and Encode (Read and Write): fat can rat fan the pat van
cat bat the man at an ban pan vat ran the mat
cat pat rat fat mat bat vat   can pan ran fan man ban van

Reading: The rat ran.   The fat rat ran.   Can the man bat?
The man can bat. Pat ran. Pat ran the fan. Can Pat pat the cat?

s	at	am	sat	Sam	**as**
h	at	am	hat	ham	**has**
d	an	Dan	-ad	dad	
	bad	had	mad	sad	
j	am	an	jam	Jan	
	-ab	-ap	cab	cap	
	-ab	-ap	tab	tap	
l	-ab	-ap	lab	lap	
g /g/	-ab	-ap	gab	gap	

1

> **RULE 1:** An a standing alone is pronounced /uh/, as in "A man ran."

Decode and Encode: Al, Hal, Sal, Pam, Sam, Pat, Dan, Jan, Nan hat, cap, tam gas had <u>has</u> a tag bad <u>the</u> cab <u>as</u> lag dad a fad gag sad gal <u>has</u> gap jab lab lap sap mad a map nab nag dab pad pal rag lad ram a <u>has</u> bag rap <u>as</u> sag tab

Reading: As a sad Jan had jam, mad Dan had a ham. Sal has a cap. Al had a hat. Pat had a tam. Dad ran the lab. Nan has a pal. The cab had gas. The cab has gas. Hal had a bad map.

◆ i	[Short /ĭ/ as in the word *it*.]			
	/ĭ/	/n/	in	
	/ĭ/	/t/	it	
	in	it	pin	pit	**is**
	in	it	fin	fit	
	in	it	sin	sit	**his**
	in	it	bin	bit	
w	in	it	win	wit	**was**
k	in	it	kin	kit	

Decode and Encode: win kin wit kit <u>is</u> <u>was</u> bid bad big bag bin ban bit bat did dad dim dam din Dan fin fan fit fat hid had him ham hit hat in an it at Jim jam lid lad lip lap mid mad nip nap pin pan pit pat rig rag rim ram rip rap Sid sad sip sap sit sat Tim tam tin tan tip tap wig wag <u>his</u> a pal <u>is</u> tag can <u>was</u> map am if him dig cab dip fib man hip pal man bib can

Reading: Is it a big can? It is a big tin can. The can had ham in it. A lad in a cab is mad. The pig had a nap. Was it his map ? The map was his. Was it Sam? It was Sam. Is the jam in a pan? The jam hit the fan! Jan has a tan pal. The rag mat is in the van. The hat hid the wig. Dan had a bad bat. Nan did a jig. Sis is in a jam.

RULE 2: The /k/ sound after a short vowel in a one syllable word is spelled -*ck*.

-ck /k/ pack   pick   lack   lick

          sack   sick   rack   Rick   **said**

          tack   tick   Mack Mick

          back   Jack   kick   wick

Decode and Encode: pick pack   lick lack sick sack Rick rack Mick Mack tick tack Dick Jack back <u>said</u> map tag hit hip fig <u>was</u>

Reading: Rick said, "Jack is sick." Dick said, "The kick was bad."

RULE 3: Q & u are always written together and are treated as one letter, *qu-*.

---

qu-   /k-w/   quit   quack quick   **are**

x   /k-s/   ax   tax   wax

y   yam   yap   yip   **you**

z   zap   zip   **your**

Decode and Encode: ax tax fax lax Max wax quip quit quiz <u>is</u> a quick kick <u>was</u> ran <u>your</u> mat map <u>said</u> fix mix six <u>has</u> fan man tan van <u>are</u> at it in <u>as</u> an <u>the</u> Zack <u>his</u> bad Jack back tack

Reading: Jack is back. Zack had a tack. The quick kick was bad. Your bag is tan. Are you sick?   Max said, "The lid is on the can." Dad quit his job.   Your pal is lax.   Are you six?   You are six. Mad Dan had a ham. Jack has a bad back. Dad is in his lab.

♦ o   [Short /ŏ/ as in the word *ox*.]

          /ŏ/   /x/   ox   fox

          /ŏ/   /n/   on   Don   <u>do</u>

          -ot   not   dot   hot   <u>to</u>

          got   lot   cot   rot

          -ob   mob   cob   rob

          -op   mop   top   cop

Decode and Encode: ox box fox on Don Ron yon cot dot got hot jot lot not pot rot tot bob cob fob gob job lob mob rob sob bop cop hop mop pop top dock hock jock lock mock rock sock <u>do</u> <u>to</u> hat hit hot pat pit pot fax fix fox   Dan din Don Bab bib bob Bob an in on bag big bog hack hick hock lab Lib lob lack lick lock Mack Mick mock   sack sick sock   tack tick tock   tam Tim Tom mom tap tip top ran Ron   rat rot   rib rob   rid rod sad sod <u>do</u> <u>to</u>

Reading: Don had to do it.   Ron has to bat.   To bat is not bad. It is hot. To wax the van is not bad. Bab has a bat. Tom has a fox. Lock the van.   Hal has to dig.   Bob did the job.   Mom got sick.

┌───┐
RULE 4: A closed syllable is one in which a single vowel is followed by a consonant. The vowel is usually short. All of the phonetic words so far are CLOSED SYLLABLES---the vowels are all short.
└───┘

➲ an in on hat hit hot sack sick sock *(These are all closed syllables.)*

◆	**e**	[Short /ĕ/ as in the name, *Ed*.]			
	/ĕ/	/d/	Ed	red	**egg**
	-ed	bed	fed	led	
	-et	let	get	yet	
	-en	ten	men	den	

┌───┐
☞   **Remember: whenever you write, you are sounding or spelling!** ✍
└───┘

Decode and encode: Ed Ben Ken Peg Ted bed beg den get hem hen led leg let men met net pen pep pet red set web wed wet yes yet pat pet pit pot Dan den din Don   bag beg big bog hack heck hick hock   red rid rod   tan ten tin <u>egg</u> not <u>his</u> zip <u>said</u>

Reading: Men met to set the fox net.   Peg said, "Do not do it." Ted has the cat on his lap.   Nan said, "Pet it."   The tin jet had gas. A gas can fit in the jet.   The jet was red hot.   It had zip, pep. The tan jet did the job.   Tim sat in the jet.   Tim got egg on the map!

RULE 5: THE FIZZLE RULE.   /f/, /s/, /z/, /l/
f, s, z, & l after a short vowel in a one
syllable word are almost always doubled.

-ff /f/	Jeff	miff	tiff	(if)			**one**
-ss /s/	hiss	mass	miss	(gas)	(yes)		
-zz /z/	fizz	jazz	razz	(quiz)			**of**
-ll /l/	ill	hill	bill	mill			**off**

⚑ **Decode and encode; Reading** are teacher generated from now on.

A common consonant combination is **-ng**. It is often combined with *i* or *a*.

-ing /ing/	sing	king	ring	wing	**Mr.**
-ang /ang/	sang	bang	fang	hang	**Mrs.**
-ink /ingk/	sink	rink	link	wink	**Ms.**
-ank /angk/	sank	rank	tank	bank	

⇨   THE "H BROTHERS": TH-, SH-, CH-, WH-

th-	that	them	then	(this)	**there**
	than	thing	think	thank	**their**
sh-	shall	shell	ship	shop	
ch-	chat	chill	chip	chop	**what**
wh-	whiff	whim	whip	(whiz)	**where**

RULE 6:   An OPEN SYLLABLE is one where the
vowel is not followed by a consonant.
The vowel then is long; it says its own
name.

🗁   EXAMPLES OF **OPEN SYLLABLES** WITH LONG VOWELS:

I	me	he	she
we	no	so	go

> **RULE 7:** [The "SILENT E" or "MAGIC E" Rule.]
> An "e" following a closed syllable makes
> the vowel long; it says its own name.

mat	mate	them	theme	
win	wine	rob	robe	**does**
mad	made	cap	cape	**goes**
plan	plane	slid	slide	

✋ The number of these pairs is surprising. See Ap. i-35.

> ☞ **Remember: whenever you write, you are sounding or spelling!** ✍

⇨ **CONSONANT "L" BLENDS:** bl-, cl-, fl-, gl-, pl-, sl-

bl-	black	bless	bliss	block	**blood**
cl-	clap	(clef)	cling	clod	**flood**
fl-	flag	fled	flick	flop	
gl-	glad	glen	glib	glob	**once**
pl-	plan	pled	plot	plod	
sl-	slab	slam	sling	slack	**only**

⇨ **CONSONANT "R" BLENDS:** br-, cr-, dr-, fr-, gr-, pr-, shr-, thr-, tr-, wr-

br-	brag	bran	brass	brat	
cr-	crab	crack	cram	crash	
dr-	drab	dress	drill	drop	**done**
fr-	frame	fresh	frill	froze	**gone**
gr-	grape	grass	grid	gripe	
pr-	prep	press	prick	pride	
shr-	shred	shrill	shrine	shrink	**any**
thr-	thrash	thrill	thrive	throb	**many**
tr-	track	trade	tribe	trick	
wr- (The *w* is silent.)	write	wrote	wreck		

6

⇨ **CONSONANT "W": BLENDS**: dw-, sw-, tw-.

dw-	dwell	dwelling		**who**
sw-	swim	swell	swish	swing	**whom**
tw-	twin	twine	twig		**whose**

◆ **u**   [Short /ŭ/ as in the word *up.*]

/ŭ/	/p/	up	(us)	
bug	bum	bun	(bus)	**put**
slug	slum	rub	(plus)	(thus)

RULE 8: The /-ch/ sound after a short vowel in a one syllable word is spelled -tch.*

-tch /ch/   catch latch patch match **two**
pitch ditch hitch botch

✋ But memorize: **rich which much such** (no *t*)

☝ **Remember: whenever you write, you are sounding or spelling!** ✍

RULE 9: G is often soft, /j/, when followed by *e, i,* or *y.*

g /j/   gem   gin   gist   gym (y = ĭ)
✋ But not: get gift girl give

RULE 10: The /j/ sound after a short vowel in a one syllable word is spelled -dge.*

-dge /j/   badge edge ledge ridge
bridge dodge lodge fudge

QUESTIONS: [What Rule applies to each of the **bold** letters?] There <u>was</u> a wre**ck** at <u>the</u> bri**dge**. <u>As</u> she spoke <u>of</u> it, <u>the</u> ju**dge** wrote a note with a **qu**ill pen. <u>The</u> <u>blood</u> red **gem** <u>was</u> <u>gone</u>! "Did he pi**tch** it in?" "**Yes**," she <u>said</u>. [What do you say when you write the <u>underlined</u> words?]

* Advanced students: See **-tch** Ap. i-39 & **-dge** Ap. i-17 for rules of when to drop the **t** or **d**.

⇨ **BLENDS BEGINNING WITH "S":** sc-, sk-, sm-, sn-, sp-, squ-, st-.

sc-	scat	scale	scope	scum	**some**
sk-	skin	skate	skit	skid	**come**
sm-	smog	smell	smack	smug	
sn-	snake	snap	snip	snug	
sp-	spell	spin	spit	spike	
squ-	squid	squish	squelch		
st-	step	stem	still	stop	

⇨ **DOUBLE CONSONANTS AT END OF WORDS:**
  -ct, -ft, -ld, -lk, -lp, -lt, -mp, -nch, -nd, -nt, -pt, -sk, -sp, -st.

-ct	fact	pact	sect	tract	
-ft	gift	left	lift	raft	
-ld	held	meld	weld	gild	**could**
-lk	milk	silk	bulk	sulk	**should**
-lp	help	gulp	pulp	scalp	**would**
-lt	belt	felt	melt	tilt	
-mp	lamp	damp	bump	jump	
-nch	bunch	lunch	drench	crunch	
-nd	land	sand	bend	bond	**bull**
-nt	lint	lent	bent	bunt	**pull**
-pt	kept	wept	crept	slept	
-sk	cask	desk	disk	dusk	
-sp	gasp	grasp	clasp	crisp	**bush**
-st	fast	last	test	wrist	**push**

⇨ **BLENDS WITH THREE CONSONANTS** ("clusters"): spl-, scr-, spr-, str-.

spl-	splash	split	splint	splotch	
scr-	scram	scrap	scrimp	script	**odd**
spr-	sprig	sprang	spring	sprint	
str-	strap	strip	strut	strand	

RULE 11: C is soft /s/ when followed by e, i, or y.

c /s/   cell   cent   cinch   cyst (y = ĭ)

☞ **a** has an /aw/ sound when followed by **-ll** as in the word **all**.

-all /awl/ all   ball   call   fall   **false**
hall   tall   wall   small   **always**

[**shall** has regular short /ă/ sound.]

☞   **ar** is pronounced as one would say the letter **R**, /are/.

ar /are/ bar   bark   far   farm
car   card   mar   mart

☞   **or** is pronounced as the word "or" is pronounced, /or/.

or /or/ or   for   form   fort   **door**
north   short   born   scorch   **floor**

☞   **ai-** & **-ay** are common spellings for long *a*, /ā/.

ai- /ā/   aim   rain   main   strain
claim   grain   saint   snail
-ay /ā/   day   may   say   pay   **says**
clay   gray   play   stray

(Note the position in word of **ai-** and **-ay**.)

☞   **ee** is a common spelling for *long e*, /ē/.

ee /ē/   bee   free   tree   three   **four**
street   sheet   deed   queen

☞   **er**, **ir**, & **ur** are pronounced /er/.

er /er/ herd   fern   germ   pert   **sure**
ir /er/ bird   girl   firm   third
ur /er/ fur   burn   turn   hurt

9

⇨ **DIPHTHONG PAIRS**: oi-, -oy;   au-, -aw;   ou-, -ow.

oi- /oi/   (As in, "**Oi, oi!** What next?")

oil   toil   soil   spoil
coin   joint   moist   point

-oy /oi/ boy   toy   joy   ploy

(Note position in word of **oi-** and **-oy**.)

au- /aw/   (As in, "**Aw!** I don't believe it!")

haul Paul   fraud   flaunt

-aw /aw/ jaw law   raw   saw

(Note position in word of **au-** and **-aw**;   **-aw-** may <u>also</u> come before **-n** and **-l**.)

lawn drawn bawl crawl

ou- /ow/   (As in, "**Ow!** This hurts!")

out   loud   ouch   found   <u>**our**</u>
count scout stout   proud   <u>**hour**</u>

-ow /ow/ how   now   cow   plow

(Note position in word of **ou-** and **-ow**;   **-ow-** may also come before **-n** and **-l**.)

down brown growl scowl

-ow is also pronounced as a long o, (ō):

-OW /ō/ own   low   show   grow   <u>**owe**</u>
snow slow   flow   throw

┌──┐
│ RULE 12:   A word usually does not end in -v, │
│   but in -ve.   │
└──┘

So, vowels may be short: live give have
solve delve twelve shelve   <u>**love**</u>

or long: live Steve five   strive
save brave Dave dive   <u>**both**</u>
cove crave clove thrive   <u>**whole**</u>

10

☞   **oo** is usually pronounced /o͞o/, as in the word ***moon***.
(As in, "**Oo!** What's that?")

oo /o͞o/   too   moon   cool   groove   **move**
          loop   noon   spoon   broom   **prove**

[Less often "oo" is pronounced /oo/, as in *good*.]

oo /o͝o/   good   book   look   foot
         took   look   cook   wood

☝ **Remember: whenever you write, you are sounding or spelling!** ✍

☞   **oa** is pronounced /ō/.

oa- /ō/   oak   boat   goal   boast
        loan   toast   loaf   coach

To separate ***oa-*** words into their own group, draw a <u>picture</u> representing all of the above words, plus as many of these as you can: boar   board   boast broach   cloak   coal   coast   coax   croak   float   foal   foam   gloat   goat groan   hoard   hoax   Joan   load   moan   moat   oaf   oar   oath   poach roach   road   roam   roar   roast   soak   soap   soar   throat   toad   toast

☞   **ea** in many words is pronounced /ē/.

ea /ē/   read   east   each   deal
        meat   leap   least   dream   **been**

[Most other times "ea"" is pronounced /ĕ/.]

ea /ĕ/   read   head   bread   sweat
       deaf   meant   health   thread   **busy**

✋ However, in four exceptions "ea" sounds /ā/.

ea /ā/   great   steak   break   yea

☞   **-igh** sounds /ī/.

-igh /ī/   high   light   tight   fight
        might   sight   fright   flight

☞ **eigh** sounds /ā/.

eigh /ā/ eight sleigh weigh weight freight

✋ Exception: **height** /hīt/.

☞ **ie** most often sounds /ē/.

ie /ē/ brief thief field shield

However, **ie** sounds /ī/ as end of short words.

ie /ī/ pie lie tie die

✋ Exception: **friend** /frend/.

☝ Remember: whenever you write, you are sounding or spelling! ✍

☞ **ear** has three pronunciations /ear/, /er/, & /air/.

ear /ear/ ear fear near <u>tear</u> **often**
ear /er/ earn earth heard learn <u>**listen**</u>
ear /air/ bear wear pear <u>tear</u>

✋ Exception: **heart** /hart/.

☞ **-ild, -ind, -old,** & **-ost** all have long vowel sounds.

-ild /īld/ mild wild child
-ind /īnd/ find kind mind blind
-old /ōld/ old bold cold mold
            sold fold hold scold
-ost /ōst/ most post host

✋ But /awst/ with: **cost** and **lost**.

☞ **Long u** may sound either /yōō/ or /ōō/.

u /yōō/ cube cute huge mute <u>**build**</u>
u /ōō/ tune rule flute crude <u>**buy**</u>
      June brute rude Luke

12

☞   **oe** sounds /ō/.

-oe /ō/   toe foe hoe doe woe o/boe   **shoe**

☞   In several common words, *o* sounds /aw/ instead of /ŏ/.
Many dictionaries mark the /aw/ sound /ô/.

o /ô/   bog   boss   cost   dog   fog   frog
frost   golf   gone   hog   honk   log   long
loss   lost   moth   off   smog   soft   song

RULE 13:   Often,   when   there   are   two
consonants between two vowels, a division
can   be   made   between   them   to   form
syllables or word parts.   For example,
d e n / t i s t   n a p / k i n
V C / C V   V C / C V

📁   **Examples of two syllable words** with the **v c / c v** pattern:

den/tist nap/kin ad/mit   hap/pen
bas/ket   sub/way un/der   trum/pet
kit/ten   pic/nic af/ter   din/ner

☞   **-ei-** may sound either /ā/ or /ē/.

-ei- /ā/   vein   veil   rein   their   heir   **toward**
-ei- /ē/   seize ei/ther nei/ther re/ceive

☞   **-ey** may sound either /ā/ or /ē/.

-ey /ā/   they   prey   hey   o/bey
-ey /ē/   key tur/key hock/ey mon/ey /mun-ē/

☞   **-ui-** sounds /o͞o/.

-ui- /o͞o/   suit   fruit   juice   bruise /bro͞oz/

13

☞   **war** sounds /wor/   Just like the word, **war**.

war /wor/   war   ward   warn   dwarf

☞   **wor-** sounds /wer/.

wor- /wer/   work   word   worm   world

✋ Exceptions: /wor/   **wore, worn, swore, sworn**

☞   **-alt** & **-alk** have an /aw/ vowel sound.

-alt /awlt/   salt   halt   malt

-alk /awk/   talk   walk   chalk   stalk   **aunt**

(Note in the **-alk** words the "l" is silent.)

☞   Some silent letters: **gn, kn, -mb**.

gn /n/   gnaw   gnash   gnat   gnome   **sign**
kn- /n/ knock   knee   know   knife
-mb /m/ dumb   thumb   limb   bomb

☞   **eu-** & **-ue** may each have both of the *long u* sounds,
/yo͞o/ & /o͞o/.

eu- /yo͞o/ feud Europe /yo͞or-up/   eulogy /yo͞o-lō-gē/
eu- /o͞o/ deuce   sleuth   neu/tral Zeus
-ue /yo͞o/ cue res/cue hue ar/gue con/tin/ue
-ue /o͞o/ true blue due clue glue Sue pur/sue

(Note position in word of **eu-** and **-ue**.)

☞   **ew** may sound /yo͞o/ or /o͞o/.   (Fine, since **w** is a *double u*.)

ew /yo͞o/   few   mew   pew   hew   **sew** /sō/
ew /o͞o/   chew   grew   flew   blew

☞   **augh** is another /aw/ sound.

Most examples can be remembered with this sentence:

"I caught my haugh/ty, naugh/ty daugh/ter
and taught her not to slaugh/ter."

14

☞ Another less common *a* sound than *short a* (mǎd) or *long a* (māde) is /ah/, in most dictionaries, /ä/, as in *ma* /mä/. This often occurs after *qu* or *w* and in some *silent l* words. Note this is also the sound of short o, /ŏ/ (lŏt).

a /ä/ father ma calm palm squad
swamp swan want wash watch

☞ **qua-** is pronounced /kwä/.

qua- /kwä/ quad quality /kwäl-i-tē/ quantity /kwän-ti-tē/
squad squash <u>Exceptions</u>: quāke, quǎck

☞ **wa-** is pronounced /wä/.

wa- /wä/ wash watch want wallet wander
Exceptions: /waw/ water walk wall walnut waltz

☞ **-ough** has the basic sound /aw/ when it is followed by *t*.

-ough thought bought brought fought **though**

✋ But notice the **Spell-words**. Try spelling them with **through**
some sort of rhythm for better retention. **thorough**

6/8 ♪|♩ ♪ ♩ ♪|♩. ; ♪|♩. ♩̆ ♪|♩ ♪ ♩.|; ♪ ♩ ♪̆|♩̆ ♪ ♪ ♪|♩. ; ‖
t-h-o-u-g-h, t-h-<u>r</u>-o-u-g-h, t-h-<u>o-r</u>-o-u-g-h.

✋ Four more Spell-words might be remembered by the saying, **enough**
"I've had <u>enough</u> of this <u>rough, tough cough</u>." **rough**
Here the **-gh** in each word sounds /f/. **tough**
cough

☞ **gh** sounds /g/ or /f/.

gh- /g/ ghōst ghastly ghetto ghoul /o͞o/
-gh /f/ enough rough tough cough **laugh**

☞ Note the position of each **gh** in the word.

15

☞   **-ly** sounds /lē/ and is added to an adjective to form an adverb. "How did the <u>slow</u> (adjective) boy (noun) walk? He walked (verb) <u>slowly</u> (adverb)." An **adjective** tells more about a **noun**; an **adverb** tells more about a **verb**.

-ly /lē/ slowly boldly loudly quickly

☞   **-tion**, sounding /shun/, is a common noun ending.

-tion /shun/ nation motion fiction friction   <u>**woman**</u>
caution action mention option   <u>**women**</u>

☝ Remember to note "open" & "closed" syllables.

☞   **quar-** sounds /kwor/.

quar- /kwor/   quart quarter quartet quartz

☝ **Remember: whenever you write, you are sounding or spelling!** ✍

☞   **-sion** (like **-tion**) usually sounds /shun/.

-sion /shun/ tension mansion pension mission
but **-sion** may also sound /zhun/: version vision

☞   *y*, in addition to being a consonant (as in *yell* and *yawn*), can act as a vowel at the end of a word, sounding /ī/ when ending one syllable words and /ē/ when ending longer words. [Verbs ending in "-fy" will be addressed later.]

-y /ī/   cry   dry   fly   shy   <u>**bye**</u>
         try   sky   why   sly   <u>**eye**</u>
-y /ē/   pity   city   duty   lady
         angry   ready   booty   history

☞   Listing **wa-, war-, qua-, quar-** together is an easy way to remember their sounds: /wä/, /wor/, /quä/, /quor/.

want   warm   quad   quart

16

> ☞ Like *soft c* and *soft g*, **sc** is soft, /s/, when followed by *e, i,* or *y*.   Tap: 2/4: ♩ ♪♪♪|♩♩ | e, i, or y. ♩ ♪♪♪|♩♩ | e, i, or y.

sc /s/ scene sci/ence scythe /sīth/

sc is still hard, /sk/, when followed by *a* or *u*: **scat, scum.**

> ☞ **ar** at the end of a word (often an adjective) sounds /er/.

-ar /er/ singular regular popular

> ☞ **or** at the end of a word (usually a noun) sounds /er/.

-or /er/ author actor doctor tractor

RULE 14: Drop a *silent* e when adding a vowel ending.

take+ing = taking make+ing= making time+ed = timed
hike + er = hiker like + able = likable *but:* like/ness

OTHER SORTS OF WORDS ENDING IN *E*:

1. **-ce** & **-ge** retain *e* to keep *c* & *g* soft: notice + able = noticeable, courage + ous = courageous, manage + able = manageable
2. In some cases "e" is not dropped in order to keep the identity of the word: dye+ing= dyeing, mile/age, canoe/ing, hoe/ing
3. Exceptions that drop "e" even with a consonant ending:
due+ly= duly, argue+ment= argument, true+ly= truly,
whole+ly= wholly
4. Special cases: lie + ing = lying, die dying, tie tying, vie vying

Spelling the Alphabet: Often the name of a letter of the alphabet is heard in a word. If one could "spell" the alphabet, this would make one less encoding step. ā bē cē dē ē ĕf gē ī jā kā ĕl ĕm ĕn ō pē ar ĕs tē ū vē ĕx zē Notice that rules of open and closed syllables apply here. (Spellings of *h, q, w, & y* are not useful.) Listen to the *letter names* as you read:

crazy being cedar decent she effort geology ice
Jake Kate elder emblem enemy zone penal car
escape tepee cube vehicle expense zebra

17

☞ **-ture** is pronounced /chur/.

-ture /chur/ capture culture denture fixture fracture future gesture lecture mixture nature nurture pasture picture posture puncture rupture structure texture

---

☞ **-age** is usually pronounced /ij/.

-age /ij/ average bandage blockage garbage manage package postage sausage shortage storage baggage cabbage cottage luggage message passage pillage rummage tonnage village
Exceptions: (French) /ahzh/ garage mirage massage (See Ap. iv-19.)

☞ One of the syllables in a multi-syllable word is usually said with a bit more stress. This is called ***accent*** and will be noted, when necessary, by underlining the accented syllable.

<u>af</u>ter <u>ban</u>dit <u>bas</u>ket <u>blis</u>ter <u>cos</u>mic <u>den</u>tist **<u>sug</u>ar**
<u>din</u>ner <u>es</u>cort <u>hap</u>pen <u>kit</u>ten <u>nap</u>kin <u>pic</u>nic **<u>min</u>ute**

Although the accent is on the first syllable in the above examples, it may be shifted if one part of the word is more important or from a Latin root. (More on Latin roots later.)

ad<u>mit</u> con<u>nect</u> de<u>tract</u> dis<u>pute</u> ex<u>ter</u>nal **<u>o</u>cean**
for<u>get</u> in<u>spect</u> pro<u>duc</u>tive re<u>turn</u> Ver<u>mont</u> **<u>view</u>**

Sometimes the accent shifts in the same word depending on its part of speech. Examples of the ***noun-verb accent shift*** are given here:

<u>con</u>flict "The <u>con</u>flict was resolved." <u>Con</u>flict is noun; sentence **subject**.

con<u>flict</u> "The two suggestions con<u>flict</u>." Con<u>flict</u> is a **verb**.

<u>pro</u>test pro<u>test</u> <u>con</u>tract con<u>tract</u> **<u>lose</u>**
<u>sub</u>ject sub<u>ject</u> <u>re</u>cord re<u>cord</u> **<u>straight</u>**

An easy way to remember these accent placements is to realize that the noun is usually the subject of the sentence: "<u>Subject comes first--accent comes first.</u>"
The verb is usually the second element in the sentence:
<u>"Verb comes second---accent comes second."</u>

18

RULE 15: The SCHWA is marked by the distinctive symbol, ə, and sounds /uh/, a sound we are familiar with as a short ŭ. Our short /ŭ/ notation, as in /shun/ for -tion, may now be noted /shən/. Any of the vowels may have this sound as in *about* /ə-<u>bowt</u>/ and *oven* /ə-vən/, but it is usually reserved for vowels in <u>unaccented</u> syllables of multi-syllable words.

co<u>nnec</u>tion /kə-<u>nek</u>-shən/ (short ĕ kept in closed accented syllable and the vowels in the unaccented syllables become **schwaed**.)

<u>prob</u>able /<u>prob</u>-ə-bəl/ <u>sev</u>en /<u>sev</u>-ən/

com<u>pat</u>ibility /kəm-<u>pat</u>-ə-bil'-ə-tē/ (**-bil** is a secondary accent.)

With the fine tuning the schwa allows, **<u>con</u>flict** (noun) and **con<u>flict</u>** (verb) are pronounced /<u>con</u>-flikt/ and /cən-<u>flikt</u>/ respectively.

☞ **-ion** is pronounced /yən/.

-ion /yən/ bunion dominion million onion opinion union

RULE 16: THE 1-1-1-V RULE. In a *1 syllable* word with *1 vowel* followed by *1 consonant* to which a *Vowel ending* (-<u>e</u>d, -<u>i</u>ng, -<u>e</u>n) is to be added, double the consonant. For example, before adding *-ing* to *run*, note that *run* is 1 syllable, has 1 vowel, *(u)*, followed by 1 consonant, *(n)* and that what is to be added begins with a Vowel, *(i)*. Therefore, double the consonant to get the word, *running*.

📁 **1-1-1-V examples:** sad + en = sadden;
rip + ed = ripped; mad + est = maddest
mad + er = madder; hit + ing = hitting
✋ But: si<u>ng</u>ing, wet<u>n</u>ess, f<u>oo</u>ting, f<u>ai</u>ling, la<u>nd</u>ed, *etc.*
(These do not fit the rule, so no doubling.)

19

THERE ARE UNVOICED AND VOICED SOUND PARTNERS!

/t/ + /d/ ☺   /f/ + /v/ ☺   /p/ + /b/ ☺   /s/ + /z/ ☺   /k/ + /g/ ☺

/ch/ + /j/ ☺   /sh/ + /zh/ ☺   /th/ + /th/ ☺   /wh/ + /w/ ☺

[Teacher may read:] To prove this to yourself hold one hand lightly on your throat while pronouncing each pair. You will notice a slight vibration only on the second of each pair; this is the voiced member. *Voiced* means that the vocal cords are in use; they are *not* used with the unvoiced member. Unvoiced (without a partner ☹) is /h/. Voiced (without partners ☹) are /n/, /m/, /l/, /r/, and /y/. <u>All vowel sounds are voiced</u>. Vowels are what is sustained in singing. Now, what is in motion, tends, or likes, to stay in motion (Newton's First Law of Motion). So once /ă/ is voiced in the word ***has***, it is easier to slip into the voiced /z/ than to stop the vocal cords and produce /s/. Try /haz/ and /has/. Which is easier? Be sure you are producing /s/ in /has/ and are not just reading a word you know. *Has* is pronounced /haz/. Well, knowing that *s* has either an /s/ <u>or</u> a /z/ sound, *as, is, has, his* can graduate from the *Spell-Word* class to being *phonetic* after all! /s/ /z/ ☺

Now **-tch** /ch/ and **-dge** /j/ are seen as related not only in sound (unvoiced and voiced) but in spelling. Before we produce /ch/, our tongue goes to a *t* position giving excuse to the **-tch** spelling. Also before we produce /j/ our tongue goes to a *d* position and thus the **-dge** spelling. /ch/ /j/ ☺ /t/ /d/ ☺

Listen to **ink** /ingk/. The voiced *n* is linked by voiced *g* to its unvoiced partner *k*. /k/ /g/ ☺

Chapter 5 on Plurals will comment on the plurals of *leaf, wife, knife*. They become *leaves, wives, knives*. /f/ /v/ ☺

Consider *tension* /-shən/; *version* /-zhən/. /sh/ /zh/ ☺

Listen to *thin* /thin/ and *that* /<u>th</u>at/ /th/ /<u>th</u>/ ☺

How do you say *water*? Most people say /<u>waw</u>-der/. It takes special care to say /<u>waw</u>-ter/, but /<u>waw</u>-der/ tumbles right out! /t/ /d/ ☺

For more on this subject see *Unvoiced and Voiced Consonants* in Ap. i-41.

☞   In **-mn**, the *n* is silent.

-mn̸ /m/   autumn column condemn hymn solemn

20

RULE # 17: Most words are made plural by adding _s_.

---

cliff cliffs   hat hats   map maps   rack racks   lamp lamps
Notice the single words listed all end in unvoiced sounds, /f/, /k/, /p/, /t/. This allows the added _s_ to take its unvoiced sound, /s/. However, the following singular words end in a voiced sound: bud buds   bag bags   pal pals   gum gums   ten tens   car cars   cave caves
The voicing tends to last through /d/, /g/, /l/, /m/, /n/, /r/, and /v/, to produce /z/. Remember all vowels sounds are voiced also, thus producing the voiced /z/ in their plurals: tree trees   solo solos   soda sodas.

RULE # 18: Words ending in _s_, _sh_, _ch_, _x_, and _z_ form their plurals by adding -es. This adds an extra syllable.

---

mess messes   dish dishes   church churches
whizz whizzes   box boxes

☞   **-ed** may sound /id/, /d/, or /t/.

-ed /id/ (after _t_ or _d_)   planted rusted ended needed
-ed /d/ (after _voiced_ sound)   banged loved seemed spilled
-ed /t/ (after _unvoiced_ sound)   blinked dumped helped looked

---

☞   More words with silent letters!

---

subtle debt doubt honor honest calf yolk   **usual**
folk answer island (See Ap.i-37 for more complete list.)   **beauty**

☞ Deliberate mispronunciation of some words aids spelling.

Wed-nes-day, Feb-ru-ar-y, _etc._

RULE: 19: To form the plural of a word ending in _vowel-Y_, add _s_ as in Rule 17, but with a _consonant-Y_, "CHANGE THE _Y_ TO _I_ AND ADD -_ES_."

---

way ways   key keys   toy toys   guy guys   play plays
lady ladies   family families   duty duties   pony ponies

21

☞   **-du-** is pronounced /jо̄о̄/.

du /jо̄о̄/ arduous   education   individual   modulate

☞   **-tu-** is pronounced /chо̄о̄/.

tu   /chо̄о̄/ actual   fortune   habitual   punctual   statue

❖ **A SET OF SPECIAL ENDINGS**: -ble /bəl/, -dle /dəl/, -fle /fəl/, -gle /gəl/, -kle /kəl/, -ple /pəl/, -tle /təl/, -zle /zəl/.

RULE 20: Immediately after a <u>short</u> vowel, double the first consonant in special *-ble*, *-dle*, *-fle*, *-gle*, *-kle*, *-ple*, *-tle*, *-zle* endings.
☝ Note: **k** doubles to **ck**.

-ble	babble dribble gobble wobble stubble
-dle	middle paddle saddle muddle
-fle	sniffle shuffle baffle muffle
-gle	wiggle jiggle juggle straggle
-kle	pickle freckle knuckle tickle
-ple	apple ripple cripple grapple
-tle	little bottle battle kettle
-zle	fizzle puzzle dazzle sizzle

again

against

✋   But,   no doubling with a long or double vowel.

-ble	able Bible cable gable noble stable table
-dle	cradle idle needle noodle
-fle	rifle stifle trifle
-gle	beagle bugle eagle ogle
-ple	couple disciple maple staple steeple
	Exception: triple /trĭp-əl/
-tle	beetle entitle title tootle
-zle	foozle

cloth

clothes

people

22

✋ And no doubling with an intervening consonant.

-ble amble assemble bumble crumble fumble gamble garble grumble humble jumble marble mumble ramble rumble stumble tremble tumble thimble

-dle bundle candle curdle dwindle fondle girdle handle hurdle kindle swindle trundle

-gle angle bangle bungle dangle gargle gurgle jingle jungle mangle mingle shingle single tangle tingle

-kle ankle crinkle sparkle sprinkle twinkle wrinkle

-ple ample crimple crumple dimple example pimple purple rumple sample simple temple trample

-tle gentle hurtle mantle myrtle startle subtle turtle

☞ **-stle** /səl/ is akin to the "-ble" group, but follows only short vowels, never uses doubling, and has a *silent t*.

-stle bristle castle gristle rustle thistle whistle wrestle

RULE 21A: When adding a suffix (whatever) to a <u>vowel-*y*</u> word, keep the *y*.

joy+ous= joyous play+ing= playing pay+able= payable
joy+ful= joyful play+ful= playful pay+ment= payment

✋ Exceptions: pay+ed= paid lay+ed= laid say+ed= said
day+ly= daily

RULE 21B: When adding a suffix (beginning with anything but *i*) to a <u>*consonant*-*y*</u> word, change the *y* to *i*.

cry+ed= cried study+ed= studied lazy+est= laziest
lazy+ly= lazily noisy+ly= noisily noisy+ness= noisiness

☞ With **-ing**, keep the *y*: cry+ing= crying studying flying buying
✋ Exception: skiing

23

☞ **ph** is another spelling for /f/, from Greek **phi**, φ (small), Φ (capital).

ph /f/ alphabet graph phase philosophy phone sphinx

RULE 22: Treat -y- in the middle of a word
as if it were an -i.

☞ *Y*, in addition to starting a word /y/ or ending a word /ē/ or /ī/, may appear within a word (medially) and act and sound exactly like an *i* would act and sound, /ĭ/ or /ī/. This medial *y* is found mostly in words of Greek origin and is a tranliteration of the Greek letter, **upsilon,** ʊ (small), Y (capital).

y /ĭ/   gym (gymnasium) myth   cyn/ic
mys/tic   mys/ter/y   hyp/no/sis   <u>iron</u>

y /ī/,   cy/cle   hy/dro/gen   type   hy/phen
dy/nam/ic   ty/phoon   ty/rant

☞ In **rh-** the *h* is silent. rh = /r/ in sound. The rh spelling comes from the Greek letter, **rho,** ρ (small), P (capital).

rh /r/   rhyme   rhap/so/dy   rhe/sus
rhyth/m   rhom/boid   Rhodes   <u>bury</u>

☞ Many **th** words derive from Greek; th is a transliteration of Greek letter, **theta,** θ (small), Θ (capital).

th /th/ theater theme theology therapy thermal

☞ **ch**, in addition to the /ch/ pronunciation *(chain, chum)*, may also sound /k/ (from Greek letter **chi** χ, X) <u>and</u> /sh/ (French).

ch /k/ (Gk.) archive anchor chasm chorus Christmas
chronic echo orchestra orchid scheme school

ch /sh/ (F) brochure chagrin Charlotte chef Chicago
chiffon chivalry chute machine Michigan mustache

☞ **Remember: whenever you write, you are sounding or spelling!** ✍

> **RULE   23:   In   syllabication,   keep   blends   and clusters together.**

re/**fresh** com/**plete** con/**struct** un/**scram**/ble in/**st**ant

---

☞   **-que** is the French spelling of *k* and sounds /k/.

-que /k/ baroque brusque mosque opaque plaque

-ique /ēk/ antique boutique critique Dominique Mozambique mystique physique technique unique

---

☞   **-gue** at the end of a word is pronounced /g/.

-gue /g/ vāgue rōgue vōgue fūgue

-igue /ēg/ fatigue intrigue   [☺ /k/ /g/ are partners.]

☞   **gu-** is pronounced /g/ in most common words.

gu- /g/ guard guest guess guilt guide guise guarantee

☞   **ou** is most often /ow/, but may be /o͞o/, /ō/, or /ə/. These four sounds may be remembered by "**C**o**u**nt **you**thful s**ou**ls d**ou**ble."

ou /ow/ crouch ground mound mouth noun round
ou /o͞o/ boutique group route soup wound you youth
ou /ō/ boulder cantaloupe four poultry shoulder soul
ou /ə/ country couple double touch tough trouble
And: **ou** /o͝o/ could should would tour detour contour

☞   Review the unvoiced and voiced sound pairs while touching throat. You can feel the vibration of the voiced partner!

/t/ + /d/ ☺	/f/ + /v/ ☺	/p/ + /b/ ☺	/s/ + /z/ ☺
/k/ + /g/ ☺	/ch/ + /j/ ☺	/sh/ + /zh/ ☺	/th/ + /th/ ☺

> **RULE 24: All vowels, except *i*, are usually long before -*tion*.**

oblig**ā**tion compl**ē**tion repet**ĭ**tion dev**ō**tion instit**u**tion (u = o͞o)

RULE 25: There are six kinds of syllables: closed, open, vowel pair, silent e, r- controlled, and "-ble" type. These may be easily remembered with the acronym, CLOVER.

CLOSED	not
-BLE TYPE	noble
OPEN	no
VOWEL PAIR	noon
E SILENT	note
R CONTROLLED	nor

RULE 26: In syllabicating when there is only one consonant between two vowels, VCV, the division may be on either side of the consonant. If the word is not immediately identifiable, divide before the consonant (first syllable open with long vowel); if this doesn't "work," divide after the consonant (first syllable is closed with a short vowel). "Cā/bin" is not a word, but "căb/in" is.

Divide <u>before</u> consonant making first syllable open with long vowel, **v**/**cv**:

ba/sic e/ven fi/nal mo/tive pu/pil ty/rant fu/sion

Divide <u>after</u> consonant making first syllable closed with short vowel, **vc**/**v**:

val/or cred/it riv/it mod/ern phys/ics

On occasion both divisions work: <u>Po</u>/lish, pol/<u>ish</u>; des/ert. de/<u>sert</u>.

RULE 27 "Protect the short vowel, for it is weak. The strong long vowel, no help does it seek."

We have already been doing this in a number of ways:
1. **Closed syllable.** red it last tin fix (The consonant following the vowel "protects" it.)
2. **Fizzle Rule.** hill mall cliff fizz mass (The double consonant "protects" the vowel.)
3. **-ck Rule.** lack pick sock nick luck (The vowel is "protected" by -ck.)
4. **-tch Rule.** catch pitch latch match (The vowel is "protected" by -tch.)
5. **-dge Rule.** judge fudge lodge (The vowel is "protected" by -dge.)
6. **1-1-1-V Rule.** running sadden (The doubled consonant is "protecting" the vowel.)
7. **-ble, -dle,** *etc.* bubble rattle muddle (The doubled consonant is "protecting" the vowel.)

26

> ☞ **-ci** and **-ti** are pronounced /sh/.
>
> An example of this has been seen in **-tion** /shən/.

-cial /shəl/ artificial crucial facial racial social special

-tial /shəl/ confidential essential initial martial partial

-cian /shən/ electrician musician physician politician

-tian /shən/ Christian Egyptian Martian Titian Venetian

-cient /shənt/ ancient efficient deficient sufficient

-tient /shənt/ dissentient impatient patient quotient

-cious /shəs/ atrocious gracious spacious vicious

-tious /shəs/ ambitious cautious fictitious infectious

-ciate /shē-āt/ appreciate associate officiate

-tiate /shē-āt/ initiate differentiate negotiate satiate

RULE 28: Often a single *i* followed by a different vowel in a suffix, is pronounced /ē/.

A beginning example list can be made by dropping the "c" from **-cial, -cian, -cient, -cious, & -ciate.**

-ial /ē-əl/ editorial material remedial trivial tutorial

-ian /ē-ən/ custodian guardian historian librarian

-ient /ē-ənt/ expedient ingredient lenient obedient

-ious /ē-əs/ curious devious notorious tedious various

-iate /ē-āt/ deviate humiliate mediate radiate

RULE 29: In syllabicating when two vowels are to be divided, usually the first one is long with the syllable accented, and the second vowel has a schwa sound with the syllable unaccented, v/v.

---

lion /lī-ən/ giant /jī-ənt/ bias client cruel dial diet fuel peon poem poet quiet riot trial Zion (See Appendix ii-15.)

> ✍ **Remember: whenever you write, you are sounding or spelling!** ✍

ONWARD AND EVER UPWARDS

Advanced Phonics and Level 3 Rules

☞ **-oll** is most often pronounced /ōl/.

-oll /ōl/ boll droll enroll knoll poll roll scroll stroll toll troll
Taking the expected short *o:* doll loll moll

> RULE 30: There are three degrees of an adjective: *positive, comparative,* and *superlative.* The comparative is formed by adding -er to the positive; the superlative is formed by adding -est to the positive.

positive:	big	fast	mean	soft	tough
comparative:	bigger	faster	meaner	softer	tougher
superlative:	biggest	fastest	meanest	softest	toughest

☞ There are a few adjective degree forms that are unusual.

positive:	good	bad	many	little
comparative:	better	worse	more	less
superlative:	best	worst	most	least

☞ Longer words might use *more* (comparative) and *most* (superlative).

positive:	comfortable	ridiculous
comparative:	more comfortable	more ridiculous
superlative:	most comfortable	most ridiculous

> RULE 31: THE <u>2-1-1-V</u> RULE. Review THE <u>1-1-1-V</u> RULE on page 19. Now, in a two syllable word the last consonant is doubled if the last syllable has one vowel followed by one consonant, the suffix to be added begins with a vowel *AND THE SYLLABLE IS ACCENTED*.

o/<u>mit</u> + ed = omitted   for/<u>get</u> + ing = forgetting

re/<u>gret</u> + able = regrettable   for/<u>got</u> + en = forgotten

✋ BUT: <u>mar</u>/ket + ing = marketing   (Accent on <u>first</u> syllable.)

per/<u>form</u> + ance = performance   *(rm* is not a <u>single</u> consonant.)

RULE 32: The principal parts of a verb are: present tense, past tense, and past participle.

---

sing sang sung are the principal parts of the verb **to sing**.
sing: Present tense. I *sing* for joy! **sang:** Past tense. I *sang* yesterday.
sung: Past participle. I *have sung* there before. I *had sung* it before noon.
(The past participle is used with compound verbs--verbs with more than one part.)

A Present participle is formed by adding **-ing** to the present tense:
singing. He *is singing* there tonight. This can also be used as a noun:
Singing is fun. When it is used as a noun it is called a gerund.
To sing is the Infinitive. This identifies the verb (Let's consider the verb, *to sing.*) and may also be used as a noun (*To sing* is the highest art!)
"Sing" is a *strong verb* (irregular) since all the principal parts are different: **sing sang sung.** "Walk" is a *weak verb* (regular) since the principal parts are not all different: **walk walked walked.** I *walk* for recreation. I *walked* to the store yesterday. I *have walked* there many times. I *had walked* there before the fire.
Weak (regular) verbs are more common than strong (irregular) verbs.
[Chapter 6 will carry the study of verbs further.]

RULE 33: Accented **ar-r** and **er-r** are pronounced /air/.

---

ar-r /air/ arrogant arrow barrel carrot carry Harry marry parrot
er-r /air/ berry cherry errand erratic error ferry merry Sherry Terry

---

RULE 34 Accented **ar** and **er** followed by a vowel are also pronounced /air/.

---

ar-V /air/ baron Carol guaranty harem Karen parent Paris vary
er-V /air/ America experiment herald heresy heritage merit peril

[Chapter 4 will provide a summary of "R" pronunciations.]

➔ An *e & i* exchange: **-less** /lis/, **-let** /lit/, **-ness** /nis/.

-less /lis/ aimless blameless careless fearless restless timeless
-let /lit/ anklet booklet bracelet droplet leaflet toilet triplet
-ness /nis/ boldness cleverness darkness fairness sickness
Also: **-et** /it/ closet blanket target; and **-ess** /is/ actress hostess

29

More *e* & *i* exchanges: **be-** /bi/, **de-** /di/, **re-** /ri/.

before below between; decay decline defend; receive recover refer

RULE 35: -ate   as a verb ending is pronounced   /āt/;   -ate   as a noun or adjective ending, /it/.

-ate /āt/ (verb) anticipate calculate celebrate dedicate demonstrate donate educate frustrate gravitate insulate investigate liberate medicate navigate obligate radiate regulate rotate separate violate

-ate /it/ (noun) barbiturate bicarbonate chocolate climate consulate directorate doctorate electorate palate pirate surrogate senate

☻ NOTE: Some words can "flip-flop" between verb and noun. Pronounce the following words alternately with /āt/ and /it/: advocate alternate* associate* degenerate* delegate duplicate* graduate* intimate* moderate* postulate predicate* repatriate subordinate* syndicate
* Also adjective.

-ate /it/ (adjective) accurate adequate affectionate celibate compassionate considerate delicate desolate desperate fortunate illiterate intimate intricate obstinate private separate temperate

RULE 36: **-ace** ending a word that can be used both as
          a   verb   and   noun,   is   pronounced /ās/;
          as a noun ending only, /is/.

-ace /ās/ (verb & noun) disgrace embrace face lace place space
-ace /is/ (noun only) furnace menace palace preface solace surface

☞ Use **-ous** /əs/ for as adjective ending and **-us** /əs/ for noun ending.

-ous /əs/ adventurous disastrous generous humorous marvelous
-us /əs/ asparagus cactus campus discus esophagus exodus rumpus

☞ **-ism** indicates a theory, doctrine or condition.   **-ist** is an adherent to a doctrine or a person who does something.

-ism /iz-əm/ capitalism communism fascism existentialism botulism
-ist /ist/ capitalist communist fascist existentialist columnist

ASSIGNMENT A: Read page 2 of Appendix v. This will give you an appreciation of English as basically a Germanic language. Look quickly at pages 3 through 10 in this Appendix to see the extent of our present-day vocabulary indebted to Old English (Anglo-Saxon).

RULE 37: It is generally true that **-y,** at the end of one syllable words *(sky, why, dry)*, is pronounced /ī/ and that **-y,** at the end of multi-syllable words *(philosophy, history)*, is pronounced /ē/ (page 16). But there are two exceptions: (1) In multi-syllable words, the suffix **-fy** is pronounced /fī/ *(amplify, purify)*. This is from the Latin verb, facere *(to make or do)*. (2) When the last syllable is accented, the **-y** is pronounced /ī/ *(deny, comply)*.

(1) beautify calcify certify classify electrify falsify fortify glorify horrify humidify identify intensify justify magnify modify pacify petrify purify qualify satisfy signify simplify solidify specify testify

(2) ally   apply   comply   decry   deny   imply   reply   supply

☞ With **-eu** assigned to an initial or medial place in a word, *eulogy, feud,* and **-ue** to the end, *continue, value,* (Page 14), there may be an assumption that a word never ends in *u*. This is not true.

beau /bō/ bureau guru Hindu Honolulu impromptu jujitsu lieu menu Peru plateau tofu Zulu <u>See</u>: "Words Ending in *u*" Ap. i-43.

ASSIGNMENT B: Read *Old Norse*, Appendix v, pages 6 & 7. This will show the Norse (Viking) influence on English. Also note the extent of words from *Old French*, Appendix vi, pages 1 through 4. These two sources were major influences on the development of *Middle English*, Appendix v, pages 7 to 9.

☞ Sometimes a letter that is silent in one form of a word, sounds in another.

gnostic agnostic   autumn autumnal   column columnist
condemn condemnation crumb crumble damn damnable damnation
design designation   hymn hymnal   limb limber   resign resignation
sign signal signature For other pairs see **Silent Letters Come To Life** in Ap. i-38.

☞ As seen on page 15, the basic sound of **ough** is /aw/ *(bought, brought, fought, ought, sought, thought);* and *though, through, thorough, enough, rough, tough, cough* have been learned as Spell-Words. Knowing these words is generally adequate for most purposes, but a listing of most **ough** manifestations is given here for your information.

ough /aw/ bought brought fought ought sought thought wrought
ough /ō/   borough dough furlough Marlborough Peterborough
          though thorough
ough /ow/ bough drought plough (plow)
ough /ōō/ through
ough /əf/ clough *(A gourge.)* enough rough slough *(A bog.)* tough
ough /awf/ cough

◆ Nouns and Pronouns in English are in a certain **Case***: Nominative, Possessive,* or *Objective.* "The boy's (Possessive) father (Nominative) threw the ball (Objective--Direct Object) to him (Objective--Indirect Object)." The *nominative* is used for the subject of a sentence or clause; the *possessive* shows ownership or relationship; the *objective* receives direct or indirect action. When studying many foreign languages, the *nominative* is still the *nominative;* the *possessive* is the *genitive;*   the *objective* is divided into *dative* (Indirect Object) and *accusative* (Direct Object).

In English, *Case* is most obvious in the use of pronouns.

nominative	I	you	he	she	it	we	they	who
possessive	my	your	his	her	its	our	their	whose
	mine	yours		hers		ours	theirs	
objective	me	you	him	her	it	us	them	whom

I gave my book to you. Now it is yours. He gave his book to her. Now it is hers. She gave her book to him. Now it is his. You gave your book to me. Now it is mine. They gave their book to them. Now it is theirs. Who gave the book? Whose book is it? To whom did you give the book?

☞ Review Rule 20 on p. 22 concerning *-ble, -dle, -fle, -gle, -kle, -ple, -tle, -zle.* Notice the absence of *-cle*. This is in a class by itself.

RULE 38: **-cle** is used in three & four syllable words(undoubled even after a short vowel).

-cle /kəl/ article barnacle carbuncle chronicle cubicle cuticle debacle icicle miracle obstacle oracle particle Popsicle receptacle spectacle tabernacle tentacle testicle vehicle ventricle

---

♦ The **-able, -ible** dilemma: unfortunately both are pronounced /ə-bəl/ and both are adjective producing suffixes. That **-able** is from the Latin *-abilis* and **-ible** is from the Latin *-ibilis* is of little help to the English speller. The **-able** suffix, in addition to its Latin relatives, has been added to many non-Latin words, so that there are almost exactly three times as many words ending with **-able** as there are in **-ible** (Guessing hint!).

1. Often **-able** is simply added to a verb: accept acceptable account accountable adapt adaptable agree agreeable depend dependable enjoy enjoyable laugh laughable reason reasonable wash washable.
2. Some **-ate** verbs are made into **-able** adjectives: appreciate appreciable communicate communicable educate educable medicate medicable
3. Many *silent-e* words drop the *e* and add **-able**: admire admirable cure curable debate debatable desire desirable dispose disposable like likable move movable solve solvable value valuable
4. Some *silent-e* words keep their *e* to retain the *soft c & g* sound: replace replaceable peace peaceable change changeable manage manageable
5. **-able** is added to words ending in *y* by changing the *y* to *i*: comply compliable deny deniable envy enviable rely reliable vary variable

---

6. The nouns horror and terror use **-ible** to form their adjectives:
horror horrible   terror terrible
7. Unlike the examples in 1-5 above, some **-ible** words have no *partners*: audible compatible credible divisible edible eligible feasible gullible incomprehensible incorrigible incredible indelible infallible intelligible legible negligible plausible susceptible tangible visible

-able, -ible cont.

8. Most roots ending in *ss* have **-ible** endings: accessible admissible discussible dismissible expressible permissible possible suppressible

9. Since some **-ible**, like **-able**, endings can be added to complete words or to *silent-e* words, some of the most common are listed here: contemptible convertible corruptible deductible digestible discernible exhaustible extendible flexible forcible perceptible perfectible resistible responsible reversible sensible suggestible
<u>See</u>: **-able** in Ap. iv-17 and **-ible** in Ap. iv-33.

RULE 39: A <u>prefix</u> (a letter group placed in front of *root* or *stem*) alters meaning. The word *prefix* is an example. The root is *fix* from Latin *fixus*. The prefix is *pre-* meaning *before*. So the meaning *fixed* is altered to *fixed before*.

PREFIXES

Our most common prefixes come from three sources: Old English, Latin, and Greek. A working group from each source is given here, but you will want to peruse Ap. iii for a more complete listing with appropriate use examples.

OLD ENGLISH Prefixes:

after- all- be- by- fore- in- mid- mis- off- out- over- step- under- up-

LATIN Prefixes:

ab- *from;* ad- *to, toward;* bi- *two;* circum- *around;* com- *with, together;* contra- *against;* de- *down; not;* dis- *apart;* ex- *out;* in- *in, not;* inter- *between;* intra- *within;* multi- *much, many;* non- *not;* per- *through;* post- *after;* pre- *before;* pro- *for, forward;* re- *again, back;* se- *apart;* sub- *under;* super- *above;* trans- *across;* tri- *three.*

GREEK Prefixes:

a- *not;* ana- *up, back;* amphi- *both, around;* anti- *against;* apo- *off, away;* cata- *down, against;* dia- *across, apart;* di- *two;* dys- *defective, difficult;* en- *in, into;* epi- *upon, beside;* eu- *good, well;* ex- *out of, from;* hemi- *half;* hyper- *above;* hypo- *under;* kilo- *one thousand;* meso- *middle;* meta- *after, beyond;* mono- *one;* neo- *new, recent;* octo- *eight;* para- *beside, beyond;* penta- *five;* peri- *around, near;* pro- *before, forward;* syn- *with, together;* tri- *three.*

Since *prefixes* are to be attached to root words, let's do so.

OLD ENGLISH Prefix + Root:

aftercare **after**noon **after**thought **al**most **al**ready **al**ways **be**fore **be**side **be**yond **by**road **by**law **by**stander **fore**father **fore**head **fore**sight **in**put **in**side **in**to **mid**land **mid**night **mid**way **mis**behave **mis**deed **mis**take **off**shoot **off**shore **off**spring **out**come **out**look **out**standing **over**load **over**look **over**time **step**father **step**mother **step**son **under**ground **under**stand **under**weight **up**hold **up**roar

LATIN Prefix + Root:

abduct **ab**sent **ab**normal **ad**aptable **ad**dress **ad**here **bi**centennial **bi**focals **bi**sect **circum**ference **circum**navigate **circum**vent **com**mission **com**pact **com**passion **contra**band **contra**dict **contra**st **de**cide **de**fend **de**jected **dis**place **dis**regard **dis**traction **ex**claim **ex**tend **ex**tract **in**complete **in**decisive **in**finite **inter**act **inter**mission **inter**national **intra**mural **intra**venous **multi**colored **multi**lingual **multi**purpose **non**profit **non**resident **non**sense **per**plex **per**spire **per**vade **post**lude **post**pone **post**war **pre**dict **pre**fix **pre**war **pro**fession **pro**ject **pro**noun **re**act **re**turn **re**tain **se**clude **se**lect **se**parate **sub**heading **sub**ject **sub**marine **super**charge **super**highway **super**power **trans**fer **trans**form **trans**mit **tri**angle **tri**dent **tri**focals

GREEK Prefix + Root:

apathy **a**theist **a**tom **amphi**bious **amphi**theater **ana**chronism **ana**lyze **ana**tomy **anti**biotic **anti**dote **anti**thesis **apo**logy **apo**strophe **apo**stle **cata**logue **cata**ract **cata**strophe **dia**gnosis **dia**meter **dia**per **di**lemma **di**oxide **di**phthong **dys**entery **dys**functional **dys**lexic **en**demic **en**ergy **en**thusiasm **epi**demic **epi**dermis **epi**sode **eu**logy **eu**phemism **eu**thanasia **exo**dus **exe**gesis **exo**rcism **hemi**algia **hemi**plegia **hemi**sphere **hyper**active **hyper**tension **hyper**thermia **hypo**dermic **hypo**thermia **hypo**thetical **kilo**cycle **kilo**gram **kilo**meter **meso**morphic **Meso**potamia **Meso**zoic **meta**bolism **meta**phor **meta**physics **mono**gamy **mono**gram **mono**tone **neo**classic **Neo**lithic **neo**phyte **octo**pod **octo**pus **para**dox **para**noia **para**phrase **penta**gon **penta**meter **penta**thlon **peri**meter **peri**od **peri**scope **pro**blem **pro**gnosis **pro**gram **syn**chronize **syn**onym **syn**opsis **tri**gonometry **tri**logy **tri**pod

> RULE 40:   A <u>prefix</u> changes a *root's* meaning, but a <u>suffix</u> usually dictates part of speech. A <u>suffix</u> *("fixed beneath")* is a group of letters added to a *root*.

SUFFIXES

Here, for example, are some common OLD ENGLISH suffixes:

-ed (verb past tense, past participle) added dented lifted needed painted

-en (verb) broaden darken lessen moisten quicken shorten tighten

-er (noun, verb) answer cluster master matter order offer slander

-ful (adj.) careful cheerful dreadful faithful joyful tasteful thankful

-ier (comparative adjective) crazier flimsier prettier soapier wackier

-iest (superlative adj.) craziest flimsiest prettiest soapiest wackiest

-ing (present participle of verb) boating crying dancing singing swimming

-ish (adj.) boyish childish feverish outlandish selfish ticklish yellowish

-less /lis/ (adj.) aimless careless endless helpless restless timeless

-ly (adv.) badly boldly commonly falsely intensely slowly softly vaguely

-most (adj.) almost foremost hindmost inmost outmost topmost utmost

-ness /nis/ (noun) business cleverness darkness happiness sickness

Look at the contents to Appendix iv. Three pages of contents and 61 pages of examples! Suffixes are indeed a large category of linguistic concern. Although the parts-of-speech-dictates of suffixes are important, our primary concern now as *readers* and *spellers* will be *pronunciation*. Recall we have already studied: **-ace** /ās/, /is/, **-age** /ij/, /ahzh/, **-ar** /er/, **-ate** /āt/, /it/, **-cial** /shəl/, **-cian** /shən/, **-ciate** /shē-āt/, **-cient** /shənt/, **-cious** /shəs/, **-ial** /ē-əl/, **-ian** /ē-ən/, **-iate** /ē-āte/, **-ient** /ē-ənt/, **-ion** /yən/, **-ious** /ē-əs/, **-ing** /ing/, **-ism** /iz-əm/, **-ist** /ist/, **-le** /əl/, (-ble, -cle, -dle, -fle, -gle, -kle, -ple, -tle, -zle), **-less** /lis/, **-let** /lit/, **-ly** /lē/, **-ness** /nis/, **-or** /er/, **-ous** /əs/, **-sion** /shən/, /zhən/, **-tial** /shəl/, **-tian** /shən/, **-tient** /shənt/, **-tion** /shən/, **-tious** /shəs/, **-ture** /cher/, **-tiate** /shē-āt/, **-us** /əs/, **-y** /ī/, /ē/.

Using this list we can get some analogous pronunciations: **-ly** /lē/, thus:

-cy /sē/ complacency fallacy inaccuracy infancy policy presidency

-ty /tē/ certainty community entity honesty loyalty purity specialty

Since suffixes are almost never accented, what might have been /ǎ/ becomes a schwa, /ə/, as in **cial** /shəl/ and **cian** /shən/.

-a /ə/ formula harmonica nova opera peninsula retina rotunda tuba
-able /ə-bəl/ adaptable available comfortable laughable measurable
-ably /ə-blē/ admirably agreeably considerably favorably notably
-acy /ə-sē/ adequacy confederacy intricacy legacy lunacy supremacy
-al /əl/ animal carnival oval radical rascal scandal survival vandal
-an /ən/ Mexican pelican puritan Roman republican sultan urban
-ance /əns/ admittance clearance entrance endurance fragrance
-ant /ənt/ accountant assistant covenant defendant pollutant servant
-ah /ə/ Allah Deborah Delilah Elijah Isaiah Jehovah Jonah Judah

Likewise, what might have been ŏ becomes /ə/ as in **-tion** /shən/.

-some /səm/ awesome burdensome foursome gruesome handsome
-son /sən/ lesson person Emerson Jackson Jefferson Johnson
-ton /tən/ carton piston Boston Charleston Hampton Princeton
-dom /dəm/ boredom freedom kingdom martyrdom officialdom
-om /əm/ axiom atom custom idiom random ransom seldom venom
-on /ən/ apron beacon beckon button carbon jargon lemon patron
✋ But in Greek words:
-on /on/ electron icon ion moron neon Parthenon Pentagon photon

In the following, *e* is pronounced /ə/ in fluid speaking. If this is not a problem and the letter *e* appears easily in spelling, fine. However, if this causes a confusion with other schwaed vowels when spelling, use the /ě/ pronunciation when spelling. You can practice this with a *read-spell* pronunciation alternation:

     cancel /kan-səl/, /kan-sěl/; system /sis-təm/, /sis-těm/.

Since we aren't spelling at the moment, read the following with /ə/.
-el /əl/ angel cancel camel duel level model novel panel travel
-em /əm/ Harlem Moslem problem Salem system tandem theorem
-en /ən/ citizen dozen hyphen mitten omen oxygen warden Yemen
-ence /əns/ absence audience coherence difference existence
-ency /ən-sē/ clemency currency delinquency emergency urgency
-ent /ənt/ accident client current deterrent incident parent resident
-ment /mənt/ ailment argument enjoyment garment instrument

As with *e, i* has an /ə/ pronunciation. If this presents spelling problems, a *read-spell* pronunciation may be helpful: pencil /p̲e̲n̲-səl/, /p̲e̲n̲-sĭl/.

-il /əl/ April civil council evil nostril pencil pupil stencil tonsil vigil
-ible /ə-bəl/   audible   credible   terrible   visible
-ibly /ə-blē/   audibly   credibly   terribly   visibly

-um /əm/ album arboretum curriculum forum minimum quantum
-us /əs/ bonus census circus discus fungus Jesus lotus Olympus

Latin Word Indicators

Most Latin words are easily recognized by a definite ***prefix, root,*** and ***suffix:*** con-fer-ence suc-ces-sion de-duc-tion This three-part system allows for much variety in words coming from a common root. Sometimes only one or two parts of the system is used; occasionally a double prefix or a double suffix appears. For example, in Latin the principle parts of the verb, *to drag, to pull,* are **traho, trahere, traxi, tractus,** (*I pull,* Present Tense; *to pull,* Infinitive; *I pulled,* Past Tense; *pulled,* Past Participle). With the English language's propensity to drop cases endings (inflections), *tractus* becomes *tract* (with the difficult /k-t/ pronunciation). *Tract* is termed the *root.* A playing with prefixes, suffixes, and the root *tract,* yields this sort of variety: abs̲t̲r̲a̲c̲t abs̲t̲r̲a̲c̲ted abs̲t̲r̲a̲c̲tion at̲t̲r̲a̲c̲t at̲t̲r̲a̲c̲tion at̲t̲r̲a̲c̲tive cont̲r̲a̲c̲t cont̲r̲a̲c̲ted cont̲r̲a̲c̲tion cont̲r̲a̲c̲tor cont̲r̲a̲c̲tual det̲r̲a̲c̲t det̲r̲a̲c̲tion det̲r̲a̲c̲tive det̲r̲a̲c̲tor ext̲r̲a̲c̲t ext̲r̲a̲c̲tion ext̲r̲a̲c̲tor intract̲a̲ble prot̲r̲a̲c̲t prot̲r̲a̲c̲ter prot̲r̲a̲c̲tor prot̲r̲a̲c̲tion ret̲r̲a̲c̲t ret̲r̲a̲c̲tion ret̲r̲a̲c̲tor retract̲ile subt̲r̲a̲c̲t subt̲r̲a̲c̲tion t̲r̲a̲c̲t t̲r̲a̲c̲tor t̲r̲a̲c̲table   A few more common LATIN roots:

dic (speak) contradiction dictation dictator dictionary indicate prediction
duc (lead) abduct aqueduct conducive deductible educate production
grad (step) degrade gradation grade gradient gradual graduation
jec (throw) conjecture dejected eject injection objection project reject
mit (send) admit commit emit omit permit remit submit transmit
port (carry) deport export import port portable porter reporting support
spect (watch) circumspect inspection introspective prospect suspect
struct (build) construction destruction instruction obstruct structure
ten (hold) contented contents intention retentive tenant tenor tenure
ven (come) adventure convene eventful intervention prevent venture
ver (turn) avert converge convertible divergence invert reversal versus
vis (see) advise envision invisible visa visionary visit visual visualize

GREEK Word Indicators

Most Greek Word Indicators come directly from the Greek alphabet:
theta θ (th), rho ρ (rh), upsilon υ (-y-), phi φ (ph), chi χ (ch), psi ψ (ps):

th theater theology theorem theory therapy thermostat thesis theta
  ✍ *th* is also Old English: than that the then there these them this those
rh /r/ rhapsody rheostat rhesus rhetoric rheumatism rhinoceros rho
-y- /ĭ/ cylinder gymnasium laryngitis mystery Olympics physical
-y- /ī/ cyclone enzyme hydrogen hyphen rhyme style type typhoid
ph /f/ alphabet atmosphere blasphemy phi photograph symphony
ch /k/ archives anchor character charisma chemistry chi chronic
  ✍ O.F. *ch* /ch/ chain chair chance; Fr. *ch* /sh/ brochure chagrin chef chute
ps /s/ psalm pseudo pseudonym psi psoriasis psyche psychology

Unusual letter combinations:
mn- /n/ (Gk. *mnāmon*, mindful) mnemonic /nē-<u>mon</u>-ik/ (aiding memory)
pn- /n/ (Gk. *pneuma*, breath) pneumatic; (*pneumo*, lung) pneumology pneumonia

Usually Greek word roots are referred to as *Combining Forms* because they can be combined or added together. Sometimes a connecting vowel is needed. This *combining* is not a feature of Latin. Thus, **tele** (distance), **phone** (sound), **graph** (write), **scope** (see), **photo** (light) can be combined to form: **telephone photograph telescope phonograph telegraph**. Since the ancient Greeks had none of these devices, as you might suspect, our word-making scientists have been very busy.

A few more common GREEK Combining Forms:
auto (self) autobiography autocracy autograph automatic automobile
bio (life) biochemistry biography biology biopsy biosphere biotron
chron (time) anachronism chronic chronicle chronology synchronize
dem (people) endemic epidemic demagogue democracy demography
geo (earth) geocentric geography geologist geometry geophysics
logy (study of) anthropology ecology musicology neurology sociology
meter (measure) barometer centimeter diameter perimeter thermometer
ortho (straight) orthodontist orthodox orthography orthopedics
path (feeling) antipathy pathology psychopath sympathy telepathy
polis (city) acropolis metropolis Minneapolis police policy politician
poly (many) polygamy polygraph polyp polyphony polyunsaturated
psycho (mind) psyche psychedelic psychiatry psychic psychology

GREEK Medical Terms

From the previous words it is obvious that Greek is alive and well in technical and scientific realms. Its terms are also especially useful in medical circles. Here are a just a few common medical combining forms:

cardio (heart) cardiac cardiogram cardiograph cardiology carditis
-ectomy (cutting out) appendectomy mastectomy tonsillectomy
hema (blood) hematology hemophilia hemorrhage hemorrhoid
-iatric (healing) geriatric gyniatric hydriatric pediatric psychiatric
-itis (inflammation) appendicitis arthritis bronchitis bursitis colitis
   conjunctivitis encephalitis gastritis gingivitis hepatitis laryngitis
   meningitis neuritis phlebitis poliomyelitis tenonitis tonsillitis
-mania (infatuation) egomania kleptomania nymphomania pyromania
-oma (cancer) carcinoma glaucoma hematoma leukoma melanoma
optic (of the eye) optic optical optician optics optometrist optometry
-osis (condition) arteriosclerosis hypnosis narcosis neurosis psychosis
osteo (bone) osteology osteomyelitis osteopathy osteoporosis
phobia (fear of) acrophobia agoraphobia claustrophobia necrophobia
therapy (treatment) chemotherapy hypnotherapy psychotherapy

FRENCH Word Indicators

-é /ā/ attaché café cliché consommé entrée passé resumé
-age /ahzh/ corsage espionage garage massage mirage sabotage
-eau /ō/ beau bureau chateau Juneau plateau Rousseau Thoreau
-que /k/ critique mystique oblique physique technique unique
-esque /esk/ burlesque grotesque picturesque statuesque
-et /ā/ ballet bouquet buffet Chevrolet croquet fillet gourmet valet
-ette /et/ briquette brunette cassette cigarette gazette majorette
   marionette novelette silhouette statuette suffragette usherette
ch /sh/ chalet champagne chandelier chagrin charade Chartres
   Charlemagne chateau chauvinism Chopin gauche machine
ç- /s/ (before a, o, u.) façade français /fran-sā/ (French) garçon
-eur /er/ carillonneur chauffeur connoisseur entrepreneur
   grandeur /gran-jer/ liqueur masseur Monsieur saboteur voyeur

See: Ap. viii-1 for more borrowed French words; Ap. i-5 for **-é, e** /ā/; Ap. i-16 for more **ch, ç-**;
Ap. i-19 for **-eau**; Ap. iv-19 for **-age**; Ap. iv-62-64 for **-que, -esque, -et, -ette, -eur.**

SPANISH Word Indicators

ñ /ny/ cañon Doña el Niño mañana piñata señor señora señorita
i (long) /ē/ amigo fiesta hacienda lariat mosquito si siesta tortilla (l=y)
e (long) /ā/ hombre mesa peyote San Diego Sierra Madre Teresa
a /ä/ adios habanera hacienda macho mañana padre papaya plaza
j /h/ Juan Guadalajara junta La Jolla /hoi-yə/ marijuana Navajo
San (Masc. *Saint.*) San Diego   San Francisco   San Jose   San Juan
Santa (Fem. *Saint.*) Santa Barbara Santa Clara Santa Fe Santa Maria

<u>See</u>: Ap. viii-5-6 for a more extensive list of borrowed Spanish words.

ITALIAN Word Indicators

c (Before *e* & *i*.) /ch/ a rivederci Botticelli ciao cello concerto da Vinci
i (long) /ē/ ballerina lira maraschino piazza pizza ravioli rialto
e (long) /ā/ Dante   il Duce /doo-chā/ forte   grave /grä-vā/   padre
a /ä/   aria a tempo bravo mafia padre pasta /pas-tə/ salami
-o (long) /ō/ alto arioso fiasco lento piano primo solo soprano trio
A good summary: a rivederci /ä rē-vā-dair-chē/ *(Until we meet again.)*

<u>See</u>: Ap. viii-4-5 for a more extensive list of borrowed Italian words.

BORROWINGS From Other Sources

African Languages banana banjo chimpanzee jumbo marimba

American Indian caucus chipmunk papoose skunk squash wigwam

Arabic algebra almanac arsenal assassin coffee cork cotton lemon

Chinese chop suey chow mein gung ho kumquat tea tycoon yen

Hawaiian aloha hula lei /lā/ luau muumuu *(A lady's gown.)* poi ukulele

Hebrew cherub cider cinnamon Eden hallelujah kibbutz kosher rabbi

Hindi bandanna bangle bungalow cheetah dungaree shampoo thug

Japanese banzai geisha hari-kari judo jujitsu kamikaze karate soy

Persian arsenic bazaar caravan check chess divan jackal khaki

Russian borscht commissar czar glasnost gulag perestroika vodka

See: Ap. x for a more inclusive listing from these and other sources.

♦ **CHAMELEON PREFIXES**: The Assimilation Process. Common prefixes often change a letter to match what it is being fixed to. The prefix is partly *assimilated* to the root or, as with a chameleon, it changes with its environment. The most prominent example is **ad-** *(to, toward, near)* which can change to **ab-, ac-, af-, ag-, al-, an-, ap-, ar-, as-,** or **at-.** Let's see how this works. Notice it doesn't always change.

---

ad-	a	adapt adaptable adaptive
ab-	**b**	abbreviate abbreviation
ac-	**c**	acclaim account accommodate accomplish accord accuse
ad-	d	address addict addition addendum adduce addiction
ad-	e	adept adeem ad extremum ademption
af-	**f**	affection affair affiliate affirm affect afflict affront affliction
ag-	**g**	aggress aggression aggrandize aggressive aggrieved
ad-	h	adhere adhesive adhesion adhibit ad hoc ad hominem
ad-	i	ad infinitum ad interim ad initium
ad-	j	adjourn adjacent adjective adjust adjudge adjunct adjutant
al-	**l**	alliance allied allege alleviate allow allowance allure
ad-	m	admire admit admission admonish administer administration
an-	**n**	announce announcement annex annihilate annul
ad-	o	adopt adoption adorn adore
ap-	**p**	appoint apparel apparent appeal appear appease applaud
ac-	**q**	acquaint acquaintance acquire acquit acquittal acquisitive
ar-	**r**	arrest arrive arrival arrange arrangement arraignment arrear
as-	**s**	assist assemble assail assault assent assess assign assert
at-	**t**	attempt attention attain attend attendance attest attire attract
ad-	u	adult adulterate adulterer adulteress adunc adust
ad-	v	adventure adverb adversary adversity advertise advice

Reading hint: if you see an *a* followed by two consonants, it most likely can be pronounced /ə/ plus the consonant sounded once: acclaim = /ə-klām/; affect = /ə-<u>fekt</u>/; allow = /ə-<u>low</u>/; announce = /ə-<u>nowns</u>; appoint = /ə-<u>point</u>/; arrest /ə-<u>rest</u>/; assert /ə-<u>sert</u>/; attain /ə-<u>tān</u>/.

> Spelling hint: often if /ə/ is heard first, write *a* and then double the consonant representing the next sound heard: /ə-klām/ = acclaim; /ə-fekt/ = affect; /ə-low/ = allow; /ə-<u>nowns</u> = announce; /ə-point/ = appoint; /ə-<u>rest</u>/ = arrest; /ə-<u>sert</u>/ = assert; /ə-<u>tān</u>/ = attain.

But Note:

1. The **accent shift from noun to verb** is still in effect.
address (noun) /<u>ad</u>-res/, address (verb) /ə-<u>dres</u>/,

2. The **beginning *a* is short** /ă/, not schwaed /ə/, when the first syllable is accented:
adage, adaptation, accurate, adequate, affluent, allegation, alloy, adolescent, apparatus, appetite, apprehend, acquisition.

3. In *ac-c* words the *a* is short /ă/ when the second *c* is soft /s/: accede, accelerate, accent, accentuate, accept, acceptable, access, accessible, accident, accidental

4. **Before *q*** , *ad-* becomes *ac-* with one /k/ sound: acquit /ə-<u>kwit</u>/ acquire.

5. In **ad-h, ad-m, ad-s, and ad-v words**, *ad* has its /ad/ pronunciation:
adhere, administer, adsorb, advise

6. In *ad-j* words the *d* is not pronounced: adjective /<u>aj</u>-ik-tiv/.

OTHER CHAMELEON PREFIXES:

com-, con-, col-, cor-, co- *(with, together)* (L)
combat command compare concede conduct confine congress connect conquer consist contest convert collect college correct corrode coerce coherent coincidence cooperate

dis-, dif-, di- *(apart; reverse; not)* (L)
disable disband disclose discuss disdain disease disfavor disgrace dishonest disinfect disjointed dislike dismiss disorder dispense disqualify disregard disrupt dissolve distance disturb disuse differ difficult digest dilute dimension direct

ex-, ef-, e- *(out of; lacking; former)* (L)
exact example exceed exempt exert exhale exit exorbitant expand exquisite effect efficient edition eject elect emerge emission enunciate erase escort extent exude evict evolve

in-, il-, im-, ir-, i- *(not, without)* (L)
inactive incapable indefinite inept infamous ingrate inhuman iniquity injury innocent inoperable insane intact invalid illegal illiterate illogical immature imbalance impatient irrational irregular irrelevant ignoble ignominious ignorance

43

in-, il-, im-, ir- *(within)* (OE, L) [A chameleon prefix only in Latin.]
inaugurate inborn incision income increase indent infection infielder ingest ingrown inhabit initial inject inland inmate innate inoculate input inquire insert inside insight intense inundate invade illuminate illusion illustrate immense immerse impede impel impetuous irrigation irritate irruption

ob-, oc-, of-, op-, o- *(toward; against; over)* (L)
obese obey obituary object oblige obnoxious obscure obtain obvious occasion occur offend offer oppose oppress omit

sub-, suc-, suf-, sug-, sup-, sur-, sus- *(under; secondary)* (L)
subbasement subcommittee subconscious subdivide subdue subgroup subheading subject sublime submarine subnormal subordinate subscribe subtract suburb subvert subway succeed successive succumb suffer sufficient suffix suggest supply support suppose surrogate surreptitious suspect sustain

syn-, syl-, sym-, sys- *(with, together)* (Gk.)
synagogue synchronize synergism synonym synthesis syllable syllogism symbolism symmetrical sympathy symphony system
<u>See:</u> Ap. iii for a more complete listing of Chameleon Prefix examples.

☞ You have probably noticed a few differences in **British and American spellings**. A basic list of such British words is given here with the American counterpart in parentheses.

---

appetiser (appetizer) arbour (arbor) ardour (ardor) armour (armor) behaviour (behavior) cheque (check) colour (color) connexion (connection) defence (defense) distil (distill) epitomise (epitomize) favour (favor) generalise (generalize) harmonise (harmonize) honour (honor) instal (install) instil (instill) kerb (curb) labour (labor) litre (liter) metre (meter) minimise (minimize) mouldy (moldy) nationalise (nationalize) naturalise (naturalize) neighbour (neighbor) offence (offense) pasteurise (pasteurize) polarise (polarize) practise (practice) pretence (pretense) programme (program) realise (realize) recognise (recognize) reconnoitre (reconnoiter) scrutinise (scrutinize) stabilise (stabilize) subsidise (subsidize) summarise (summarize) sympathise (sympathize) synthesise (synthesize) temporise (temporize) terrorise (terrorize) theatre (theater) theorise (theorize) tranquillise(tranquilize) tyre (tire) valour (valor) vapour (vapor) vigour (vigor) visualise (visualize) vulgarise (vulgarize)   What sort of regularities do you see here?

◆　　　　　　More thoughts on "i" sounding /ē/.

Rule 28 (page 27) stated that single "i" followed by a different vowel in a suffix, is pronounced /ē/ . Why should this be? Compare /ī/ & /ē/. /ē/ is one pure sound /ee/ as in *bee*. /ī/, however, is a diphthong (Gk. *two sounds*): /ah-ee/ or /ä-ē/. Try saying "trivial" /<u>triv</u>-ī-əl/. This is really /<u>triv</u>-ä-ē-əl/. Difficult? Certainly. Three unaccented vowel sounds are not appreciated by speakers of English. Perhaps the *i* in question should be a schwa; it is unaccented. Well, try /<u>triv</u>-ə-əl/. Again, two successive schwas are difficult to say. This is why we don't say "a oven", but "an oven." So "trivial" pronounced /<u>triv</u>-ē-əl/ works just fine!

❖　　　Here are the instances where *i* is pronounced /ē/:

1. When *i* is followed by a different vowel (sound) in a suffix:
-ial /ē-əl/ material,　**-ian** /ē-ən/ historian,　**-ient** /ē-ənt/ lenient,
-ious /ē-əs/ tedious,　**-iate** /ē-āt/ mediate,　**-ior** /ē-or/ superior,
-ia /ē-ə/ media,　**-iance** /ē-əns/ radiance,　**-ience** /ē-əns/ audience,
-ium /ē-əm/ radium, **-iatric** /ē-<u>at</u>-ric/ psychiatric, **-iet** /ē-et/ Soviet,
-iator /ē-āt-er/ mediator, **-iot** /ē-ət/ idiot, **-iasm** /ē-az-əm/ enthusiasm,
-iose /ē-ōs/ grandiose,

2. Before **-que** and **-gue**.
-ique /ēk/ antique clique critique oblique physique technique unique
-igue /ēg/ fatigue intrigue

3. When a final *y* with an /ē/ pronunciation is changed to *i* to form a new suffix, the *i* retains the original /ē/ sound.
(a) Forming Degrees with <u>adjectives</u> ending in *y*. /ē/, /ē-er/, /ē-est/.
cozy cozier coziest　sleepy sleepier sleepiest　pretty prettier prettiest
✋ But where *y* is sounded /ī/, keep the /ī/ sound. (One syllable adjectives.)
dry /drī/, drier /drī-er/, driest /drī-est/; shy shier shiest; sly slier sliest
(b) Forming plural <u>nouns</u> from *consonant-y* words. /ē/, /ēz/.
army armies cavity cavities city cities remedy remedies sixty sixties
✋ But where *y* is sounded /ī/, keep the /ī/ sound. (One syllable nouns.)
fly flies　sky skies　spy spies　try tries

45

I Sounding E cont.

(c) Forming 3rd person singular <u>verbs</u> from those ending in *consonant y*.

/ē/, /ēz/ carry carries hurry hurries study studies worry worries

🖐 But where *y* is sounded /ī/, keep the /ī/ sound (Accented syllables as in **comply, rel<u>y</u>, supp<u>ly</u>** and in **-fy** words such as **fortify, glorify, petrify**.) <u>See</u>: Rule 37, page 31.

/ī/, /īz/ comply complies rely relies; fortify fortifies glorify glorifies

4. Generally a final *i* is pronounced /ē/.

Biloxi broccoli da Vinci Capri Fiji Gandhi Garibaldi Hawaii
Helsinki Hindi Marconi martini Medici merci mi Miami Mississippi
Missouri Mitsubishi Nazi pastrami Pulaski ravioli si Suzuki suki
yaki Swahili Tahiti Tivoli Watusi

5. In French, Spanish, and Italian long *i* is pronounced /ē/.

chic /shēk/ cliché fiancée; amigo fiesta siesta; antipasto pizza ravioli

---

◆ You probably have been living happily with many ***word contractions***: can't for cannot; I'm for I am; that's for that is, *etc.* The apostrophe (') takes the place of what has been dropped. Check page 5 of Ap. xi to see if you have missed any other *contractions*.

◆ Many words in English derive from people's names or geographical places. A few are listed here. You might be interested in exploring others in Ap. xii.

Names: atlas August braille Cadillac Eiffel (Tower) diesel (engine) ferris (wheel) Freud(ian) Hudson (River) Jupiter levi(s) lynch Marx(ism) maverick Mercury Nobel (prize) pan(ic) Pasteur(ize) ritz(y) Titan(ic)

Places: airedale ammon(ia) angora babel badminton bikini champagne china cologne duffel (bag) hamburg(er) lima (bean) mecca

---

☞ Some pronunciations just don't seem to make sense! Memorize:

boatswain /bō-sən/   colonel /ker-nəl/   corps /kor/
corpsman /kor-mən/ coxswain /kok-sən/ coyote /kī-ō-tē/
ensemble /än-säm-bəl/ Gloucester /glos-ter/ indict /in-dīt/
rendezvous /rän-dā-voo/ sergeant /sar-gənt/ victul /vit-l/
women /wim-in/ Worcester /woos-ter/

R'S ARE EASY

Rules of "R" Pronunciation

> **1. Any vowel with an r may be pronounced /er/.**

-ar /er/ [Note position in word.] burglar cellar collar dollar grammar lunar particular
   pillar popular regular scholar similar solar sugar vulgar; <u>See</u>: **-ar²** Ap.i-12.

er /er/ after butter clerk concert converse expert darker faster fern finger germ
   her jumper laughter letter lumber manner modern nerve number offer
   percent perfect permit player renter term tiger verb verse; <u>See</u>: **er** Ap.i-21-22.

ir /er/ birch bird birth chirp circumstances circle circus confirm dirt fir firm first
   girl quirk shirk sir skirt squirm squirt swirl third thirst twirl; <u>See</u>: **ir** Ap.i-26.

-or /er/ [Note position in word.] actor author color doctor favor flavor labor major
   mayor minor motor odor rumor sector tractor tutor vapor; <u>See</u>: **-or** Ap.i-29.

ur /er/ blur burn blurt burden burlap burn burp burst church curb curl curse curve
   fur hurt murder murmur nurse purple purse sturdy surf turn; <u>See</u>: **ur** Ap.i-42.

-yr /er/ martyr myrrh myrtle satyr zephyr;   <u>See</u>: **yr** Ap.i-46.

> **2. However, ar is usually pronounced /are/.**

ar- /are/ ark arm army art artist bark car cargo cart carve chart dark dart far
   hard hark harm harp harvest lard large marble market mart pardon park
   scar scarf scarlet smart snarl spark star start tar tardy yard; <u>See</u>: **ar-** Ap.i-11.

> **3. And or is usually pronounced /or/.**

or- /or/ accord afford assort border born cord cork corn corner dorm for force
   fork forlorn form fort forty horn hornet horse lord more morn morning
   pork port shore short sort stork storm thorn torment York; <u>See</u>: **or¹** Ap.i-29.

> **4. Silent e still makes preceding vowel long.**

-are /air/ aware bare beware blare care dare declare ensnare fare flare
   glare hare mare pare rare scare share snare spare square stare tare ware

-ere /ear/ adhere ampere cohere here inhere mere revere sere severe sphere we're
   <u>Note</u>: cereal /<u>sear</u>-ē-əl/; <u>Exceptions</u>: ere /air/ there /thair/ where /whair/ were /wer/

-ire /ī-er/ admire afire aspire attire conspire desire dire empire entire expire fire
   hire mire quire rehire retire satire shire sire spire squire tire umpire wire

-ore /or/ adore afore ashore before bore chore core encore /äng-kor/ fore galore
   gore ignore lore more pore score shore snore sore spore store swore tore wore

-ure / o͞or/ abjure adjure allure assure endure ensure lure manure velure;
   /yo͞or/ cure demure immure impure inure pure secure;
   <u>Exceptions</u>: /er/ azure injure;   /yer/ figure tenure;   <u>And</u>: sure /sher/

-yre /ī-er/ lyre pyre;   <u>See</u>: **Silent-e Pairs and Unpaired Examples** in Ap.i-35-36.

---

5. Accented ar-r and er-r are pronounced /air/.

---

ar-r /air/ arrogant arrow barracks barrel barren carrot carry carriage carried Harris
Harry marry marriage narrow parrot tarry wheelbarrow; <u>See:</u> ar-r Ap.i-12.
Note when *ar-r* is part of an *unaccented Chameleon Prefix*, ar<u>rest</u> /ə-rest/, on page 42.

er-r /air/ berry cherry error errand errant erratic ferry merry Terry Sierra
<u>See:</u> er-r Ap.i-23.

---

6. Similarly, accented ar and er followed by a vowel, are also pronounced /air/.

---

ar-V /air/ barely barium baron Carol carols familiarity garish guaranty harass
harem Karen Mary parent Paris parish parity parody pharaoh planetarium
primarily sharable rarity tariff Sarah varied varies vary; <u>See:</u> **ar-V** Ap.i-12.

er-V /air/ American America Cheryl clerical emeritus experiment generic gerund
herald heresy heritage heroin Jeremy merits perils seraph sheriff verify verity;
<u>See:</u> **er-V** Ap.i-22. <u>Remember:</u> -ere still generally follows *Silent e Rule.* See #4.
<u>But:</u> the *unaccented* suffix er-y is pronounced /er-ē/: archery bakery battery
delivery discovery nursery pottery recovery surgery; <u>See:</u> -ery in Ap. iv-30.

[Note: Because of regional differences, some may hear and make a difference in the
pronunciation of *Mary, marry,* & *merry.* These fine distinctions are beyond the scope of this book.
Happily, regional speakers will make these and other "adjustments" easily and automatically.]

---

7. ir-r is pronounced /ear/.

---

ir-r /ear/ cirrus irritation irregular irrational irrelevant irreplaceable irresistible
irresponsible irreverence irrigation irritate irruption mirror; <u>See:</u> ir-r Ap.i-26.

---

8. -yr- followed by a vowel (not e) also sounds /ear/.

---

yr-V /ear/ lyrics myriad pyramid Syria syringe syrup tyranny; <u>See:</u> -yr-V Ap.i-46.
<u>But:</u> if the *y* is in a separate accented syllable, it follows open syllable rule: (ī) gyrate pyrite
styrofoam thyroid tyrant; <u>And:</u> lyre /līr/ & pyre /pīr/ follow the Silent E Rule.

---

9. or-r and ur-r keep their usual sounds.

---

or-r /or/ borrow corral horrible horrid horrify horror lorry Morris morrow
sorrow sorry torrent torrid; <u>But:</u> the unaccented prefix cor- is often /kə/: correct
correction corroborate corrode corrosion corrupt; <u>See:</u> cor/r in Ap. iii-9.

ur-r /er/ burro burrow burr currant current curry currier furry furrier
furrow hurrah hurry hurried purr surreal surrealism surrey surround turret

48

---

10. After a *w*, -or takes its /er/ sound.

---

wor- /wer/ word work workbook worker world worldly worm worry worse worship worst worth worthy; Exceptions: sword worn; See: **wor** Ap. i-43.

---

11. After a *w* or *qu*, -ar takes a new /or/ sound.

---

war- /wor/ dwarf swarm thwart warble ward warden war warfare warrior warble warbler warm warmth warn warp warrant Warsaw wart; See: **war** Ap. i-42.

quar- /kwor/ quark quarrel quarry quart quarter quartet quartz; See: **qua** Ap. i-32.

---

12. -ear has three pronunciations: /er/, /air/, & /ear/.

-ear /er/ early earn earnest earth earthly heard learn pearl rehearse search yearn

-ear /air/ bear bearing bearer pear swear tear wear

-ear /ear/ clear dear ear fear gear hear near rear tear year; See: **-ear** in Ap. i-19.

---

13. -er-, when followed by the vowel *i* whose pronunciation has been changed to /ē/ since it is followed by another vowel, has the sound /ear/.

-er-i /ear-ē/ anterior arterial bacterial deleterious experience exterior hysteria imperial imperialism imperious inferior interior managerial material mysterious posterior serial serious superior ulterior; See: **er-i + vowel** in Ap. i-23.

---

14. aer- is a Greek combining form meaning *air*. It is pronounced /air/.

---

aer- /air/ aerate aerial aerodynamics aeronautics aerospace; See: **aero-** in Ap. ix-5.

---

15. -eur, from French, is pronounced /er/ in English and is usually accented.

-eur /er/ carillonneur chauffeur connoisseur entrepreneur liqueur masseur Monsieur saboteur restaurateur voyageur voyeur /vwä-yer/;
But: amateur /am-ə-choŏr/; grandeur /gran-jer/ See: **-eur-** in Ap. iv-63.

Be careful that the *r* and *vowel* are a unit. For example, the above rules do not apply to *de/ride, be/reave, re/run, by/road, etc.*

Ch. 5.   *PLURALS*

Just How Many Are There?

1. Most English words form their plural by adding "s":   bat *bats*   building *buildings*
hall *halls*   projection *projections*   string *strings*. This includes most "silent -e" words:
frame *frames* gate *gates* joke *jokes*   tape *tapes*;
The ending does not add another syllable.

2. However, words ending in "s", "sh", "ch", "z", or "x" need to add "es" to distinguish a plural
sound.   This "es" ending does add another syllable: guess *guesses*   bush *bushes*
arch *arches* buzz *buzzes* tax *taxes*.   The plural of "silent -e" words ending with /j/, /s/, or
/z/ also add an extra syllable: ledge *ledges*   collapse *collapses*   size *sizes*

3. When a final "y" is preceded by a vowel, "s" is added to form the plural just as in #1:
tray *trays*   decoy *decoys*   relay *relays*.

4. However, when a final "'y" is preceded by a consonant, **change y to i and add es.**
baby *babies*   sixty *sixties*   copy *copies*   enemy *enemies*   lady *ladies*.

   Nota Bene: 3rd person singular present tense verbs follow these same rules:
   (1) *I bat. You bat. He bats*   (2) *I blush. You blush. She blushes.*
   (3) *I stay. You stay. It stays.*   (4) *I pity. You pity. She pities.*

5. Six Old English words have vowel changes (ablaut) to indicate plural:
foot *feet*   tooth *teeth*   man *men*   woman *women*   mouse *mice*   louse *lice*.

6. A few nouns keep their Old English inflections:
child *children*   ox *oxen*   brother *brethren*

7. Some words from Old English with a final /f/ sound change the "f" to "v" and add "es":
calf *calves* elf *elves* half *halves* hoof *hooves* knife *knives* leaf *leaves* life *lives*
loaf *loaves*   scarf *scarves*   self *selves*   sheaf *sheaves*   shelf *shelves*   thief *thieves*
wharf *wharves*   wife *wives*   wolf *wolves*;
Remember that unvoiced "f" and voiced "v" are partners. ☺

8. Some words have the same form for plural and singular: *deer fish fowl sheep trout;*
and those ending in "-ese": *Chinese Japanese Maltese Portuguese Sudanese,* etc.

9. Some words are plural in form but are used as if they were singular: *barracks bellows
bloomers gallows goods means measles mumps odds pains pants scissors slacks
small pox* (Sing. pock.) *species tactics trousers* and many "-ics" words: *acrobatics
aerodynamics aesthetics athletics civics ethics genetics gymnastics linguistics
mathematics Olympics physics politics thermodynamics*

10. Words ending in "o":

(a) If the "o" is preceded by a vowel, add "s": cameo *cameos* radio *radios* studio *studios.*

(b) If the "o" is preceded by a consonant, usually "es" is added: echo *echoes* hero *heroes* Negro *Negroes* no *noes* potato *potatoes* tomato *tomatoes* veto *vetoes.*

(c) However, in some words where final "o" is preceded by a consonant, common usage allows either an "s" or "es" ending: buffalo *buffalos buffaloes.* This is true for: *banjo bravo calico cargo domino halo innuendo motto mulatto proviso tobacco tornado zero,* but for many just "s" seems less awkward and is preferred.

(d) Add only "s": Eskimo *Eskimos* Filipino *Filipinos* silo *silos*

(e) Musical terms from Italian add only "s": allegro *allegros* alto *altos* crescendo *crescendos* decrescendo *decrescendos* diminuendo *diminuendos* fortissimo *fortissimos* largo *largos* oratorio *oratorios* presto *prestos* scherzo *scherzos** soprano *sopranos** staccato *staccatos* solo *solos** tremolo *tremolos* trio *trios* vibrato *vibratos;* *See # 14.

11. LATIN words often keep their original plural inflections.

(a) Masculine nouns: [-us /əs/; -i /ī/] alumnus *alumni* bacillus *bacilli* cactus *cacti* fungus *fungi* gladiolus *gladioli* locus *loci* radius *radii* nucleus *nuclei* stimulus *stimuli* syllabus *syllabi* terminus *termini*; and index *indices* vertex *vertices* vortex *vortices*

(b) Feminine nouns: [-a /ə/;-ae /ē/] alga *algae* alumna *alumnae* amphora *amphorae* antenna *antennae* axilla *axillae* (Armpit.) fascia *fasciae* (Connective tissue.) formula *formulae* larva *larvae* macula *maculae* (Spot on skin.) mamma *mammae* maxilla *maxillae* (Jawbone.) minutia *minutiae* nebula *nebulae* nova *novae* palestra *palestrae* (Gk., *palaistra,* exercise area.) patella *patellae* (Kneecap bone.) persona *personae* placenta *placentae* tenebra *tenebrae* tibia *tibiae* trachea *tracheae* ungula *ungulae* (A claw.) vertebra *vertebrae* vibrissa *vibrissae* (Nose hair.) vita *vitae* (Résumé.) and appendix *appendices* matrix *matrices*

(c) Neuter nouns: [-um /əm/; -a /ə/] addendum *addenda* agendum *agenda* continuum *continua* curriculum *curricula* datum *data* erratum *errata* (An error.) medium *media* memorandum *memoranda* momentum *momenta* moratorium *moratoria* ovum *ova* quantum *quanta* referendum *referenda* rostrum *rostra* spectrum *spectra* stadium *stadia* stratum *strata* substratum *substrata* trivium *trivia*; Used only in plural: (dejectum) *dejecta* (Excrements.) (impedimentum) *impedimenta* (ingestum) *ingesta* (Injested food.) (insigne) *insignia*

12. GREEK words, too, often keep their original plural inflections.

 (a) Masculine nouns: [-os /os/; -oi /oi/] mythos *mythoi;* Some are used only in singular: *asbestos chaos cosmos eros ethos logos pathos* and Atlas *Atlantes* (Thus: *Atlantic.*)

 (b) Feminine nouns: [-is /is/; -es /ēz/] analysis *analyses* basis *bases* crisis *crises* diagnosis *diagnoses* emphasis *emphases* exegesis *exegeses* hypothesis *hypotheses* nemesis *nemeses* neurosis *neuroses* oasis *oases* parenthesis *parentheses* prognosis *prognoses* psychosis *psychoses* synopsis *synopses* synthesis *syntheses* thesis *theses.*

 (c) Neuter nouns: [-on /ən/; -a /ə/] criterion *criteria* noumenon *noumena* phenomenon *phenomena;* Used only in plural: *erotica* (phylon *phyla* & podion *podia* become Latin neuter phylum *phyla* & podium *podia*); also: anathema *anathemata* schema *schemata* stigma *stigmata* stoma *stomata* (Opening.) trauma *traumata.*

13. FRENCH words with retained plurals: [-eau /ō/; -eaux /ōz/] beau *beaux* bureau *bureaux* chapeau *chapeaux* chateau *chateaux* plateau *plateaux* rondeau *rondeaux* tableau *tableaux* trousseau *trousseaux;* and madame *mesdames* mademoiselle *mesdemoiselles* monsieur *messieurs.* But it is quite common to Anglicize these plurals: beau *beaus* bureau *bureaus* plateau *plateaus, etc.*

14. ITALIAN musical terms may keep their Italian inflections: [-o /ō/; -i /ē/] concerto *concerti* libretto *libretti* primo *primi* scherzo *scherzi* solo *soli* soprano *soprani* tempo *tempi* virtuoso *virtuosi;* and opus *opera.*

15. HEBREW: cherub *cherubim* seraph *seraphim*

16. OLD FRENCH die *dice*

Oh, By the Way---

 You have probably heard somewhere, sometime: *"I before e, except after c, unless they sound long a, as in neighbor and weigh."* Most often this is the case.
1. *I before e:* /ē/ belief believe brief chief field grief niece piece priest relief relieve retrieve shield shriek siege thief yield; /e/ friend; See: **ie¹** Ap. i-25; /ī/ die lie pie tie; See: **ie²** Ap. i-25;
2. *Except after c:* conceive deceive perceive receive ceiling conceit deceit; See: **ei²** Ap. i-20; Verb to noun: drop *i.* conception deception perception reception;
3. *Unless they sound long a, as in neighbor and weigh.* /ā/ eight freight neighbor sleigh weigh weight; See: **eigh** Ap. i-21
/ā/ beige /bāzh/ feign feint heinous heir lei reign rein Seine skein surveillance their veil vein; See: **ei¹** Ap. i-20;
4. However, exceptions are: *ei* /ē/ either Keith Leif leisure Neil neither protein seize seizure sheik weird; See: **ei²** Ap. i-20

 And *ei* /ī/ (Mostly German words.) eiderdown Einstein Eisenhower Frankenstein Fraulein Geiger gesundheit Guggenheim Heidelberg **height** Heifetz Holstein Leipzig leitmotif Meistersinger Oppenheimer poltergeist Reich Schweitzer; See: **ei³** AP. i-21

VERBS

Let's Do or Be Something.

Ch. 6.

CONJUGATION OF THE VERB, TO SING

PRINCIPAL PARTS: **sing,** *present tense;* **sang,** *past tense;* **sung,** *past participle;* **singing,** *present participle;* **to sing,** *infinitive*

PRESENT TENSE

	Singular	Plural
1st Person:	I sing.	We sing.
2nd Person:	You sing.	You sing.
3rd Person:	He, she, it sings.	They sing.

Note: 3rd Person Singular Present Tense adds **-s.**

PAST TENSE

	Singular	Plural
1st Person:	I sang.	We sang.
2nd Person:	You sang.	You sang.
3rd Person:	He sang.	They sang.

FUTURE TENSE

	Singular	Plural
1st Person:	I shall sing.	We shall sing.
2nd Person:	You will sing.	You will sing.
3rd Person:	He will sing.	They will sing.

PRESENT PERFECT

	Singular	Plural
1st Person:	I have sung.	We have sung.
2nd Person:	You have sung.	You have sung.
3rd Person:	He has sung.	They have sung.

Note: the *past participle* **sung** is used in all Perfect Tenses.

PAST PERFECT

	Singular	Plural
1st Person:	I had sung.	We had sung.
2nd Person:	You had sung.	You had sung.
3rd Person:	He had sung.	They had sung.

FUTURE PERFECT

	Singular	Plural
1st Person:	I shall have sung.	We shall have sung.
2nd Person:	You will have sung.	You will have sung.
3rd Person:	He will have sung.	They will have sung.

PRESENT PROGRESSIVE

	Singular	Plural
1st Person:	I am singing.	We are singing.
2nd Person:	You are singing.	You are singing.
3rd Person:	He is singing.	They are singing.

PAST PROGRESSIVE

	Singular	Plural
1st Person:	I was singing.	We were singing.
2nd Person:	You were singing.	You were singing.
3rd Person:	He was singing.	They were singing.

FUTURE PROGRESSIVE

	Singular	Plural
1st Person:	I shall be singing.	We shall be singing.
2nd Person:	You will be singing.	You will be singing.
3rd Person:	He will be singing.	They will be singing.

PRESENT PERFECT PROGRESSIVE

	Singular	Plural
1st Person:	I have been singing.	We have been singing.
2nd Person:	You have been singing.	You have been singing.
3rd Person:	He has been singing.	They have been singing.

Note: the *present participle* **singing** is used in all Progressive Tenses.

PAST PERFECT PROGRESSIVE

	Singular	Plural
1st Person:	I had been singing.	We had been singing.
2nd Person:	You had been singing.	You had been singing.
3rd Person:	He had been singing.	They had been singing.

FUTURE PERFECT PROGRESSIVE

	Singular	Plural
1st Person:	I shall have been singing.	We shall have been singing.
2nd Person:	You will have been singing.	You will have been singing.
3rd Person:	He will have been singing.	They will have been singing.

Ch. 6. Verbs

A **verb** is one of the eight parts of speech (noun, pronoun, verb, adverb, adjective, conjunction, preposition, interjection) and expresses existence *(I am.)*, state of being *(She is happy.)*, action *(He ran quickly.)*, or occurrence *(It all happened yesterday.)*. A verb has five properties: *tense, person, number, mood,* and *voice*.

From the ***conjugation*** (an ordered presentation of verb forms) of ***to sing*** on the previous page, it is obvious that there are twelve tenses of an English verb. **Tense** indicates time. Is something happening now? Did it happen yesterday? Will it happen tomorrow? Was it a single event or an ongoing event? All these positions in time are indicated by a verb's *tense*. Although the use of present, past, and future tenses are obvious, comments on the perfect and progressive tenses may be useful. "Present Perfect happened before Present; Past Perfect happened before Past; Future Perfect happened before Future." But maxims are never enough; they are made meaningful by examples: "I have come here *(Present Perfect)* so that I can make a statement *(Present)*." "I had arrived *(Past Perfect)* long before he came home *(Past)*." "He will have finished his presentation *(Future Perfect)*, a few minutes before her plane will arrive *(Future)*." Progressive Tenses show continuing action. "She is speaking now." "She was speaking yesterday." "She will be speaking tomorrow." "He has been speaking so that they can make an agreement." "He had been speaking well before the storm interrupted him." "He will have been speaking on the subject, days before his opponent will be ready."

A verb has **person:** oneself *(First Person, indicated by* **I**), the person being talked to *(Second Person, indicated by* **you**), the person, thing, or event being talked about *(Third Person,* **he, she, it**, Bob, Sue, bread, kite, inflation, *etc.)*. Each of these three *singular* persons may be *plural: First Person Plural,* **we**; *Second Person Plural,* **you** (same as singular); *Third Person Plural,* **they**, boys, flowers, teams, successes, *etc.* A verb's **number** property refers to whether the subject of a verb is *singular* or *plural*. **Person** and **number** can cause a verb change: *I am, you are, he is, we are, you are, they are.* In every case *Third Person Singular, Present Tense*, ends in *-s: I hit, you hit, he hits, we hit, you hit, they hit. I have, you have, he has, we have, you have, they have.*

Verbs may be in one of three **moods:** *indicative, imperative,* or *subjunctive*. All the above examples are in the *indicative mood*. This is the most common *mood*; it deals with actuality or negation; most English sentences are in the *indicative mood*. It is called the *"fact" mood*; it *indicates* what is the case. "I am the person you are looking for." "I'm not the person you are looking for." "There are twelve inches in a foot." The *imperative mood* is used in commands and exhortations: "Go to the store now!" "Love thy neighbor." The *subjunctive mood* is used in hypothetical, wishful, imaginative, or parliamentary situations. "If that were true, we would have to start again." "Long live the king." "If only I were president; things would be different." "I move that Mac be elected unanimously."

Ch. 6. Verbs

Most verbs are in **active voice**; the subject is doing the action. However, if the subject is being acted upon, the verb is in **passive voice**. "He sang a merry tune." <u>Active voice</u>, *he,* the subject, is doing the action: *singing a merry tune.* "The sad melody was composed shortly after World War I." <u>Passive voice</u>, the subject, *melody,* is not doing the action, it is being acted upon: *being composed.*

A verb may be *transitive,* takes an object, or *intransitive,* doesn't take an object. *Sing* may be either. "I sing Schubert songs." Here *sing* is a <u>transitive verb</u>, it takes an object. *Songs* is the *direct object;* it receives the action of the verb. However in, "I sing loudly!" *sing* is an <u>intransitive verb</u>; it does not act on an object. *Loudly* is an <u>adverb</u>, not a direct object; it modifies the verb. A dictionary might abbreviate *transitive verb,* **v.t.** and *intransitive verb,* **v.i.**

The *infinitive* (not limited by person, number, or tense) is a verb preceded by *to. To sing, to run, to stop, to apologize* are all <u>infinitives</u>. The infinitive may be used to merely identify the verb being considered: "Let's conjugate the verb, **to sing**." Or it may be used as a subject noun: "<u>To sing</u> professionally is my life long ambition." or as a predicate noun: "My life long ambition is <u>to sing</u> professionally."

When a *present participle* (ends in *-ing*) is used as a noun, it is called a *gerund.* "The <u>singing</u> of the fourth graders was surprisingly good." "<u>Dancing</u> is fun." "The greatest sport is <u>rowing</u>!"

It is the nature of a *participle* to have both verb and adjective qualities. The past participle of 'freeze' is 'frozen'; the present participle is 'freezing'; thus, "He was nearly frozen (verb) when he got home." "The frozen (adjective) chicken was finally thawed." "They've been freezing (verb) in that house for a long time." "The freezing (adjective) drizzle spoiled our hike."

There are two classes of verbs: *regular (weak)* and *irregular (strong). Regular verbs* are the most common; their past tense and past participle are the same. Present: "I <u>talk</u>." Past: "I **talked**." Past Participle: "I have **talked**." Present Participle: "I am <u>talking</u>." Similarly with most of our verbs: walk, walked, walked, walking; negotiate, negotiated, negotiated, negotiating; apologize, apologized, apologized, apologizing, *etc.*

Some of our most common verbs are irregular. *To sing* with its *sing, sang, sung* vowel changes is an excellent example. This vowel change *(Ger. ablaut)* is characteristic of Indo-European languages. Closest to home, of course, is German with its *singen, sang, gesungen* which also left its mark on Dutch *zingen, zong, gezongen*; Danish & Norwegian *synge, sang, sunget;* and Swedish *sjunga, sjöng, sjungit.*

To be is our most highly inflected irregular verb:
PRESENT TENSE: I *am.* You *are.* He *is.* We *are.* You *are.* They *are.*
PAST TENSE: I *was.* You *were.* He *was.* We *were.* You *were.* They *were.*
FUTURE TENSE: I *shall be.* You *will be.* He *will be.* We *shall be.* You *will be. etc.*
PRESENT PERFECT: I *have been.* You *have been.* He *has been.* We *have been. etc*
PAST PERFECT: I *had been.* You *had been.* He *had been.* We *had been. etc*
FUTURE PERFECT: I *shall have been.* You *will have been.* He *will have been. etc*

IRREGULAR VERBS (PRESENT TENSE, PAST TENSE, PAST PARTICIPLE)

Three Different Vowels
begin began begun
drink drank drunk
ring rang rung
shrink shrank shrunk
sing sang sung
sink sank sunk
spring sprang sprung
swim swam swum
swing swang (dial.) swung

Unusual
come came come
do did done
go went gone
run ran run

Past Participle with -n
bite bit bitten
blow blew blown
break broke broken
choose chose chosen
draw drew drawn
drive drove driven
eat ate eaten
fall fell fallen
fly flew flown
forbid forbade forbidden
forget forgot forgotten
forgive forgave forgiven
freeze froze frozen
get got gotten
give gave given
grow grew grown
hide hid hidden
know knew known
lie lay lain
ride rode ridden
rise rose risen
see saw seen
shake shook shaken
slay slew slain

speak spoke spoken
steal stole stolen
swear swore sworn
take took taken
tear tore torn
throw threw thrown
wake woke waken
wear wore worn
weave wove woven
write wrote written

Same Past & Past Participle
bend bent bent
bleed bled bled
bring brought brought
build built built
catch caught caught
creep crept crept
dig dug dug
dream dreamed dreamed
feed fed fed
feel felt felt
fight fought fought
grind ground ground
hang hung hung
has had had
hear heard heard
hold held held
keep kept kept
kneel knelt knelt
lay laid laid
lead led led
leap leapt leapt
leave left left
lend lent lent
light lit lit
lose lost lost
make made made
mean meant meant
mow mowed mowed (mown)
say said said
saw sawed sawed (sawn)

sell sold sold
sew sewed sewed (sewn)
shine shone shone (shined)
shoot shot shot
show showed showed (shown)
sit sat sat
sleep slept slept
slide slid slid
sow sowed sowed (sown)
spend spent spent
spin spun spun
stand stood stood
stick stuck stuck
sting stung stung
strike struck struck
string strung strung
sweat sweated sweated
sweep swept swept
swing swung swung
teach taught taught
tell told told
think thought thought
weep wept wept
win won won
wind wound wound

All Parts the Same
bet bet bet
burst burst burst
cost cost cost
cut cut cut
hurt hurt hurt
let let let
put put put
read /rēd/ read /rĕd/ read /rĕd/
set set set
shed shed shed
shut shut shut
spit spit spit
split split split
spread spread spread
wet wet wet

Ch. 7.

GENDER

Masculine, Feminine, or Neuter?

Why *island* is feminine in Latin, *river* masculine in Greek, *maiden* neuter in German, and in French *train* is masculine, but *trainstation* is feminine, we may never know. Nevertheless, gender is still an important aspect of the English language; we would not give a *girl's* name to a *boy*, refer to *her* as *him*, or call a *sidewalk, she*. We reserve *masculine* (he) for anything *male, feminine* (she) for anything *female,* and *neuter* (it) for anything else: *box, toy, idea, mismanagement, etc.* If we have grown up speaking English, we manage **gender *and* person *and* number *and* case** with little trouble. "*He* (masculine, third person, singular, nominative) is here." "*His* (masculine, third person, singular, possessive) book fell." "It is *his* (same)." "I gave the book to *him* (masculine, third person, singular, objective *[indirect object]*)." "The bully hurt *him* (masculine, third person, singular, objective *[direct object]*) only psychologically." Similarly, with the *feminine* gender: "*She* is here." "*Her* book fell." "It is *hers*." "I gave the book to *her*." "The bully hurt *her* only psychologically." And with the *neuter* gender: "*It* (neuter, third person, singular, nominative) happened right here." "*Its* (neuter, third person, singular, possessive) impact will be felt for a long time." "This book! To *it* (neuter, third person, singular, objective *[indirect object]*) I owe my new insight." "Careful of that chair; you might break *it* (neuter, third person, singular, objective *[direct object]*)."

A given name might have both a <u>masculine</u> and *<u>feminine</u>* form:

Albert, *Alberta* (Ger.)	Eric, *Erica* (ON)	Julius, *Julia* (L)
Alex, *Alexis* (Gk.)	Ernest, *Ernestine* (Gmc.)	Justin, *Justina* (L)
Alexander, *Alexandra* (Gk.)	Eugene, *Eugenia* (Gk.)	Leo, Leon, *Leona* (Gk.)
Alfred, *Alfreda* (OE)	Fernando, *Fernanda* (Sp.)	Louis, *Louise* (Gmc.)
Alphonso, *Alphonsine* (Ger.)	Francis, *Frances* (Gmc.)	Lucius, *Lucia* (L)
Alvin, *Alvina* (Ger.)	Frederick, *Frederica* (Gmc.)	Lucretius, *Lucretia* (L)
Andrew, *Andrea* (Gk.)	Gabriel, *Gabrielle* (Heb.)	Marcus, *Marcia* (L)
Anthony, *Antonia* (L)	George, *Georgia* (Gk.)	Max (Maximilian), *Maxine* (L)
Antoine, *Antoinette* (F)	Georges, *Georgette* (F)	Nicolas, *Nicole* (F)
Augustus, *Augusta* (L)	Gerald, *Geraldine* (Gmc.)	Octavius, *Octavia* (L)
Bernard, *Bernadette* (F)	Giovanni (John), *Giovanna* (It.)	Patrick, *Patricia* (L)
Carlo (It.), Carlos (Sp.), *Carla*	Glenn, *Glenna* (Cel.)	Paul, *Paula, Pauline* (L)
Charles, *Charlene* (Ger.)	Harry (Harold), *Harriet* (OE)	Paul, *Paulette* (F)
Cecil, *Cecilia* (L)	Henri (Henry), *Henriette* (F)	Philip, *Philippa* (Gk.)
Christian, *Christiana* (Gk.)	Henry, *Henrietta* (Gmc.)	Ramón, *Ramona* (Sp.)
Claude, *Claudia* (L)	Hermes, *Hermione* (Gk.)	Robert, *Roberta* (Gmc.)
Clement, *Clementine* (L)	Isidore, *Isadora* (Gk.)	Simon, *Simone* (Heb.)
Constantine, *Constance* (L)	Jacques (Jacob), *Jacqueline* (F)	Stephen, *Stephanie* (Gk.)
Cornelius, *Cornelia* (L)	Jean /zhän/ (John), *Jeannette* (F)	Theodore, *Theodora* (Gk.)
Dennis (Dionysius), *Denise* (Gk.)	Jesse, *Jessica* (Heb.)	Valerius, *Valeria* (L)
Dominic, *Dominique* (F)	John, *Joan* (Heb.)	Virginius, *Virginia* (L)
Edwin, *Edwina* (OE)	Joseph, *Josephine* (Heb.)	Virgilius, *Virgilia* (L)
Emil, *Emily* (L)	Juan (John), *Juanita* (Sp.)	Wilhelm, *Wilhelmina* (Ger.)

Ch. 7. Gender

One of the most common feminine producing suffixes in English is *-ess.* Thus: actor, *actress;* auditor, *auditress;* adulterer, *adulteress;* adventurer, *adventuress;* author, *authoress;* baron, *baroness;* conductor, *conductress;* count, *countess;* deacon, *deaconess;* duke, *duchess;* emperor, *empress;* god, *goddess;* governor, *governess;* host, *hostess;* hunter, *huntress;* janitor, *janitress;* mister, *mistress;* poet, *poetess;* priest, *priestess;* prince, *princess;* protector, *protectress;* sculptor, *sculptress;* seducer, *seductress;* songster, *songstress;* traitor, *traitress;* waiter, *waitress.*

A class of *-tor* masculine nouns in Latin have a *-trix* feminine ending: administrator, *administratrix;* aviator, *aviatrix;* executor, *executrix;* inheritor, *inheritrix;* testator, *testatrix.*

Although *-ette* is a French suffix usually meaning small (e.g. *kitchenette),* in a few cases it is a feminine indicator: *bachelorette, coquette, farmerette, majorette, suffragette, usherette;* Names: *Antoinette, Bernadette, Claudette, Georgette, Henriette, Paulette.*

More obvious masculine-feminine endings are *-man, -woman*: congressman, *congresswoman*; policeman, *policewoman,* sportsman, *sportswoman,* salesman, *saleswoman*; etc.

Unique is the pairing of widower, *widow*; where for once the female term seems to have preceded the male term, probably due to there being more widows than widowers!

There are etymologically unrelated gender couplings that should be noted: father, *mother;* pa, *ma;* papa, *mama;* daddy, *mammy (mommy);* dad, *mom;* son, *daughter;* brother, *sister;* bro, *sis;* boy, *girl;* lad, *lass;* guy, *doll;* gentleman, *lady;* uncle, *aunt;* nephew, *niece*; grandfather, *grandmother*; gran'pa, *gran'ma*; grandson, *granddaughter;* groom, *bride;* groomsman, *bridesmaid;* best man, *maid of honor;* masculine, *feminine;* Mr., *Mrs.;* husband, *wife;* ♂ (Mars, masculine), ♀ (Venus, feminine).

There are distinctions to be made in the animal kingdom too: buck, *doe* (deer, antelopes, goats, rabbits); bull, *cow;* dog, *bitch;* drake, *duck;* drone, *worker, queen* (bee, ant, termite) gander, *goose;* hog, pig, swine, *sow;* horse, *mare;* lion, *lioness;* rooster, cock, *hen, chicken;* tiger, *tigress, etc..* Gender is usually not a distinction for the young: calf, chick, cub, fawn, filly, kid, pup, *etc.*

Often knowing the gender of a **Latin** noun will aid in forming its plural. **Masculine** singular *-us* becomes *-i* in the plural: alumnus, *alumni;* radius, *radii;* stimulus, *stimuli.* **Feminine** singular *-a* becomes *-ae* in the plural: alumna, *alumnae;* larva, *larvae;* persona, *personae;* vertebra, *vertebrae.* **Neuter** singular *-um* becomes *-a* in the plural: addendum, *addenda;* continuum, *continua,* medium, *media;* referendum, *referenda.*

Remembering that *-os* is a **Greek masculine** singular, it is easy to recognize the derivation of *chaos, cosmos,* and *pathos.* **Feminine** singular *-is* becomes *-es* in the plural. Knowing this makes spelling the plural of several common Greek words easy: analysis, *analyses;* crisis, *crises;* diagnosis, *diagnoses;* emphasis, *emphases;* hypothesis, *hypotheses;* neurosis, *neuroses;* psychosis, *psychoses;* synthesis, *syntheses;*

thesis, *theses.* The **neuter** singular ending *-on* aids us in identifying the derivation of *chameleon, colon, demon, dragon, epsilon, horizon, icon, ion, melon, moron, neon, neuron omicron, pantheon, paragon, pentagon, photon, Poseidon, proton, siphon, skeleton.* The neuter plural *-a* explains: criterion, *criteria;* phenomenon, *phenomena.*

Some **French** masculine-feminine couples have come into English usage unchanged: blond, *blonde;* brunet, *brunette;* comedian, *comedienne;* couturier, *couturière;* divorcé, *divorcée;* fiancé, *fiancée;* Monsieur (Mr. abbr. M.), *Madame* (Mrs. abbr. Mme.); *Mademoiselle* (Miss, abbr. Mlle.), père (father), *mère* (mother); naif, *naive; née* (born with the name of); protége, *protégée;*

Spanish: padre (father), *madre* (mother); San (Saint), *Santa;* Señor (Mr. abbr. Sr.), *Señora* (Mrs. abbr. Sra.), *Señorita* (Miss, abbr. Srta.)

Italian: ballerino (dancer), *ballerina;* bambino (baby), *bambina;* padre, *madre* Santo (Saint), *Santa;* Signore (Mr.), *Signora* (Mrs.), *Signorina* (Miss)

Portuguese: Santo (Saint), *Santa,* São (abbr.); Senhor (Mr. abbr. Sr), Senhora (Mrs. abbr. Sra), Senhorita (Miss); pai (father), mãe (mother)

Often Hindi middle names are: *masculine* Singh *(lion)* and *feminine* Kaur *(princess).*

The middle name in Russian names usually indicates the father's name. *-ovich* indicates *son of* and *-ovna* the daughter of; thus, Ivanovich *(son of Ivan)* and Ivanova *(daughter of Ivan).*

And finally: male, *female.*

AND WHAT NEXT? SUGGESTIONS:

1. Continue **Syllabication** practice. (Ap. ii.)
2. Do the **Latin Short Course**. (Ap. vii.)
3. Do the **Greek Short Course**. (Ap. ix.)
4. Learn more about the **History of English.** (Ap. xv.)
5. Become familiar with English's many **Homophones** a few at a time. (Ap. xi.)
6. Get into **Prefixes** a bit further. (Ap. iii.)
7. Is there an **American English**? (Ap. xiii.)
8. Have you missed any of the **Phonics** bits? (Ap. i.)
9. Explore the **Romance Language** contribution to English. (Ap. viii.)
10. Use **Suffix** listings for reference as needed. (Ap. iv.)
11. Look at the many **Borrowings** from other languages from around the world. (Ap. x.)
12. Study the concept **MIND** by seeing how the word is used in English. (Ap. xiii.)
13. Compare **Black English Vernacular** and Standard English. (Ap. xiv.)
14. Learn more English words deriving from **Names and Places.** (Ap. xii.)
15. Check through **Odds and Ends** for items of interest. (Ap. xi.)
16. Use main **Latin & Greek** listings. Learn the **Greek Alphabet.** (Ap.vii, Ap. ix.)

basic ă, ĕ, ĭ, ŏ, ŭ, ... Ap.i- 3

ă, +ă, ă+, +ă+, ä, ā, ... Ap.i- 4
   (<u>Note</u>: +ă = blend before ă; ă+ =blend after ă; +ă+ = blend before & after ă.)

ĕ, +ĕ, ĕ+, +ĕ+, é, e /ā/, ... Ap.i- 5

ē, ĭ, +ĭ, ĭ+, +ĭ+, ... Ap.i- 6

i /ē/, ī, ... Ap.i- 7

ŏ, +ŏ, ŏ+, +ŏ+, ô, o /o͞o/, ō, ... Ap.i- 8

ŭ, +ŭ, ŭ+, +ŭ+, u /o͞o/, u /w/, ū, ... Ap.i- 9

aa, ae, aer-, -age /ij/, -age /ahzh/, ai /ā/, ... Ap.i-10

ai /ī/, air, -alk, al(l), -alt, -ang, -ank, ar /are/, ... Ap.i-11

-ar /er/, ar-r, ar (+ vowel), ... Ap.i-12

au /aw/, au /ow/, au /ō/, augh, aw, ... Ap.i-13

ay, -ble (-dle, -fle, -gle, -kle, -ple, -tle, -zle), ... Ap.i-14

-cle, c /k/, c /s/, c /ch/, ... Ap.i-15

ç, -cc- /k-s/, ch /ch/, ch /sh/, ch /k/, ch /kh/, ... Ap.i-16

-ck, -dge, ... Ap.i-17

Diacritical Marks, -du-, ea /ē/, ea /ĕ/, ... Ap.i-18

ear /er/, ear /air/, ear /ear/, eau, -ed /id/, -ed /t/, -ed /d/, . Ap.i-19

ee, -eer, ei /ā/, ei /ē/, ... Ap.i-20

ei /ī/, eigh, er (Within a word.), -er (Noun or pronoun ending.), . . . Ap.i-21

-er /verb/, -er /adj./, -er (Comparative), ere, er (+ vowel other than *e*.), . . Ap.i-22

er-i (+ vowel), er-r, -et /ā/, eu /yo͞o/, eu /o͞o/, ew /yo͞o/, ew /o͞o/, ey /ā/, ey /ē/ Ap.i-23

g /g/, g /j/, g /zh/, -gg- /g-j/, gh /g/, gh /f/, gn, gu, -gue (-igue), . Ap.i-24

ie /ē/, ie /ī/, -igh, -ild, -ind, -ing, ... Ap.i-25

-ink, -ion, ir, -ire, ir-r, ir (+ vowel other than *e*.), j /h/, kn-, -ly, Ap.i-26

-mb, -mn, n /ng/, ñ, oa, oe, ... Ap.i-27

oi, old, -oll, oo /o͞o/, oo /o͝o/, ... Ap.i-28

or /or/, or /er/, -ost /ōst/, -ost /awst/, ou /ow/, ... Ap.i-29

ou /o͞o/, ou /ō/, ou /ə/, ou /o͝o/, ough, -our, ... Ap.i-30

Outrageous Pronunciations, -ow /ow/, -ow /ō/, -oy, ph, . . . Ap.i-31

ps, qua, quar, -que (ique), rh-, s /s/, s /z/, ... Ap.i-32

sc /s/, sc /sk/, sch /sk/, sch /sh/, -sci- /sh/, ... Ap.i-33

Schwa, scr-, sh, ... Ap.i-34

Silent-E Pairs, ... Ap.i-35

Silent-E (Unpaired Examples), ... Ap.i-36

Silent Letters, ... Ap.i-37

Silent Letters Come To Life, -sion, spl-, spr-, -stle, str-, . Ap.i-38

-tch, th (unvoiced), th (voiced), th /t/, -tion /shən/, ... Ap.i-39

-tion /chən/, -tu-, -ture, ue /o͞o/, ue /yo͞o/, ... Ap.i-40

ui, "umlaut", -ung, -unk, Unvoiced & Voiced Consonants, Ap.i-41

ur, -ve, wa, war, wh, ... Ap.i-42

wor, Word Pairs (Long Vowel, Short Vowel), ... Ap.i-43

Words Ending in *U*, wr, ... Ap. i-43

x /k-s/, x /z/, y /y/, -y /ī/ (One syllable words), -y /ē/ (verb), -y /ē/ (noun), . Ap.i-44

-y /ē/ (adj.), -y- /ī/ (Greek), ... Ap.i-45

-y- /ĭ/ (Greek), -yr (+ vowel other than *e*.), z /z/, z /s/ . . . . Ap. i-46

Note: The most common words (first to teach) are in **bold print**.

ă basic	Al	am	an	as	at	ax	bad	bag	ban	bat	cab
	can	cap	cat	dab	dad	dam	Dan	fad	fan	fat	Fax
	gag	gal	gap	gas	had	Hal	ham	has	hat	jab	jam
	Jan	lab	lad	lag	lap	lax	mad	man	map	mat	Max
	nab	nag	Nan	nap	pad	pal	Pam	pan	pat	rag	ram
	ran	rap	rat	sad	sag	Sal	Sam	sap	sat	tab	tad
	tag	tam	tan	tap	tax	van	vat	wag	wax	yam	zap

ĕ basic	bed	beg	Ben	bet	den	Ed	fed	get	hem	hen	jet
	keg	Ken	led	leg	let	men	met	net	peg	Peg	pen
	pep	pet	red	set	Ted	ten	web	wed	wet	yes	yet

ĭ basic	bib	bid	big	bin	bit	did	dig	dim	din	dip	fib
	fig	fin	fit	fix	hid	him	hip	his	hit	if	in
	is	it	jig	kit	lid	lip	lit	Liz	mid	mix	nip
	nix	pig	pin	pit	rib	rid	rig	rim	rip	sin	sip
	sis	sit	six	Tim	tin	tip	vim	wig	win	wit	zip

ŏ basic	bob	Bob	bog	box	cob	cod	cog	cop	cot	don	Don
	dot	fox	gob	god	God	got	hop	hot	job	jog	jot
	lob	lot	mob	mom	mop	nod	not	on	ox	pod	pop
	pot	pox	rob	rod	Ron	rot	sob	sod	Tom	top	tot

ŭ basic	bud	Bud	bug	bum	bun	bus	but	cub	cup	cut	dub
	dud	dug	fun	gum	gun	gut	hub	hug	hum	hut	jug
	jut	lug	mud	mug	mum	nun	nut	pun	put	rub	rug
	rum	run	rut	sub	sum	sun	sup	tub	tub	up	us

Test words for short vowels: **at Ed it ox up**.

ă add Al am an Ann as ash ass at ax back bad badge bag ban bash bass bat batch bath Bess cab cad cam can cap cash cat catch Chad Chan chap chat chaff dab dad dam Dan dash fad fag fan fat Fax gab gad gaff gag gal gam gap gas gash gat hack had hag Hal ham Han hap has hash hat hatch hath have jab jack Jack jag jam Jan jazz lab lack lad lag lam lap Lapp lash lass latch lath lax mad Madge man map mash mass mat match math Matt Max nab nag Nan nap Nat pack pad pal Pam pan pap pass pat patch path Pax quack rack rag ram ran rap rash rat razz sac sack sad sag Sal Sam sap sash sass sat sax shad shag shall sham shack tab tack tad tag tam tan tap tat tax than that van vat wag wax whack wham yak yam yap Zack zag zap

+ă blab black blat brad Brad brag bran brash brass brat clack clad clam clan clap claque clash class crab crack crag cram crap crash crass drab drag dram drat flab flack flag flak flam flap flash flat flax frap Fran frat glad glass gnash gnat grab grad gram graph grass Klan knap knock plan plaque plash plat pled pram scab scam scan scat scrag scram scrap scratch slab slack slag slam slap slash slat smack smash snack snag snap snatch Spam span spat splash splat sprat stab stack staff stag Stan stash strap swam thrash track tram trap trash wrap wrath

ă+ act adz aft Alps amp and ant apt ask asp band bang bank bask camp canst cant can't cask cast caste champ chance Chang chant daft damp dang dank fact fang fast gang gasp Hadj haft half halve hand hang hank hasp hast jamb lamb lamp lance land lank lapse last manse mask mast pact pang pant pants past raft ramp ranch rand Rand rang rank rant rapt rasp salve sand sang sank shaft shalt shank tact Taft tamp tang tank task thank valve vamp vast waft yank

+ă+ blanch bland blank blast branch brand clamp clang clank Clark clasp craft cramp crank draft drank flange flank flask franc France frank Frank Franz glance gland graft gramp grand grant Grant grasp kraft plank plant prance prank scads scalp scamp scant shrank slang slant spank splint stand strand sprang stamp stance stanch stand stank swank tract tramp trance twang

ä /ah/ /ä/ Bali balm calm father Graf khan ka Kant kas la ma Maya palm Prague psalm quality quantity schmaltz schnapps schwa shah squad swab swamp swan swap swash swat swatch swath wad waff waft wallaby wallet wan wand wander want wash wasp watch wigwam; See: qua-. Ap. i-32, wa-, Ap. i-42.

ā   1. In open accented syllable: agent apron David nation patron vacant vagrant
    2. Before undoubled -ble, -dle, -gle, etc.: able cable fable maple staple table
    3. In a Silent-e word: bake base cape Dane fake gale lame male sale
    4. In dropped Silent-e word with vowel ending added: caning scaring taping taming
    5. Before -tion: carnation donation elation fixation frustration relation

ĕ   bed beg bel bell ben Ben Bess bet cell check chef cheque chess deck dell den ebb Ed edge ef egg el ell em en es etch ex fed Fed. fell fen fetch fez gel gem get guess heck hedge hell hem hen hep het hex Jebb Jeff jell Jess jet kedge keg ken Ken ketch led ledge leg less let lex Meg mel Mel men mesh mess met neck Ned Nell ness net peck peg Peg pen pep pet quell red rep Rep. rem ret retch rev Rex sedge sell set Seth sex shed shell Ted tell ten Tex them then vet vex web wed wen wet when whet yell yen yep yes yet well Zen

+ĕ   bleb bled bless blet bred clef crèche crème cress crest Czech dredge dreg dress dwell fleck fled fledge flesh flex Fred fresh fret glen Glenn Greg pleb pled pledge prep press prest shred skep sketch sled sledge smell speck sped spell stem step stet stress stretch swell thresh tress wreck wren wretch

ĕ+   belt bench bend bent best Celt cense cent chest deft delve dent depth desk elf elk elm else end felt fence fend fest geld gelt gens gent guest heft held helm help hemp hence jest kelp Kent kept left lend length lens lent Lent lest meld melt mend nest next pelf pelt pence pend pent pest quench quest rend rent rest scent sect self send sense sent sext shelf shelve tempt tend tent test text theft thence vend vent vest weft weld Welsh welt wench wend went wept west whelp whence yelp zest

+ĕ+   blend blest Brent cleft clench crept crest dregs drench dwelt flense French knelt prest skelp slept smelt spend spent squelch stench swept trench trend twelve wrench wrest

é   /ā/ (e with an acute accent---French) André aérogramme animé apéritif appliqué attaché auto-da-fé blasé bourrée broché café canapé Cézanne chassé cliché communiqué consommé coupé déclassé décor dégagé déjà vu déjeuner démarche dénouement détente distingué divorcé (m) divorcée (f) dragée Elysée éclair éclaircissement éclat école égalité élan élite émigré entrée étape étude exposé Fauré fiancé (m) fiancée (f) flambée fléchette frappé frisé glacé habitué Héloise idée fixe ingénue lycée macramé malgré mélange naiveté née outré papier-mâché passé pâté piqué plié /plē-ā/ précis protégé purée raison d'état Renée répondez repoussé résumé retroussé risqué rissolé sauté séance soirée soufflé touché velouté

e   /ā/ (In French, Spanish, Italian, etc.) Allegheny Beowulf crepe duce /dōō-chā/ Ebert eta (Greek letter, η H) fete /fāt/ forte /for-tā/ Galileo Hegel Koine mesa omega (Greek letter, ω Ω) Ortega Pareto peyote peso Pieta /pyā-tä/ Ponce /pôn-sā/ Puerto /pwair-tō/ Rico re (do, re, mi) Realpolitik /rā-äl-pō-li-tēk/ rendezvous /rän-dā-vōō/ Rivera Riviera Robespierre roble /rō-blā/ San Diego /dē-ā-gō/ shillelagh /shi-lā-lē/ Sierra Sudetenland suede /swād/ Tenochtitlan /tā-nōkh-tē-tlän/ Teresa theta (Greek letter, θ Θ) torero /tō-rā-rō/ ukulele /yōō-kə-lā-lē/ zeta (Greek letter, ζ Z)

ē   1. In open syllable: be <u>be</u>ing com<u>ple</u>tion <u>cre</u>dence <u>Gre</u>cian he <u>Le</u>o <u>ne</u>on she
        2. In a *Silent-e* word: Pete concede convene Crete delete theme these
        3. In dropped *Silent-e* word with vowel ending added: conceding convening deleting
        4. Usually before *-tion:* completion deletion depletion excretion secretion

ĭ bib bid big bill Bill bin bit chick chill chin chip chit Dick did dig dill dim
din dip dish ditch fib fid fig fill fin Finn fish fit Fitch fix fizz gib gid gig gill
gin give hick hid hill him hip his hiss hit hitch ick id if ill in inn is it itch jib
jig Jill Jim kick kid kill Kim kin Kip kiss kit kith kid lick lid lip lit live Liz mib
Mick mid midge Midge miff mig mil mill Mill miss Miss Mitch mitt mix nib
nick Nick nil nip nit nix pick pig pill pin pip pish! piss pit pitch pith pix
quick quid quill quip quit quiz rib rich Rick rid ridge Rif riff rig rill rim rip
shill shim shin ship shiv sib sic sick Sid sill sin sip sis sit six thick thin this
tic tick tiff till Tim tin tip tit Vick vim which whiff Whig whim whip whish whit
whiz wick wig will win wish wit witch with yin yip zig zip

+ĭ blip bliss brick bridge brig brill brim Brit click cliff cling clip crib crick
drill drip flick flip flit flitch frill frit frizz glib glim gliss glitch grid grig grill
grim Grimm grin grip grit knit prick prig prim scrip scrim shtick shrill skid
skiff skill skim skin skip skit slick slid slim slip slit smith Smith sniff snit spiff
spill squib snip spin spit split sprig squib squid squish stick stiff still stitch switch
strip swig swill swim swish Swiss switch trick trig trill trim trip twig twill twin
twit twitch writ

ĭ+ bilge bilk binge chimp chink chintz cinch cinque dibs ding dink dint disc
dished disk fifth filch film filth finch find fink fist gift gild gill gilt gimp gist
guild guilt hilt hinge hint hissed hist! ilk imp inch ink its it's jilt jinx kiln kilt
king kink kitsch lift lilt limb limp Lind link lint lisp list Liszt midst milch
milled milk milt Milt mince Ming mink Minsk minx mint mist mixed Pict pimp
pince ping pinch pink quilt quince quint rift ring rink rinse risk schist shift sift
silk silt simp since sing singe sink sixth sixths ting think thing tilt tinge tint
whisk whist width wilt wince winch wind wing wink wisp zinc zing

+ĭ+ blink blimp blink blitz bring brink brisk clinch cling clink crimp cringe crisp
drift drink flinch fling flint fringe frisk glint grist grits plink plinth primp prince
prink print scrimp script shrift shrimp shrink skimp sling slink splint spring sprint
squint stilt sting stink stint strict string swift swing twinge twist wring wrist

i /ē/ (From French, Spanish, Italian, Hindi, Japanese, etc.) acquiesce adios Adriatic alias ami ani **antique** Aparri ashanti Aurelius Azerbaijani Bali beriberi Bernoulli bijou bikini Biloxi bise Botticelli Bragi Brindisi broccoli Burundi Capri casino Cellini chariot charivari charqui chianti chic /shēk/ chichi /shē-shē/ chili Cincinnati Corelli Costa Rica Dali diabolo Dias diva Dostoevski Eliot Fascisti **fatigue** fiasco fiesta Fiji Gallipoli Galvani Gandhi Garibaldi Ghiberti Gobi Desert Gorki Hawaii Helsinki hibachi Hindi Hopi Houri Iago Ibo idiom idiot Iliad illuminati incognito indri Israeli jinni Joliet Juliet kaki kami Kali kepi Kiev kiva kiwi kris Lanai Laski li liaison **machine** Machiavelli Malawi Mali Marconi martini Mascagni Medici mediocre Menotti merci mi Miami Mississippi Missouri Montessori Monteverdi mosquito Nagasaki naive /nä-ēv/ Naomi Nazi obi ocarina olio oriel origami oriole Paganini Pahlavi Palestrina Pali palomino Paoli parcheesi pastrami patriot Pergolesi peri Periander Petri Phidias pianissimo pianist **piano** Picasso piccalilli Pima piquant pistachio **police** Pontiac Potawotomi potpourri primo Pulaski Punjabi ravioli ragi Riga Resphighi Rialto Rio Grande Rivera Riviera Robespierre Rossetti Rossi Rossini safari salami salmagundi saluki San Diego sardine sari satori Scarlatti Scipio Scorpio Scriabin secretariat Shansi Shensi Shiah Shiism Shiite **si** Siena Sierra siesta Sikh Siva **ski** satori Sofia Somali Soviet spaghetti spermaceti Stradivari Stradivarius subito Sufi sukiyaki Suribachi Suzuki Swahili Swami Swazi Tahiti tapioca **taxi** Tel Aviv tiara Tiki Timor Titikaka Tito Tokushima Tommasini topi Torricelli Toscanini Trieste Tupi tuti Ubangi **via** Vienna Vietnam viola vis-à-vis /vē-zə-vē/ viva Vivaldi vive Wakiki wapiti Watusi Yaqui yeti yogi Ypsilanti Zambezi zucchini; **See:** **-gue** (-igue), Ap. i-24 and **-que** (-ique), Ap. i-32.

---

i /ē/ (Where *i* precedes a suffix beginning with a vowel.) audience devious exterior jovial lenient media median mediate radiance radium radius studio suppliant, *etc.*
See: **-ia, -ial, -iance, -iant, -iate, -ian, -ience, -ient, -io, -ious, -ior, -ium, -ius** in Appendix iv.

---

i /ē/ (Where adjective *-y* /ē/ ending is changed to *i* when adding *-er* or *-est*.) happy happier happiest   lucky luckier luckiest   crazy crazier craziest

---

ī
1. In open accented syllable: client compliant dial giant lion silent tirade
2. Before undoubled *-ble, -dle, -gle*, etc.: Bible   bridle   idle   rifle   title   trifle
3. In a *Silent-e* word: bite   dime   dine   file   grime   mile   pile   ride   slide
4. In dropped *Silent-e* word with vowel ending added: diner   filing   griping   riding
5. In *-ild, -ind* words: child   mild   wild   blind   find   grind   kind   mind
6. In *-igh* words: fight   high   light   might   night   right   sigh   sight   slight
7. Where *-y* /ī/ is changed to *i* to add *a* or *e* suffix: fry fried; dry drier driest; appliance
8. In some common *spell-words*: climb   iron   island   ninth   pint   sign
9. The Greek letters (open syllables): chi (χ, X)   phi (φ, Φ)   pi (π, Π)   psi (ψ, Ψ)

Ŏ bob Bob bog bop bosh botch box chock chop cob Cobb cock cod cog con cop cot dock dodge doff dol doll Dom don Don dot fob fox fop gob gog god God gosh got Goth hob hock hod hop hot job jock jog John josh Josh jot lob loch lock lodge loll lop lot lox mob mock mod moll mom mop nob nock nod nog non- not notch od odd on Oshkosh Oz pock pod pog pop posh pot pox rob Rob rock rod Ron Rosh rot shock shod shop shot sob sock sod Sol sop sot Sox tock Todd tog Tom top tot whop Yom yon; <u>Exceptions:</u> /ə/ son, ton, won, wont; /ō/ Job won't (contraction of Middle English *woll not.*)

+Ŏ blob bloc block blot blotch clock clod clop clog clot crock crop crotch drop dross flock flog flop frock frosh glob grog grot knob knock knot Knox plod plop plot prod prog prom prop Scot scotch Scotch Scott scrod shroff slob slog slop slosh slot sloth smock snob snot splotch spot stock stodge stop strop trod trot

---

Ŏ+ bomb bond Bosch bosk chomp conch conk copse Copt fond font gosh hong nonce odds opt pomp pond pons prong romp solve yond

---

+Ŏ+ blond blonde Bronx bronze croft flong frond prompt rhomb sconce stomp; <u>Exception:</u> /ə/ front

---

Ô /aw/ /ô/ along belong bog bong boss broth cloth coffee conk cost cross dog dross floss fog frog frost froth furlong gloss glost golf gone gong hog honk lacrosse LaCrosse loft log long loss lost moss moth oblong off offer oft often ostrich ping-pong pog prong Ross sarong scoff smog soft song strong thong throng tong toss troth wrong; <u>Exceptions:</u> /o͝o/ wolf, woman; /ĭ/ women /wĭm-in/.

O /o͞o/ lose prove reprove who whom whose womb

Ō
1. In open accented syllable: frozen go hobo no Noah noble pro so solo
2. In many unaccented final syllables: halo Leo Oslo piano polo silo studio
3. In a *Silent-e* word: choke code hope joke note poke rode slope spoke
4. In dropped *Silent-e* word with vowel ending added: choking coding hoping joking
5. In *-old, -ost* words: bold cold gold hold sold told ghost host most post
6. In *-oll* words: droll enroll poll roll scroll stroll toll troll
7. In some common *spell-words:* clothes comb don't folk goes only owe own
8. Before undoubled *-ble* and *-gle:* noble ogle
9. Before *-tion:* commotion devotion locomotion lotion motion notion potion

ŭ bub buck bud Bud budge buff bug bum bun bus but butt buzz chub chuck
Chuck chug chum cub cud cuff cull cup cuss cut cutch dub duck dud dug duff
dull dun Dutch fudge fun fuss fuzz guck guff gull gum gun gush gut hub Huck
huff hug huh hull hum Hun hush Huss hut hutch judge jug jus jut luck luff lug
lull Lum lush lux much muck mud muff mug mull mum mush muss mutt nub
nudge null nun nut pub puck pug puff pun pup pus putt rub ruck rudd ruff
rug rum run rush rut shuck shun shush shut sub such suck sudd sum sun sup
thud thug thus tub tug tun tup tut Tut tux up us

+ŭ bluff blush brush club cluck clutch crud crus crush crutch crux drub
drudge drug drum flub fluff flush flux glum glut grub grudge gruff Krupp pluck
plug plum plus plush scrub scruff scud scuff scull scum scut scutch shrub shrug
skull slub sludge sluff slug slum slush slut smudge smug smut snub snuck snuff
snug spud spun strum strut stub stuck stud stuff stun swum thrush truck trudge truss

ŭ+ bulb bulge bulk bump bunch bund bung bunk bunt busk bust chump chunk
culch culm cult cusk cusp duct duds dumb dump dunce dung dunk dusk dust
fund funk gulch gulf gulp gunk gust hulk hump humph hunch hung hunk hunt
husk jump junk just lump lunch lung lunge Lunt lust mulch mulct mumps
munch musk must numb nuts pulp pulse pump punch pung punk punt rump rung
runt rush rusk rust shucks shunt suds sulk sump sung sunk thumb thump tuft tusk

+ŭ+ blunt brunch brunt clump clung crumb crunch crust drunk flump flung
flunk frump grump grunt plumb plump plunge plunk rhumb scurf shrunk skulk
skunk slump slung slunk sprung spunk struck strung stump stung stunk stunt
swung thrust trump trunk trust wrung

U /oo/ bull bush full Jung pull push puss put sugar sure /sho͝or/

U /w/ (Often Spanish or Italian.) anguish assuage Buena Vista Buenos Aires dissuade
distinguish guano Guadalajara Guadalcanal Guadeloupe Guam guanaco
Guantánamo Guarani Guarnerius Guatemala Guelph Guenever Guido Guinevere
jaguar Juan /hwän/ Juárez /hwä-räs/ LaGuardia language languid languish linguist
liquid penguin persuade pueblo Pueblo Puerto Rico suave suede /swād/ suite

ū (Long "u" may sound either /yo͞o/ or /o͞o/.)
   1. In open accented syllable: brutal bugle Cuba cupid human Judy pupil
   2. In a *Silent-e* word: cure cute duke fuse Luke mule plume tune
   3. In dropped *Silent-e* word with vowel ending added: curable cuter cutest tuning
   4. In some closed syllables: Hugh Ruth truth
   5. Before undoubled *-ble* and *-gle:* bugle duple scruple scruples
   6. Before *-tion:* constitution evolution pollution revolution solution substitution

y See -y & -y- listings on pages 44 through 46 of this Appendix for *y* used as a vowel.

aa /ah/ /ä/ Aachen aardvark Afrikaans **bazaar** Haarlem Kaaba Kierkegaard kraal laager Saab Saar /zär/ Spaak Taal Transvaal Vaal; Exceptions: /ā/ Baal; /air/ Aaron; /ə/ Kwanzaa Canaan /kā-nən/ Canaanite /kā-nən-īt/

ae /ē/ (Mostly from ancient history; often written "æ".) Aeacus aedile Aegeus aegis Aegyptus Aeolian Aeolic Aeolus **Aesop** Antaeus **Caesar** daedal daemon Lacedaemon maenad **Nicaea** Mycenae paean **Piraeus** Plataea praedial praefect praenomen praetor propylaeum taenia; Exceptions: /ĕ/ Aeschylus aesthete **aesthetic** Aetna; /ĭ/ **Aegean** Aeneas Aeneid caesura praetorian; /ā/ Gaelic, Israeli maelstrom, Mae; /ə/ **Michael** propaedeutic; Note: Phaethon /fā-ə-thon/; See: Latin feminine nouns Ch. 5, Page 51 where -a singular becomes -ae in the plural: *alumna, alumnae; nebula, nebulae;* etc.

aer- /air/ aerate aerator **aerial** aerialist aerie aerification aerify aerobatics aerobe aerobiology aerodynamics aerodyne aerogenic aerogram aerography aerolite aerology aerometer aeronaut aeronautic aeroneurosis aerophagia aerophysics aeroplane aerosol aerospace aerosphere aerostat aerostatics aerotropism

-age[1] /ĭj/ advantage average **baggage bandage** beverage blockage **cabbage** cottage courage coverage **damage garbage** heritage **hostage image** language **luggage manage message** mileage orphanage outage **package passage** percentage pilgrimage portage **postage** sausage savage scrimmage shortage storage **village** voyage **yardage;** Exceptions: age page rage; (More in Ap. iv-19.)

-age[2] /ahzh/ (French) barrage corsage garage massage sabotage; (More in Ap. iv-19.)

ai[1] /ā/ Agail abstain acclaim acquaint affair afraid **aid** aide **ail aim** ain't **air** Alsace-Lorraine appertain appraise Aquitaine arraign assail assailant attain attaint avail await **bail** bailiff Baird **bait** baize bewail blain Blaine Blair **braid** brail Braille **brain** braise Cain caisson campaign **chain chair** chaise /shāz/ claim Claire cocaine cocktail complain complaint complaisant (cf. complacent) constraint corsair curtail daily dainty dairy daisy Daisy declaim delaine derail despair detail detain detrain disclaim disdain distrain domain **drain** Douai Elaine entail entertain entrails exclaim explain **fail** fain **faint faith fair** fairy flail **flair frail** fraise gaiety **Gail** gaily **gain** gait gaiter Germaine glair grail **grain** Grainger Haig **hail hair** Haiti hollandaise impair ingrain inlaid **jail** Jamaica **laid lain** lair laity legerdemain liaison Lorain Lorraine **maid mail** maim **main** maintain maintenance Maine Maisie maize malaise maitre d' mayonnaise migraine mohair Montaigne Montclair moraine mortmain naiad **nail** Novocain obtain ordain **paid pail pain** Paine **paint pair** Paisley parfait peneplain pertain Pitcairn Island **plain** plaint plaintiff plait polonaise prairie praise prevail proclaim quail quaint Rabelais **raid rail** raiment **rain** rainbow raise raisin reclaim refrain regain remain remains repair restrain restraint retail retain romaine **sail sailor saint** Sinclair slain **snail Spain** sprain staid **stair** stairs **stain** straight strain strait sustain swain **tail tailor** tain taint terrain **trail train** traipse trait traitor travail twain Twain vain vainglory Valparaiso Voltaire waif wail wain **waist wait waiter** waitress waive **wait** wraith; <u>See</u>: **-tain** in Ap. iv-44.

ai² /ī/ aisle /īl/; Ainu Azerbaijan bonzai Cairo Chou En-lai daimio daimon daiquiri Dalai Lama haifa haik haiku Hawaiian Jainism Jaipur Kaiser Kuwait Mainz Molokai Olduvai Rubaiyat Saigon Saipan samurai Shanghai Sinai Taipei Taiping Taiwan Thai Thailand Tschaikovsky Versailles /ver-sī/;
<u>Exceptions</u>: /ă/ plaid; /ĕ/ **again against** laissez faire /lĕs-ā-fair/ raison d'etat raison d'etre **said** saith; /ə/ bargain Bougainville renaissance wassail

air /air/ **air** Blair **chair** Claire dairy **fair** fairy **flair** glair **hair** lair mohair Montclair **pair stair**

-alk /awk/ /ôk/ balk calk **chalk** stalk **talk** walk

al(l) /awl/ /ôl/ Albany albeit Alcott Alden alderman **all** almighty **almost already** also altar alter alteration alternate **although** altogether **always** almanac appall asphalt **bald ball** balsam Balkan Baltic caldron **call** cobalt enthrall exalt **fall false** falter gall **hall halt** halter **mall** malt Maltese pall palsy paltry **salt scald** scall **small** smalt squall **stall** stalwart **tall** thrall **wall** waltz;
<u>Exceptions</u>: /ă/ Al Alan Albania albatross Albert albino album albumen Alcatraz alchemy alcohol alcove Alexander algebra Algeria Algiers alibi alkali allegory alligator alleluia Allen alloy aloe Alpine Alps Alsace altitude Altoona altruism alum alveolar

-alt /awlt/ basalt cobalt exalt **halt malt salt**

-ang /ang/ bang clang fang gang hang pang rang sang slang sprang

-ank /angk/ bank blank clank crank dank **drank** embank embankment flank frank Frank hank Hank lank plank prank rank sank shank spank stank **tank** yank Yank

ar¹ /are/ afar ajar alarm arbiter arbitrary arbor arc arcade Arcadia arcane **arch** archaic archer architect archives arctic Arctic Arden ardent **are** Argentina argon argue argument Argus Argyle **ark** Arkansas Arles Arlington **arm** armada armature Armenia armistice armor armory **army** Arnold aromatic arpeggio arsenal arsenic arson **art** arterial artery arthritis Arthur article articulate artifice artillery artist **bar** barb **Barb** Barbados Barbara barber barcarole Barcelona bard bargain barge **bark** barley Barlow Barkley barm **barn** barter Barth Bartholomew Bartlett Bart Bartók Barton bazaar Bismarck **car** carbine carbon carcass **card** cargo Carl carp carpenter **carpet** Carson **cart** carte Carter cartilage Cartesian cartography carton cartoon cartridge **carve** Carver char chard **charge charm chart** cigar Clark commissar czar darb **dark** darling darn **dart** Denmark depart discard discharge Eckhart escarp **far** farce **farm** fart gar garb garçon garden gargle gargoyle garland garlic garment garner garnet garnish garter gnarl go-kart guard guardian harbor **hard** **hardly hark** Harlem Harlequin Harley **harm** harmonic harness **harp harsh** hart Harte harvest Harvey Ishtar jaguar **jar** jargon Karl karma knar Lamarck larceny larch **lard large** larghetto largo **lark** larkspur **mar** margrave marl **marble** Marburg marc **march March** Margaret margin **mark market** marl marlin marmot Marne Mars marble marvel **marsh mart** martial marten martin martyr Marx nard nark Palomar par parcel parch pardon **park** parlance parlay parley parliament parlor parse parsnip parson **part** partake pulsar quasar quark radar **regard** registrar samovar sarcasm sard **scar scarf** scarlet scarp seminar shard **shark sharp smart snarl** sonar **spar spark** Spartan **star** starch stark starling **start** startle starve **tar tardy** tarn tarp **tart** tzar upstart **yard yarn** Zanzibar zarf; <u>Careful</u>: aroma /ə-r̄o-mə/, Laredo /lə-r̄a-do/, *etc.* <u>See</u>: **quar-**, Ap. i-32 and **war-**, Ap. i-42.

-ar² /er/ (At end of word) (adjective) angular cellular circular familiar granular lunar molecular muscular **particular** peculiar perpendicular polar **popular** rectangular **regular** secular **similar** singular solar spectacular stellar triangular **vulgar**; (noun) altar **beggar burglar** calendar caterpillar **cedar cellar** **collar** cougar **dollar grammar hangar** liar molar mortar nectar Oscar **pedlar** (peddler) **pillar** scholar **sugar** vinegar; <u>Exceptions</u>: /are/ afar **bar** bazaar **car** cigar **far** jaguar **jar** mar **star**; <u>See</u>: **-ar**, Ap. iv-23 and **-ard**, Ap. iv-61.

---

ar-r /air/ (Accented.) arrogant **arrow** barracks barracuda barrel barren barrier Barrow Barry carriage Carrie carried carrier carrion carrot **carry** garret Harriman Harris **Harry** marriage married **marry narrow** Parrot tarry wheelbarrow

---

ar³ (+ vowel) /air/ Aaron Arab arabesque Arabic arable Aragon Aramaic Ararat area Ares Arian arid Ariel Aries aristocracy Aristotle Arizona aromatic Aryan **bare** Baring baritone barium baron blare blaring **care** caring Carol Cary chariot **dare** daring declare declaring Delaware fare faring flare flaring Gary glare glaring guarantee guaranty harass hare harem Harold **Karen** mare Marion **Mary** Ontario pare **parent** paring **Paris** parish parity parody pharaoh proletariat rare raring rarity Sarah **scare** scaring similarity **stare** staring tare **tariff** varied ware; <u>Exceptions</u>: are garrote; <u>See</u>: **-ary**, Ap. iv-24.

au^1 /aw/ /ô/ applaud applause assault astronaut Argonaut auburn Auckland auction audacious audacity audible audio **audit** audition auditor auditorium auditory Audubon auger augment augur august **August** Augusta Augustine auk aura aural Aurelius aurora auspices austere Austin Australia Austria authentic author authority autism **auto** autocrat autograph automat automobile autonomy autopsy autumn autumnal auxiliary bauxite **because** cauliflower **caucus** cauldron caulk causation **cause** caustic cauterize caution Chaucer clause claustrophobia dauphin daub debauch **default defraud** Esau **exhaust** **faucet fault** faun fauna **flaunt fraud** fraudulent gaudy Gaul gaunt gauntlet gauze **haul haunch haunt** holocaust hydraulic jaundice **jaunt** jaunty juggernaut **laud launch** laundress laundry Laura laureate laurel leprechaun maraud maudlin mausoleum maul Milwaukee Morgenthau Nassau nautical nautilus **Paul** paucity **paunch** pauper **pause** plaudit plausible raucous **sauce** saucer **staunch** Sauk Saul sauna saunter sausage saucy somersault tarpaulin **taunt** tautology trauma traumatic **vault vaunt** Waukegan Waukesha Wausau Wauwatosa Winnepesaukee;   Exceptions: /aw/ or /ə/ because;   /ā/ gauge;   /ǎ/ or /ǒ/ aunt; /er/ restaurant;   King Saud /sä-o͞od/ Saudi Arabia /sä-o͞o-dē/

au^2 /ow/ (German) ablaut Aufklärung Auschwitz Ausgleich Austerlitz autobahn Braun Clausewitz Dachau Faust Moldau Oberammergau Rathaus sauerbraten sauerkraut Schopenhauer Straus Strauss umlaut   **tau** (Greek letter τ, T)

au^3 /ō/ (French)   au gratin   au jus   baba au rhum   chauvinism Daumier /dō-myā/ Port-au-Prince   réchauffé   Sault /so͞o/ Sainte Marie   sauté   sauterne   taupe vaudeville;   (sauté & sauterne also with /ô/)

augh /aw/ /ô/ caught daughter distraught fraught **haughty** naught **naughty** onslaught **slaughter taught**

aw /aw/ /ô/ (at end of word) aw caw claw coleslaw craw **draw flaw** gnaw guffaw haw **jaw law** Mackinaw maw naw paw **raw saw** Shaw slaw straw squaw taw **thaw** yaw;   But otherwise when followed by "l" or "n": awl awning **bawl brawl** brawn **crawl dawn** Dawn drawl **drawn** fawn **lawn pawn** Pawnee prawn **scrawl** scrawny shawl shawm Shawnee spawn **sprawl** trawl trawler tawny yawl **yawn**; Exceptions: awe awesome **awful** awkward bawdy Crawford dawdle Dawson gawk **hawk** Hawkins Hawthorne Lawrence **lawyer** mawkish Mohawk sawyer Sawyer squawk tawdry;   Note: /aw/ sound within word usually spelled *au*. See: au^1 above.

ay /ā/ <u>At end of word</u>: allay array assay astray away **bay** betray Biscay Bombay bray cay **clay day** decay defray delay disarray dismay display dray essay **Fay** flay foray fray **gay** Gay **gray hay** hooray jay Jay Kay lay Mandalay **may May** Maylay moray **nay** Norway okay parlay **pay play** portray **pray** prepay **ray** relay repay **say** sashay seaway shay slay spay splay **spray stay stray sway tray way** yay; <u>Within word</u>: bayonet Bayonne Clayton crayon Hayward Haywood Kayo (K.O.) maybe mayhem mayonnaise Mayo mayor Payne rayon Taylor Thayer Wayne; <u>Exceptions</u>: /ī/ kayak, Haydn; /ē/ Murray

---

-ble, -dle, -fle, -gle, -ple, -tle, -zle with long or double vowel.
/bəl/, /dəl/, /fəl/, /gəl/, /pəl/, /təl/, /zəl/

---

able beagle beetle Bible bridle bugle **cable** couple cradle dawdle disciple doodle double duple eagle entitle fable foible foozle gable **idle** ladle Mable **maple needle noble noodle** ogle people **rifle** sable scruple sidle stable **staple** steeple stifle **table title** tootle treadle trifle tweedle wheedle; <u>Exceptions</u>: label libel hazel

---

-ble, -dle, -fle, -gle, -kle, -ple, -tle, -zle doubled with short vowels:

[<u>Note</u>: "k" doubles to "ck".] addle **apple** babble **baffle battle** boggle **bottle** brickle **brittle bubble buckle** cackle **cattle chuckle** cobble cockle coddle **crackle** cripple cuddle dabble **dazzle** diddle draggle dribble **drizzle** duffle embezzle fickle fiddle fizzle frazzle **freckle** frizzle fuddle gaggle **giggle** gobble goggle grackle grapple griddle guzzle hackle haggle **heckle** hobble huckleberry **huddle** jiggle joggle **juggle** kettle **knuckle little** meddle **middle muddle** muffle muzzle nettle nibble nipple **nozzle** nuzzle **paddle pebble peddle pickle** piddle piffle prattle prickle **puddle puzzle** quibble rabble raffle ramshackle **rattle** razzle-dazzle **riddle** riffle **ripple** rubble ruffle saddle schnozzle **scrabble scribble** scuffle scuttle **settle** shackle shuffle **shuttle** sickle **sizzle** skittle **smuggle sniffle** snuffle snuggle spackle speckle spittle squabble squiggle stickle straddle **straggle struggle** stubble suckle supple swaddle swizzle **tackle tattle** throttle **tickle** tittle toddle toggle topple **trickle** truffle twaddle twiddle waddle waffle waggle whiffle Whipple **whittle wiggle** wobble; <u>Exceptions</u>: model, nickel

---

-ble, -dle, -fle, -gle, -kle, -ple, -tle, -zle after different consonant:

---

amble ample angle ankle bangle bramble **bumble bundle bungle candle crimple** crinkle **crumble crumple curdle** dangle dimple dwindle example fondle **fumble gamble** garble gargle **gentle** girdle **grumble** gurgle **handle humble** hurdle hurtle **jingle** jumble **jungle** kindle mangle mantle **marble** mingle **mumble** myrtle pimple purple ramble rankle **rumble** rumple **sample** scramble shamble shingle simple single spangle **sparkle sprinkle startle** strangle **stumble** subtle swindle tangle temple thimble tingle tinkle **trample tremble** trundle **tumble** turtle twangle **twinkle** wangle warble wrangle wrinkle; <u>Exceptions</u>: mantel pretzel snorkel

-cle is used in three & four syllable words (even after a short vowel):

article barnacle canticle carbuncle chronicle cubicle cuticle debacle icicle manacle miracle monocle obstacle oracle **particle** pinnacle Popsicle receptacle spectacle tabernacle tentacle testicle tubercle **vehicle** ventricle versicle; <u>Exceptions</u>: circle corpuscle /<u>cor</u>-pəs-əl/ cycle muscle /<u>mus</u>-əl/ uncle

C[1] /k/ ("<u>hard c</u>") cab cabin cable cactus cadet **cage cake call** calm calve cam came camp can candy cane cap cape caption car card care carnation cartoon carve **case cash** cask cast castle **cat catch** caution **cave** cavern claim clam clamp **clap clash** clasp class claw clay **clean** clear clench clerk clever clew **click** climb clinch cling clink clip cloak **clock** clod clog cloth cloud clove clown **club** clump clutch clutter coach coal coast **coat cob** cock cod code cog coin coke cold colt comb come cone cook cool coop cop cope copy cord core cork corn corner cost **cot** cough could coy crab crack craft crag **cram** cramp crane crank **crash** crass crate crave crawl craze cream crease creek creep crest crew crib crime crimp cringe crisp croak crock crook croon crop cross crow crowd crown crude crumb crunch **crush crust** crutch cry cub cube cud cue cuff cull cult **cup** cur curb cure curl curse curve **cut**; [Celt /selt/ or /kelt/]

C[2] /s/ [C is soft when followed by *e, i,* or *y.* ♩ ♪ ♪ | ♩ | e, i, or *y.* ♩ ♪ ♪ | ♩ |

<u>At beginning of word</u>: cease Cebu Cecil Cecilia cedar cede cedilla ceiling celebrate celery celesta celestial celibacy **cell** cellar cellophane cellular cellulose Celt cement cemetery censor censure census **cent** centaur **center** centigrade centimeter centipede central century ceramics cereal cerebellum cerebral cerebrum ceremony **certain** certify certitude Cervantes cesspool Ceylon cicada Cicero **cider** cigar **cinch cinder** cinema cinnamon cipher circa **circle** circuit circular circulate circum– circumference circumstance **circus** cirrus cisco cistern citadel citation cite citizen citron citrus **city** civic civil cyanide cycle cyclone Cyclops cylinder cynic cypress Cyril Cyrus cyst;
<u>At end of word as -ce</u>: absence **ace** advance advice apace askance avarice balance **bounce brace** cadence **chance choice** coerce **dance** deduce deface deuce **device dice** dunce efface entice evince **face farce fence** fierce fleece **force** France **glance grace** Greece hence ice induce **juice** lace lance malice menace **mice** mince **nice** niece notice nuance **office** once ounce pace palace peace pence piece pierce **place** police pounce prance **price prince** pumice **race** reduce rejoice **rice** sauce scarce seance seduce **since slice** sluice solace **source** space spice splice spruce stance thence thrice trace trance trice truce twice vice voice whence wince, *etc.*

C[3] /ch/ (Before "e" & "i" in **Italian** words.) a rivederci /ä-rē-vä-<u>der</u>-chē/ Botticelli Cellini **cello** concerto da Vinci duce /<u>doo</u>-chā/ Lucia /loo-<u>chē</u>-ə/ Medici Torricelli trecento veloce

ç /s/ (A **cedilla** used in **French** words to indicate an /s/ sound of "c" before a, o, & u.)
aperçu façade français garçon soupçon

-cc- /k-s/ accede accelerando accelerant accelerate **accent** accentuate **accept** acceptable **access** accession accessory **accident** eccentric flaccid floccilation occident **succeed success** succinct **vaccinate vaccine**;   Exception: soccer /<u>sok</u>-er/

ch[1] /ch/ (Old English, Old French, Latin)   arch archduke archer attach belch bench birch blanch **branch** brunch chafe chaff **chain chair** chalice cha<u>l</u>k **challenge** chamber **champ** champion **chance** chancel chancellor **change** channel chant chanter chantey chantry **chap** chaplain chapel **chapter** char chard **charge** chariot charity Charles **charm** charnel charry **chart** charter Chartism **chase** chaste chastise **chat** chattel **chatter cheap cheat check** Cheddar **cheek cheese cheer** cherish cherry **chess** chest Chester chestnut **chew chick chicken** chide **chief** chigger **child chill chime** chimney **chin** China chink **chip** chipmunk **chirp** chisel chit chitchat chive **choice choke choose** chop **chore chose chow chub** chubby **chuck** Chuck chuckle **chug chum chump chunk church churn cinch clinch** conch **crunch** discharge **drench** enchant enrich entrench **finch flinch** franchise grinch **gulch** henchman **hunch inch lunch** lurch lynch **march** March merchant **much** mulch **munch** orchard ostrich parch parchment penchant **perch pinch** poncho **punch quench** ranch **rich** sandwich **scorch search squelch starch** stench **such** surcharge **torch trench** trenchant urchin wench **which** winch

ch[2] /sh/ **(French)** brochure **cache** chaconne **chagrin** chalet chamois champagne Champagne chancre chandelier chanson chanterelle chapeau **charade** charades charlatan Charlemagne Charlotte Chartres chartreuse chassis chateau chauffeur Chautauqua chauvinism **chef** chenille **Cher** Cherbourg chevrolet **chevron** Cheyenne chic **Chicago chiffon** chivalry Chopin **chute** douche echelon embouchure gauche **machine Michigan mustache nonchalant** panache

ch[3] /k/ **(Greek)** (Chi: χ, X) Achilles **archive** anchor chameleon chaos character charisma **chasm** chemistry **chi** chimera chiropractic chlorine choir cholera cholesterol **chord** choreography **chorus** Chris Christ Christian **Christmas** chromatic chromium chromosome **chronic** chronicle **echo** epoch eunuch mechanical melancholly Nicholas orchestra **ocher orchid** pachysandra paschal psyche psychology schedule **scheme school synch** synchronize technical technology

ch[4] /kh/ **(German)** (A "throat-clearing" sound, but often /k/ in English.) Ausgleich Bach Cranach Dachau Ehrlich Fichte Koch Offenbach Reich Reichstag Tillich; **(Scotch)** loch; **(Hebrew)** Chanukah (Hanukkah)

-ck /k/ (Word end after short vowel.) Adirondack alack amuck attack **back beck black block** Braddock **brick** brock **buck Buck** burdock buttock Chadwick **check chick** chock chuck Chuck clack **click clock cluck cock** cossack **crack crick crock deck** derrick **Dick dock duck** flack **fleck flick flock** Frederick frock geck gimmick Gluck guck **hack** haddock hammock hassock heck **hick hock** hoick hummock **jack Jack jock kick knack** knickknack kopeck **lack lick** limerick **lock luck Mack** maverick McCormick Merrimack **mock** Monadnock **muck** mullock **neck** niblick **nick Nick** nock **pack** paddock Patrick peacock **peck pick** Planck **pluck** pock politick **prick puck quack quick rack** ransack **Rick rock** ruck **sack shack** shamrock Sherlock **shock** shtick Shylock **sick slack slick smack smock snack** snick **sock speck stack** spick-and-span **stick stock struck stuck suck tack** tamarack **thick** thwack **tick** tick-tock **track trick truck tuck** tussock Warwick whack wick wrack; <u>Exceptions:</u> frolic picnic traffic & Gk. **-ic** suffix words: <u>See:</u> Ap. iv-54.

-ck /k/ (Medially before **-et**.) becket Becket bracket **bucket cricket** crocket Crockett docket **jacket** locket Nantucket **packet** Pawtucket **picket** Pickett placket **pocket racket** rickets rickety **rocket** socket sprocket **thicket** ticket wicket

-ck /k/ (Medially before **-er**) bicker **cracker checker** crockery dicker flicker locker mackerel pickerel pucker slicker **snicker** wicker

-ck /k/ (Medially before **-ey**) dickey hickey **hockey jockey** lackey rickey

-ck /k/ (Substitute for **k** doubling in **-ckle**.) crackle **freckle** grackle heckle knuckle pickle prickle shackle sickle spackle speckle stickle suckle **tackle** tickle trickle

-ck /k/ (Others) beckon Becky bracken buckeen Bruckner Buckingham buckram **chicken** cuckoo Dickens Jackson Kentucky Mackinaw mackintosh nickel Pickford Pickwick pumpernickel **reckless** Rickenbacker rickrack rickshaw speckled **sticky stocking stocky** stricken tacky ticking **wacky**; <u>Note:</u> To keep **c** hard add **k**: frolic / frolicking   mimic / mimicking   picnic / picnicking   traffic / trafficking

-dge /j/ acknowledge **badge badger bridge budge** budget Coolidge curmudgeon dodge dredge drudge edge fidget fledge fledgling fridge **fudge** gadget **grudge hedge** hodgepodge **judge** kedge knowledge **ledge** ledger **lodge** Madge midge Midge **nudge** partridge **pledge** porridge **ridge** Rutledge sedge sledge **sludge** smidgen smudge stodge trudge wedge; <u>Note: with another consonant after the short vowel (to "protect" it), "d" is not needed:</u> barge bilge bulge cringe dirge flange forge hinge indulge large Marge merge Norge plunge purge serge splurge surge twinge urge verge; <u>Nor is the "d" needed when the vowel is long:</u> age huge oblige page rampage stage wage; <u>Note:</u> **d** keeps **g** soft in: abridgment acknowledgment judgment

Diacritical Marks: (Pronunciation aids.)

macron (From Greek, *macros* = long.) ā, ē, ī, ō, ū indicates long vowel. *ate, he, hi, so, mute*

breve (From Latin, *brevis* = short.) ă, ĕ, ĭ, ŏ, ŭ indicates short vowel. *bat, bet, bit, bot, but*

schwa (From Hebrew, the sign ":" a vowel sound.) ə /ŭ/. in unaccented syllables. *son, from, love*

dieresis (From Greek, *diairesis* = a division.) ä /ah/ *father, calm, ma, want, squat*

circumflex (From Latin, *circumflexus* = bend around.) ô /aw/ *dog, off, cost, gone, cloth*

acute accent (Found in French words.) é /ā/ *André, blasé, café.*

cedilla (From Greek, *zeta;* in French words.) ç /s/ *façade , garçon*

tilde (Spanish from Latin, *titulus* = superscription.) ñ /ny/ *cañon, mañana, señorita.*

umlaut (German, change of sound.) ü (See umlaut Ap. i-41.) *gemütlich, flügelhorn, Fräulein, ländler*

-du- /jōō/ arduous **educate education gradual graduate individual** modulate modulation residual Sadducee; **Exceptions:** /jŏō/ adulate credulous pendulous, pendulum sedulous stridulate; /jə/ fraudulent incredulous procedure verdurous; /dōō/ fiduciary credulity

---

ea[1] /ē/ anneal appeal appear appease arrear **beach** beacon **bead** beagle **beak** beaker **beam bean** beard **beast beat** beaver beleaguer beneath bequeath bereave bleach bleachers bleak bleary bleat breach breathe cease **cheap cheat clean clear** cleat cleave cleaver colleague conceal congeal creak **cream** crease creature deacon **deal** dean **Dean** dear decease decrease defeasance defeat demean demeanor disease **dream** dreary **each** eager eagle **ear ease** East Easter easy easel **eat** eaves endear entreat **fear** feasible **feast** feat feature flea freak gear gleam glean grease **heal** heap **hear heat** heath heathen heave heaves impeach increase jeans **Jean** Keats knead lea leach **lead leaf** leaflet league **leak lean leap** Lear lease leash **least leave** leaves malfeasance mead Mead Meade meager **meal mean** meantime measles **meat** neap near **neat** 'neath ordeal **pea** Peabody **peace peach** peacock **peak** peaked peal Peale peanut Pearse peat plea plead please pleat preach queasy reach **read real** ream reap rear reason release repeal repeat retreat reveal **sea seam seal** sear Sears season **seat scream** Shakespeare sheaf sheath sheathe sheaves sleazy sneak sneaker **speak** spear **squeak** squeal squeamish **steal steam** steamer **streak stream** streamer sublease **tea teach teacher** teal teak **team** teamster tear tease teat treason **treat** treatise treaty tweak upheaval veal **weak** weal wean weary weasel weave **wheat** Wheaton wreak wreath wreathe year yeast zeal Zealand; **See: ear**[3], Ap. i-19.

---

ea[2] /ĕ/ abreast ahead behead **bread** breadth breakfast breast **breath** cleanse **dead deaf** dealt **death dread** dreamt endeavor **feather head heading health** heather heaven heavy homestead **instead** jealous **lead** leapt leather leaven meadow **meant** measure peasant pheasant pleasant pleasure **read** ready realm

spread stead steady stealth **sweat** sweater **thread threat** treacherous treachery
tread treadle treasure unsteady unthread **wealth** weapon weather zealot;
<u>Exceptions</u>: /ā/ great steak break yea Yeats; /ə/ ocean pageant sergeant /sar-jənt/,
vengeance yeah /yä/ /yah/;   <u>Note</u>: lead read; (Each has the two *ea* pronunciations.)

---

ear[1] /er/ dearth earl **early earn earnest earth** earthen earthly **heard** hearse
Hearst **learn** pearl rehearse research **search** yearn

---

ear[2] /air/ bear bearing bearer pear swear tear wear

---

ear[3] /ear/ appear beard **clear dear** disappear dreary ear fear gear hear near
rear sear Sears Shakespeare shear smear spear tear weary year;
<u>Exception</u>: heart /hart/;   <u>Note</u>: tear (Has both /air/ & /ear/ pronunciations.)

---

eau /ō/ **(French)** aboideau bandeau bateau **beau** Beaumont Beauregard
Bordeaux bordereau **bureau** chalumeau **chapeau** chateau Clemenceau Cointreau
coteau couteau **Eau Claire** flambeau Fontainebleau fricandeau jambeau **Juneau**
Lambeau manteau Martineau Mirabeau morceau nouveau **plateau** portmanteau
réseau Rochambeau **rondeau** rouleau **Rousseau** tableau **Thoreau** tonneau Watteau;
<u>Exceptions</u>: /yo͞o/ beaut beautiful **beauty**

-ed[1] /id/ (After *t* & *d* ; pronounced as separate syllable.)   acted added belted blasted
bonded booted coated   dated deeded drafted drifted dusted elated ended fated
folded footed frosted gifted granted guarded handed haunted headed hinted hooded
hunted jointed   landed lasted lifted loaded masted melted minded mounted needed
nested painted panted parted planted plated pointed printed punted rusted sainted
salted sanded   seated sided sifted slanted stated stilted sweated talented tended
tented tested tilted tinted tufted vested voided waited wanted, *etc.*   (More in Ap. iv-4.)

-ed[2] /t/ (After all unvoiced letters but *t* .)   arched asked backed banked blinked
blocked bucked bumped camped checked clamped cocked corked cracked cranked
cursed cussed dumped finished fixed flocked fluffed flunked forced forked gulped
helped honked hooked hoped huffed hushed iced jumped kicked kissed limped
linked lucked marked masked missed mixed paced packed passed picked puffed
risked shaped toothed touched versed vexed voiced yanked, *etc.* (More in Ap. iv-4.)

-ed[3] /d/ (After all voiced letters but *d* .)   aged agreed armed banged barbed bared
blamed called clanged drilled dulled edged egged filled filmed fumed fused
ganged grilled hanged happened healed heeled horned hued hulled hushed informed
involved jelled keyed killed learned lettered lived lobed longed loved lulled mailed
mended milled mouthed mulled nerved peeved pickled raised reasoned refined
reformed removed robbed screamed seemed served sized skilled smelled spelled
spilled stilled stoned strained tired traveled used willed yelled, *etc..* (More in Ap. iv-4.)

ee /ē/ Aberdeen **absentee addressee agree** alee alienee allotee **amputee** apogee appellee **appointee** asleep assignee **bee** beech **beef beet beetle** beseech between **bleed bootee** breech breed breeze **canteen** careen **cheek** cheep cheese Cherokee chickadee chivaree coffee **committee** conferee consignee coulee Cree creed creek Creek **creep** decree **deed** deem **deep** degree deportee designee devotee disagree discreet divorcee donee **draftee** Dundee dungaree eel **eighteen** emcee (M.C.) **employee** endorsee enfeeble epopee **escapee** esteem evacuee examinee exceed **fee feeble feed feel feet fifteen flee** filigree fleece fleet **fourteen free freeze** fricassee Galilee garnishee gee geek geese geezer genteel Genesee glee goatee grantee **greed** Greece **Greek** Greeley **green greet** guarantee Halloween **heed heel indeed** inductee internee jamboree jeep jeer jubilee keel keen **keep** Kleenex **knee kneel** lee **Lee** lees leech leek legatee lessee levee licensee Machree marquee Maureen **meek meet** Menominee Milwaukee mortgagee **need needle** Needham **nineteen nominee** ogee parakeet parolee patentee **payee** Pawnee pedigree **peek peel** peen peep peeve peevish peewee perigee Pharisee preen presentee proceed promisee Pyrenees **queen** redeem **reed** reef reek reel reeve **referee refugee** repartee rupee Sadducee **see** sateen **screen screech** Seabee **seed seek seem seen** seep seethe selectee **settee seventeen sixteen** Shawnee sheen **sheep** shivaree skeet sleek **sleep** sleet sneer **sneeze speech speed** spleen spree squeegee squeeze standee steed **steel** Steele Steen **steep** steeple Streep **street** succeed suttee Swanee **sweep sweet** Tallahassee tee teem **teen** teeny **teeth** te-hee Tennessee tepee thee **thirteen three** Toynbee **trainee** Tralee transferee **tree** trochee **trustee** tureen tweed Tweed Tweedle (Dum & Dee) 'tween tweet tweezers upkeep usee vee velveteen **Yankee warrantee** wee **weed week** Weems **weep** weevil wheedle **wheel** Wheeler wheeze whoopee wildebeest Winnepesaukee Zee; <u>Exceptions</u>: /ā/ Klee matinee melee negligee soiree toupee; <u>See</u>: **-eer.**

-eer /ear/ auctioneer **beer** career charioteer **cheer** cheerio **deer** domineer domineering electioneer **engineer jeer leer** leery musketeer mutineer **peer pioneer** profiteer puppeteer **queer** racketeer rocketeer sheer **sneer steer** veer **volunteer weaponeer**; <u>Exception</u>: seer /sē -er/; (More in Ap. iv-62.)

ei¹ /ā/ beige /bāzh/ Beirut chow mein deign Eire feign feint geisha heinous **heir** lei Nisei /nē sā/ obeisance reign rein reindeer Seine Sinn Fein skein Suleiman surveillance Taipei /tī pā/ **their** Trondheim veil vein; <u>See</u>: **eigh** on next page.

ei² /ē/ caffeine **ceiling conceive** codeine **conceit deceit deceive either** Keith keister Leif Ericson leisure Leith Madeira Monseigneur **Neil** Neilson Neiman's **neither perceive** Pleiades **protein** receipt **receive** Reims seize seizure seignior sheik **weir weird**; <u>Exceptions</u>: /ĕ/ heifer; /ĭ/ counterfeit; /ə/ reveille

ei³ /ī/ feisty height heist Oneida; **(German)** Braunschweig Dreiser eiderdown Eiffel Einstein Eisenhower Epstein Fahrenheit Frankenstein Fraulein Freiburg Gauleiter Geiger gesundheit Guggenheim heil Heidelberg Heilbronn Heifetz Heine Heisenberg Holstein Keitel Klein Kreisler Leiden Leipzig leitmotif Lorelei Mein Kampf Meissen Meistersinger Mundelein Oppenheimer poltergeist Reich Reims Reinhardt Rheingold Rubinstein schrecklichkeit Schumann-Heink Schweitzer Zeitgeist zum Beispiel (for example) zollverein; **(Greek)** eidetic Peisistratus Poseidon seismic; **(Dutch)** apartheid; **(Irish)** Eileen; **(Arabic)** Leila

---

eigh /ā/ eight freight inveigh neigh neighbor sleigh weigh weight;
Exceptions: /ī/ heigh heigh-ho height sleight; /ē/ Raleigh

---

er /er/ **(Within a word; followed by a consonant.)** adverb adverse advert alert Antwerp artery assert avert bakery berg Bergen Bergson Berlin berm Bern berserk berth cavern celery cistern checkers **clerk commerce concern concert conserve** converge converse **convert** covert culvert derby desert dessert discern disperse diverge diverse divert erg ersatz erst excerpt **expert** fern fertile fervent fervid fervor **germ** German germane **govern herb** Herb Herbert Herculean Hercules herd herl hermit hertz Hertz inert **insert interest** intern inverse **invert jerk** jerkin kerchief kerf kern kernel **lantern** lectern merge **modern** nerd **nerve** obverse opera overt pattern **percent perch perfect** perfume **perhaps** perk Perkins perky **permit** perplex **persist person** pert Perth revert Robert serf sermon serpent **serve** sperm sterling **stern** sternum superb swerve tavern **term** termite tern terse **verb** verbose verdant verdict vermin Vermont **verse** versus **western**

-er (Noun or pronoun ending.) anger answer archer backer badger baker banker banner barber bather batter beater beaver beeper biker binder blazer bleacher blender blinker blister blocker blotter blunder boarder boiler bomber booster border bother boxer breather brother bubbler bumper burger burner Buster butcher butler butter buyer buzzer caller camper cancer catcher center chapter checker cleaner climber clover cluster clutter coaster cooker cooler copper corner counter cover cracker crater crisper cutter dancer danger daughter dealer decker Denver digger dimmer diner dinner dipper dither diver dodger doer Dover drawer dreamer dresser drifter driller drinker driver dropper drummer duster Easter eater elder ember eraser farmer father feeder feeler fencer fender fever fiber fibber fielder fighter filler filter finger fisher fixer flicker flower folder freezer gardener garter gender ginger girder giver glider glimmer glitter goer goiter golfer goner grocer grounder grower gunner gusher gutter hamburger hammer hamper hamster hanger healer heater helper her hiker hitter holder hotter hunger hunter informer inhaler insider jailer jester jogger joker jumper keeper kicker killer ladder lather laughter leader letter lever liver lobster locker lodger loser lover lumber luster maker manger manner marker master matter member merger meter milker miner mister mixer monster mother mover murder nearer neither November number oiler opener order other ouster oyster owner packer paper partner passer pauper payer pepper Peter picker pitcher planner planter plaster platter player plunger pointer poker popper porter poster powder power printer punter quarter quitter racer rafter raider rambler rancher ranger rapper reader renter reporter revolver rider river roaster robber rocker roller roofer roomer rooster rooter roster rover Rover rower rubber rudder ruler runner rusher saver scorcher scraper sealer seeker seller semester sender September server shaker shaver shelter shipper shiver shooter shopper shower shudder silver singer sister sitter skater slaughter slipper sliver slower slumber smoker sneaker soccer sparkler speaker speeder speller spider splinter starter sticker stinger stranger streamer stretcher striker summer super supper surfer sweater taker talker tanker tamer taster teacher teenager teller temper tender tester thinker thriller thunder tiger timber timer toaster tower trader trailer trainer trapper trigger trooper trucker twister usher usurer voter voucher waiter walker washer watcher water weeper wheeler whimper whisker whisper winner winter wonder worker writer zipper;   (More in Ap. iv-5.)

-er (Verb) alter anger answer banter barber barter blister blunder bluster bolster border bother center chatter cluster clutter confer corner cover enter filter flicker flounder flower fluster flutter foster gather glimmer glitter hammer hamper hinder hunger lather letter linger litter lower lumber master matter murder muster mutter neuter number offer order pamper paper plaster plunder ponder powder prefer refer remember render scamper scatter shatter shelter shiver shower shudder slander slaughter slobber slumber smother snicker spatter splatter stagger stammer stutter suffer swelter tamper taper tinker trigger usher utter wager wander waver whimper whisper wonder; (Adverb) ever never;   (More in Ap. iv-6.)

-er (Adjective) bitter clever either inner other tender upper; (More in Ap. iv-7.)

-er (Comparative form of adjective.) better blacker bluer blunter braver brighter calmer cleaner closer cooler crisper damper darker dimmer duller dumber elder farther faster fatter firmer fitter greater greener harder higher hotter later lesser lighter longer lower madder milder moister nearer older quicker redder riper rougher sadder sharper shorter sicker slicker slower smarter softer sooner sounder stronger swifter tamer tanner thinner weaker wetter whiter younger; (More in Ap. iv-7.)

ere /ear/ adhere ampere cereal cohere coherent **here** interfere mere merely revere sere severe sphere we're; <u>Exceptions:</u> /er/ were; /air/ ere heresy Jeremy there where

er (+ **vowel** other than *e*.) /air/ America Bering cherish Cherokee cherub Cheryl clerical emeritus **era** ferric gerund generic Heracles Heraclitus herald heritage heroin heron kerosene Kerry **merit peril perish** posterity seraph sheriff steroid verify verity;   <u>Exceptions:</u> /ear/ hero Nero **zero**

er-i + **vowel** /ear-ē/ (Where "i" is pronounced /ē/ since it is followed by another vowel.) anterior arterial bacterial deleterious **experience** exterior hysteria imperial imperialism imperious **inferior interior** managerial **material mysterious** posterior serial **serious** superior ulterior

er-r /air/ berry **cherry** errand errant erratic error **ferry merry** Perry Sherry Sierra terra **Terry**

-et /ā/ (French) ballet buffet cabaret crochet fillet gourmet valet; <u>See</u>: -et³, Ap. iv-62.

eu¹ /yōō/ Beulah Euboea eucalyptus Eucharist euchre Euclid eudemonia Eugene eugenics **eulogy** eunuch euphemism euphonium euphoria eureka Euripides **Europe** European Eurydice eurythmics Eustachian euthanasia **feud** feudal heuristic therapeutic; **(Eu- is a Greek prefix meaning "well" or "good.")**

eu² /ōō/ Aleutian Betelgeuse **deuce** Deuteronomy leukemia maneuver neume neural neurologist **neuron neurotic neuter** neutral Pentateuch pharmaceutical pneuma pneumatic propaedeutics pseudo **Reuben** Reuters Reuther rheum rheumatic rheumatism Seleucus **sleuth** Steuben Teuton Theseus **Zeus**; <u>Exceptions</u>: **(In German "eu" = /oi/.)** Deutschland Freud.

ew¹ /yōō/ askew curfew ewe ewer **few hew** hewn Matthew **mew** nephew **pew** pewter phew! sinew skew skewer **spew** thew **whew!**

ew² /ōō/ Agnew Andrew Andrews anew **blew brew** cashew **chew crew** crewel **dew** Dewey **drew** eschew **flew grew** Hebrew **Jew** jewel lewd Lewis mildew **new** news newt renew Renfrew **screw** sewer sewerage shrew shrewd **slew stew** steward strew Tewkesbury threw yew; <u>Exception</u>: /ō/ sew

ey¹ /ā/ bey convey dey disobey fey frey Grey Keynes **hey** heyday Heywood Leyte Monterrey **obey** prey purvey Reykjavik survey **they** trey whey

ey² /ē/ abbey alley attorney Audrey Barkley Barnsley Bentley Berkeley **barley** chantey **chimney** Copley covey Dewey dickey Disney **donkey** doohickey dopey Dudley hackney Halley Harley Harvey Henley hickey **hockey** hokeypokey **honey** Humphrey Jeffrey **jersey Jersey jockey** journey **key** kidney Kinsey lackey lamprey malarkey Massey McGuffey McKinley **medley mickey Mickey money monkey** Morley Moseley mosey Mosley Nutley Odyssey Orkney Paisley Paley parley **parsley** Pompey Priestley pulley Riley Rodney Romney Shelley Shirley Sidney Stanley surrey Surrey Sydney **trolley turkey Turkey valley volley** Wellesley **whiskey** Wolseley Wesley; <u>Exceptions</u>: /ĭ/ Boleyn Ceylon; /ĕ/ Reynolds

g¹ /g/ (Is always "hard" before a, o, u, & consonants.) gasp go gum glad grape, *etc.*
(Sometimes "hard" before e & i.) gear geek **geese** Gehena Geiger geisha geld
gemsbok gemütlich Gesundheit **get** Getysburg geyser gibbon Gibbons Gibson
giddy **gift** gig giggle Gilbert gild gill Gilman gilt gimlet gimmal gimmick
gimp gingham gink ginkgo gird girder girdle **girl** girth gismo **give** gizzard

g² /j/ (Often soft before e, i, & y.) age agent aging agitate allege angel apogee
barge change **gem** Gemini gender gene genealogy genera general generator
generic generous genesis Genesis genet genetics Geneva genial genitals genitive
genius Genoa gens genteel Gentile **gentle** gentleman gentry genuflect
genuine **genus** geography geology geometry George geranium gerbil geriatrics
germ German germane Germany gerontology gerund gesso gestate gesture
giant gibber gibberish gibbet gibe giblet Gibralter Gibran giga– /jig-ə/ gigantic
gigolo Giles Gillette **gin ginger** ginseng Giotto giraffe Girard gist **gym**
gymkhana gymnasium gymnast gypsum Gypsy gyrate gyration gyro gyroscope
hydrogen large oxygen, *etc.*   See: **-age¹**, Ap. i-10; **-dge**, Ap. i-17.

g³ /zh/ **(French)** gendarme Genêt genre Gide gigolo gigue Gironde

-gg- /g-j/ suggest **suggestion** suggestive

gh¹ /g/ aghast ghastly Ghent gherkin ghetto Ghiberti **ghost ghoul** sorghum
spaghetti;   But: Van Gogh /van gō/ or /van gôkh/

gh² /f/ cough **enough** laugh **rough** slough sough **tough**

gn /n/ align alignment arraign assign assignment benign campaign champagne
Charlemagne coign condign consign deign /dān/ **design** ensign feign /fān/ foreign
gnar **gnarl** gnarled gnash **gnat gnaw gnome** gnostic Gnostic gnu impugn
malign Monseigneur oppugn reign /rān/ **resign sign** sovereign

gu-¹ /g/ guarantee guarantor guaranty **guard** guardian Guernica guernsey
Guernsey guerrilla **guess guest** guidance **guide** guild guile guillotine **guilt**
guilty guimpe guinea Guinea guise guitar languor

gu-² /gw/ distinguish Guadalcanal Guadeloupe Guam guano Guantanamo
Guarani Guarnerius Guatemala Guenever Guido language languid languish
lingua linguist penguin

-gue /g/ **-igue** /ēg/ brogue catalogue chaise longue /shāz lông/ colleague
dialogue disembogue **fatigue fugue** gigue The Hague harangue **intrigue** league
meringue /mə-rang/ morgue plague Prague **prologue** prorogue rogue tongue vague
vogue;   Note how *n* "subdues" the *-gue* /-ng/;   Exceptions: argue /ar-gyōō/ dengue /deng-gē/

ie¹ /ē/ (Within word.) achieve afield Algiers **belief believe** besiege bier Brie **brief** brigadier cashier cavalier chandelier **chief** debrief diesel Diesel disbelief Enfield fief **field** fiend **fierce** frieze glockenspiel **grief** Grieg **grieve** hygiene Kiel Kierkegaard Krieg Liederkranz lief liege lien mien **niece** Nielson Nieman Niemoller Nietzsche **piece** Piedmont **pier pierce** premier premiere **priest** Priestly rabies **relief relieve** reprieve retrieval **retrieve** schlemiel Schliemann series **shield shriek siege** Siegfried Singspiel spiel Tangier **thief thieve** wield wiener **yield** Ziegfeld (At end of word.) (Some are **Scottish**) anomie **auntie** beanie beastie **birdie** bogie bookie boogie woogie bourgeoisie Bowie **brownie Brownie caddie** calorie Curie Erie goalie jalousie mashie mealie menagerie movie Muncie muskie **pinkie pixie** Poughkeepsie **prairie** reverie **rookie** rotisserie sharpie sheltie Skokie sortie specie stymie smoothie sweetie Valkyrie walkie-talkie wedgie weenie weirdie Willkie **zombie** (First names.) Barbie Leslie Lizzie Lottie Maisie Mamie Margie Marie Marjorie Melanie Minnie Natalie Nettie Queenie Sadie Scottie Stacie Stephanie Trixie; <u>Exceptions:</u> friend /frĕnd/; lingerie /<u>län</u>-zhə-rā/ Pieta /pyā-tä/; (Careful when *i* & *e* are divided as in *Vi-en-na*.)

ie² /ī/ applied belie complied cried **die died** dried fie fiery **fried** hie lie lied **pie** pied plied pried shied **spied tie tied tried** vie zwieback; <u>Exceptions:</u> /ĭ/ kerchief mischief mischievous sieve; (Careful when *i* & *e* are divided as in *di-et, pi-e-ty*.)

-igh /ī/ blight bright Brighton **delight** Dwight **fight flight fright high** insight knight **light might** nigh **night** plight **right sigh sight slight thigh tight** upright Wight wright Wright

-ild /īld/ child mild wild; <u>Exception:</u> gild /gild/

-ind /īnd/ behind bind blind find grind hind kind mind remind rind wind

-ing /ing/ (One syllable.) Bing bring ding king Ming ping ring sing sling spring sting string swing ting wing wring zing (Multi-syllable.) acting ailing airing alarming amazing arching backing balding banking batting being belonging bidding billing bowling boxing breaking burning calling camping charming clearing clothing coating coloring coming covering crossing dashing distressing doing drawing dressing drilling during eating failing falling farming feeling fighting filling fishing flowing frosting going greeting hanging heading helping holding hunting incoming interesting keeping killing knowing landing lasting laughing leading leaning learning lettering living loading loving making meeting missing morning opening outing outstanding picking printing pushing railing ranking running seating seeing seeming shooting singing sitting smashing sneaking spanking speaking speeding spelling standing stinging sweeping swelling swimming talking teaching telling tempting Thanksgiving thinking trucking trusting trying turning waiting wanting warning washing writing; (More in Ap. iv-9.)

-ink /ingk / blink brink chink clink **drink** fink kink **link** mink **pink** prink rink shrink **sink** slink stink **think** **wink**

-ion /yən/ billion bunion champion communion companion dominion medallion million onion opinion rebellion reunion trillion union;   (More in Ap. iv-36.)

ir /er/ affirm birch **bird** birl Birmingham **birth** chirm chirp circa Circe **circle** circuit circulate circumference circumspect circumstance circumvent **circus** confirm dirge dirigible dirk **dirt** Dunkirk elixir fir **firm** **first** flirt gird girder **girl** girth infirm Irving Irwin irk kirk **Kirk** Kirsch **mirth** nadir Nirvana **quirk** quirt **shirk** shirr **shirt** **sir** sirloin **skirt** smirch **smirk** spirit squirm squirt **stir** stirrup **swirl** tapir triumvir **twirl** **third** **thirst** Virgil virgin virginal Virginia Virgo virtual virtue virtuoso whir whirl; **Exceptions**: /ear/ amir emir souvenir Vladimir.

-ire /īr/ acquire admire aspire conspire desire dire empire esquire expire **fire** **hire** inquire inspire **ire** Ireland mire perspire quagmire quire require **retire** sapphire satire shire sire **spire** **tire** transpire **umpire** vampire **wire**

ir-r /ear/ cirrus irreducible irreligious irremediable irremissible irremovable irreplaceable irrepressible irreproachable irresistible irresolvable irrespective irresponsible irretraceable irretrievable irreversible irrigate irrigation irritable irritant irritate irritation **mirror**; **Exceptions**: /i-r..../ irrational irreconcilable irrefutable irregular irrelevant irreparable irreverent irruption

ir- (+ **vowel** other than "e") /ear/ Hirohito Hiroshima Iroquois lira miracle Miriam nirvana pirouette virile virulent

j /h/ **(Spanish)** Guadalajara **junta** La Jolla /hoi-yə/ **Mojave** Navajo San José; /wh/ Don Juan San Juan marijuana

kn- /n/ knack knap knapsack knar knave knead **knee** kneel knelt knew Knickerbocker knickers knickknack **knife** knight knit knob knock knoll knop knot knout **Knox** Knoxville **know** knowledge **known** **knuckle** knur knurl

-ly /lē/ (Usually an adverb)   barely certainly chiefly cleanly cleverly closely coldly constantly costly daily darkly deadly dearly directly dryly earthly easily exactly fairly fatherly fondly formerly freely frequently friendly fully ghostly gladly greatly happily honestly hotly hourly instantly jointly kindly lately likely luckily lonely mainly monthly mostly nearly overly presently promptly properly publicly quickly rarely really richly rightly sickly simply slightly softly spotlessly surely timely truly unsightly weakly weekly yearly;   (More in Ap. iv-11.)

-mb /m/ aplomb bomb **climb** comb coomb coulomb **crumb** dithyramb **dumb** entomb gamb jamb **lamb** lambda **limb** **numb** plumb plumber succumb **thumb** tomb womb

-mn /m/ autumn column condemn contemn damn hymn solemn; Note: mnemonic /nē-<u>mon</u>-ik/ Mnemosyne /nē-<u>mos</u>-ə-nē/

n /ng/ (Before /k/ and /g/.) Algonquin anchor **anger** /<u>ang</u>-ger/ angle Anglican Anglo-Angola Angora **angry** anguish angular Angus ankh **ankle** anklet bank banquet **blink** /blingk/ bunco buncombe bungalow **bungle bunk bunker chunk** chunky **clank clinker** Concord conga Congo congruous conk dinghy dingo dinky **drank drink drunk dunk** embankment England /<u>ing</u>-glənd/ **English** /<u>ing</u>-glish/ **finger** flank **flunk frank** Frank Frankfort Franklin funk gangling gink ginkgo gringo hank hanker **honk hunger hungry hunk** Inca incongruous indistinguishable ingot **ink** inkling inky jingle jingo jinx junk Junker junket junkie kink kinky language languid languish languor lanky larynx Lincoln linger lingo lingual linguist linkage **longer** Mencken monger Mongel mongoose **monkey** pinkie puncture rancor Rangoon **ranking rink sanction** sanctum Sanctus sanguine shingle shingles **shrunk sink sinker slink spank** sprinkler sprinkling **spunk** spunky **stink strength** stunk succinct **sunk** sunken tango **tank** tankard **tanker tankful thank think thinker thinking tinker** tranquil unco unction vanquish wrangler Yankee Yonkers, *etc.*

ñ (Tilde) /ny/ **(Spanish)** compañero *(Comrade.)* cañon Doña el Niño mañana piña piñata piñon Porteño señor señora señorita

oa /ō/ aboard afloat approach bemoan bloat boar board **boast boat** broach charcoal cloak **coach coal** coarse **coast coat coax** croak cockroach cocoa encroach **float** foal **foam** gloaming gloat goad **goal goat groan** hoar hoard hoarse hoax Joan **load loaf** loafer loam **loan** loathe loaves **moan** moat oaf **oak** Oakland Oakley oar **oath** poach reproach roach **road** roadster **roam** roan roar **roast** shoal skoal Sloan **soak soap** soar **throat** toad **toast** whoa; Exception: broad /brawd/

oe /ō/ aloe Boer Coe Crusoe Defoe **doe** floe **foe** froe Glencoe **goes** Joe hoe mistletoe Moe Monroe oboe Poe roe Roebuck Roscoe sloe Tahoe throes tiptoe **toe woe** Zoe; Exceptions: /ē/ Croesus oenomel onomatopoeia; Phoebe Phoebus phoenix Phoenix subpoena; /ĕ/ Oedipus roentgen Roentgen; /ə/ does, Phoenicia Phoenician; /o͞o/ canoe, shoe.

oi /oi/ adjoining adroit anoint appoint asteroid avoid Beloit **boil boiler** Boise boisterous broil celluloid **choice** cloister coif **coil coin** coir counterpoint deltoid despoil Detroit devoid disappoint disjoin disjoint doily embroider embroil enjoin exploit foible foil foist goiter groin Hanoi hoick hoi polloi **hoist** hoity-toity Illinois introit invoice **join** joinder **joint** joist loin loiter mastoid **moist** moisture noise **oil ointment** paranoia paranoid parboil poi poignant poinsettia **point** poise poison purloin quoin quoit recoil reconnoiter rejoice rejoinder roil sequoia sirloin **soil spoil** St. Croix steroid **tabloid** tenderloin thyroid **tinfoil toil** toilet trapezoid troika turmoil turquoise typhoid **voice void** yoicks;   Exceptions: /ə/ tortoise, connoisseur;   See: -oid, Ap. iv-57.

old /ōld/ behold **bold cold** enfold **fold gold hold mold old** retold **scold sold told** unfold unsold untold uphold wold

-oll /ōl/ atoll **boll** droll enroll knoll **poll roll scroll stroll toll** troll; Exceptions: /ol/ doll loll moll; /ôl/ atoll

oo¹ /ōō/ afternoon aloof Altoona baboon balloon bamboo bamboozle bassoon bazooka behoove **bloom** bloomers blooper boo boob boo-boo **boohoo** booby boom boomerang boon **boost boot booth** bootleg booty booze brood **broom** buffoon bugaboo caboodle caboose Cameroon cartoon cesspool Chattanooga Chinook choose cockatoo cocoon coo **cool** Coolidge coolie coolly coon coop cooper Cooper coot croon cuckoo **doodle** doohickey Doolittle **doom** dragoon drool droop festoon floozy **food fool** forsooth galoot **gloom** goober gooey goof googol goon goop goose groom groove harpoon hooligan hooch hoodlum hoof **hoop** hoosegow Hoosier hoot Hoover hullabaloo igloo kangaroo kazoo Kickapoo koodoo lagoon lampoon loo looby **loop** loophole **loom loon** loose **loot** macaroon maroon monsoon **moo** mooch **mood** moolah **moon** moor Moore moose moot mushroom **noodle noon** noose oodles oolong oomiak **oops** ooze palooka pantaloon papoose picaroon platoon poltroon pontoon pooch **poodle** pooh **pool** poop **proof** quadroon raccoon Rangoon rood **roof room** roost rooster **root** saloon Saskatoon Sassoon schmoose **school** schooner **scoop** scoot scooter Scrooge shampoo shoo **shoot** skiddoo skookum sloop smooch **smooth** snood snook snoop snoopy snoot snooty snooze **soon** sooner sooth soothe spittoon spoof **spook spool spoon** stooge stool **stoop** swoon swoop taboo tattoo tomfoolery **too tool** toot **tooth** tootle **troop** Tuscaloosa tycoon typhoon uproot vamoose voodoo wahoo walloon Waterloo whoop whoopee Witherspoon woo woozy yahoo yoo-hoo **zoo zoom**; Exceptions: /ō/ brooch; /or/ door, floor

oo² /ŏŏ/ afoot boogie-woogie **book** booklet **brook cook** cookie cooky **crook** foot gobbledygook **good** hood hoof hook hooky hooray kookaburra manhood **look** nook Norwood oomph partook **poor** rook Sherbrooke Sherwood **shook** soot **stood** took toots tootsy **wood** woof wool; Exceptions: /ə/ blood, flood

or[1] /or/ (Initially or medially.) absorb accord acorn afford afore assort border bore born borrow borscht chord chorus clavichord cord corduroy core Corfu cork corn corner cornet coronation corpse corral deport distort divorce dorm dormant dormer encore /ä́ng-kor/ endorse escort enforce explore export extort Florence Florida for forage force forceps ford Ford fore foreign forest forge fork forlorn form fort forte forth forty forum forward gore gory horde hormone horn hornet horrible horrid horrify horror horse Hortense Horton ignore Jordan lord Lord lore Lorelei lorn Lorraine lorry morbid more Morgan morgue Mormon morn morning Morris morrow morsel Mort mortal mortar mortgage mortify Morton mortuary nor Nordic Norfolk norm Norm normal Norse north Norway or oracle oral orange orb orbit orchard orchestra orchid ordain ordnance ordeal order ordinary Oregon organ orgy orient ort orator ornate pork port scorch score scorn shore shorn short snort sordid sorrow sorry sort stork storm thorn torment torso tort torte vortex Waldorf whore whorl York

---

-or[2] /er/ (At end of word.)   actor ancestor anchor arbor armor ardor auditor author calculator captor censor clamor collector color commentator competitor conductor contractor corridor detector director doctor donor editor educator elevator emperor equator error factor favor fervor flavor generator governor harbor honor horror humor impostor indicator inspector instructor inventor investigator janitor judicator juror labor legislator major mayor mentor minor mirror moderator monitor motor navigator neighbor odor operator orator parlor pastor predictor prior proctor professor projector protector protractor rancor razor reactor receptor reflector regulator rigor rotator rotor rumor sailor savor sculptor sector selector senator spectator splendor sponsor supervisor tailor tenor terminator terror tormentor tractor traitor transgressor translator tremor tumor tutor valor vapor vector ventilator victor vigor visitor visor; (More in Ap. iv-39.)

-ost[1] /ōst/ almost ghost host impost inmost most post utmost

---

-ost[2] /awst/ /ôst/ accost cost frost lost

---

ou[1] /ow/ abound about account aground all-out aloud amount announce around arouse astound blouse bounce bound boundary bounty bout carouse cloud clout compound confound couch council counsel counselor count countenance counter countless county crouch denounce devour devout discount doubt dour douse dumfounded encounter espouse expound flounce flounder flour flout foul found founder foundry fount fountain gadabout gouge grouch grouse ground grout hound hour house Housman impound jounce joust knout loud lounge lousy lout mound mount mountain Mountbatten mouse mouth noun ouch ounce our oust out outing outline outwit pouch pounce pound pout

Ap. i-29

profound pronoun pronounce propound **proud** recount redoubt redoubtable redound remount renounce resound **round** roundup rouse **roust** rout scoundrel **scour scout scrounge shout** shroud **slouch** snout **sound** sour souse **south spouse spout sprout stout** stroud surround surmount tantamount **thou** thousand tousle tout **trounce** trousers **trout vouch voucher** vouchsafe zounds

ou² /o͞o/ acoustic Anjou bayou Bernoulli bijou bivouac boudoir boutique brouhaha caribou cougar Coulee coup coupe coupon courant couteau **croup** crouton debouch denouement double-entendre dénouement douche froufrou ghoul goulash Gould Gounod **group** Joule Louis Louise louver Louvre Manitou nougat noumenon nous pouf Proust recoup rouge roulette **route** routine Scaramouch silhouette sou **soup** Sousa souvenir toucan Toulon toupee troubadour trousseau uncouth Vancouver **wound you youth youthful**; /yo͞o/ Houston

ou³ /ō/ **boulder** bouquet cantaloupe poultry shoulder **soul**

ou⁴ /ə/ adjourn /ə-**jern**/ bourbon camouflage carousel **country couple courage** cousin **double** Douglas **enough** flourish glamour journey Monmouth moustache (mustache) nourishment Plymouth Portsmouth Poughkeepsie redouble retouch **rough** scourge sojourn tambourine **touch tough** tournament **trouble young**

ou⁵ /o͝o/ boulevard Bourbon bourdon bourg contour **could** courier **detour** embouchure entourage gourmet jalousie paramour **should** tambour **tour tourist** would

ough¹ /aw/ /ô/ ("t" ending.) bought brought fought ought sought thought wrought

-ough² /ō/ borough dough furlough Marlborough Peterborough **though** thorough

-ough³ /ow/ bough drought plough (plow); Exception: /o͞o/ through

-ough⁴ /əf/ clough **enough** rough slough **tough**; Exceptions: /awf/ cough trough; ["I've had <u>enough</u> of this <u>rough</u>, <u>tough cough</u>."]

-our /or/ concourse **course court** discourse **four fourth** gourd intercourse mourn pompadour **pour** recourse resource source troubadour **your**; Exceptions: **ou¹**: devour dour flour hour our sour; **ou²**: courante; **ou⁴**: bourbon courage flourish scourge; **ou⁵** contour courier detour entourage **tour tourist**

Outrageous Pronunciations: boatswain /bō-sən/   colonel /ker-nəl/
corps /kor/   corpsman /kor-mən/   coxswain /kok-sənt/   coyote /kī-ō-tē/
ensemble /än-säm-bəl/   Gloucester /glos-ter/   indict /in-dīt/   rendezvous /rän-dā-voo/
sergeant /sar-jənt/   victual /vit-l/   women /wim-in/   Worcester /woos-ter/

-ow¹ /ow/ allow allowance avow **bow** bowel bower Bowery browse **brow**
brown **chow** chowder **clown** cow coward cower cowl Cracow **crowd** **crown**
disallow disavow Dow dowager dowdy dowel dower **down** Downs dowry dowse
drown drowse drowsy Eisenhower endow **flower** fowl frown frowsy glower
gown growl **how** Howard Howe howitzer **howl** Jowell jowl kowtow MacDowell
meow Moscow mow **now** **ow!** owl pandowdy **plow** pow powder Powell **power**
powwow prow prowess **prowl** renown row rowdy scow **scowl** **shower** sow
towel tower town trowel uptown **vow** vowel wow wowser yowl;
Note: -ow is at end of word or often before *l* or *n* within a word.

-ow² /ō/ afterglow arrow Barlow bellow bellows below bestow billow **blow**
blown borrow **bow** bowl bungalow burrow **crow** crowbar disown elbow escrow
fallow farrow fellow **flow** **flowing** **flown** **follow** furrow gallows **glow** **grow**
grown **growth** hallow Halloween harrow **know** **low** Lowell **lower** Marlowe marrow
marshmallow meadow mellow minnow **mow** narrow owe Owen **own** pillow
rainbow **row** sallow shadow shallow **show** **shown** **slow** **snow** sorrow sow sown
sparrow stow swallow tallow **throw** **thrown** tomorrow **tow** towhead wallow
wheelbarrow **widow** **willow** **window** winnow Winslow **yellow**; Note: bow, mow,
sow, & row, depending on their meaning, may have either pronunciation.

-oy /oi/ ahoy alloy annoy arroyo **boy** boycott boysenberry buoy clairvoyance
cloy convoy corduroy **cowboy** **coy** Doyle **decoy** deploy **destroy** disloyal **employ**
enjoy envoy flamboyant Floyd foyer gargoyle hoy Hoyle **joy** Joyce Lloyd loyal
Loyola McCoy **oyster** ploy royal royalty Savoy Savoyard soy Tolstoy **toy**
Toynbee troy **Troy** voyage; <u>See:</u> -oi, Ap. i-28.

---

ph /f/ (Most from **Greek** letter *phi* φ Φ.)   alpha alphabet Alphonso atmosphere
blasphemy camphor cellophane diphthong dolphin **graph** **humph** **lymph** Memphis
morpheme morphine neophyte nymph orphan pamphlet phalanx phallus
phantom Pharaoh Pharisee pharmacy **phase** phew Phidias Philadelphia
philanthropy Philippines philter phlebitis phlegm phlox phobia Phoebe Phoenicia
phoenix phoneme phonetics **phonics** **phonograph** **phi** **Phil** Phillips **philosophy**
phone phosphate phosphorus **photo** photogenic **photograph** photosynthesis
phrase phrenic Phyllis phylum physical **physics** physique sapphire **sphere**
sphincter **sphinx** sulphur (sulfur) symphony sylph **telephone** **triumph**

---

ps- /s/ (From Greek letter *psi* ψ Ψ.)   psalm Psalms psalter psaltery pseudo pseudonym psi psoriasis psyche psychic psychedelic psychiatry psychology psychosis

qua /kwah/ /kwä/ quad quadrangle quadrant quadratic quadriceps quadrillion quadrivium quadruple qualification qualify **quality** quanta quantify **quantity** quantum Quapaw **quash** quasi quatrain **squash**;   Exceptions: /kwă/ quack quaff quagmire;   /kwā/ quail **quaint quake** Quaker quasar quaver;   /kwĕ/ quaestor; /kwə/ quadrille;   /kē/ quay

quar /kwor/ quarantine quarrel quarry **quart** quartan quarter quarterback quarterly quartern **quartet** quartile quarto **quartz**;   Exception: /ar/ quark

-que /k/ **ique** /ēk/ antique brusque clique critique discothèque mosque Mozambique mystique oblique opaque physique plaque technique torque unique; Note: "-esque" /ĕsk/ means *"in the style of"*, thus: arabesque burlesque grotesque humoresque picturesque statuesque;   See: **-esque**, Ap. iv-62 and **-que**, Ap. iv-64.

rh- /r/ (From Greek letter *rho*, ρ P.) rhapsody rheostat rhesus **rhetoric** rheumatism Rh factor Rhine rhinitis rhinoceros Rhodes rhododendron rhomboid rhombus Rhone **rhubarb rhyme rhythm**

S¹ /s/ (The most common pronunciation of *s*.)   sad sat Saturn second seed set sidewalk similar sit size small smoke sneeze sound spring stable stump sun, *etc.*

S² /z/ (Often when *s* follows a vowel or a voiced consonant, it is voiced to a *z*.   Here when there is more than one "s" in a word, the one pronounced /z/ is underlined.) abuse (v) accuse Achilles Adams advertise advise adviser AIDS **always** Andes Andrews appease applause appose appraise apprise arise arms arose arouse ashe<u>s</u> avoirdupois Barnes **because** bruise bruiser caries causative **cause** causing Cervantes charades charisma Charles chasm chasti<u>s</u>e **cheese choose** choosy chose chosen **clause** Clausewitz **close** closet clothes confuse cosmic cosmo- cosmos cousin cruise cruiser cuisine daisy damsel depose deposit desert dessert devise diesel diffuse di<u>s</u>aster disclo<u>s</u>e di<u>s</u>ea<u>s</u>e disgui<u>s</u>e dismal Disney displea<u>s</u>e dispo<u>s</u>e di<u>ss</u>olve di<u>ss</u>olvent divers divisor **does doesn't** doings Dresden drowse drowsy duds **ease** easel **easy** emphase<u>s</u> (pl) enclose espou<u>s</u>e exorcise falsie<u>s</u> fasce<u>s</u> feces fives follies fraise franchise Fresno fuse fusil gallows genitals gens gismo Gesundheit geyser **goods** gosling grisly Hades **has** herdsman **hers he's** hesitate **his** his'n hosanna Hosea house (v) housing husband impose imposing incise incised incisor incuse indispose indisposed indivisible indoors infuse Inquisition inquisitor **is** Isaac Isabella Isaiah Islington Israel Israelite −ism James Jamestown Japanese Jeffreys Jersey Jesuit Je<u>s</u>us

Johnstown Joseph Kaiser Kansas kismet knives Lisbon Louise lousy malaise measles mosey musette **music** musing muse Muslim muslin nasal **noise** noisy **nose** Osman palsy pansy panties peasant pheasant **phrase** physical **physics** **physique** pilsner pincers Pisces **plasma** pleasant **please** poison **pose** posit possess posy presence **present** **preserve** **preside** **presume** prism **prison** prosit quasi queasy quinsy quisling rabies **raise** raised **raisin** raising Ramsay Ramses **reason** **refuse** **remains** repose represent reprise **resent** **reserve** **reside** **resign** resin **resort** **resound** **result** **resume** **revise** Reynolds Rhodes **riches** **rise** riser **rising** Rockies Rosa **rose** rosette rosin rosy rouse rousing runners Saar sarcasm schism scissors **season** seismic series **she's** Shingles shiftings Sousa species spousal Stevens **suds** sudsy summons **suppose** surmise **surprise** tease teaser testes **thousand** **Thursday** tidings tousle transpose trousers **Tuesday** tweezers unties unused unwise vespers visa visage **visit** **visor** vitals Wales **was** **ways** weasel **weighs** Wellesley whimsy Windsor Winslow **wisdom** **wise** Withers Wolsey Wordsworth Xerxes Youngstown zounds;   (Both /s/ & /z/ depending on use in sentence: abuse, close, house reserve resort resound reside use.) Exceptions: /zh/ Asia Asian casual closure Frisian **measure** Persia pleasure treasure usual unusual; See: **-sion**[2] /zhən/, Ap. i-38 and **-sure**, Ap. iv-44.

---

sc[1] /s/ (When followed by *e, i* or *y*.) scenario **scene** scenery scenic **scent** scepter sciatic **science** scintillating scion Scipio scission **scissors** Scylla Scythia **scythe**

---

sc[2] /sk/ scab scads scaffold **scald** **scale** scallop **scalp** scalpel **scamp** scamper scan scandal Scandinavia **scant** scapegoat **scar** scarab Scarborough **scarce** **scare** **scarf** **scarlet** scat scathing **scatter** scavenger sclerosis scoff **scold** sconce scoop scoot **scooter** scope scorch score scorn Scorpio scorpion Scot scotch Scotch Scott **scoundrel** **scour** scourge scout scowl scrabble **scratch** scram scramble Scranton **scrap** scrape scratch scrawl **scream** screech **screen** screw scribble scribe scrim scrip **script** scrod **scroll** Scrooge scrotum **scrounge** **scrub** scruple scrupulous **scuffle** **sculptor** sculpture **scum** scumble scurrilous scurry scurvy scuttle

---

sch[1] /sk/: **schedule** schema Schenectady **scheme** scherzo schipperke schism schizophrenia Schofield **scholar** **scholastic** **school** schooner

---

sch[2] /sh/: (German & Yiddish) Schacht Scharnhorst Schaumburg Scheherezade **Schelling** Schick Schiller schilling Schlegel Schleiermacher schlemiel Schleswig-Holstein Schliemann schmaltz schmelze Schmidt schmo schmoose Schnabel schnapper schnapps schnauzer Schnitzler schnorrer schnozzle schottische Schrecklichkeit **Schubert** **Schumann** Schumann-Heink Schurz Schuschnigg schuss Schutzstaffel **schwa** Schwab Schwarzwald **Schweitzer**

-sci- /sh/: conscience conscious consciousness;   /shē/ conscientious

---

Schwa

(The schwa is the shortest and most common of vowel sounds, sounding like a short *u,* /ŭ/, and marked by ə in most dictionaries. A vowel is usually pronounced this way in unaccented syllables, often in prefixes or suffixes. It is also found in many very common words. Only a sampling of words containing the schwa sound can be given here since it is pervasive in the English language. For convenience, and here only, the schwa sound will be marked with a dot above the affected vowel.) about above abyss acclaim adapt affect affirm ago aggression agree akin alarm alas alert alight align alike alive allegro alliance allotment alone along aloof aloud amaze announce ancient apart appoint around arouse arrive ascend assert attack audible avenge benevolence brother cafeteria canvas changeable civil cogent collapse come comma company complexion contract correct custom Dallas dietitian dictation distant done does dove effervescence emergency escape essential even excitabilaty experience fearsome fictitious Finland focus formative from general glove gullible habitual historical hydrogen inertia initial instrument integration Jackson judicial kennel laudatory legacy levity librarian local lotion love lowest Mexican mindful monk Montana month mother musician Nebraska nebula nirvanna none notably nothing obedient object occasion o'clock of offend once /wəns/ one /wən/ opponent optimum other oven pagoda parted pilot plowman pollutant Princeton pupil quicken quotient radium rhinoceros scallop seven shove shovel silence smother some son substance suspicion system tension tomato ton union was what, *etc.* **Note: An *e* in an unaccented prefix is often /ĭ/ rather than a schwa:** because before decline deduce effect eject ellipse embody employ enjoy enlarge erase event exam extend;
<u>See</u>: **be-,** Ap. iii-2; **de-,** Ap. iii-9; **ex-,** Ap. iii-11; **en-,** Ap. iii-26.

---

scr- /skr/ (Consonant cluster) ascribe prescribe prescript proscribe scrabble scraggy scram scramble scrap scrape scratch scrawl scream screech screen screw scribble scribe scrim scrimmage scrimp scrip script Scripture scroll Scrooge scrotum scrounge scrub scruff scrumptious scruple scrutiny subscribe subscript transcribe unscrew

---

sh /sh/ ash blush brash brush burnish cash clash crush dash dish English fish flash flesh flush gash hash harsh hush mash marsh marshal mesh mush Oshkosh plush publish rash rubbish rush sash selfish shack shad shaddock shade shaft shag shake shalt sham shame shamrock shank shan't shanty shape share shark sharp shatter shave she shelf shell shellac shelve sherbet sherry shift shim shimmer shin shindig shine ship shirt shock shod shop shore shorn short shot shuck shudder shut shutter shrank shrapnel shred shrift shrill shrimp shrine shrink shrub shrug shrunk shudder shun shunt shush shut shy slash slosh slush smash splash squash swish trash tush vanquish varnish wash Welsh worship; <u>See</u>: **-ish,** Ap. iv-10 and **-ship,** Ap. iv-13.

Silent-E Pairs

( ) = c and g become soft with added e.

add ade ag age Al ale at ate Bab babe back bake bad bade ban bane bar bare
bass base bast baste bat bate bed Bede Bick bike (bice) bid bide bill bile
bin bine bit bite byte black Blake block bloke bod bode brack brake (brace)
breath breathe cad cade cam came can cane cap cape car care Cass case
chaff chafe Chang (change) chap chape chin chine chock choke cloth clothe
cock coke cod code con cone cop cope cot cote crack crake crud crude
cub cube cur cure cut cute dam dame Dan Dane demur demure Dick dike (dice)
dim dime din dine dyne diplomat diplomate dog (doge) doll dole Dom dome
dot dote duck duke dud dude dun dune Eck eke envelop envelope fad fade
fan fane far fare fat fate fill file fin fine fir fire flack flake flam flame fuss fuse
gal gale gam game gap gape gat gate German germane gib gibe glad glade
glob globe grad grade grid gride grim grime grip gripe had hade hack hake
Hal hale ham hame hast haste hat hate her here hick hike hid hide Hyde
hip hype hop hope hug (huge) hum Hume human humane ick Ike (ice)
Jack Jake jams James Jan Jane jib jibe jock joke Judd Jude jut jute kit kite
lack lake (lace) lad lade lamb lam lame lat late lath lathe lick like (lice)
limb lime lĭve līve lĭves līves lob lobe log (loge) Lon lone lop lope luck Luke
lung (lunge) Lynn line Mac Mack make (mace) mad made mal- male man mane
mar mare mat mate met mete mill mile Mick Mike (mice) Mim mime Min mine
miss mise mitt mite mod mode moll mole mop mope mull mule muss muse
mutt mute nab nabe Nam name nap nape nick Nick (nice) nit nite nod node
not note odd ode pack (pace) pal pale pan pane par pare past paste pat pate
pet Pete pick pike pill pile pin pine pip pipe plan plane plat plate pleb plebe
plum plume pock poke pop Pope prick (price) prim prime quack quake
quit quite rag (rage) rack rake (race) rang (range) rap rape rat rate razz raze
red rede regal regale Rick (rice) rid ride rill rile rim rime rip ripe rob robe
rod rode Ross rose rot rote rub rube rudd rude run rune Russ ruse
Sabin Sabine sack sake sag (sage) Sal sale Sam same sat sate scar scare
scrap scrape sever severe shack shake shad shade shall shale sham shame
shin shine shiv shive Sid side sin sine sir sire sit site slack slake slat slate
Slav slave slick (slice) slid slide slim slime slop slope snack snake snip snipe
sock soke spat spate spill spile spin spine spit spite Spock spoke stack stake
stag (stage) stall stale star stare still stile style stock stoke strip stripe
swag (swage) tack take tam tame tap tape tar tare tat Tate than thane
them theme thin thine tick tyke till tile Tim time tin tine Tyne ting (tinge)
tip type Tom tome ton tone top tope tot tote track (trace)
trick trike (trice) trip tripe trod trode truck (truce) tub tube tun tune
twin twine unit unite urban urbane us use Val vale van vane vas vase
Vick (vice) vill vile wack wake wag (wage) wad wade wan wane whin whine
whit white will wile win wine with withe wok woke war /wor/ ware writ write

Silent-E   (Unpaired Examples)

abide Abilene ablaze abode absolute Academe accuse **ace** ache acute alive
allude **alone** Alpine Alsace amaze Ambrose amuse anecdote anode antecede
antelope **ape** arise arrive ascribe aside assume astride athlete atone attire
awake aware awoke bale became behave beside beware blade blame
blaspheme blaze blithe **bone brace brake brave** braze **bribe bride brine** Brisbane
brocade Bruce brume **brute cage cake** capote **cave** centrifuge **change chase**
chaste chide chime chive **chose** chute chromosome chyme Clare clime cline
close clove Clyde cole complete concave concede condone conduce confuse
connote console conspire consume contravene contribute contrite contrive
contuse convene convoke cosine costume cove crane crate crave craze
cremate Crete **crime** crone cyclone **dale Dale** Danube **dare date daze** debate
decide declare decline decode decompose deduce defame defile define delete
delude deluge demote denote denude deprave derive describe desire despise
despite device devise devote diatribe diffuse dilate dire discrete disgrace
dispose dispute **dive** divide divine dole **dope dose doze** drake **drape drive**
drome **drone drove** Druse **dupe** dyne effete electrocute elope elude embrace
emote encage encase enclave enclose encode engage enquire enrage enshrine
enslave ensnare enterprise enthuse entice entire Eocene erase erode escapade
escape Essene estate esthete evade eve **Eve** evoke excite exclave excrete
excuse execute **exhale** exhume exile expire explode expose extreme **face fake**
fame fanfare **faze** female **fife five** flare fluke flume **flute** franchise fume
gave gaze gene Gene glare **glide** gnome gore **grace Grace** grange **grape grate**
grave graze grope grove guide guile guise hare haze Hellene hire **hive hole**
home hone **hose** imbibe impale impede implode implore impose impute incite
incline include indispose induce inflate infuse inhale inhume inmate innate
insane inscribe **inside** insole institute intercede interlope interlude intrude
invade invite invoke involute irate jade jive Jove June knave **knife lane** lave
laze legume **life** lithe lode lute lyre mange **maze mime** mire morpheme
mote naked nave nide **nine** Nome **nope nose nude** oblige ope ozone **page**
parole partake **pave phase phone** phoneme **phrase place** pole Pole polite pone
pore **pose** prate precede prescribe **pride prize** profane profile promote **prone**
propane propose proscribe **prose** prosecute proselyte prostate prostyle protyle
provide provoke prude prune puce pule **quote** rare **rave** rebuke recede recite
refuse refute remote replete repute requite resale reside resole resume
retrocede revive revoke rewrite Rhine Rhodes rhyme **rise** rive **role Rome** rope
rove rule safe sane **save scale** scape scathe **scene scheme** scone **scope score**
secede seclude secrete semaphore Seminole severe **shape** share **shave** shire
shone shore shrine shrive sine size smile smote snare snide snore sole sore
space spade spare sphere **spice spike** spire **splice** spline spore sprite **spruce**
spume square squire stampede stave **stone stove** strafe **stride strife strike**
strive strobe **strode stroke** strove stupe style sublime subscribe subsume

surprise **Swede** swine swipe syne tadpole **tale** Tamerlane **these those** Thrace
throne thyme **tide** tirade tore **trade** transcribe transpose trapeze **tribe** trice
trine trireme **trite** tritone triune trombone trope trove update upgrade
upstage velocipede velure **vile** vole volume **vote** wale **waste wave whale while**
whole wide wife wipe wise wove writhe wrote Yale yoke Yule zone
zyme; **Also: -ate & -ize**; <u>Exceptions</u>: above come done give gone have once one prove

Silent Letters

<u>Silent b</u>: **debt doubt** lambda subpoena subtle
<u>Silent c</u>: arctic Connecticut indict **muscle** Tucson victual yacht
<u>Silent d</u>: adjacent adjective adjoin adjourn adjudge adjudicate adjunct adjure
adjust adjutant hadj Gounod **handsome** Rembrandt Reinhardt **Wednesday**
<u>Silent e</u>: omelet
<u>Silent g</u>: apothegm benign bologna Bologna campaign cognac cologne Cologne
diaphragm foreign imbroglio lorgnette malign Pagliacci paradigm passacaglia
phlegm poignant signor /sēn-yor/ vignette
<u>Silent h</u>: ankh dinghy Durham **exhaust** exhume Gandhi graham Graham heir **herb**
hombre **honest honor hour John** Johnson Lockhart sahib shepherd vehement vehicle
<u>Silent l</u>: almond alms balk balm becalm behalf **calf** calk **calm** calve caulk
chalk **could** Falkland **Falkner folk half** halve halves haulm holm Holmes
lambkin Lincoln Norfolk Norwalk palm Polk psalm psalmody qualm Salk
salmon salve **should** sol solder stalk **talk walk would yolk**
<u>Silent m</u>: mnemonic mnemonics Mnemosyne
<u>Silent p</u>: Campbell corps coup hasenpfeffer pneuma pneumatic pneumectomy
pneumococcus pneumonectomy pneumothorax **pneumonia** Pnom-Penh Pnyx **psalm**
Psalms Psalter psaltery **pseudo** pseudonym pshew! **psyche** Psyche **psychedelic**
psychiatry psychic psychoanalysis psychoanalyst psychoanalyze psychodrama
psychological psychologist **psychology** psychometry psychoneurosis **psychopath**
psychopathology **psychosis** psychosomatic psychotherapy **psychotic** psychrometer
pteridology pterodactyl Ptolemy ptomaine ptosis ptyalism raspberry **receipt**
<u>Silent qu</u>: lacquer   *<u>Silent r</u>:* sarsaparilla
<u>Silent s</u>: **aisle** apropos Arkansas bas-relief Carlisle corps debris DesCartes
islet Illinois Iroquois **island** isle Mardi gras pas rendezvous viscount
<u>Silent t</u>: argot ballet **cents** chasten christcross christen Christmas **debut depot**
ducts escargot **facts fasten** glisten gormet hasten **listen moisten** mortgage
mot /mō/ Nietzsche **often** pacts parfait picot Pierrot ragout **rapport** sects
soften tarot tracts *<u>Silent th</u>:* asthma *<u>Silent w</u>:* answer sword
<u>Silent z</u>: Liszt rendezvous

**Also see: -alk, -augh, -ck, -dge, -eigh, -et, gn, gu-[1], -igh, -kn, -mb,
-mn, -ough, -ps-, rh-, -stle, -tch, -wr-** in this Appendix.

Silent Letters Come To Life.

assign assignation
autumn autumnal
ballet balletomane
benign benignant
column columnist
condemn condemnation
crumb crumble

damn damnable damnation
design designation
diaphragm diaphragmatic
dithyramb dithyrambic
gnostic agnostic
hymn hymnal
impugn impugnation

limb limber
malign malignant
oppugn oppugnant
phlegm phlegmatic
resign resignation
salmon salmonoid salmonella
sign signal signature

-sion[1] /shən/ admission commission compassion compulsion confession convulsion declension depression dimension discussion expansion expression expulsion extension fission impression intermission mansion mission omission passion pension permission percussion possession profession progression regression repression repulsion revulsion session submission succession suppression suspension tension torsion transmission; (More in Ap. iv-42.)

-sion[2] /zhən/ collision conclusion confusion conversion decision delusion diversion division erosion evasion exclusion excursion explosion fusion illusion immersion inclusion incursion intrusion invasion inversion occasion persuasion precision provision reversion revision seclusion submersion supervision television transfusion version vision; (More in Ap. iv-42.)

spl- /spl/ (Consonant cluster.) splash splat splatter splay spleen splendid splendor splice splint splinter split splotch splurge splutter

spr- /spr/ (Consonant cluster.) sprain sprang sprat sprawl spray spread spree sprig sprightly spring sprinkle sprint sprite sprocket sprout spruce sprung spry

-stle /səl/ apostle bristle bustle castle epistle gristle hustle jostle mistletoe nestle pestle rustle thistle trestle whistle wrestle; Exceptions: hassle tousle tussle

str- /str/ (Consonant cluster.) abstract constrain maelstrom minstrel monstrous obstruct restrain restraint straddle Stradivarius strafe straggle straight strain strait strand strange stranger strangle strangulate strap strapping Strasbourg stratagem strategic strategy Stratford stratify stratosphere stratum Strauss Stravinsky straw strawberry stray streak stream streamer street strength strenuous streptococcus streptomycin stress stretch stretcher stretto strew striate stricken strict stricture stride strident strife strike striker string stringendo stringent stringer strip stripe stripper strive strobe stroboscope strode stroke stroll stroller Stromboli strong strontium strop stroud strove struck structural structure struggle strum strumpet strung strut strychnine unstrap unstring unstrung

-tch /ch/ batch bewitch bitch botch blotch Butch butcher catch clutch crotch crutch ditch Dutch escutcheon etch fetch Fitchburg fletch Fletcher glitch hatch hatchet hitch hutch Hutchins Hutchinson itch ketch ketchup kitchen latch match Mitchell Natchez notch patch pitch pitcher ratchet retch Saskatchewan satchel Satchmo Scotch scratch sketch snatch snitch splotch stitch stretch stretcher swatch switch thatch twitch vetch watch witch wretch; **Note: with another consonant after the short vowel, "t" is not needed:** belch bench birch blanch blench branch brunch bunch church cinch clench clinch conch crunch drench filch finch flinch French gulch haunch hunch larch launch lunch lurch lynch march March mulch munch parch paunch perch pinch porch punch quench ranch scorch search smirch starch staunch stench torch trench wench winch wrench; **Nor is "t" needed after a vowel pair:** beach beech bleach breach breech broach coach couch crouch grouch leach leech mooch pooch pouch preach reach roach slouch speech teach touch vouch

th[1] /th/ (Unvoiced.) aftermath anthem anthrax Arthur athlete bath beneath birth both Carthage death depth earth enthusiasm ethnic fifth filthy fourth Goth health hundredth Kathryn Kenneth lath length mammoth math menthol mirth month moth mouth myth north oath panther path Sabbath sixth Smith strength tenth thank theft theme thermal thermos thick thin thing think third thirst thirty thong Thor thorn thrash thresh thrice thrift thrill thrive throb throne throng thrush thrust thud thug thump thunder thwart troth truth width with worth

th[2] /th/ (Voiced.) another bathe blithe breathe brethren brother clothe clothier clothing dither either farther farthest farthing father fathom feather further furthermore furthest gather heathen heather lathe lithe northern rather scathe scythe seethe sheathe slither smoothie smother soothing swarthy swathe teethe tether than that the thee their them then thence there these they thine this thither those thou though thus thy tithe tithing weather whether whither wither Withers worthy wreathe wuthering; **See:** **-the** in Ap. iv-14.

th[3] /t/ discothèque /dis-kə-tek/ Esther Goethe Kathmandu *(Capital of Nepal.)* Thai Thailand Thames /tĕmz/ Theresa Thomas Thomism Thompson Thomson Thor /tor/ or /thor/ Thun thyme

-tion[1] /shən/ [Notes on -a-tion, -e-tion, -i-tion, -o-tion, -u-tion follow.] action caption caution correction corruption deception deduction defection deflection dejection deletion depletion description desertion destruction detection detention detraction diction digestion direction disruption distinction distortion distraction ejection election exception exertion exhaustion extinction extraction faction fiction fraction friction function gumption induction infection inflection infliction infraction injection injunction inscription insertion inspection instruction invention junction mention objection obstruction option perception perfection portion prediction prescription presumption prevention production projection proportion

protection   reaction   reception   reduction   reflection   rejection   restriction
resumption   retention   retraction   section   selection   subjection   subscription
subtraction   suction   traction   transaction   transcription

---

1. *a* is always long in **-a-tion** /ā-shən/: carnation citation combination decoration donation
   formation location nation notation operation relation rotation station vacation
2. *e* is usually long in **-e-tion** /ē-shən/: completion deletion depletion excretion secretion
   However, *e* is short in discretion   indiscretion.
3. *i* is always short in **-i-tion** /ĭ-shən/: addition ambition audition condition definition
   edition ignition nutrition partition petition position tradition transition tuition
4. *o* is always long in **-o-tion** /ō-shən/: devotion emotion lotion motion notion potion
5. *u* is always long in **-u-tion** /ōō-shən/ or /yōō-shən/: constitution contribution diminution
   distribution evolution institution pollution resolution revolution solution

---

For a more extensive example listing see **-tion** (**-ation**) (**-etion**) (**-ition**) (**-otion**) (**-ution**),
Ap. iv 44-47 and **-faction, -fication**, Ap. iv-31.

-tion² /chən/ (following *s*)   combustion question suggestion;   <u>See</u>: -tion², Ap. iv-47.

-tu-   /chōō/ accentuate **actual** actually actuate anfractuous botulism capitulate
congratulate contemptuous effectual effectuate estuary eventually eventuate
fatuous **fluctuate fortune** fortunate fructuous **habitual** habituate impetuous
incestuous **infatuate** intellectual mortuary **mutual natural** obituary perpetual
perpetuate petulant Portugal postulate presumptuous punctual punctuate
punctuation **ritual** sanctuary saturate septuagenarian Septuagint situate **situation**
spatula spiritual spirituous statuary **statue** statute statutory sumptuous
tarantula tempestuous textuary tortuous tumultuous unctuous **virtue** virtually
virtuosity virtuous voluptuous;   <u>Exceptions</u>: /chə/ century   fortunate   Portugal
rapturous;   /tōō/   fortuitous   gratuitous   gratuity   multitudinous   perpetuity
pituitary;   /chŏŏ/ botulism fistula flatulence gratulant maturate pustulate tarantula

---

-ture   /cher/   adventure   agriculture   architecture   capture   creature culture
curvature   denture   departure   expenditure   feature   fixture   fracture   furniture   future
gesture   juncture   lecture   legislature   literature   manufacture   mixture   moisture   nature
nurture   overture   pasture   picture   posture   puncture   rapture   rupture   scripture
sculpture   signature   stature   structure   suture   temperature   texture   tincture   torture
venture   vulture;   <u>But</u>: mature /mə-tyŏŏr/;   (More in Ap. iv-49.)

---

ue¹   /yōō/   ague   **argue**   barbecue   **continue   cue**   detinue   discontinue   Fuehrer
(Führer)   **hue** imbue   Montague   recue   **rescue**   revue   queue /kyōō/   **value** venue

---

ue²   /ōō/   accrue   avenue   **blue clue   construe**   due   endue   ensue   flue   fondue glue
imbrue   issue /ĭsh-ōō/   Purdue   **pursue**   residue   retinue   revalue   revenue   **rue** slue
sprue   statue /stăch-ōō/   **subdue   sue   Sue** tissue /tĭsh-ōō/   **Tuesday   true** undue
untrue   vendue   virtue /ver-chōō/;   <u>Exceptions</u>:   desuetude /des-wə-tōōd/
marguerite /mar-gə-rēt/   Puerto Rico /pwer-tō rē-kō/   suede /swād/   Brueghel /brŏ-gəl/

ui /o͞o/ bruise bruit cruise cruiser fruit juice nuisance pursuit recruit sluice suit suitor;   Exceptions: /ē/ beguine ennui /än-wē/ Guiana, suite /swēt/; /ī/ beguile disguise guide;   /ĭ/ biscuit, build;   /ū/ puisne /pyo͞o-nē/

umlaut /o͝om-lowt/ (ä , ö, ü)

(An umlaut is used to modifiy vowel sounds in **German** words.)
flügelhorn /flo͞o-gəl-horn/   Fräulein /froi-līn/   Führer /fyo͝or-er/   ländler /lent-ler/
langläufer /lahng-loi-fer/;   For ö round the lips for ō and say ā: Möbius strip /mö-bē-o͝os/
In the next three words for ü round the lips for o͞o and say ē: gemütlichkeit Müller
Übermensch

-ung /ung/ clung dung flung hung lung rung slung sprung stung sung swung wrung

-unk /ungk/ bunk chunk debunk drunk dunk flunk funk hunk junk plunk
Podunk punk shrunk skunk slunk spunk stunk sunk trunk

Unvoiced and Voiced Consonants

UNVOICED	VOICED	
p	b	bilabial (both lips)
	m	"
wh	w	"
f	v	labio-dental (lower lip to upper teeth)
th	th	inter-dental (between the teeth)
t	d	alveolar (where teeth and roof of mouth meet)
	n, l, r	"
s	z	"
sh	zh	palatal (roof of mouth--hard palate)
ch	j	"
	y	"
k	g	velar (roof of mouth--back--soft palate)
	ng	"
h		glottal (back of throat)

Note: 1. p, b, t, d, k, & g are further characterized as *stopped* consonants because the air flow is actually interrupted or stopped as they are articulated.

2. f, v, th, th, s, z, sh, & zh are also termed *fricative* because their sound is due to the friction the air produces as it moves through various narrowed mouth passages.

3. ch & j are termed *affricative* (against friction) because a *t* tongue position temporarily blocks the *ch* (unvoiced) utterance and a similar *d* tongue position temporarily blocks the *j* (voiced) utterance.   This no doubt accounts for the **-tch** /ch/ & **-dge** /j/ spellings.

4. m, n, & -ng are *nasal* (produced through the nose); this can be proven by holding the nose and attempting to produce these sounds.

5. For their own aesthetic reasons, the ancients termed **l** & **r** *liquids* and **y** & **w** *glides*.

6. All vowels sounds are voiced and can be prolonged when sung.

ur /er/ absurd Arthur blur blurb blurt bur burly burden burg burlap burl burlesque Burlington Burma **burn burnt burp** burr burro burrow burse **burst** Burton **church** churl **churn** churr concur **cur curb** curd **curl** currant current curry currier **curse** cursive **curt Curtis** curtsy **curve** disburse disturb flurry **fur furrier furl** furrow furry furtive gurgle Hapsburg Homburg **hurdle hurl** hurrah **hurry hurt** incur incursion kookaburra Kurd **lurch lurk murder murk** murmur Murphy Murray nocturne **nurse** nurture occur perturb purl purge **purple** purpose purr **purse** purser scurry **slur slurp spur spurn spurt sturdy sulfur surf surge** surmise **surplus** surprise surreal surrey **survive** turban turbid **turf Turk** turkey Turkey **turn** turnip turret urban **urge urn** Ursa ursine Ursula usurer usurp usury **yogurt yurt;**   <u>See</u>: **-burg** in Ap. iv-4.

-ve /v/ An English word almost never ends in -v, but in -ve. This makes it impossible on first sight of a **-ve** word to know if a single vowel is long or short. This can be learned only through experience; fortunately many of them are common words. **The Silent E Rule** applies only where there is an underlined <u>e</u>. A few have a long vowel sound because of a <u>vowel pair</u>. abov<u>e</u> absolve abusive ach<u>ie</u>ve active alcov<u>e</u> aliv<u>e</u> approve arriv<u>e</u> behav<u>e</u> behoove bel<u>ie</u>ve ber<u>ea</u>ve brav<u>e</u> breve captive carve cav<u>e</u> cl<u>ea</u>ve clov<u>e</u> conc<u>ei</u>ve conclav<u>e</u> conniv<u>e</u> conserve contriv<u>e</u> cov<u>e</u> crav<u>e</u> cursive curve dative Dav<u>e</u> dec<u>ei</u>ve delve deprav<u>e</u> depriv<u>e</u> deriv<u>e</u> deserve dissolve div<u>e</u> dov<u>e</u> driv<u>e</u> drov<u>e</u> elusive emotive enclav<u>e</u> engrav<u>e</u> erosive evasive evolve festive fiv<u>e</u> forgive gav<u>e</u> give glove grav<u>e</u> gr<u>ie</u>ve gr<u>oo</u>ve grov<u>e</u> halve have h<u>ea</u>ve hiv<u>e</u> improve involve knav<u>e</u> l<u>ea</u>ve live liv<u>e</u> love massive missive motive move naive native nav<u>e</u> negative nerve observe octave olive passive pav<u>e</u> p<u>ee</u>ve pensive perc<u>ei</u>ve preserve prove rav<u>e</u> rec<u>ei</u>ve rel<u>ie</u>ve reliv<u>e</u> remove repr<u>ie</u>ve reserve resolve retr<u>ie</u>ve reviv<u>e</u> revolve rov<u>e</u> salve sav<u>e</u> serve shav<u>e</u> shelve shov<u>e</u> sieve slav<u>e</u> sl<u>ee</u>ve solve starve Stev<u>e</u> stov<u>e</u> striv<u>e</u> suave surviv<u>e</u> swerve th<u>ie</u>ve thriv<u>e</u> twelve valve verve votive w<u>ai</u>ve wav<u>e</u> w<u>ea</u>ve wov<u>e</u>   **Note: A few words do end in -v:** Pavlov slav; <u>**v**</u> **is seldom doubled:** civvies divvy flivver improvvisatore savvy skivvy skivvies

---

wa /wah/ /wä/ schwa swab swamp swan swap swat wacky wad waff waft wallaby Walla Wala wallet wallop wallow walrus **wan wand wander want** wanton **wash wasp watch** Watson Watt Watteau wigwam;   <u>Exceptions</u>: /waw/ /wô/ water **walk wall** walrus walnut **waltz;**   /wă/ wag wagon wacky wangle.

---

war /wor/ dwarf **swarm** swarthy **thwart war** warble warbler **ward Ward** warden warfare **warm warmth warn** warp warrant warranty warren Warren warrior Warsaw **wart** Warwick;   <u>Exceptions</u>: toward /tord/, Edward /ĕd-werd/

---

wh /wh/ whack whale wham whammy whang wharf wharves **what** whatever whatnot whatsoever **wheat** Wheaton wheedle **wheel** wheeler Wheeler **wheeze** whelm whelp **when whence where** whereas whereby wherefore wherein wheresoever wherever wherewithal wherry whet whether whetstone whew whey **which** whichever **whiff** whiffet whiffle Whig **while** whilst **whim** whimper

whimsical whimsy whin **whine** whinny **whip** whippet whipping Whipple whippoorwill whipstitch whir **whirl** whirligig whirlpool whirlwind whirlybird whish whisk whiskbroom whiskers whiskey **whisper** whist whistle Whistler whit **white** Whitman Whitney Whitsun Whittier whittle **whiz** whoa whoop whoopee whooper whop whopping whorl whort **why**;
Exceptions: /h/ who whoever whole whom whose whore

===

wor /wer/ Ellsworth word wording Wordsworth work workable workaday workbook workday worker working workload workman workmanship workshop world worldly worldwide worm wormhole worry worse worsen worship worst wort worth worthless worthwhile worthy; Exceptions: sword /sord/ worn /worn/ worsted /wŏŏs-tid/.

Word Pairs (Long Vowel, Short Vowel)

baring barring   bated batted   biding bidding   biter bitter   boner Bonner   bony bonny caning canning   caper capper   chafer chaffer   coble cobble   coder codder coma comma   coping copping   cuter cutter   Daly dally   dimed dimmed   dimer dimmer dined dinned   diner dinner   doting dotting   doty dotty   fated fatted   fiber fibber filer filler   filing filling   fogy foggy   gable gabble   gaping gapping   griping gripping hater hatter   hoper hopper   hoping hopping   loping lopping   mating matting miler miller   moping mopping   paling palling   pilar pillar   pining pinning   planer planner plater platter   primer primmer   raper rapper   raping rapping   rater ratter   rating ratting riding ridding   riper ripper   rober robber   robing robbing   scared scarred scaring scarring   scraper scrapper   scraping scrapping   shaming shamming slating slatting   shiny shinny   sloping slopping   sniper snipper   sparing sparring spiting spitting   stager stagger   staring starring   striped stripped   striper stripper striping stripping   super supper   taping tapping   tiler tiller   tiny tinny   title tittle tody toddy   toper topper   wading wadding   wager wagger   winer winner

---

Words Ending in *U.*

ainu Anu aralu Attu Baku Bangweulu Bantu **beau** Bornu **bureau** Cebu cheju cordon bleu Corfu Cornu coypu Danu Diu ecru feu fichu genu Gifu gnu **guru** habu **Hindu Honolulu impromptu** Isuzu Jehu jujitsu juju Kathmandu **lieu** Malibu Manchu **menu** Nehru Oahu ormolu parvenu perdu **Peru plateau** Ryukyu Islands Snafu *(Situation normal; all fouled up.)* Sou Subaru **Thou** Timbuktu **tofu** Urdu Vishnu Yalu **you** zebu Zulu;   See: -eau, Ap. i-19.

===

wr /r/ wrack wraith wrangle wrangler wrap wrapper wrapping wrap-up wrath wrathful wreak wreath wreathe wreck wrecker wren wrench wrest wrestle wrestler wretch wretched wriggle wright Wright wring wrinkle wrist writ write writer writhe writing written wrong wrongful wrote wrought wrung   wry

X-1 /k-s/ (Within and at end of word.) boxer fixture maxim mix oxen tax text wax, *etc.*

X-2 /z/ (At beginning of word.) Xanthippe xanthoma Xavier xebec Xenocrates xenogenesis xenolith xenomorphic xenon Xenophanes xenophobe xenophobia Xenophon xeric xeroderma xerography xerophthalmia xerosis **Xerox** Xerxes **xi** (Greek letter ξ Ξ) xiphoid Xuthus xylem xylograph xyloid xylophagous **xylophone** xylotomy xyst xyster

y-1 /y/ (As a consonant at the beginning of word.) yacht /yaht/ **yes** yah yahoo Yahweh **yak** **Yale** Yalta Yalu **yam** Yamamoto Yamashita **yammer** yang ("yin & yang") Yang Yangtze **yank** **Yank** Yankee **yap** Yaqui **yard** Yarmouth yarmulke /yah-məl-kə/ **yarn** yashmak yaw yawl **yawn** yawp yaws yay yea yeah yean **year** **yearn** **yeast** Yeats yegg **yell** **yellow** yelp Yemen yen yeoman **yes** yeshiva **yesterday** **yet** yew Yiddish **yield** yin yip yodel yoga yogi yogurt yoicks! yoke Yokohama Yokosuka **yolk** Yom Kippur **yon yond yonder** Yonkers yoo-hoo yore **York** Yorkshire Yorktown Yoruba Yosemite Yoshihito **you young Young youngster** Youngstown younker **your yours yourself youth youthful yowl** yo-yo yuan yucca Yuga Yugoslavia **yuk** Yukon Yule Yuma Yuman yummy Yunnan yurt

-y2 /ī/ (As a vowel at the end of one syllable words.) by dry fly fry guy my ply pry shy sky sly spry spy sty thy try why wry   (At end of two syllable word with accent on last syllable.) ally apply comply decry deny espy imply reply supply (With -fy suffix, **Latin,** "to make.") dignify glorify specify, *etc.* <u>See</u>: **-fy**, Ap. iv-32.

-y3 /ē/ (As a vowel at the end of multi-syllable verbs.) bandy bury carry curry embody disembody marry shilly- shally study tarry vary worry

-y3 /ē/ (As a vowel at the end of multi-syllable nouns.) ability amnesty anchovy apology **army** artery assembly **baby** balcony barony **beauty** belfry **belly** bevy biography biology blackberry **body** bogy booby bounty **buggy bully** bunny butchery **caddy candy** cannery **cavity** celery **city** clergy company **copy county** country cranny dairy daisy dally **dandy** deary deputy derby **destiny** discovery ditty doggy dormitory dowry drudgery **dummy duty** eighty elderberry enemy **energy entry envy** factory faculty fairy **family** fanny felony ferry **fifty** flurry folly **forty** frenzy gallery **gravy** gully harmony hickory **history honesty** industry infantry **injury** ivory ivy **jelly lady liberty** library lily lobby lottery majesty **mastery** melody **memory modesty mummy** mutiny **mystery navy ninety** organdy **penny** philosophy **pity** pixy **plenty** pony **poppy** potty **puppy putty rally** remedy rhapsody **rowdy ruby** rugby **safety** sally scurvy **seventy sixty** skulduggery strategy subsidy symphony **taffy tally** testimony therapy **thirty** tragedy treaty

trophy **twenty unity** worry; Andy Anthony Antony Ashley Audrey Barney Barry Becky Betsy Betty Beverly Billy Bobby Bonny Charity Chauncey Cicely Cindy Charity Daisy Davy Dolly Dorothy Dotty Eddy Emily Emmy Fanny Gary Gregory Harley Harry Henry Hetty Hilary Humphrey Ivy Jeffrey Jenny Jerry Jimmy Johnny Judy Kathy Kitty Letty Libby Lily Lucy Mandy Margery Mary Mercy Molly Nancy Nicky Pansy Patsy Penny Perry Polly Poppy Rodney Ronny Rosemary Ruby Sally Sammy Sandy Shirley Sidney Stanley Tilly Timmy Timothy Toby Tommy Tony Trixy Trudy Wendy Willy; *etc.* Last Names: Daly Kerensky Koussevitzky Murphy Mussorgsky, *etc.* **Place Names:** Albany Bowery Burgundy Calvary Germany Kentucky Saxony Schenectady Tuscany, *etc* Others: Epiphany, Romany, Tory, *etc.*
See: **-y** (Latin), Ap. iv-53 and **-y** (Greek), Ap. iv-60.

-y³ /ē/ (As a vowel at the end of multi-syllable adjectives.) (Remember the 1-1-1-V Rule: bag + y = baggy.) airy angry any arty baggy batty bossy brainy brawny breathy bulky bumpy bushy busy catchy cheery chewy chilly choppy chummy chunky clammy classy cloudy cozy crabby crafty cranky crazy creaky creamy creepy crispy crusty curly dainty dewy dirty dizzy drafty dreamy dressy dusty easy empty every fancy faulty filthy foamy foggy frisky funny fussy fuzzy glassy gloomy goofy grassy greedy grouchy grumpy hairy happy hardy haughty healthy hearty hefty hilly holy husky icy inky itchy jerky jolly jumpy lazy leafy lengthy lofty loony lucky lumpy lusty many marshy mighty milky misty moldy moody muddy murky nasty naughty needy nifty nutty peppy petty pretty puffy rainy risky rocky roomy rusty salty sandy sassy shadowy shaggy showy silly silky silvery sketchy skimpy skinny sleepy sloppy smelly snappy sneaky snippy snoopy snowy soapy sorry soupy speedy spooky sporty spotty spunky squeaky starry steady steamy steely sticky stingy stocky stormy streaky stringy stuffy sturdy sulky sunny swampy swanky tardy thirsty thorny thrifty tidy tiny touchy tricky ugly unlucky wacky watery waxy weedy woody worthy; See: **-y** (Old English), Ap. iv-15.

-y-⁴ /ī/ (As a vowel from Greek letter upsilon, υ Y; long because of *open syllable* or *silent e.*) acolyte analyze asylum cryogenics cyanide **cycle cyclone** Cyclops **cypress** Cyprus **-cyte** cytogenics cytology Dionysus dyad dynamic dynamite dynamo dynasty dyne encyclopedia **enzyme** glycol gynecology **gyrate** gyroscope hyacinth hybrid hydra hydrangea hydrant hydraulic **hydro** hydrogen hygiene hygrometry hymen **hype hyper** hyperactive hyperbole **hyphen** hypochondriac hypodermic hypotenuse hypothesis (Pl.: hypotheses) kylix lyceum lyre lysis myalgia myopia Myron papyrus proselyte prostyle protyle psyche psychiatry psychology pylon **pyre Pyrex** pyrexia pyromaniac **python rhyme style** stylus thyme thymus **thyroid type typhoid typhoon** typhus tyrant Tyre xylem xylophone zygote zyme zymosis

-y-[5] /ĭ/ (As a vowel from Greek letter upsilon, υ Y; follows closed syllable rule.) abysmal abyss acronym Aeschylus agrypnotic analysis analytic anonymous antonym apocalypse apocryphal arrhythmia asphyxia bicycle Babylon Byzantine clamys coccyx **crypt** crystal cygnet **cylinder** cymbal **cynic** Cynthia **cyst** dialysis diptych dithyramb dysentery dysfunction dyslexia dyspepsia dysphagia dysphasia dystrophy ecosystem **Egypt** Elysian Elysium ethyl etymology eucalyptus glyph **gym** gymnasium gymnast gypsum gypsy homonym hymn hypnosis hypocrisy hypocrite hysteria idyl labyrinth **laryngitis** larnyx **lymph lynx lyric mystery mystic myth** myxoma **nymph** Odysseus Odyssey **Olympics** Olympus onyx oxygen pachyderm pachysandra paralysis paronym paroxysm pharynx physical physician **physics** Pnyx polyglot **polygon polygraph polyp** presbyter Presbyterian prophylactic prophylaxis propylaeum propylon pseudonym pterodactyl Pygmalion **pygmy** pyknic Pythagoras pyx pyxie **rhythm** Sisyphus styptic sycamore sycophant syllable syllabus syllogism symbiosis symbol symmetrical symmetry sympathy symphony symposium symptom synagogue synapse synchronize syncopate syndrome synod synonym synopsis syntax synthetic **system** Thermopylae Thucydides triglyph triptych tricycle tympani typical xyst; /ē/ (Before another vowel.): embryo halcyon presbyopia;

Note: Most of the time when a **-y-** is in the middle of a word, the word derives from Greek. However, here are a few examples from other sources: /ī/: Bryan Bryant Bryce **bye** byte Clyde **dye eye** geyser **lye** Lyon myna **rye** Shylock shyster stymie styrofoam **tycoon tyke Tyler** Tyre Tyrol Wyatt Wycliffe Wyeth Wyoming; /ĭ/: Goldwyn Gwyn **lynch** Lynch **Lynn** sylvan Pennsylvania Pyrenees Plymouth **sylph** Tennyson Tyndale **tryst** Wycliffe

---

-yr /er/ martyr myrrh myrtle satyr **zephyr**;   **Exception**: Pyrrhic /pear-ik/

-yr- (+ vowel other than *e*.) /ear/ Cyril lyrics myriad myriapod panegyric pyramid Syria Syrian syringe syrinx *(A bird's song organ.)* syrup tyranny Valkyrie; **Follow Silent E Rule**: lyre /līr/ pyre /pīr/

---

z[1] /z/ (Its usually sound.)   Amazon amaze Aztec bazaar blaze Brazil buzzer cozy crazy daze dazzle dizzy dozen enzyme fez fizzle freeze fuzzy gauze gaze gazebo gizzard glaze graze guzzle haze jacuzzi jazz lazy lizard nozzle ooze ozone pizazz plaza prize puzzle razor size unzip wizard zebra zeal zero zest zip zone zoology

---

z[2] /s/ (Usually German.) blitz chintzy Danzig eczema ersatz Hertz Kreutzer

| Appendix ii | The Cutting Edge (Syllabication) | CONTENTS |

Compound Words . . . . Ap.ii -2

Syllabication Tips . . . . Ap.ii -6

<u>VC</u>-CV . . . . Ap.ii- 8

VC-<u>CV</u> Ap.ii-14

<u>V</u>-V . . . V-<u>V</u> Ap.ii-15

<u>V</u>-CV Ap.ii-16

V-<u>CV</u> . . . . Ap .ii-18

<u>VC</u>-V Ap.ii-20

VC-<u>V</u> . . <u>V</u>-CCV . . V-<u>CCV</u> . . <u>VC</u>-CCV Ap.ii-22

VC-<u>CCV</u> . . . <u>VCC</u>-CV Ap.ii-23

VCC-<u>CV</u> . . . . <u>VCC</u>-CCV . . . VCC-<u>CCV</u> Ap.ii-24

<u>VC</u>-CCCV . . . VC-<u>CCCV</u> . . . <u>VCC</u>-V Ap.ii-24

V-<u>CCCV</u> . . . . <u>VCCC</u>-CV Ap.ii-24

VCC-<u>V</u> . . . . . <u>V</u>-CCCCV Ap.ii-24

Multi-Syllable Compound Words Ap.ii-25

Hyphenated Words Ap.ii-27

"X" Divided Between Syllables Ap.ii-30

Accent Shift Words Ap.ii-31

"Silent E" in Base Word Ap.ii-31

Syllables With No or Equal Accent Ap.ii-31

Let's Do the Big Ones! . . . . Ap. ii-32

Syllable Written without a Vowel but Pronounced with a Vowel Ap. ii-33

Syllable Written with a Vowel which is not Pronounced . . . . Ap. ii-33

Compound words divide easily and are a good introduction to syllabication.

on/set knock/out lines/man lip/stick nut/brown north/east half/way, etc.

a ageless aimless airborne airbrush aircraft aircrew airdrop airfield airflow airless airlift airlike airline airman airplane airport airproof airship airsick airspace airstream airstrip airtight airway anthill archway armband armchair armhole armpit awesome

b backache backbone backdoor backfield backfire background backhand backlog backpack backrest backside backstage backstairs backstop backstroke backtrack backwoods badlands bagpipe ballroom bankbook barbell bareback barefoot barmaid barnstorm barnyard barroom baseball baseboard bathhouse bathrobe bathroom bathtub Batman beachhead beadwork beanbag beanpole beanstalk bearskin bedbug bedrock bedroll beehive beeline beeswax bellboy bellhop bestman bighorn bighouse bigwig billboard birdbath birdcall birdhouse birthday birthmark birthplace birthright birthstone blackball blackbelt blackbird blackboard blackhead blackjack blacklist blackmail blackout blacksmith blacktop blastoff blindfold blockhead blockhouse bloodhound bloodline bloodshed bloodshot bloodstain blowgun blowout blowtorch blowup bluebell bluebird bluegill bluegrass blueprint boardwalk boathouse bobcat bobsled bobtail bobwhite boldface bolthead bombproof bombshell bombsight bondsman bonehead bookcase bookmark bookplate bookrack bookshelf bookstack bookstall bookstand bookstore bookworm bootleg boundless bowleg bowstring boxcar brainstorm brainwash breakdown breakfast breakthrough breakup breastbone breastpin breastplate breathless breezeway brickwork brickyard bridegroom bridesmaid bridgehead briefcase broadcast broadside Broadway broomstick brushoff brushwork buckskin buildup bulldog bullfight bullfrog bullhead bullpen bullring bullwhip bunkhouse burnout bushland Bushman busman byroad byway

c cakewalk calfskin callboard campfire campground camshaft cannot cardboard cardsharp carefree careless careworn carfare carhop carload carport cartwheel caseload casework castiron castoff catbird catboat catcall catchall catchword catfish catlike catnip cattail catwalk causeway caveman charcoal cheapskate checkbook checkmate checkoff checkout checkroom checkup cheekbone cheesecake cheesecloth chessboard chessman childbirth childlike choirboy choirgirl chopsticks churchman churchyard clambake clamshell clansman classmate classroom cleanup clipboard cloakroom clockwise clockwork clothesline clothespin cloudburst clubhouse coalyard coastline cockpit cockroach codfish cogwheel comeback comedown cookbook cookout corkscrew corncake corncob corncrib cornhusk cornfield cornmeal cornstalk cornstarch countdown countless courthouse courtroom courtyard cowbell cowboy cowhand cowhide cowlick crackdown crackpot crackup craftsman crankcase crankshaft crossbar crossbeam crossbow crosscheck crosscut crosseyed crossfire crossroad crossroads crosswalk crossway crosswind crowbar crownwork curbstone cupboard cupcake cutback cutoff cutout cutthroat cutup

d darkroom dashboard daybreak daydream daylight daylights daytime deadbeat deadhead deadline deadlock deadpan deadwood deathbed deathblow deathtrap deckhouse deepfreeze deerskin dewdrop dewfall dimwit dipstick dishcloth dishpan dishrag dockyard doeskin dogcart dogfight doghouse doomsday doorbell doorknob doorman doorpost doorstep doorstop doorway doubtless doughnut dovetail downbeat downcast downfall downgrade downhill downpour downright downspout downstage downstairs downstream downtown draftsman dragnet drainpipe drawback drawbar drawbridge drawstring dreamland driftwood driveway dropout drumbeat drumhead drumstick duckbill duckpin dugout dumbbell dustcloth dustpan dustproof **e** earache eardrum earmuff earphone earplug earring earshot earthborn earthbound earthquake earthworm earthwork earwax eastbound eavesdrop edgewise egghead eggplant eggshell elsewhere endless eyeball eyebolt eyebrow eyecup eyeglass eyehole eyehook eyelash eyelid eyepiece eyesight eyesore eyestrain eyetooth eyewash **f** fairground fairway fallout fanfare fantail farewell farmhouse farmyard fathead feedback feedbag fieldwork filmstrip firearm fireboat firebox firebug firefly firehouse firelight fireman fireplace fireplug fireproof fireside firetrap firewall firewood fireworks fishbowl fishhook fishline fishnet fishpole fivespot flagman flagship flagstone flareup flashback flashboard flashlight flatcar flatfoot flatiron flattop flatwork flaxseed fleabite flintlock floodgate floodlight floorboard flyleaf flyspeck flytrap flyweight flywheel fogbound foghorn folklore folkways foodstuff foolproof football footboard footbridge foothill foothold footlights footnote footpad footpath footprint footrest footstep footstool footwear footwork forthright fourscore foxhole framework freehand freestyle freeway freewill freshman frostbite fruitcake fullback **g** gallstone gangplank gangway gasman gasworks gatehouse gatepost gateway gearbox gearcase gearshift gemstone glassworks globefish glowworm goatskin godchild godson goldbrick goldbug goldfinch goldfish goldsmith gooseneck grandchild grandpa grandma grandson grandstand grapefruit grapevine grassland grassroots gravestone graveyard greenback greenbelt greenhouse greyhound grindstone grownup guardhouse guardrail guardroom guesswork guidebook guideline guidepost guiderope gumdrop gumtree gumwood gunboat gunfire gunman gunshot **h** hacksaw hailstone hailstorm hairbrush haircut hairdo hairline hairpin halfback halftone halfway hallmark hallway hamstring handbag handball handbook handclasp handcuff handgrip handgun handmade handout handrail handsaw handshake handspring handwork hangnail hangout hardhat hardtop hardware hardwood hatbox hatchway hatpin hayfork hayloft hayrack hayride haystack haywire headache headband headboard headdress headfirst headgear headlight headline headlock headlong headphone headrest headroom headset headstone headstrong headway hearsay heartache heartbeat heartbreak heartburn heartfelt heartland heartsick heartstrings heartthrob heartworm heatwave hedgehog hedgehop helmsman hemline hemstitch henceforth hencoop helpless helpmate herdsman herself hideout highbrow highchair highland highlight highroad highway hijack hillside hilltop himself hindmost hindsight hipbone hitchhike hobnob hockshop holdup homeland homeless homemade homesick homespun homestead homestretch homework hoodwink hoofbeat hookup hopscotch hornpipe horseback horsefly horselaugh horseman horseplay horseshoe horsetail horsewhip hotfoot hothead hothouse hourglass houseboat housecoat housedress housefly household housewife housework hubcap

i iceberg iceboat icebox icebound icecap icehouse Iceland iceman inboard inborn inbound inbred inbreed inchworm income indeed indent indoors infield inlay inland inlet inmost input inroad inset inside insight instep intake into intone invoice itself

j jackknife jackpot jailbird jawbone jaywalk jigsaw jockstrap junkman junkyard

k keepsake keyboard keyhole keynote keystone kickback kickoff kidnap kidskin kinfolk kingbird kingfish kingpin kneecap kneehole knockdown knockout knothole

l lacework lambskin lamppost landlocked landlord landmark landscape landslide laptop larkspur latchkey lawman lawsuit layoff layout leadoff leapfrog leeway legwork letdown letup lifeblood lifeboat lifeguard lifelike lifelong lifetime lifework liftoff lighthouse lightweight limelight limestone lineman lipstick livestock lockjaw lockout locksmith lockup logbook logjam logroll longboat longhair longhand lookout loophole lovebird lovesick lowbrow lowdown lowland lukewarm lunchroom

m madhouse madman mailbag mailbox mailman mainland mainmast mainsail mainstay mainstream makeshift manhole manhunt mankind manmade marksman markup matchbook matchbox maybe mealtime meantime meltdown midair midday midland midnight midpoint midships midstream midterm midtown midwatch midway midweek Midwest midwife milestone milkmaid milkman milktoast milkweed millpond millstone millstream millwork minefield mixup molehill moonbeam moonlight moonrise moonstruck mopboard mousetrap mouthpiece mouthwash myself

n namesake nearby neckband necklace neckline necktie neckwear needn't network newborn newsboy newscast newsman newsprint newsreel newsstand nickname nightclub nightfall nightgown nighthawk nightmare nightshirt nightspot nightstand nightstick nighttime nightwear nitwit nohow noonday northbound northeast northwest nosebleed notebook noway nowhere numbskull nursemaid nutshell

o oarlock oarsman oatmeal offbeat offhand offset offshoot offshore offside offspring oilcan oilcloth oneself onrush onset onshore onto ourselves outback outbid outbreak outburst outcast outclass outcome outcry outdate outdo outdoors outfield outfit outgrowth outguess outhouse outland outlast outlaw outlay outline outlive outlook outpost outpour output outrank outreach outride outrun outsell outset outshine outshoot outside outskirts outsmart outweigh outwit outwork

p packman packsack padlock paintbrush pancake parkland parkway passbook passkey passport password patchwork pathway pawnshop payday payload payoff payroll peacetime peanut peephole pegboard penknife pickax piecemeal piecework pigpen pigskin pigtail pillbox pinball pinhole pinkeye pinpoint pinup pinwheel pinworm pipeline pitchfork pitfall plainchant playback playbill playground playhouse playmate playoff playpen plaything playtime playwright plywood pockmark pointblank polecat polestar pondweed poolroom poorhouse popcorn popgun porthole pothole potluck pressroom proofread puffball pullback pullout pushcart pushpin putoff putout

r racecourse racehorse racetrack raceway ragtime ragweed railroad railway rainbow raincoat raindrop rainfall rainproof rainstorm ramrod ranchman ransack rattail rattrap rawhide rearview redbird redbreast redcap redcoat redhead redneck redskin redwing redwood ringside ringworm ripsaw riptide roadbed roadblock roadhouse roadside roadway roadwork rollback roommate rosebud rosebush rosewood roughhouse roughneck roundup rowboat rowlock rubdown rundown runoff runway

S safeguard sagebrush sailboat sailcloth sailfish salesclerk salesgirl salesman salesroom saltworks sandbag sandbar sandblast sandbox sandhog sandman sandstone sandstorm sapwood sawdust sawhorse sawmill scapegoat scarecrow schoolbook schoolboy schoolgirl schoolroom schoolyard scrapbook screenplay screwball seacoast seafood sealskin seaman seaplane seaport searchlight seashell seashore seasick seaway seaweed seesaw sellout sendoff setback setscrew setup shakedown shakeup sharkskin sheepfold sheepskin shellfire shellfish shellproof shinbone shipboard shipload shipmate shipshape shipwreck shipyard shoehorn shoelace shoeshine shoestring shopman shoptalk shopworn shoreline shortbread shortcake shortchange shorthand shorthorn shortstop shotgun shouldn't showboat showcase showdown showman showoff showpiece shutdown shuteye shutoff shutout sickbay sickbed sickroom sideboard sidekick sideline sidestep sideswipe sidetrack sidewalk sideways signboard silkworm sinkhole sketchbook skullcap skylark skylight skyline slapstick slingshot slipknot slipshod slowdown slowpoke slugfest slumlord smallpox smalltime smashup smokehouse smokestack snakebite snakeskin snapshot snowball snowbank snowblow snowbound snowcap snowdrift snowfall snowflake snowman snowplow snowshoes snowslide snowstorm snowsuit soapbox soapstone soapsuds softball software softwood someday somehow someone someplace something sometime sometimes someway somewhat somewhere songbird sorehead soundboard soundproof soupspoon sourdough southbound southeast southwest soybean spacecraft spaceman spaceport spadework spareribs sparkplug spearfish spearhead spearmint speedboat speedup speedway spellbound spendthrift spillway spitball spitfire splashboard spoilsport spokesman spoonbill sportsman sportswear spotlight springboard Springfield springtime spyglass stagecoach stagecraft stagehand staircase stairway stairwell stalemate standby standoff standout standpat standpoint standstill standup starboard starfish stargaze starlight statecraft stateroom stateside statesman steadfast steakhouse steamboat steamship steelworks steelyard stemware stepchild stepson stickball stickpin stickup stillbirth stillborn stinkweed stockboy stockpile stockroom stockyard stonewall stoneware stonework stopgap stoplight stopwatch storehouse storeroom stormbelt stormbound stormproof stovepipe straightarm straightedge straightway strawman streamlined streetcar stretchpants strikebound striptease strongarm strongbox stronghold strongman strongroom suitcase sunbeam sunburn Sunday sundown sunfish sunglass sunlight sunlit sunrise sunroom sunset sunshade sunshine sunspot sunstroke sunup surfboard swampland sweatband sweatbox sweatshop sweepstakes sweetheart swimsuit switchblade switchboard swordfish

t tadpole tagboard tailgate taillight tailspin takedown takeoff tapeworm taproom taproot teacup teahouse teammate teamwork teapot tearoom teardrop teaspoon telltale tenpin textbook themselves thenceforth thereby therefore therein thereof thereon thereto therewith thighbone thindown threadbare threefold throughout throwback thruway thumbnail thumbprint thumbscrew thumbtack tideland tideway tieback tightlipped tightrope tightwad timepiece timeworn tinfoil tinhorn tinsmith tintype tinware tinworks tipoff tiptoe tiptop toadstool today toehold toenail toilworn tollbooth tollgate tollhouse tombstone tomcat toothache toothbrush toothpaste toothpick topcoat topmast topmost topnotch topsail topside topsoil

torchlight tossup touchback touchdown touchup towrope trackman trademark
tramway treadmill treetop trueblue truelove tryout tugboat tunesmith turncoat
turndown turnoff turnout turnpike turnstile twofold typecast typewrite
u upbeat upbraid update updraft upend upgrade upgrowth uphill uphold upkeep
upland uplift upon upraise upright uprise uproar uproot upset upshot upspring
upstage upstart upstate upstream upsurge upsweep uptake uptight uptown upturn
v viewpoint voiceless voiceprint vouchsafe
w waistcoat waistline walkout walkup walkway wardrobe wardroom warehouse
warfare warhead warlord warmup warpath warplane warship wartime washboard
washbowl washcloth washday washout washrag washroom washstand washtub
wasteland watchcase watchdog watchman watchword wavelength waylay wayside
webfoot weekday weekend weeklong wellspring westbound wetback whaleboat
whalebone whatnot wheelchair wheelhouse wheelman wheelwork whereas whereby
wherein whipcord whiplash whirlpool whirlwind whiskbroom whitecap whitefish
whiteout whizbang wholesale widespread wildcat wildfire wildlife wildwood
windbag windbreak windburn windfall windpipe windmill windshield windsock
windstorm wineglass winepress wingback wiretap wisecrack wishbone witchcraft
withdraw withdrawn withhold within without withstand wolfhound woodblock
woodchuck woodcraft woodcut woodhouse woodland woodpile woodscrew
woodshed woodsman woodwinds woodwork wordbook Wordsworth workbench
workbook workbox workday workhorse workload workman workout workroom
worksheet workshop workweek worldwide wormwood worthwhile wristband
y yachtsman yardarm yardbird yardman yardstick yearbook yourself Yuletide

SYLLABICATION TIPS:

1. Syllabication is only concerned with what goes on <u>between</u> vowels. In the word, *prospect,* the division is to be made between the **o** and the **e**. When there are only two consonants between the vowels, the most usual division is between them: pr**os**/**pe**ct.

This will be noted as vc-cv (vowel consonant/ consonant vowel).

2. There may be no consonants between the vowels or as many as four. The possible divisions are: **V-V** (li/on),   **V-CV** (la/dy),   **VC-V** (cab/in),
   V-CCV (re/fresh),   **VC-CV** (in/form),   **VCC-V** (hang/ing),
   VC-CCV (con/trol),   **VCC-CV** (most/ly),   **V-CCCV** (re/strict),
   VC-CCCV (con/strict), **VCC-CCV** (gangster), **VCCC-CV** (Hunts/ville)

3. Keeping *consonant blends* (bl, br, dw, cl, cr, dr, fl, fr, gl, gr, ng, pl, pr, sc, shr, sk, sl, sm, sn, sp, squ, st, sw, thr, tr, wr, tw,) and *consonant clusters* (spl, scr, spr, str) together as units, will, in most cases, assign a given word to the appropriate division pattern as listed above. See *re/fr̲esh, hang̲/ing, con̲/tr̲ol, mos̲t/ly, re/str̲ict, etc.* above.   However, an isolated blend may divide: *fas-ter.*

4. Treat *ch, -ck, -dge (-dg-), gh, ph, qu, sh, -tch, th, wh,* each as <u>one consonant</u>:
ca<u>tch</u>/er = **vc-v**,   cra<u>ck</u>/er = **vc-v**,   wi<u>th</u>/stand = **vc-ccv**,   ship/<u>sh</u>ape = **vc-cv**

Ap. ii-6

5. Treat *ai, au, augh, aw, ay, ea, ee, ei, eigh, eu, ew, ey, ie, igh, oa, oe, oi, oo, ou, ough, ow, oy, ue, ui,* as <u>one vowel</u>. n**eigh**/bor = **v**-cv, keep/ing = vc-v, *etc.*

6. Open syllable (long vowel or vowel pair) and closed syllable (short vowel or vowel pair) are important concerns on <u>accented</u> syllables: lō/cal = <u>v</u>-cv, lōō/sen = <u>v</u>-cv, lĕv/er = <u>vc</u>-v, hăb/it = <u>vc</u>-v, h<u>ea</u>v/y = <u>vc</u>- v.

7. The vowel sound in an unaccented syllable is often the sound of the <u>schwa</u> (ə), /ŭ/: a/<u>bout</u> = **v**-<u>cv</u>, /ə-<u>bowt</u>/, fr<u>e</u>/quent = <u>v</u>-cv, /frē-kwənt/.

8. The same consonant doubled is usually divided: at/tract = vc-<u>ccv</u>, but only one of the pair is pronounced, /ə-<u>tract</u>/. Notice again that the unaccented vowel is a schwa.

9. Sometimes a word like **contract** may be a noun or a verb depending on accent: **con/tract** is a noun; **con/*tract*** is a verb. These will be marked (n) or (v). Notice that **con-** is pronounced /cŏn/ when accented and /cən/ when unaccented. (See the end of this appendix for a list of these *Accent Shift Words*.)

10. Not all examples of each prefix and suffix are included in this appendix. See Appendices i, iii, & iv for more complete listings.

11. Note the difference between *hyphenating* a word by putting a part on each of two lines for space economy, *peel-ing*, and *syllabicating* a word to aid in its decoding and encoding, *pee/ling*. The first retains meaning parts, the second respects phonics aids. No harm is done in using a combination of these, if it aids the student in decoding and encoding. In many cases these are the same.

12. Examples of -ble, -dle, -fle, etc. are not given here. Usually each is a single syllable. Examples of these may be found in appendix i, *ta/ble, pad/dle, etc.*

13. Although the general rule is to divide between two like consonants (slop/py, sput/ter, *etc.*), usually **Fizzle-rule** words keep the consonants together: jazz/y hell/ish hill/y hiss/ing kill/er kill/ing mill/er miss/ing press/ing roll/er roll/ing tell/er tell/ing thrill/ing till/er truss/ing, *etc.* These are listed under **vc-v.**

14. At the end of this appendix can be found: "X" DIVIDED BETWEEN SYLLABLES; LONG VOWEL, SHORT VOWEL WORD PAIRS; ACCENT SHIFT WORDS; SILENT E IN BASE WORDS; and SYLLABLES WITH NO OR EQUAL ACCENT.

15. This appendix is mostly two syllable words. However, once familiar with common two syllable divisions and **prefix-root-suffix** word structure, longer words give little trouble: reconstruction = re/con/struc/tion, cor/re/spon/dent, par/a/psy/chol/o/gy, *etc.*

16. Henceforth as pronunciation aids in this appendix: s /z/ = <u>s</u> (outdoor<u>s</u> /owt-<u>dorz</u>); n /ng/ (before /k/) = <u>n</u> (la<u>n</u>ky /<u>lang</u>-kē/); n /ng/ (often before /g/) = <u>n</u> (fi<u>n</u>ger /<u>fing</u>-ger/); silent letter = strikethrough (p̶salm̶s̶ /sämz/).

VC-CV den/tist nap/kin hap/pen bas/ket lim/pid af/ter din/ner, *etc.*

a abbey abbot acrid acting action active adder addict Adler after aglet Albert album alcove alder alga alley alloy ally almond alpha alpine altar alter amber ambit ambush anchor Andes angel anger Angus Anjou Anna annals ante anthem anti- antic anvil arbor archon ardent ardor Argo argon argue arming Arnold arrant arrow arson Arthur artist arty aspect aspen asphalt asset aster Astor athlete atlas Atlas Atman attic Auckland Austin awkward   **b** Balfour Balkan ballad ballast Baltic Balzac bandage bandit banjo banker banking banquet banshee bantam banyan bargain barker barley Barlow barracks barrel barrow Bartók Barton basket basset basso bastard beatnik bedlam Belfast Belgian Belgium bellow bellows Belsen bencher Bendix Bennett Bentham Benton benzine Berber Bergen better billet billiards /bil-yerdz/ Billings billion /bil-yən/ billow binder binding bingo /bing-gō/ biscuit Bismarck bittern bitters bladder blanket blender blinder blinker blister blizzard bluster boarder bobbin Bobby bombard bombast bonded bonnet Bonny booster border Borgia borrow Boston bottom bouffant bouillon /bool-yon/ boulder bounty Bourbon bourdon bourgeois /boor-zhwah/ boycott Braddock Bradford Bradley braggart Brahma Brahman brandish brandy bratwurst Brennan Brenner brethren Bretton brightness brilliance /bril-yəns/ brilliant /bril-yənt/ brimful brisket Britten Brockton buddy bugger buggy builder building bumkin bumper bumpy bunco bunting Burbank burden burgeon burger burgess burgher burlap burlesque burly Burma burner Burney burning burnish burrow Burton busby /buz-bē/ buskin buster Buster butler Butler butter button buzzard   **c** cabbage cactus Cadmus cadre caffeine caisson callow callus Calvert Calvin camber cannon canto canton cantus canvas canyon capsize capsule /kap-səl/ captain /kap-tən/ carbine carbon carcass Cardiff cargo Carlos Carmel carnage carnal carpet carpus carrel carriage Carroll carrot Carson Carter Carthage carton Carver Casbah cascade cashmere casket Caspar Casper Cassatt castor catchment Caxton cello /chel-ō/ Celtic censure census centaur /sen-tor/ certain /ser-tən/ cession Chadwick challenge chamber Chambers champagne /sham-pān/ Champaigne chancy channel chanson /shan-sən/ chaplain /chap-lin/ Chapman Charlotte /shar-lət/ charnel chassis /shas-ē/ chattel chauffeur /shō-fer/ Chelsea Cherbourg /sher-boorg/ cherry Chester chevron chieftain chipmunk chirrup chimney chunky circuit /ser-kit/ circus cirrus cistern citron citrus cittern Clinton cockney coffee coffin cognate collie combat (n) combine (n) combo comma common comrade concern (n) concert (n) Concord condom condor Congo contact (n) content (n) contest (n) convert (n) convict (n) copper cordon corner cornice corpus corset cortex cosmic cosmos Cossack coastal costume cottage cotton council counsel counter couplet Cranmer Crassus crescent crimson Cromwell crumpet crystal culvert Cummings currant current cursive cuspid custard Custer custom cutlet **d** dactyl daddy daffy Dallas damsel dandy Danzig Daphne Darwin Delphi delta deltoid dental dentist Denver derrick dervish despot destine /des-tin/ dictate dictum dilly dingo /ding-gō/ dinner diphthong diptych disco discord discus dismal distant ditto ditty dobber dobbin doctor doggone dolce /dōl-chā/ dogma dollop dolly dolphin Donna dormant dorsal Douglas drachma Dresden Dublin ductile /duk-təl/ Dudley duffel Dulles dummy Dunbar Duncan dungeon /dun-jən/ Dunkirk Dunlop Durban **e** earful early earnest earthy Easter eastern eddy Edgar Edna Edward effort Egbert Eiffel Elba elbow elder eldest Elgar Elgin Ellis ember Emma Emmy empire encore /äng-kor/ engine ennui /än-wē/ enter envoy envy enzyme Epsom ergo ermine errand errant error escort (n) esquire essay essence Essex Esther /es-ter/ esthete ethnic **f** fabric faction factor Fairbanks Fairfax Fairfield fairly Fairmont faithful faithless falcon fallow falter fancy fanfare fanny Farley farmer farming farrow farther farthest farthing Fascist /fash-ist/ fasting fatling fatten fatty faulty fearful fearless fearsome feisty fellow fencer fencing fender fennel ferment (n) fermi Fermi ferret ferric ferrous ferry fertile fervent fervid fervor festal fester festive fetter fiction fifteen fifteenth fifty figment filbert filter filthy finder finding finger /fing-ger/ Finland fiscal fission fissure Fitchburg fitful fitting fixture flaccid flagging Flanders flannel flapper flatter fledgling flimsy flippant flipper flitter flivver flogging floppy flotsom flounder flunky flurry flutter fodder foggy follow folly forfeit formal format former forte /for-tā/ fortune forty forward Fosdick fossil foster Foster foulness fountain foursome fourteen fraction fracture fragment franchise Frances Francis Franco frantic frenzy fresco Fresno fretful friction Friesland frisky frightful frontage frontal frosty fructose fruitful fruitless frumpish Fulton Fundy fungal /fung-gəl/ fungus /fung-gəs/ funnel funny furbish furlough furnace furnish furrow furry **g** gaffer gainful gallant galley galliard /gol-yerd/ gallon gallop gallows Gallup Galton Galway gambit gamma gammon gander Ganges garbage garden Garfield gargoyle garland garlic garment garner garnet garnish garret garter Gaskell gasket Gaspar gelding gendarme /zhän-darm/ gender genre /zhän-rə/ Gentile Georgia /jor-jə/ Georgian gerbil German gesso gesture gherkin ghetto gibber gibbon Gibbon Gibbons Gibson giddy gifted Gilbert gilding gimmick ginger gingham ginseng Giotto /jôt-tō/ girder gismo gizzard gladly Glasgow Glendale glimmer Glinka glitter glottis glutton gnostic goblet goblin goddess godly golden golly goodness gorgeous /gor-jəs/ Gorgon Gorki gosling gospel Gospel gossip grammar granny granted grantor grasping greatly gremlin griffin Griffith grinder gringo /gring-gō/ grisly gritty groggy grotto grubby grumpy guilty Gullah gullet gully gummy gunner gunny Gunther guppy Gustaf gusto gutsy gutter gymnast gypsum **h** haddock Hadley haggard haggis Halley hallow halter halyard Hamburg Hamden hamlet Hamlet hammer hammock Hammond hamper Hancock handed Handel handy hanker Hannah hansome hapless happen happy harbor harden hardy Hardy harken Harlem harlot harness harpist harpy Harris harrow Harvard harvest Harvey haslet hasn't /haz-ənt/ hassock Hastings hāsty haunted haunting hawkshaw Haydn /hīd-n/ healthy hearten /har-tən/ hearty hectic Hector heedful heedless heirloom Hellas Hellene hellion helmet helper helping hemlock Hendon Henley henna Henry heptad herbal Herbert Herder Herman Hermes hermit herpes herring hiccup hidden hinder Hindi /hin-dē/ Hindu hippie hippo Hitler Hittite hoarder hoarding hobby hobnob Hoffman hoggish Holbein holder holding Holland holler hollow holly Holyoke Homburg hoodlum hoopla Hopkins hoplite hopper Hopper hormone Hormuz hornet horny horrid horror horsy hospice hostage hostel hostess hostile hourly Housman

Houston Hubbard hubbub Hudson huffy hulking Humbolt humbug humming humpy hunger /hung-ger/ hunter hunting hurry husband husky hussy Huxley Hypnos hymnal **i** ictus iffy igloo immy impact (n) impasse /im-pas/ import (n) impost impulse inboard inborn inbound Inca incense (n) incest income incurve (n) indent (n) indoor indoors Indus Indy infant infarct infield ingot /ing-gət/ injure inky inlaid inland inlaw inlay (n) inlet inner inning inquest insect insert (n) inset (n) insight insole insult (n) inter- intern invert (n) invite (n) invoice inward Ishtar island issue /ish-ōō/ it'll /it-l/ itself **j** jabber Jackson Jaffa jagged Janesville Jansen jargon jasmine Jaspers jaundice jaunty jello jelly jenny Jenny jerkin jerky Jerry jersey Jersey Jesse jester Jethro jetsam jetty jiffy jigger jimmy Jimmy jingo jitters jobless joinder jointed jolly Joplin Joppa Jordan journal /jer-nəl/ journey judgment jumbo jumper jumpy Junker /yoong-ker/ junket junta /hōōn-tə/ justice Justin Jutland **k** Kaddish /kä-dish/ Kafka /käf-kä/ Kansas kappa karma Karnak Kaufman kegler keister Keller kennel Kenya Kepler kerchief /ker-chif/ kernel Kerry Khartoum Khrushchev /krōōsh-chawf/ kidnap kidney Kilmer kilter kinship Kipling kipper kismet kitten kitty Klondike knapsack knighthood knitting knobby knotted knotty Knoxville Kreisler Kremlin Krishna krypton kumquat Kwanzaa **l** lacquer ladder laggard lagging Lambeth lancer landed landing language /lang-gwij/ languish Lansing lantern lanyard Lapland lapsus larder largo larva lassie lasso lasting latter lattice laughter /laf-ter/ launcher launching launder leaflet learned /ler-nid/ learning lectern lector lecture leftist lefty legging leggy Leibnitz /līb-nits/ Leipzig lemma lemming Lennox Lenten lentil lento lesson lessor letter lettuce /let-is/ lightning lignite limber limbo Limburg limpid Lincoln linden linger /ling-ger/ lingo /ling-gō/ lingual /ling-gwəl/ linguist /ling-gwist/ linkage linnet linseed linty lippy Lipton Lisbon lissome listen Lister listing litmus litter lobby lofty logger logging Lombard London /lən-dən/ lorry lotto lubber Luddite Ludlow Ludwig luggage Lully lumber lummox lumpy luncheon luster lusty **m** madden madder maddest madness maggot magma magna magnate magnet magnum magpie Magyar mahjong Mahler mainly mallard mallet mallow Malta malted Malthus mambo mammal mammon mammoth mammy mandate manger /mān-jer/ mango mangy /mān-gē/ manhood manly manna manner mannish mansion manta mantel mantis Marburg Marcus Marcy Marduk margin market marking marlin marmot marriage /mair-ij/ married marrow marshal marshy marten Martha martial Martian martin martyr marvel mascot massage massive master mastiff mastoid matted matter Matthew /math-yōō/ matting mattock matzo /mät-sə/ maudlin maunder Maundy Maxwell meanness measly Mecca Medford medley Melba Melbourne Mellon mellow Melrose Melville member Memphis Mencken Mendel Menlo Mensa mental menthol /men-thawl/ mention mentor merchant mercy merger Merlin mermaid merry mescal message messy metric metro mezzo /met-sō/ middy Midland midriff midship midterm midtown midwatch midway Midway Midwest midwife midyear Milton mincing minded minnow mirror mischief /mis-chif/ misfit (n) mishap Mishnah missal missile /mis-əl/ mission /mish-ən/ missive missy Mister misty Mithras mitten mixture mizzen moisten moisture molding moldy mollusk Molly molten /mōl-tən/ molto momma Monday /mən-dā/ monger /mong-ger/ Mongol /mong-gəl/ mongoose /mong-gōōs/ monkey Monmouth

VC-CV *continued.*

montane moppet morbid mordant mordent Morgan Morley Mormon morning
Morris morsel mortal mortar mortise Morton Moscow motley motto mountain
mounted mounting Mounty mourner mourning mouthful muddy muffin mugger
muggy mugwump mukluk mullah multi- mummer mummy murder murky murmur
Murphy Murry mushroom musket musky Muslim muslin mussel mustache /mus-tash/
mustang mustard /mus-terd/ muster musty mutter mutton mystic **n** nagger Nancy
nanny naphtha napkin narrate narrow narthex Nashville Nassau /nä-sow/ Nasser
nasty natty nearly nectar Needham Nehru /nā-roo/ Neilson Nelson Neptune
nervous nervy Nestor netting niblick nicknack nickname Nielsen nifty niggard
nightly nimbus Nimrod ninny nocturne noggin noncom Nordic Norfolk Norma
normal Norman Norris Norwich (England) /nor-ij/ Norwich (Connecticut) /nor-wich/
Norwood nudnik nugget number nurture Nutley nutmeg nutty **o** Oakland Oakley
object (n) oblate oblong Ockham octad octane octant octave /ok-tiv/ offer office often
Ogden only /ōn-lē/ onward optic optics option orbit orchard orchid /or-kid/ order
organ orgy Orlon orphan orphic ortho- Orwell Oscar Oshkosh Osler /ōs-ler/ Oslo
/os-lō/ Osman otter Otto outlet outward oxford Oxford oyster **p** padding paddock
paddy padlock painful painter painting Paisley pallet pallid pallor palsy pampas
pamper panda pander pansy panther panties panzer pappy parboil parcel pardon
parka Parker parlance parley parlor Parma parrot parry parson Parsons parted
partial parting partite party paschal passage passim passion passive pastime pastor
pasture pasty Patmos Patrick patsy patter pattern Patton patty Pavlov Pearson
pectin pellet pelvis pencil pendant pending penguin pennant pennon penny pension
pensive pentad pepper peppy pepsin percept Percy perfect perjure Perkins perky
permit (n) Perry Pershing Persia /per-zhə/ Persian /per-zhən/ person pervert (n) pesky
pester petrol petrous petty phallic phallus phantom philter Phyllis Pickford Pickwick
picnic picture Piedmont piggish piggy pigment pilfer pillage pillar pillow pincers
Pinchot /pin-shō/ Pindar pinkie pinnate Pinta pinto Pisces /pī-sēz/ pistil pistol piston
pittance pizza /pēt-sə/ plaintiff plaintive Plainview plantar planter plasma plaster
plastic platform platter plenty plodder plotter plunder plunger Pnom-Penh pointed
pointer polka pollack pollen Pollock pommel Pompey /pom-pē/ pompon pompous
poncho pontiff poplar poppa popper poppy porgy porky porpoise /por-pəs/ porridge
portage portal portent porter Portia /por-shə/ portion posse possum postage postal
poster posture potlatch potsherd pottage potted potto potty poultis practice
pregnant Prescott pressure presto Preston pretty pretzel /pret-səl/ prickly priestess
princess printer printing prissy pristine /pris-tēn/ problem proctor proffer progress (n)
pronto prospect prosper prostate Prussia psalter public publish pudding pueblo
/pweb-lō/ pullet pulley pulpit pulsar pulsate pundit pungent Punjab puppet puppy
Purcell purchase /per-chəs/ purpose /per-pəs/ purser Pushkin pussy pustule Putnam
putter putty pygmy **q** quadrant quagmire quantum quarrel queenly question
/kwes-chən/ quickly quilting Quincy quinsy quisling quitter quitting Quonset **r** rabbet
rabbi rabbit rafter ragged raglan rally rampage (n) rampant rampart Ramsay /ram-zē/
Ramses rancher rancho rancid rancor Randolph random Randy ranger ransack
ransom rapture rascal rasping Rathaus /rät-hows/ ratty really rearward reckless recluse

rectal recto rector rectum rectus redden reindeer Reinhardt remnant render rental renter reptile rescue respite /res-pit/ resting restive Rheingold rhombic rhomboid rhombus rhythmics ribbing ribbon Richfield richly Richmond riddance rigger rightful rightly Rilke rinsing Ripley ripper risky rissole ritzy /rit-sē/ roaster robber Rockford Rollo Romberg Rommel romper rondo rooster roster rotten rotter rounded rounder Rousseau rubber rubbish rudder ruddy Rugby rugged rumba rummage rummy rumpus runner running rupture Rushmore Ruskin Russell russet Russia /rush-ə/ Russian /rush-ən/ rustic rusty Rutledge **s** Sabbath sackbut sadden sallow sally Sally salted salty salvage salvo samba sampan Samson sandal sanded sander sandy Sandy Sanford sanguine /sang-gwin/ sapling sapphire Sappho /saf-ō/ sappy Sardis sassy savvy scabbard scaffold scallion scallop scalpel scamper scandal scansion scanty scarlet scepter scherzo /sker-tsō/ Schiller schilling Schleswig schnozzle Schonberg schottische /shot-ish/ scissors Scottish scraggy Scranton scrappy scrimmage scrimpy Scripture scrubby scummy scurvy searching section sector seemly segment seismic seldom Selma sensate sensor sentence sergeant /sar-jənt/ sermon serpent serrate servant service servile session setter setting sextant sexton shabby shafting shaggy shallow shamrock Shannon shanty sharpen shatter Sheffield sheikdom Shelby Shelley shelter shelving shepherd sherbet sherlock Sherman sherry shielding shifty shilling shimmer shimmy shindig Shinto Shirley shirting shoddy shopper shortage shorten shoulder shrapnel shudder shutter shyster /shīs-ter/ sibling sickly sickness Sidra Siegmund siftings sigma Sigmund signal signet silken silky silly silver simmer simper Sinbad sinful sinner sirloin sissy sister Sistine /sis-tēn/ sixteen Sixtus sixty skeptic skillet skimmer skimpy Skinner skinny skipper skirmish skittish skivvy slander sledding slender slightly slippage slipper slobber sloppy slothful slugger sluggard sluggish slumber sluttish smarten smatter smelter smitten smolder smutty snapper snappy snifter snippy snobbish snorkel snotty soccer softy soggy soldier /sol-jer/ solvent somber Somnus sonnet sonny /sən-ē/ sopping sordid sordine /sor-dēn/ sorrel sorrow sorry sounder sounding sparrow spastic spatter Spencer spender spiffy spinner spinning splatter splendid splendor splinter splitting sponger spongy sponsor spoonful sporting sportive sporty spotted spotter spotty sprightly sprinter Sputnik sputter squander squatter squirrel staffer stagger stagnant stagnate stallion stalwart Stamford stammer stanchion standard standee standing Standish Stanford Stanley stanza starchy starlet starling starry starter stealthy steenbok Steinbeck stellar stencil stentor sterling sternum Stetson stickler stigma stilted Stilwell Stimson stingy stirring stirrup Stockholm /stok-hōm/ Stockton stopper Strafford stranger strapper strapping Strasbourg Stratford stretto stricture stringent structure strumpet strychnine /strik-nin/ stubborn stubby stucco studding stunner stunning sturdy sturgeon stutter styptic subject (n) sublease (n) subplot subsoil subway succor suckling suction sudden sudsy suffer suffix (n) Suffolk sulfate sulfide sulfur sulky sullen sully sulphur summa summer summit summon summons Sumner sundae /sən-dē/ Sunday sunder Sunni sunny supper surcharge (n) surface surfeit /sur-fit/ surgeon /sur-jən/ surname surrey surtax survey (n) suspect (n) Sussex swagger swallow swarthy swelter swifter swimming Sydney sylvan symbol syntax system **t** tabby tableau /tab-lō/ tablet tabloid tactic tactile /t̲a̲k̲-til/ taffy talcum tallow tally Talmud tambour Tampa tamper tampon tandem tangent ta̲n̲go /t̲a̲n̲g̲-gō/ tanner tanning tappet tapping tardy target tarmac tarnish tarpon Tarquin tarry Tarsus tartar Tarzan tassel taster tasty tatter tatting tattoo tearful teddy Teddy Teflon telly temper tempest tempo tender tendon tennis tensile /t̲e̲n̲-sil/ tension tenter termite terra terrace terror terry Terry testate testes̲ testy tetrad Tetzel /t̲e̲t̲-səl/ textile /t̲e̲k̲s̲-til/ texture thickness thinner thirty thorny thoughtful thrombus thumping thunder Thurber tickler ticklish tilde Tillich timber tinder tinsel tippy tipsy tissue /t̲i̲s̲h̲-o͞o/ titter tizzy toaster toddy Tommy tom-tom Tonkin tonnage tootsy topper topping Topsy torment torpid torpor torrent torrid torsion torso tortoise /t̲o̲r̲-təs/ torture totter tourney traction tractor traffic trammel tranquil transept transient transit transom trapper trapping̲s̲ Trappist treatment trellis trenchant Trenton trespass trigger trillion trimmer trimming trolley trollop trotter trousseau /t̲r̲o͞o̲-sō/ trumpet truncheon trusting trusty truthful tsetse /t̲s̲e̲t̲-sē/ tubby Tucson /t̲o͞o̲-son/ Tue̲s̲day tufted tunnel turban turbid turbine turbo- turgid turkey Turkey turmoil turnip turret Tuscan tutti /t̲o͞o̲-tē/ twenty twister twitter **u** ugly ulcer ulna umber umlaut /o͝o̲m̲-lowt/ umpire u̲n̲co under undie̲s̲ unguent upper uppish upward urban urchin Urdu /o͝o̲r̲-do͞o/ urgent Ursa ursine Urtext /o͝o̲r̲-tekst/ utmost utter Uzbek **v** valley vampire vandal vanguard va̲n̲quish vantage varmint varnish vassal vaulting vector vellum velvet vender vengeance venter venture verbal verdant verdict Vergil vermin vernal Verner version verso versus vertex vespers vesper̲s̲ vessel Vesta vested vestige victim victor villa village villain Vinci /v̲e̲n̲-chē/ Vinland vintage Virgil virgin Virgo virtu /v̲e̲r̲-to͞o/ virtue /v̲e̲r̲-cho͞o/ viscid viscount /v̲ī̲-cownt/ viscous Vishnu vista vitric vodka Volga volley volta volti /v̲a̲w̲l̲-tē/ vortex Vulcan vulgar vulgate vulture vulva **w** wadding Wagner /v̲ä̲g̲-ner/ Waldo Wałker Wallace wallet Walloon wallop wallow walnut Walpole walrus Walter Walter (German) /v̲ä̲l̲-ter/ Waltham Walton wampum wander wanting wanton (wɑr = /wor/) warden warlock warmer warming warning warrant Warren Warsaw War̶wick wa̲s̲n't /w̲u̲z̲-ənt/ waspish wassail /w̲ä̲s̲-əl/ waster wasting watchful wattage Watteau weakling weakly weakness wealthy webbing wedded wedding Wedgwood wedlock weekly weirdie welcome welfare welter Wendell Wessex western wetting Wexford whammy whimper whim̲s̲y whinny whippet whipping whisker whiskey whisper Whitman Whitney Whitsun wholly whopper whopping wigwam Wilcox wilder William /w̲i̲l̲-yəm/ willow Wilson Wilton winded winding window windy winker winner winning winnow winsome winter wi̲s̲dom wishful witness witty Wol̲s̲ey wonder wonky wonted woolly Worcester /w̲o͝o̲s̲-ter/ wordage wording worker working wormy worry worsen worship worthy wri̶tten w̶rapper w̶rapping w̶rathful Wycliffe **x** xyster /z̲i̲s̲-ter/ *(Surgical instrument.)* **y** Yahweh /y̲ä̲-wē/ yammer Ya̲n̲kee yardage Yarmouth yearling yearly yearning yeasty yellow Yiddish yielding yonder Yo̲n̲kers youthful yucca yummy **z** Zeitgeist Ziegfeld zigzag zipper zippy zombie

VC-CV

a account acquit adhere adjust admit advice affect affirm ally allow almost although announce antique appear appoint arrest arrive artiste /ar-tēst/ assent assign Aswan attempt attain augment (v) **b** balloon bamboo barrage bassoon Bastille Bastogne berceuse Berlin berserk blaspheme Bombay buffet /bŏo-fā/ buffoon Burmese Burnett **c** campaign Candide /kän-dēd/ canteen cartel Cartier /car-tyā/ cartoon cassette chassé /sha-sā/ chastise chiffon collect collide combat (v) combine (v) command commit compel contend content (v) contest (v) Corfu Cornell cornet corral correct corrode corsage /kor-säzh/ cortege /cor-tezh/ Cortés corvette croissant /krwä-sän/ curtail **d** Descartes /dā-kart/ discard disdain disguise dislike dislodge dismay dismiss dispatch dispel dispense distend distill Dundee **e** effect ellipse embalm enchant encode enforce engage enjoy enlist ersatz /air-säts/ enlist escape escort (v) espy excite **f** ferment (v) festoon fondue forbid forget forgive forgo forgot forlorn forsake forsooth frappé fulfill **g** garçon genteel germane Gibran /joob-rän/ Gillette gourmet /gŏor-mā/ guffaw **h** halloo harpoon hello hurrah **i** ignore immense immune impact (v) impart impeach import (v) impose impound impure incense (v) incite incur incurve (v) indeed indent indict /in-dīt/ induce induct indulge infect infer infest infirm infix infold inform infuse ingest inhale inhere inject inlay (v) innate inquire insane insert (v) inset (v) insist insult (v) insure intact intend intense intent inter intone invade inveigh invent inverse invert (v) invest invite (v) invoke involve Islam **k** kibbutz /ki-bŏots/ Kildare Knesset **l** lampoon largess Lorraine **m** Macbeth MacLeish maintain Maltese Manchu marcel marquee Marquette marquis /mar-kē/ masseur McCoy miscount miscue misdeal misfire misfit (v) misjudge mislay mislead misrule mistake Monroe monsieur /mə-syer/ monsoon montage /mon-täzh/ mundane mystique /mis-tēk/ **n** nonwhite **o** object (v) observe obsess obtain obtuse obverse occult occur octet offend offense oppose oppugn ordain ordeal ornate **p** parfait parlay parquet /par-kā/ partake partook Pascal passé pastel Pasteur percale perceive percent perchance perform perfume perfuse perhaps permit (v) persist persuade pertain perturb pervade perverse pervert (v) Pierrot /pye-rō/ pollute Pompeii /pom-pā/ pontoon possess Poussin /pŏo-san/ prestige /pres-tēzh/ purloin purport pursue pursuit purvey **q** quartet quintet **r** raccoon rampage (v) Rangoon /rang-gŏon/ rappel rapport /rə-por/ risqué /ris-kā/ **s** sardine /sar-dēn/ Sassoon septet septum settee sextet shampoo shellac sincere skiddoo stampede subject (v) sublease (v) sublet submerge submit subside subsist subsume subtend subvert succeed success succinct succumb suffice suffix (v) suffuse suggest supply support suppose supposed surcharge (v) surmise surmount surpass surround survey (v) survive suspect (v) suspend suspense sustain suttee **t** Tangier tarboosh technique /tek-nēk/ terrain trombone trustee **u** unbolt uncap uncouth /un-cŏoth/ uncut undo unfair ungird unhook unjust unkind unless unlock unmask unnerve unpack unreal unseal untie until unto unveil unwind unyoke uplift (v) upset (v) upsurge (v) upturn (v) urbane **v** vaccine /vak-sēn/ Vandyke vendee vendue verbose Verdun Vermont vermouth /ver-mŏoth/ Versailles /ver-sī/ Voltaire **w** Wilmette **y** yashmak /yäsh-mäk/ (See Ap. iii for more examples with ac-, ad-, af-, ag-, al-, an-, ap-, ar-, as-, at-, col-, com-, con-, cor-, dis-, ef-, em-, en-, ex-, im-, in-, and un-.)

V-V (First vowel is long or a diphthong & accented; second vowel short or schwaed, /ə/.)

b bayou /bī-ōō/ being bias bio- blower bluing bluish boa bowel boyish brewing brier Bryan Bryant Buick buoyant /boi-ənt/ **c** chewy Chios cion clayey client co-opt coward cower crayon creole Creole Creon Croat cruel cruet crying **d** dais dial diet diode doer /dōō-er/ doing doings dowel dower drawer drawing druid dryad drier driest drying duad dual duel duet duo dyad **e** eon Eos **f** fiat flier flower flowage flowing fluent fluid flying foyer Freon friar fryer frying fuel **g** giant glower /glow-er/ glowing /glō-ing/ gluey gnawing goer going gooey graying grayish grower growing gruel **h** hewer hewing Howard **i** iamb Io ion **j** jewel Jewish Joab Joel joyous **k** kayak /kī-ak/ kiosk /kē-osk/ knowing **l** Laos layer layette laying Leon Lewis liar lion Louis Lowell lower lowest loyal lying Lyon Lyons **m** mayor Moab mowing myope **n** neon neo- Noah nuance **o** Owen **p** paean /pē-ən/ peon pious Pius player playing pliant pliers plowing poem poet power preempt Priam prior prowess **q** quiet **r** rayon riot royal ruin **s** sayid /sī-id/ saying science séance /sā-äns/ seeing sewage sewer sewing /sō-ing/ Sheol /shē-ōl/ Shiah /shē-ə/ shier shower showing skewer skier /skē-er/ skiing /skē-ing/ sleighing steward Stewart stoa stoic stowage stria striate Stuart suet Suez **t** theo- towage towel tower triad trial trowel truant trying **v** via vial viand viewer viol vowel voyage **w** wooer Wyatt Wyeth **z** Zion;

(Second vowel <u>not</u> short or schwaed.) hooey joey kayo (K.O.) Leo luau /lōō-ow/ Mayo meow Rio /rē-ō/ Shiite /shē-īt/ showy trio /trē-ō/

V-<u>V</u> Cheyenne /shī-<u>en</u>/ coerce create Kiev (kē-<u>ev</u>/ Louise /lōō-<u>ēz</u>/ naive /nä-<u>ēv</u>/ Noël react rearm Siam /sī-<u>am</u>/

MULTI-SYLLABLE WORDS WITH V-V: a Aïda /ä-<u>ē</u>-də/ alien aorta Aramaic area aria ariel Aryan atheism **b** Balboa biopsy biology Borneo brewery **c** cameo chariot coalition coexist coincide cooperate coordinate **d** deodorant diaper diarrhea diary diocese Diogenes Dionysia Dionysus Diogenes diorama **e** embryo **f** fealty fiasco fiesta folio **g** Genoa **h** hiatus Hialeah Hiawatha hierarchy hieroglyphic hyena **i** idea idiot Iliad ingenuity innuendo intuit intuition iodine Ionia Ionic iota Iowa Ishmael /ish-mē-əl/ Israel **j** Joshua Josiah Judea **k** Korea **l** laity Laocoon /lā-<u>ok</u>-ə-won/ Leopold leotard leviathan liable liaison /lē-ā-<u>zon</u>/ **m** Macao maestoso maestro meander Meander Medea Miami Minoan mosaic **n** Naomi Nashua nausea Neapolitan Niagara **o** oasis Ohio Orion Orpheus **p** Paleolithic panacea Paoli peony Peoria Phaethon piety pioneer poetic poetics propriety prosaic puerile **r** radio Rialto /rē-<u>al</u>-tō/ Roanoke rodeo Romeo **s** Sabaoth Samoa Scipio Seattle Siamese Siena studio suicide Syria **t** tuition torii /tor-i-ē/ trivia truism tuition **v** Vietnam /vē-et-<u>näm</u>/ viola violate violence violent violet violin;

(<u>See</u>: **-ia, -ial, -ian, -iance, -iant, -iate, -ience, -ient, -ior, -ious, -ium, -ius** in Ap. iv.)

V̲-CV (First syllable open and accented with long or double vowel.)

a acorn agent Amen Amos anus apex aphid Asia /ā-zhə/ auburn audit auger august August autumn Avon **b** Babel basin basis bebop Beirut /bā-ro͞ot/ beta /bā-tə/ biceps bijou /bē-zho͞o/ binal biped bisect bison blatant blazer blazon bleacher̲s̲ bloomer̲s̲ blooper bogey bogus Boi̲s̲e bola bolo bonus boudoir /bo͞o-dwar/ bravo /br̲ä-vō/ brooder broody blooper broiler Brueghel brutal Buber butane Byron **c** cadence Caesar /s̲ē-zer/ Cairo /k̲ī-rō/ cajun Caleb caliph calix Canaan /k̲ā-nən/ canine capon caucus Cayman ceiling Cézanne /sā-zän/ Chaucer cheetah Cheka chichi /s̲h̲ē-s̲h̲ē/ China Chopin /s̲h̲ō-pan/ claimant climate climax Clovis cobalt coca codeine cogent colon coma Conant coolant Coolidge coolie cootie cosine costar coupon covert Crawford credence credo /kr̲ä-dō/ cremate crisis crocus Cronus crouton Cuba Cuban cubit cupid curate Curie cylix cypress Cyrus **d** dada Dagon Dali /d̲ä-lē/ Damon dative David Davis Dawson decal decent décor demon Dido didy digest (n) dilate diode dipole diva /d̲ē-və/ Dnieper /d̲n̲y̲e̲-per/ docent dodo /d̲ō-dō/ dolor donate doodad dotage Dover dowel Draco drama /dr̲ä-mə/ Dreiser Dreyfus Drusus Dryden duce /d̲o͞o-chā/ Duma Dürer duty **e** eager eagle easel easy eating Edam edict ego Egypt eider eighteen eighty either emu equal equine Esau eta /ā-tə/ ether ethos étude Eugene eunuch Europe even evil **f** facial failing famous fatal father faucet favor feature fecal feces fecund feeder feeler feeling feline female femur fetal fetus fever fiber fighter fighting Fiji /f̲ē-jē/ final finance finite flavor flawless fleeting flighty floater floating floozy focal focus fogy foolish Fräulein /fr̲oi̲-līn/ Frazer freedom freely freezer Freiburg freighter freightage Fremont frequent Fribourg Friday frighten frowzy frozen frugal fruity fu̲s̲ee fu̲s̲ion futile futon future **g** gaily gala Galen Gaucho /g̲ow̲-chō/ gaudy gawky Gaza /g̲ä-zə/ geezer Geiger geisah /gā-s̲h̲ə/ genie genus gey̲s̲er /g̲ī-zer/ Ghana glacial glacier glazing gleeful glider gliding gloaming gloomy glucose goalie goatee Gobi /g̲ō-bē/ Goethe /g̲ö-tə/ goiter Gómez goober goofy googol gopher Goshen goulash gracious gradate grader gra̲h̲am grainy grating gravy grazing greasy Grecian greedy Greeley greeting grievance grievous grimy grocer groovy grouchy groupy gruesome guano /g̲w̲ä-nō/ guidance guru gyral gyrate gyro **h** hades Hades hafiz /h̲ä-fiz/ Hagar Hagen /h̲ä-gən/ Haifa /h̲ī-fə/ haiku /h̲ī-ko͞o/ Haiti /h̲ā-tē/ halo haughty hawker Hawthorne hazel Hazel hazy healer heaping heater heathen heehaw Hegel /h̲ā-gəl/ Heifetz /h̲ī-fits/ heighten Heine /h̲ī-nə/ heinous /h̲ā-nəs/ helix hemic heyday /h̲ā-dā/ hijack hobo hocus Hogarth hokum holism holy homer Homer homey Homo Honan Hoosier Hoover Hopi /h̲ō-pē/ hora housing howdy howler hula human humid humor humus Hunan Huron hymen hyper hyphen hypo **i** ibex ibis icing icon icy Ida ideal idem idol ilex irate iris Irish iron /ī-ern/ Isaac iso- item Ivan ivy **j** Jacob jailer Jason Jesus jocose /j̲ō-caws/ joiner joker Jonah Joseph joyful juba Judah Judas Judith judo Judy juicy juju julep Juneau /j̲o͞o-nō/ junior /j̲o͞o-nyer/ Juno **k** kaiser /k̲ī-zer/ Kama /k̲ä-mə/ keeper keeping keno kewpie kibosh kiva /k̲ē-və/ kiwi /k̲ē-wē/ Kleenex Kodak kopeck kosher Koto kowtow Kruger kuchen kudos kulak **l** laager /l̲ä-ger/ label labor lacing lacy lady lager /l̲ä-ger/ Lagos /l̲ä-gōs/ lama /l̲ä-mə/ la̲s̲er latent later latex lava /l̲ä-və/ lawful lawyer lazy leader leafy leakage leaning leavings̲ legal legion Leiden leisure /l̲ē-zher/ lemur Lena lethal Levi

Levis /lē-vīz/ Levite Leyden /lī-dən/ Leyte /lā-tā/ Lhasa /lä-sä/ libel license lichen Lido /lē-dō/ lifer lighten lighter lighting lilac Lima /lē-mə/ *(Lima, Peru.)* /lī-mə/ *(Lima, Ohio & lima bean.)* liner lining liter /lē-ter/ liven llama /lä-mə/ loaded loading loafer local locate loci loco locus locust Logan logos loiter Lomax loony loosen loser losing lotion lotus lousy loutish louver lowly Lübeck /loo-bek/ Lucan lucent lucid Lucite Luger lulu lumen Luna lunar lupus Luther Lysol **m** Magi /mā-jī/ maiden mailing major maker making Malay Mali /mä-lē/ mama mason mating meager meaning meaty meeting melee /mā-lā/ Menes /mē-nēz/ mesa /mā-sə/ meson meter mica Micah /mī-kə/ Michael /mī-kəl/ Midas mighty miner mining minor Minos minus miser miter mobile /mō-bəl/ mocha /mō-kə/ modish modus mogul mohair Mohawk molar moment monad moody moolah Mooney Moses mosey motion motive motor mousy mouthy mover /moo-ver/ movie /moo-vē/ moving Mozart /mō-tsart/ mucous Munich /myoo-nik/ music musing mutant mutate myna Myra Myron **n** nadir naked napalm nasal natal Nathan nation native nature naughty naval navel navy nazi /nä-tsē/ needy neighbor neither neuter neutral neutron Newton Nicene Niebuhr Nieman Niger /nī-jer/ nighty nihil Nike Niña /nē-nyä/ nisi noisome noisy nomad notice notion nougat nova nudist nuisance numen nylon **o** obi /ō-bē/ oboe ocean /ō-shən/ ocher Oder Odin odor oily Okie Olaf Oman omen oolong oozy opal open opus Osage otic Otis Ouija /wē-jə/ outer outing oval ovate over overt ovum owlish owner oyer oyez ozone **p** pagan Paley papa papal paper papist pater pathos patience patient Pauline Pauling pauper paving peachy peeling peevish peewee pekoe penal penis peso /pā-sō/ Peter Petri /pē-trē/ pewee pewter phalanx phenol Philip Phoebe /fē-bē/ Phoenix phoneme phony photo photon phrasing phylum pica piker Pilate /pī-lət/ piling pilot piña /pē-nyä/ piper piping pirate /pī-rit/ Pisa /pē-sä/ placate plagal Plato plaudit playlet plaza /plä-zə/ pleading pleasing pleater plenum plumage Pluto pneuma poacher poco /pō-kō/ Podunk poison poker poky Poland polar Polish polo pony posy potent potion Poulenc /poo-länk/ pouter powder powwow praetor /prē-ter/ praline /prā-lēn/ preacher precept precinct precis /prā-sē/ prefab prefect pretext preview primal primate primer /prī-mer/ primo /prē-mō/ private /prī-vit/ probate profile prolapse prologue pronoun propane prorate prosit protest (n) proton proven Provo prudent prudish pseudo psyche /sī-kē/ psychic psycho- ptomaine ptosis pubic puma Punic puny pupa pupil pylon Pyrex pyro- python **q** Quaker quinine quota quotient **r** rabies /rā-bēz/ racer racy radar radon railing rainy raisin raising rajah /rä-jə/ rakish Rama /rä-mə/ rating ratio /rā-shō/ raucous raven raving razor reader reading reamer reason rebate rebec recall (n) recast (n) recent recess (n) recoil (n) recourse reedy reefer reeky refill (n) refund (n) regal regent region rehash (n) reject (n) relay rematch (n) remount (n) Remus renal Reno rerun (n) research (n) reset (n) retail (n) retake (n) retard (n) retouch (n) Reuben Reuter /roi-ter/ rhesus rhino rhubarb rider riding Riga /rē-gə/ Riley riser rising rival robot rodent Roland Roman romance roofer roofing roomer roomy Rose rosy rotate rotor rousing Rover rowdy ruby Rudolf rueful ruler ruling rumen rumor rupee Rupert Ryder **s** saber Sabin saga /sä-gə/ sahib /sä-ib/ Saigon /sī-gon/ sailing sailor Saipan /sī-pan/ sake /sä-kē/ Salem saline /sā-lēn/ sapor sari /sä-rē/ Satan saucer saucy sauna sausage saving savor Sawyer scalene scathing scenic schema Schliemann schnauzer /shnow-zer/ schooling schooner Schubert Schumann scooter scraper scraping scrawny screaming scrotum sealer seamy season seating secant Seder /sā-der/ seedy seeming seepage seizure semen senile Sepoy sequel sequence sequin shading shady shaker Shaker shaky shaman /shä-mən/ shaver shaving Sheba sheeting Shiloh /shī-lō/ shiner shining shiny Shiva /shē-və/ shofar shogun shoji /shō-je/ shooting Shriner shylock siding Sidon sighted silage silence silent silex silo Simon Sinai /sī-nī/ sinus siphon siren Siva /sē-və/ sizing skater Skokie slalom /slä-ləm/ slaughter Slavic sleazy sleeper sleepy slighter slimy slogan Slovak Slovene smoky smoothie sneaker sneaking sneaky sniper snoopy snooty sober social soda sofa sojourn solar solo Solon solus soma sonant sonar sooner soothing sopor Sotho soupy spacing spacious spatial speaker speaking specious speeder speeding speedy spicy spider spinal spiral spoilage spoken spooky squeaky squeegee staging Stalin /stä-lin/ stamen station statist status steamer steamy Stephen /stē-vən/ Stevens stipend stogy stoker stolen stoma stony strainer straiten stratum streaky streamer strident striker striking strobic strudel student Stuka stupid stupor stylish stylist stylus suitor sumac super supine suture swami /swä-mē/ Sweden Swedish sweeping sweeten sweetie **t** tabor Tahoe /tä-hō/ tailor Taipei /tī-pā/ Taiwan /tī-wän/ taker taking taper tapir tawny Taylor teacher teaching teaser teeming teeny teeter telic tepee Teuton Thales thesis theses /thē-sēz/ theta /thā-tə/ thousand Thracian throaty thyroid Tiber tidal tidings tidy tiger tighten timer timing Timor /tē-mor/ tirade Titan tithing Tito /tē-tō/ Titus toby Toby toga Togo toilet Tojo token tonal tony Tony tooling toothy topaz toper topi /tō-pē/ total totem toucan tracer tracing trailer trainee trainer training traitor trauma trawler treason treatise /trē-tis/ treaty tribal triceps trident trochee troika Trojan trooper trophy trouper trousers truly Truman tuba tuber tubing Tudor tulip tumid tumor tumult tuna tuner tunic Tunis tutor tweeter tweezers twilight Tyler typhoid typhus typist typo tyrant tyro Tyrol **u** Udall ukase uni- unit **v** vacant vacate valence Valens vapor Veda /vā-də/ Vegas /vā-gəs/ velar velum venal venous Venus veto Vichy /vē-shē/ viking vinyl viper viral virus visa /vē-zə/ visor vital vitals viva /vē-vä/ vocal voided volant volar voodoo votive voucher **w** Waco wader wafer wager waiter waiting waiver waken water Wausau waver wavy Wayland wayward weaken weasel weaver Weber (Ger.) /vā-ber/ weeder weedy weenie weeny weeper weeping weepy weevil weighty Weimar /vī-mar/ whaler whaling Wheaton Wheeler Wheeling wheezy whiten whiting whitish whoopee whooping widen wiener wiper Woden woeful woozy ~~writer~~ ~~writing~~ **x** /z/ xebec xenon Xhosa /kō-sä/ xylem xyloid **y** Yaqui /yä-kē/ yeoman /yō-mən/ yeti /ye-tē/ yodel yoga yogi /yō-gē/ yogurt yokel Yukon Yuma **z** zany Zealand zebu zenith zeta /zā-tə/ Zola zonal Zulu Zuñi /zoo-nyē/ zwieback /zwī-bak/ zygote

V-**CV** (a- = /ə/) abase abate abed abet abide aboard abode abort abound above aboard abuse abut abyss acute adapt adept adopt adore adorn adult afoot afoul again ago agog ahem ahoy akin alarm alert alight align alike aloft along aloof amass amaze amend amid amidst amiss among amount amour Amoy amuck

amuse anoint apart apiece arose around arouse ashamed ashore aside athirst atone avail avenge aver averse avert avoid avow await awake award aware awash away aweigh awhile awhirl awoke **b** baboon baroque Bataan baton (be- = /bĭ/) becalm became because become bedeck befall befit before befoul began beget begin begone begot beguile beguine begun behalf behave behead beheld behest behind behold behoove belie belief believe Belize /bə-lēz/ belong below bemean bemire bemoan bemused beneath benign benumb bequeath bequest bereave beret /bə-rā/ beseech beset beside besides besiege besought beware bewitch beyond Bizet /bē-zā/ bouquet /bō-kā/ boutique Brazil brigade briquette brocade /brō-kād/ brochure /brō-shŏŏr/ **c** cabal caboose cachet /ka-shā/ cadet cahoots cajole Camus /kə-mōō/ canal canard carafe /kə-raf/ careen career caress Casals /kä-säls/ café /ka-fā/ catarrh cavort Cavour Cebu /sā-bōō/ cement Ceylon /si-lon/ chaconne /shə-kôn/ Chagall /shə-gahl/ chalet /sha-lā/ charades /shə-rädz/ chateau /sha-tō/ chemise /shə-mēz/ chicane /shə-kān/ Chinese chinook Chinook cigar cliché /klē-shā/ cocaine cocoon cohere /cō-hear/ coupé courante croquet /krō-kā/ croquette crusade cuisine /kwi-zēn/ culottes **d** Dachau Daumier /dō-myā/ (de- = /dĭ/) debar debase debate debut /di-byōō/ debase debate decay decease deceit deceive decide decline decode declare decree deduct defense defend degree depend desire device devise digest (v) dinette direct divan divine domain donee dragoon Dubuque /də-byōōk/ Duluth duress **e** (e- = /ĭ/) eject élan /ā-län/ elapse elate elect elide élite /ā-lēt/ elope elude emerge emir enough **f** façade fatigue Fauré /fō-rā/ filet /fi-lā/ finesse foment /fō-ment/ **g** galoot galore galosh garage /gə-räzh/ Gauguin /gō-gan/ gavotte gazette giraffe Girard Gironde glacé Gounod /gōō-nō/ gravure grenade grotesque guitar **h** Hanoi harangue harass hooray hotel Houdon /ōō-dawn/ **i** Imam /i-mäm/ Iran Iraq **j** Jerome jihad /ji-häd/ July **k** kabob kaput /kä-pŏŏt/ kazoo Koran /kō-rän/ Kuwait /kōō-wīt/ **l** lagoon lament Lamont lapel legit Levant liqueur /li-ker/ locale Lorain Lucerne lunette Luzon lycée /lē-sā/ **m** Macao /mə-kow/ macaque /mə-käk/ macaw machine /mə-shēn/ malign Malone Manet /ma-nā/ manure /mə-nŏŏr/ maroon mature Maurice /mə-rēs/ Mekong /mā-kong/ menage /mā-näzh/ meringue /me-rang/ Milan milieu /mē-lŭ/ minute /mī-nōōt/ mirage /mi-räzh/ Miro /mē-rō/ molest Moline /mō-lēn/ Monet /mō-nā/ moraine morale /mə-ral/ morass morel morose motel /mō-tel/ motet /mō-tet/ motif /mō-tēf/ moulage /mōō-läzh/ musette /myōō-zet/ **n** negate Nepal névé Nobel **o** obese obey obit O'Keefe omit O'Neill opaque opine Oran **p** papoose parole pâté /pä-tā/ pavan Pawnee pecan Perón /pā-rōn/ Peru peruse Pétain /pā-tan/ petite /pə-tēt/ physique Pieta /pyā-tä/ pilaf piqué /pē-kā/ plateau /pla-tō/ platoon police /pə-lēs/ polite potage /pō-täzh/ (Unless marked otherwise, pre- = /prĭ/ & pro- = /prə/.) precede precise predict prefer prējudge premier /pri-mear/ premiere prepare prēpay presage (v) present (v) preserve preside presume pretend pretense prevail prevent proceed prōcure produce /v/ profane profess profound profuse project (v) prolong promote pronounce propel propose propound protect protest (v) provide provoke purée /pū-rā/ **q** Quebec **r** Racine /rə-sēn/ ragout /rə-gōō/ Rainier /rā-near/ Ravel ravine /rə-vēn/ (Unless marked otherwise, re- = /rĭ/.) rebel (v) rēbirth rēborn rebound rebuff rebuke rebut recall (v) recant rēcap rēcast recede receipt receive recess (v) recite recoil (v) record (v) recount recoup recur redact redeem redound redress (v) reduce refer rēfill (v) refine rēfit reform refund (v) refu_s_e refute regain regale regard regime /ri-_zhēm_/ rēhash (v) rehearse rēheat reject (v) rējoin relapse relate relax release relent relief relieve rēlive rely remain remain_s_ remark rēmatch (v) remind remiss remit remorse remote rēmount (v) remove renege /ri-_nig_/ renew renounce renown repair repast repay repeal repeat repel repent rēphra_s_e replace replete reply report repo_s_e repulse repute request require requite rērun (v) rescind research (v) rēsell rēsend re_s_ent re_s_erve rēset (v) rēship re_s_ide re_s_ign resist re_s_olve re_s_ort re_s_ound resource re_s_ult re_s_ume resurge retail (v) retain rētake (v) retard (v) retire retort rētouch (v) rētry return rēvamp reveal revenge revere /ri-_vear_/ Revere reverse revert review revile revi_s_e revive revoke revolt revolve revue reward rēwind rēwire rēword rēwrite (v) riposte robust ro_s_ette rotund roulette routine /r$\overline{oo}$-_tēn_/ **s** salaam /sə-_läm_/ salon saloon salute saran sarong sashay sateen Satie sauté sauterne savant /sə-_vänt_/ Savoy (se- = /sĭ/) secede secure sedan sedate seduce select señor /sā-_nyor_/ serene severe Seville shebang /shi-_bang_/ Smōlensk snafu soiree /swä-_rā_/ soubrette /s$\overline{oo}$-_bret_/ Spokane /spō-_kan_/ stockade Sudan superb synapse **t** taboo Tibet today to-do Tokay /tō-_kā_/ tonight touché /t$\overline{oo}$-_shā_/ Toulon /t$\overline{oo}$-_lawn_/ Toulouse /t$\overline{oo}$-_l$\overline{oo}$z_/ toupee /t$\overline{oo}$-_pā_/ trapeze travail traverse tureen tycoon typhoon **u** unique unite upon usurp **v** valise /və-_lēs_/ vamoose velure veneer vizier voilà /vwä-_lä_/ voyeur /vwä-_yer_/

VC-V   (In "fizzle" *words treat -_ff_, -_ss_, -_zz_, -_ll_ each as one consonant.)

a acid Adam Adams aloe alum anode arid atoll atom aura avid axis azure **b** baron Becket beckon Bering bevel bevy bezel bigot *billing bishop boron bo_s_om /b$\breve{oo}$z-əm/ bracket Breton brigand British Briton brothel bucket budget bureau /by$\breve{oo}$r-ō/ bushel buxom buzzer **c** cabin Cabot Calais /_kal_-ä/ caller camel canon carat carob carol Carol carom Cary cashew cathode cavern Cecil /_ses_-əl/ chili /_chil_-ē/ *chilling chi_s_el choral chorus civic civics civil Clarence claret clement cleric clo_s_et colic column comet comic conic coral Corinth cou_s_in covet Cracow credit crevice cricket critic Crockett cuckold cudgel cushion cynic Cyril **d** dahlia /_dal_-yə/ damage damask Daniel /_dan_-yəl/ Danube debit decade denim de_s_ert /_dez_-ert/ devil Dicken_s_ digit docile /_dos_-əl/ Doris dozen dragon ducat **e** echo Eden /_ēd_-n/ edit eerie Eire /_air_-ə/ ephor epic epoch era /_ear_-ə/ Erie /_ear_-ē/ Eros etching ethic ethics ethyl Evans ever **f** facet facile failure fairy famine famished fashion fathom feather felon fetching fetid fetish feudal fidget figure finis finish fisher fishy *fizzing flashing flashy flaxen Fleming Flemish fleshy Fletcher flexor flicker flooring flora floral Florence floret florid florist flourish fluky Flushing forest forum foxy fragile freakish freaky freshen frigate frigid frolic frothy furor *fussing **g** gadget gamut gamy garish gather gavel genius /_jēn_-yəs/ gerund given glamour glaring globule glory goner goody gory Gotham Gothic govern granite granule gratis gravel grovel *guessing Guinea /_gin_-ē/ gusher gushy **h** habit hairy harem hashish /_häsh_-ēsh/ hatchet hatching havoc hawkish hazard headed heading hearing heather heaven heavy heifer /_hef_-er/ *hellish helot Helen Hera /_hear_-ə/ herald hero /_hear_-ō/ hickey *hilly *hissing hither hoary hockey homage ~~honest~~ honey ~~honor~~ hooded hoofer hooker hooky Horace Horeb Horus hovel hover *huffing   **i** image itchy   **j** jackal jacket Janet Java *jazzy jealous Jekyll jockey jurist juror jury   **k** karat kepi /kep-ē/ ketchup khaki /kak-ē/ kibitz kicker *killer *killing kitchen ~~knickers~~ knowledge /nol-ij/ **l** lackey larynx /lair-ingks/ lashing lather Latin laughing Laura laurel lavish Lawrence leaden leather leaven lecher ledger leering legate /leg-it/ legend legume lemon Lenin leopard /lep-erd/ leper *lesser levee level lever levy licit licking Lilith lily limit linen lipid liquid /lik-wid/ liquor /lik-er/ lira lithic liver livid living Livy lizard lockage locker locket lodger lodging logic looker loran lover loving lozenge lucky lurid lyric **m** madam magic malice manage manor many /men-ē/ Mary masher mashie Mather matin meadow medal medic mega- melic melon memo memoir /mem-war/ menace menu merit meso- /mes-ə/ meta /met-ə/ metal methane method methyl Mickey midget *miller mimic mini- minion /min-yən/ minute /min-it/ *missing Mitchell mocking model modern modest monarch money /mən-ē/ mono- mooring moral moray mores /mor-āz/ moron mother /muth-er/ mucky mural mushy mythos **n** Natchez nephew Nero /near-ō/ never nickel Nimitz nonage nothing /nəth-ing/ nourish novel novice **o** olive onion onyx oral orange /or-inj/ orate other oven Ovid oxide **p** packer packet packing pageant /paj-ənt/ palace palate /pal-it/ palette panel panic para- parent paring /pair-ing/ Paris parish patchy paten patent peasant pedal pedant penance peril petal Pharaoh /fair-ō/ pheasant Philip phonics phrenic physics picket picking pidgin pigeon /pij-ən/ pinion pitcher pithy pity pivot placard placid placket planet platen pleasant pleasure Pliny plover plucky plural plushy Plymouth pocket polish poly- polyp pomace porous posit potash prairie preface prelude /prel-yood/ premise presage (n) presence present (n) *pressing primer /prim-er/ prison privy process produce (n) product profit project (n) promise proper prophet proverb Proverbs province prudent /prood-nt/ pucker pudgy *puffy pumice punish purist pusher pushy **q** query quicken quiver quorum **r** rabid racket radish rapid raring ratchet rather ration /rash-ən/ ravage ravel ravish *razzing ready rebel (n) reckon record (n) refuge relic relish resin revel Reynolds /ren-əldz/ ribald Richard riches rickets rickey rigid rigor river rivet roaring Robert robin rocker rocket Rockies Rocky Roger *roller *rolling rookie rosin rural rusher **s** salad sapid Sarah satchel satin satire Saturn satyr savage Saviour /sāv-yər/ scarab scary scavenge scholar scourer scouting second *seller *selling semi Semite Senate /sen-it/ senior /sen-yer/ seraph series serum /sear-əm/ seven seventh sever sexy shadow shako Sharon shekel Shepard sheriff shiva shiver shocker shocking shovel shrivel shucking sibyl sicken sicker sickish sinew sketchy slacken slacker slicker slither sliver smacking smashing smidgen smudgy snicker snivel socket /sok-it/ Sodom solace ~~solemn~~ solid sonic sooty sophist sovereign /sov-rən/ Spaniard /span-yerd/ spaniel /span-yəl/ Spanish sparing species spheric spheroid spigot spinach /spin-ich/ spinet /spin-it/ spirit splashy spreader sprocket squalid squalor stacker stalag static statue stature /stach-er/ statute /stach-oot/ steady steerage sterile /ster-əl/ steroid sticker sticky stitching stocking stocky stodgy stolid stomach /stəm-ək/ storage stormy story stretcher stricken study suburb sucker sugar sweater swivel synod syrup **t** tacet tacit tacky talent talon tariff tarot /tar-ō/ Taurus tauten tavern tele- *teller *telling tenant tenet tenor tenure tepid tether thatching thicken thicket thither Thomas /tom-əs/ thorax thorough /ther-ō/ thrasher threaten *thrilling ticker ticket ticking *tiller timid tonic topic Torah Tory touching touchy toughen /tuf-ən/ tourist tragic trashy travel treasure tremor tribune tribute tricky trivet tropic trucker **u** union Ural uric /yŏor-ik/ urine usage usher **v** valance valet /val-ā/ valid valor value valued vanish vapid varied vary veining Venice venom venue very vicar vigil vigor virile /vear-əl/ visage visit vivid vixen vizard voidance volume vomit **w** wacky wagon wary washer washing watcher weapon wearing /wair-ing/ weary /wear-ē/ weather Weber wedgie whacking whether whither wicked wicker wicket widow wiring wiry wither Withers wizard wizen woman /wŏom-ən/ women /wim-in/ woofer woolen wreckage wrecker wrecking wretched **x** Xerox **y** Yemen **z** zealot zealous zephyr zero zither Zurich

VC-V

cockade disarm disown enact foray inane inapt inept inert malaise /mal-āz/ unearth unused upend

V-CCV

April apron biplane Brueghel cobra costar cypress Cyprus Dacron digraph duplex egress egret euchre Euclid febrile fibrous flagrant froufrou hasten hatred Hebrew hubris hybrid hydra hydrant hydro Koblenz Louvre /loo-vr/ lucre /loo-ker/ macron matrix matron measles micro- micron migraine migrant migrate Naples nascent Negro neutral neutron nitrate nitric nitro- ogre /ō-ger/ okra padre /pä-drā/ patron Petrarch pogrom program putrid (re- = /rē/) redress (n) reflex (n) regress (n) reprint (n) retread (n) rewrite (n) rubric sacral sacred sacrum satrap Schweitzer /shvī-tser/ secret stapler sucrose sutra tawdry tigress Tigris triglyph vagrant vibrant vibrate waitress zebra

V-CCV (Keep blends together: a/burped, a/blaze, be/friend, pro/greases, *etc.*)

abrupt ablaze abreast abridge across adrift adroit aflame afloat afraid afresh aghast agree agreed ascend ascent askance askew aslant asleep asperse aspire astern astound astride astute athwart (be- = /bĭ/) befriend begrudge besmear besmirch bestir bestow betray betroth between betwixt Capri /kä-prē/ caprice /kə-prēs/ chablis /shə-blē/ chagrin /shə-grin/ éclair eclipse estate esteem gestalt /gə-shtält/ LaCrosse /lə-craws/ latrine /lə-trēn/ machree Madrid neglect oblige oblique o'clock patrol preclude prōclaim progress (v) prōtract quadrille (Unless otherwise marked, re- = /rĭ/) reclaim recline recruit reflect reflex (v) refract refrain refresh regress (v) regret repress reprieve rēprint (v) reprise reproach reproof reprove respect respire respond response rēstate restore retrace retract rētread (v) retreat retrench retrieve (se- = /sĭ/) seclude secrete sublime supreme

VC-CCV

a Alfred amply André Andrew answer anthrax astral **b** belfry Belgrade bistro bolster Buddha burglar buttress **c** Cambridge cancroid capstan cartridge castrate Castro central centric centrist centrum chancre /shang-ker/ complex (n) Comstock

VC-CCV *continued.*

conclave concrete conflict (n) congress conscious conscience Constance constant contra- contract (n) contrast (n) country Cranston culprit **d** dandruff doctrine Doppler Dunstan **e** Einstein emblem empress entrance (n) entrant escrow estrus **f** Falstaff Flagstad fortress frustrate fulcrum **g** Gandhi gangling /gang-gling/ gantry gastric gentry giggly Gladstone Godfrey **h** hamster Hausfrau /hows-frow/ hipster Holstein holster hombre /om-brä/ hopscotch huckster humdrum Humphrey hundred hundredth hungry /hung-grē/ **i** impress (n) imprint (n) incline (n) increase (n) Indra indrawn ingrate Ingres /an-gr/ ingress ingrown instance instant intra- intrigue (n) intro- istle /is-lē/ **j** Jeffrey juggler **k** kindred **l** lamprey laundress laundry lobster lustrous **m** maestro /mīs-trō/ mandrake mandrill margrave mattress membrane middling misprint (n) mistress mobster mongrel monster muffler Munster **n** Nevski nostril numskull **o** Oersted osprey ostrich **p** paltry pamphlet pantry pastry piddling pilgrim plectrum portrait /por-trit/ poultry prostrate puddling punster **q** quipster **r** rambler rambling rattler rattling Rembrandt Renfrew roadster rostrum **s** saffron sampler sampling Sartre /sar-tr/ scoundrel scraggly scrambler semblance sempre /sem-prä/ sentry settler Siegfried simply Sinclair smuggler smuggling solstice sorghum sparkler sparkling spectral spectrum spinster sprinkler sprinkling squiggly straggly substance suffrage sultry sundry surplus swindler syndrome **t** tangly /tang-glē/ tangram tantrum tattler teamster Telstar template /tem-plit/ tendril tipster Tolstoy transcend trickster Trotsky tumbler tundra **u** Ulster ultra umbra umbrage upgrade (n) upstart (n) upsweep (n) upswing (n) **v** ventral vestry **w** wainwright wastrel Webster wiggler Winston Winthrop wintry worsted wrangler

VC-CCV (Keep blends together.)

a acclaim address (v) afflict affray affront aggrieve applaud applause apply appraise apprise approach approve **c** Champlain complain complete complex (adj) comply compress (v) comprise conclude conflict (v) confront conspire contract (v) contrast (v) contrite contrive control **d** discreet displace display **e** embrace employ enthrone entrance (v) /in-trans/ entrap entrench esprit /es-prē/ **f** forswear **i** imbrue implant implied implode implore imply impress (v) imprint (v) improve incline (v) include increase (v) incrust inflame inflate inflect inflict infract infringe ingrain inspect inspire install instead instep instill intrigue intrude **l** lorgnette /lor-nyet/ **m** maltreat misplace misprint (v) misspell misstep **o** obscene obscure obtrude occlude oppress **p** perplex perspire portray **s** soufflé subtract supplant suppress surprise **t** transpire **u** unclose unclothe unwrap

VCC-CV

a antler Antwerp artful **b** Baldwin bankrupt Bartlett beastly Benchley Bently Bergson Berkshire blintze /blint-sə/ boastful breadthwise Brunswick bumpkin **c** Caldwell chintzy Christmas chutzpah /hoots-pə/ Crompton curtsy **d** dachshund dinghy /ding-gē/ Durkheim **e** earthly Elmhurst empty England /ing-glənd/ English /ing-glish/ **f** Faulkner faultless fistful fondly fondness formless foundling Frankfort Franklin frankly frankness friendly friendship function **g** gantlet /gawnt-lit/ gauntlet gemsbok   ghastly   ghostly   girlhood   Goldberg   guernsey   guiltless   gumption **h** Hampshire Hampton handful handsel handsome Hapsburg hardly hardness hardship harmful harmless Hartford healthful heartless helpful hurtful **i** inkling Ipswich irksome **j** Johnny Johnson jointly juncture **k** kindling kindly kindness kingdom kingly kingship **l** lambda lambkin ländler /lent-ler/ Lardner lastly lengthy /lengk-thē/ Lindbergh Lindsay lustful **m** Mansfield mindful monthly mortgage /mor-gij/ mortmain mostly mournful **o** ointment **p** parchment pardner parsley parsnip partly partner pilsner Piltdown plankton pointless portly postlude Potsdam Priestley pumpkin puncture **r** restful rustler **s** sainthood sanction sanctum Sanctus sandwich scrumptious sculptor sculpture seltzer /selt-ser/ Shanghai /shang-hī/ shortly singsong Springfield startling strengthen /strengk-thən/ Strindberg Stuttgart **t** tactful tankful thankful thirsty Thompson /tomp-sən/ Thursday tincture transfer (n) transport (n) **u** unction **v** vestment Vicksburg **w** warbler Wartburg Westfield westward Whistler windlass Windsor Winslow wistful worldly wouldn't wrestler wrestling wrongful **y** Yorkshire /york-shear/ Yorktown **z** zestful Zwingli /tsving-lē/

VCC-<u>CV</u> transfer (v) transfix transform transfuse translate transmit transmute transport (v)   transpose Transvaal transverse

<u>VCC-CCV</u> (Double blend)   Blitzkrieg Cartwright gangster Hampstead Hempstead Johnston Jungfrau /yoong-frow/ Kingston singspiel songster transplant (n) tungsten Yangtze /yang-tsē/ youngster

VCC-<u>CCV</u>   Montclair   transgress   transplant (v)

<u>VC</u>-CCCV   abstract (n) Bradstreet conscript (n) construct (n) maelstrom /māl-strəm/ minstrel monstrous Sanskrit subscript transcript upstroke

VC-<u>CCCV</u> (Keep clusters together: scr, spl, spr, str.)
abstract (v) abstruse conscript (v) constrain constraint constrict construct (v) construe inscribe instruct obstruct subscribe transcribe unscrew unstrap unstring unstrung

<u>VCC</u>-V christen hadji /haj-ē/ hangar hanger hanging impish kinky longing nursing poignant /poin-yənt/ ranking ringer scorcher seignior /sēn-yer/ singer sinker slangy slinky solder spanking springer springing spunky stinker stringer stringy sunken surfer surfing swinger swinging tangy tankard tanker thinker thinking tinker victual /vit-l/ wolfish wringer yachting /yot-ing/ younger /yung-ger/ youngish /yung-ish/

V-<u>CCCV</u> (Keep cluster together.) ascribe astray bestride prescribe proscribe (re = /rĭ/) restrain restraint restrict

<u>VCCC</u>-CV Ellsworth erstwhile Huntsville marksman Pittsburg Pittsfield Plattsburg Youngstown; **VCC-<u>V</u>** transact vignette /vin-yet/; **<u>V</u>-CCCCV** Nietzsche /nē-chə/

MULTI-SYLLABLE COMPOUND WORDS

a aboveboard afterbirth aftercare afterdeck afterglow afterimage afterlife aftermath afternoon afterpains aftershock aftertaste airsickness allover alongshore alongside altarpiece amidships angelfish angleworm anklebone another anyone anyplace anything anyway anyways anywhere applejack applesauce Appleseed arrowhead **b** backbreaking backhanded backwater baffleplate baggagemaster Bakersfield baldheaded ballcarrier bandmaster bandwagon bantamweight barbershop barehanded bareheaded barelegged barkeeper barleycorn barnstorming bartender basketball battlefield battleship battlewagon beachcomber beaverboard Beaverbrook bedcover bedfellow bedridden bedwarmer beforehand beforetime Bellflower bellyache bellyband bellybutton bittersweet blabbermouth blackberry blameworthy blindstory blockbuster bloodletting bloodmobile bloodthirsty blueberry bluejacket bobbysoxer bodycheck bodyguard bondholder bookbinder bookbinding bookkeeper bookkeeping bookmaker bottleneck brainwashing breadbasket breadwinner breakwater breathless breathtaking brokenhearted bulletproof bullheaded businessman busybody butterball buttercup butterfat butterfingers butterfly buttermilk butternut butterscotch buttonhole bystander **c** cablegram camelhair candleholder candlelight candlepower candlestick candlewick cardplayer caretaker carpetbagger carryall cedarwood centerboard centerpiece chairwoman chambermaid chapelmaster Charlottetown chatterbox checkerboard cheeseburger childbearing choirmaster chokecherry churchgoer cliffhanger clockmaker clodhopper cloverleaf cobblestone coffeepot coldhearted collarbone colorfast comeuppance cornerstone cottonseed cottontail cottonwood countryfolk countryside countyseat coveralls cowpuncher crackerjack crapshooter crosscurrent crossover crybaby customhouse cutaway cutover **d** dairymaid daredevil dogcatcher doodlebug doorkeeper downhearted dragonfly dressmaker dumbwaiter dunderhead **e** easygoing eiderdown elderberry evenhanded evenminded evergreen everlasting everybody everyday everyone everything everywhere evildoer extracurricular extramural extraordinary extraphysical extrasensory extraterritoriality **f** farseeing farsighted fatherland featherbrain feathercut featheredge featherweight ferryboat fiddlesticks figurehead fingerboard fingernail firecracker firefighter firepower firewater flashlight flatiron floorwalker flowerpot flyover flypaper foolhardy footlocker foulmouthed fountainhead fourflusher freehearted freestanding freethinker freewheeling freshwater furthermore furthermost **g** gadabout gatecrasher gatekeeper getaway ghostwriter gingersnap giveaway globetrotter goalkeeper godfather godforsaken goodhearted grandfather grandmother grasshopper gravedigger gunpowder **h** hairdresser hairsplitting halfcocked halfhearted hammerhead handwriting handyman hangover harbormaster hardheaded hardhearted Haymarket hazelnut headmaster headquarters headwaters heartbroken heavyset heavyweight hereafter herringbone heretofore hideaway highflying highhanded highliner hinterland hitchingpost hitherto hobbyhorse holdover hollyhock Hollywood homebody homecoming homemaker honeybee honeydew honeymoon honeysuckle horsepower hotheaded housebroken householder housekeeper housemother housewarming however howsoever hummingbird hushpuppy **i** icebreaker incoming infielder innkeeper ironbound ironclad Ironside Ironwood ironworks **j** jackhammer jawbreaker jellybean jellyfish jerkwater **k** kindhearted knockabout knucklebone **l** laborsaving lackluster ladybug ladyfinger landholder landlady landlubber landowner latecomer lattermost latticework lawabiding lawbreaker lawgiver lawmaker layover leatherneck leftover letterhead letterman levelheaded lifesaver lightheaded lighthearted linebacker Livingstone lopsided lowermost lumberjack **m** manhandle manpower manslaughter Marblehead Maryland mastermind masterpiece masterstroke masterwork matchmaker meadowlark meaningless merrymaking middleman middleweight midsummer midwinter minesweeper mockingbird moneybag moneylender moneymaking moonlighting moreover mortarboard motherland motorbike motorboat motorcycle motorman muddleheaded mudslinger muttonhead muzzleloader **n** nearsighted needlework nevermore nevertheless Newfoundland nightingale nightrider nobody noisemaker notwithstanding nowadays nutcracker **o** Oceanside oftentimes onlooker openhanded openhearted orangewood outdated outdistance outermost outgoing outnumber outpatient outsider outstanding overabundance overactive overcast overcautious overcoat overcompensate overconfidence overcook overdose overdress overdue overhaul overjoyed overheat overload overlook overnight overpass overpopulate overpower overproduction overrate overrule overrun oversee overshadow oversight oversleep overstate overstay overstep oversupply overtake overthrow overtime overturn overwork **p** pacemaker painkiller painstaking panhandler paperback paperhanger paperknife paperweight paperwork Passover pathfinder pawnbroker paymaster peacemaker peashooter penholder peppercorn peppergrass pickpocket pigeonhole piggyback pigheaded pillowcase pilothouse pineapple pinfeather playgoer playwright pocketbook pocketknife policeman policyholder popover porterhouse potbelly potboiler powerhouse praiseworthy pullover pushover **q** quarterback quartermaster quicksilver **r** radarscope radioactive radiobroadcast railroader rainmaker rainwater rattlebrain rattlesnake rattletrap razorback redbaiting redblooded ringleader riverside rollaway roughrider roundabout roustabout rubberneck runaround runaway **s** saddlebag safecracker safekeeping salesperson saltshaker sandpaper sapsucker scaremonger scatterbrain schoolmaster schoolteacher scoutmaster screwdriver scriptwriter seaworthy secondhand selectman shadowbox shantytown sharecropper shareholder sharpshooter sheepherder shipbuilder shipowner shoemaker shopkeeper shoplifter shortcoming shortsighted sidesaddle sidesplitting sidewinder sightseeing silverfish silversmith silverware skydiving skyscraper skywriting slaphappy slaughterhouse slaveholder sleepwalking sleepyhead slipcover slipover slowwitted slumberland snapdragon softhearted somebody songwriter soothsayer sousaphone speakeasy spellbinder spillover sportscaster sportswoman stableboy stationmaster steamfitter steamroller steeplechase steeplejack stepfather stepladder stepmother steppingstone stockbreeder stockbroker stockholder stonecutter stopover storekeeper storybook storyteller stowaway straightaway strawberry strikebreaker stumblebum summerhouse summertime sundial sunflower sunglasses **t** tablecloth tableland tablespoon tableware tailgunner takeover taleteller tarpaper taskmaster tattletale taxicab taxpayer teddybear tenderfoot tenderhearted thanksgiving theatergoer thereabout thereafter thereupon thoroughbred thoroughfare thoroughgoing throwaway thunderbolt thundercloud thunderhead thunderstorm thunderstruck ticktacktoe tidewater tightfisted timberland timesaver tinderbox titleholder toastmaster tomfoolery tommyrot tomorrow toolmaker toothpowder torchbearer towaway townspeople trailblazer trainmaster trelliswork trestlework triggerman troublemaker trustworthy tumbleweed turnabout turnaround turnbuckle turnover turntable turtledove typesetter typewriter **u** underachiever underage underclassman undercover underfed undergraduate underhanded undermine undershirt undershoot undershrub understanding upbringing upcountry upperclassman upriver upstanding uttermost **v** vainglory volleyball **w** wageworker wagonload walkaway wallflower wallpaper wanderlust warmhearted wastebasket wastepaper watchmaker watchtower watercress waterfall Waterford waterfowl waterfront waterlogged watermark watermelon waterpower waterproof watershed watertight Watertown waterway waterworks weathercast weatherproof weightlifter whatever whatsoever wheelbarrow whenever wherewithal whichever whodunit whoever wholehearted whomever whosoever wickerwork wildflower windbreaker windowpane winegrower wintergreen wintertime woebegone wonderland woodcarving woodpecker workaday worktable wraparound wrongdoer **y** yardmaster Yellowstone; <u>See</u>: Ap. iii prefixes **after-, be-, by-, for-, in-, mid-, off-, out-, over-, under-, up-, with-**; Ap. iv suffixes **-burg, -field, -fold, -land, -less, -like, -man, -most, -some, -town, -way, -woman, -work, -worthy, -wright**.

HYPHENATED WORDS (Hyphenated words are often verbs: *"In this situation, he would drop-kick."* But -- *"The drop kick failed."* Hyphenated words also act as adjectives: *"The teen-aged boy fell."* But not as predicate adjectives: *"She is the one who is teen aged."* Hypenated words may also serve as nouns: *battle-ax, by-product,* etc.

a able-bodied about-face about-ship above-cited above-named absent-minded after-dinner air-condition air-cool air-driven air-dry air-filled air-raid shelter all-around all-American all-fired all-out all-purpose all-round all-star at-home ax-hammer **b** baby-sit bachelor's-button ball-and-socket joint Band-Aid bang-up battering-ram battle-ax battle-scarred big-hearted bird-watch black-and-blue blood-red blue-chip blue-collar blue-pencil boom-and-bust brain-injured bread-and-butter breast-feed bringing-up broad-gauge broad-minded broken-down brother-in-law bug-eyed built-in bull's-eye by-path by-product **c** carry-over cast-iron cat's-eye cave-in cell-block chicken-hearted chicken-livered city-bred city-state clean-cut clean-handed clear-cut clear-eyed clear-headed clearing-house clear-sighted close-fisted close-fitting close-lipped close-mouthed cold-blooded color-blind come-as-able coming-out cool-headed cop-out cost-plus cotton-picking country-dance cracker-barrel cross-examine cross-eyed cross-index cross-legged cross-town crow's-feet cure-all custom-built custom-made cut-rate **d** deep-fry deep-rooted deep-sea deep-seated deep-set devil-may-care devil's-food (cake) die-hard dim-out dirt-cheap dog-eared do-gooder do-nothing double-barreled double-breasted double-cross double-date double-dealer double-decker double-edged double-faced double-header double-jointed double-park double-quick double-reed double-stop double-time double-tongue down-bow dressing-down drip-dry drive-in drop-kick dry-eyed duck-footed duty-free dyed-in-the-wool **e** eagle-eyed end-all evil-minded **f** face-off face-saving fact-finding fade-in fade-out fail-safe fair-haired fair-minded fair-trade fair-weather fancy-free far-flung far-off far-out far-reaching father-in-law fat-soluble fighter-bomber fill-in fine-cut fine-grained fine-toothed finger-marked fire-and-brimstone first-born first-class first-hand first-rate five-and-ten-cent store flea-bitten flesh-colored flip-flop fly-by fly-by-night fly-fish follow-up foot-and-mouth disease foot-candle foot-pound force-out fore-and-aft four-bagger four-footed four-leaf clover four-letter word four-masted four-poster fourth-class four-wheel fox-trot frame-up free-and-easy free-for-all free-lance free-throw line freeze-up fresh-air fresh-water front-page full-blooded full-blown full-bodied full-dress full-faced full-fledged full-grown full-length full-scale **g** gentleman-farmer get-up gilt-edged give-and-take go-ahead god-fearing goggle-eyed gold-filled gold-star mother good-by good-fellowship good-for-nothing good-humored good-looking good-natured good-sized good-tempered good-will ambassador goose-step grant-in-aid gray-headed great-granddaughter great-grandfather great-grandmother great-grandson green-eyed grief-stricken ground-hog day gun-shy **h** hail-fellow hair-raiser hair-trigger half-alive half-and-half half-asleep half-baked half-blooded half-breed half-day half-dead half-done half-dozen half-eaten half-full half-hour half-inch half-joking half-length half-mast half-moon half-mile half-open half-serious half-sole half-truth half-wit hand-knit hand-me-down hand-to-hand hand-to-mouth hanger-on happy-go-lucky hard-boiled hard-core hard-fisted hard-nosed hard-shell has-been have-not hawk-eyed head-hunting heal-all heart-rending heart-stricken heart-to-heart heavy-duty heavy-handed heavy-hearted heel-and-toe hell-bent he-man hen-and-chickens hide-and-seek hide-out hi-fi High-Church high-class higher-up high-flown high-grade high-hat high-minded high-muck-a-muck high-necked high-pitched high-pressure high-proof high-rise high-sounding high-spirited high-strung high-tension high-test high-toned high-up high-water mark hit-and-run hit-or-miss hoe-down holier-than-thou hollow-eyed home-brew hook-and-ladder hot-blooded house-raising a fine how-do-you-do hush-hush **i** ice-cold ice-skate ill-advised ill-bred ill-defined ill-fated ill-founded ill-humored ill-kept ill-mannered ill-matched ill-mated ill-natured ill-placed ill-spent ill-starred ill-suited ill-tempered ill-timed ill-treat ill-use ill-wisher in-law **j** jack-in-the-box jack-in-the-pulpit jack-of-all-trades jack-o'-lantern jam-packed jet-black jim-crow laws joint-stock company **k** knee-deep knee-high knife-edge knock-kneed know-how know-it-all know-nothing **l** ladder-back lady's-slipper land-grant land-poor lap-joint latter-day lead-in lean-to leave-taking left-handed leg-of-mutton letter-perfect lickety-split life-sized lighter-than-air light-fingered light-footed light-year like-minded lily-livered lily-of-the-valley lily-white line-up lip-read loan-word long-awaited long-delayed long-distance long-drawn-out long-established long-expected long-forgotten long-held long-kept long-lived long-playing long-range long-standing long-suffering long-term long-time long-winded look-see loose-jointed loose-leaf lotus-eater loud-speaker Low-Church low-down lower-case low-key low-minded low-necked low-pitched low-pressure low-spirited low-test low-water mark **m** machine-gun made-up mail-order house make-believe make-up man-eating man-hating man-hours man-of-war man-sized matter-of-course matter-of-fact mealy-mouthed merry-go-round mid-course mid-life mid-ocean middle-of-the-road milk-white morning-glory moth-ball mother-in-law mother-of-pearl **n** name-dropping narrow-guage narrow-minded native-born ne'er-do-well nerve-racking newly-wed nickel-plate night-light nit-picking north-northeast north-northwest nose-dive no-show no-trump **o** off-Broadway off-color off-stage off-white oil-fueled oil-producing oil-soaked old-fashioned old-line old-style old-time old-timer old-world once-over one-base one-horse one-night stand one-sided one-step one-time one-track one-way on-the-job open-air open-and-shut open-door open-ended open-eyed open-faced open-minded open-mouthed out-and-out out-group out-of-date out-of-doors out-of-the-way **p** part-time pedal-pushers peg-top penny-wise and pound-foolish pent-up pepper-and-salt picked-over pick-me-up pinch-hit pip-squeak pistol-whip pitch-black pitch-dark plain-dealing plain-spoken play-by-play pole-vault poor-spirited Port-au-Prince poverty-stricken print-out punch-drunk push-button push-up put-on **q** quarter-deck quarter-final quarter-hour quick-firing quick-freeze quick-tempered quick-witted **r** rabble-rouser rail-splitter rare-earth element rat-a-tat-tat ready-made ready-mix ready-to-wear ready-witted red-handed red-hot red-letter day right-angled right-handed right-minded right-to-work law ring-necked rip-roaring rock-and-roll rock-bound roller-skate roll-top rose-colored rough-and-ready rough-and-tumble round-bottomed round-faced round-shouldered round-the-clock rubber-stamp run-down run-in runner-up run-of-the-mill run-on run-over **s** safe-conduct safe-deposit box salt-water sand-lot save-all sawed-off saw-toothed say-so scot-free second-best second-class second-guess second-rate second-string self-centered self-confidence self-conscious self-control self-defense self-educated self-employed self-esteem self-evident self-help self-interest self-love self-made self-pity self-reliance self-respect self-sufficient self-taught self-winding Seventy-Six seven-up shaggy-dog story sharp-eyed sharp-sighted sharp-tongued sharp-witted she-wolf shoo-in short-circuit short-cut short-handed short-lived short-tempered short-term shot-put shut-in sight-reading silk-screen silk-stocking silver-tongued simple-minded single-breasted single-handed single-minded sister-in-law sit-down strike sit-in six-shooter skin-deep skin-dive sky-high slack-off slip-on slip-up smack-dab small-minded small-scale smooth-faced smooth-shod smug-faced snow-clad snow-white so-and-so soft-boiled soft-pedal soft-shelled soft-soap son-in-law soul-searching space-time Spanish-American spin-off spoon-fed spread-eagle square-dance square-rigger squint-eyed stage-struck standard-bearer stand-in starry-eyed star-spangled States-General step-down step-in step-up stick-in-the-mud stock-still stone-blind stone-broke storm-swept storm-tossed straight-laced stream-of-consciousness strong-bodied strong-minded strong-smelling strong-spirited strong-willed stuck-up sun-baked sun-bathe sun-dried sun-heated sun-kissed sure-enough sure-fire sure-footed swallow-tailed sway-backed **t** tail-heavy tailor-made take-home pay take-up talking-to tap-dance tear-dimmed tear-filled tear-stained tear-jerker teen-age teen-ager ten-strike theater-in-the-round thick-skinned thick-witted thing-in-itself thin-skinned third-rate thought-out three-base hit three-color three-decker three-mile limit three-phase three-ply three-point landing three-ring circus tie-in tie-up time-consuming time-honored time-lapse time-out time-tested tin-plate to-and-fro tom-tom tone-deaf tongue-and-groove tongue-lashing tongue-tied top-drawer top-dressing top-heavy top-secret touch-and-go touch-me-not tough-minded trade-in tree-covered trigger-happy trouble-shooter true-false tumble-down tune-up Twelfth-day Twelfth-night twenty-one twice-told two-base hit two-bit two-by-four two-cycle two-faced two-edged two-fisted two-handed two-phase two-ply two-spot two-step two-stroke two-time two-way **u** under-expose up-bow up-and-coming up-and-down upside-down up-to-date **v** vest-pocket vice-chairman vice-principal vice-admiralty vice-chancellor vice-consul vice-president vice-regent **w** walk-on wall-eyed war-god warm-blooded wash-and-wear washed-out washed-up waste-water water-resistant water-color water-cool water-repellent water-ski water-soaked water-soluble watt-hour way-out weak-eyed weak-kneed weak-limbed weak-minded weak-voice weak-willed weather-beaten weather-bound weather-strip weather-wise web-footed well-balanced well-being well-bred well-built well-done well-fed well-fixed well-fought well-founded well-groomed well-grounded well-heeled well-intentioned well-kept well-known well-liked well-loved well-made well-mannered well-meaning well-off well-read well-rounded well-spoken well-thought-of well-timed well-to-do well-wisher wet-nurse wheeler-dealer white-collar white-headed white-hot whole-wheat wide-angle lens wide-awake wide-eyed wide-open wide-screen wild-goose chase will-o'-the-wisp wind-blown wind-borne window-dressing window-shopping wind-up wine-colored wine-skin wing-footed winter-feed wire-draw wire-haired terrier with-it wonder-stricken wonder-work wool-dyed world-famous world-renowned worldly-minded worldly-wise world-shaking world-weary worm-eaten worn-out would-be wrap-up write-in write-off write-up wrong-headed **y** yarn-dyed year-round yellow-bellied

"X" DIVIDED BETWEEN SYLLABLES

x = /k-s/, Texas /tek-səs/

anorexia anoxia axiom axon Baxter boxer boxing complexion crucifixion dexter dextrose Drexel epoxy expand execute exegesis exercise exorcise expect expedient expedite expel expend expense experience experiment expert expire explain expletive explicit explode exploit explore explosion exponent export expose expound express expulsion extant extend extension extent exterior external extinct extinguish extort extra extract extraordinary extreme extrinsic fixate foxing flaxen klaxon Luxor Marxist maxim mixer nexus noxious pixy plexus praxis proxy Saxon sexy taxi taxis Texas toxic toxin waxen waxy Xerxes /zerk-sēz/

Sometimes /k-s/ is voiced to /g-z/: exact exaggerate exalted examine example exasperate executive exemplary exempt exhaust exhibit exhilarate exhort exile exist existence exodus exonerate exorbitant inexhaustible exit /eg-zit/ or /ek-sit/

ACCENT SHIFT WORDS (Usually the accent on the first syllable indicates a noun and the accent on the second syllable indicates a verb. "This object is heavy." "I object to that statement." Each of the following words can be pronounced these two ways.)

absent addict address affect attribute augment combat combine commerce commune compact compound compress concert conduct confect conflict conscript consort construct construe content contest contract contrast converse convert convict convoy digest discord discount discourse escort excerpt excise exploit export extract ferment impact import impress imprint incense incline increase incurve indent inlay insert inset insult invert invite misfit misprint object permit pervert prefix premise presage present primer produce progress project protest purport rampage rebel recall recess recoil record redress refill refund regress rehash reject rematch remount reprint rerun research reset retake retouch retread rewrite subject sublease suffix surcharge surmise surname survey suspect transplant transport transfer upgrade uplift upset upstart upsurge upswing upturn

No accent shift: acclaim control comfort command comment compromise concentrate concern consent contact contour corral defeat effect embrace index influence neglect process program prospect recruit regret

Of interest: (Often different meanings.) [s = /z/] abuse (n) abuse (v) agape agape /ä-gä-pā/ August (n) august (adj) busyness business close close console console desert desert dessert deviate /dē-vē-it/ (n) deviate /dē-vē-āt/ (v) entrance entrance /in-trans/ house (n) house (v) inter- inter invalid invalid mama mama minute minute polish /pol-ish/ Polish /pō-lish/ ravel Ravel really re-ally recreate re-create refuse refuse re-sign resign resume résumé sake sake /sä-kē/ salve salve /sal-vē/ (L. *Hail!*) use (n) use (v)

Some noun and verb pairs have different forms: constrain (v) constraint (n); constrict (v) constriction (n); contain (v) container (n); retain (v) retention (n); *etc.*

SILENT "E" IN BASE WORD (Divide between base word and suffix: *age/less* . Note that all the suffixes here begin with a consonant.)

ageless barely basement boneless careful careless casement comely cuteness dateless direly direness dukedom faceless fateful finely fineness gameness hateful homeward hopeful hopeless lamely lameness lately lateness lifeless likely likeness lonely lovely loveless merely movement nameless namely nicely nineteen Norseman oneness paleness pavement peaceful placement purely rarely Rhineland ripeness rudely safely safety sameness sanely scarcely senseless sorely soreness spiteful squarely statement stalemate stately surely sureness tamely timeless timely tireless tubeless tuneful useful useless vengeful viceroy vileness voiceless wakeful wasteful widely wireless wisely (**Note:** When adding a suffix beginning with a vowel, the "e" is dropped. Review Rule #14, page 17 in Chapter 1.)

SYLLABLES WITH NO OR EQUAL ACCENT

thirteen fourteen fifteen sixteen eighteen nineteen; amen emcee (M.C.) nonstop upstate upstream uptight uptown; carte blanche /kärt bländsh/ (F); Yalu (River in N. Korea); Japanese: Kyoto /kyō-tō/ Meiji /mā-jē/ Nisei /nē-sā/ Sansei /sän-sā/ Tojo /tō-jō/

LET'S DO THE BIG ONES!

18 Letter Words

anthropomorphizing
commercializations
constitutionalisms
counterrevolutions
denationalizations
electrocardiograms
extemporaneousness
hydroelectricities
impracticabilities
inconsequentiality
indiscriminatingly
interchangeability
internationalities
irresponsibilities
monochromaticities
oversimplification
photolithographies
proletarianization
representativeness
subclassifications
transcendentalisms
ultraconservatives

autobiographically
compartmentalizing
constitutionalists
decriminalizations
disenfranchisement
electrocardiograph
extraterritorially
hypersensitivities
inappreciativeness
inconsiderableness
individualizations
intercommunicating
interrelationships
maladministrations
noncooperationists
particularizations
photolithographing
psychoanalytically
roentgenologically
tachistoscopically
transcendentalists
ultranationalistic

bureaucratizations
comprehensibleness
contradistinctions
dematerializations
disproportionately
establishmentarian
fractionalizations
impersonalizations
incommensurability
indestructibleness
industrializations
intercommunication
irreconcilableness
misinterpretations
noninterventionist
phenomenologically
photosynthetically
psychopathological
semiprofessionally
telecommunications
transubstantiating
unconscionableness

characteristically
congregationalists
conversationalists
demythologizations
distinguishability
evapotranspiration
gastroenterologist
imperturbabilities
inconceivabilities
indiscriminateness
institutionalizing
internationalizing
irreproachableness
misrepresentations
overcapitalization
photolithographers
photosensitivities
psychopathologists
sentimentalization
territorialization
transubstantiation
unconstitutionally

19 Letter Words

anthropomorphically
constitutionalities
counterintelligence
electrocardiographs
establishmentarians
gastroenterologists
indestructibilities
intercommuications
multidimensionality
parthenogenetically
representationalist
transubstantiations

chromatographically
contemporaneousness
departmentalization
electrocardiography
evapotranspirations
historiographically
individualistically
interdenominational
noninterventionists
phenomenalistically
sentimentalizations
unconstitutionality

cinematographically
contradistinctively
disadvantageousness
electromagnetically
expressionistically
incomprehensibility
intellectualization
interdepartmentally
overcapitalizations
photoconductivities
straightforwardness
unexceptionableness

circumstantialities
conventionalization
disenfranchisements
electromechanically
extraterritoriality
incompressibilities
interchangeableness
irreconcilabilities
oversimplifications
representationalism
territorializations
unintelligibilities

20 Letter Words

antiauthoritarianism · compartmentalization · conventionalizations · counterrevolutionary
counterrevolutionist · departmentalizations · electrocardiographic · existentialistically
incommensurabilities · incomprehensibleness · indistinguishability · institutionalization
intellectualizations · internationalization · microminiaturization · noninterventionalist
representationalisms · representationalists · ultraminiaturization · uncharacteristically

21 Letter Words

compartmentalizations · counterrevolutionists · electroencephalograms
electroencephalograph · electroencephaloscope · establishmentarianism
incomprehensibilities · indistinguishableness · ultraminiaturizations

22 Letter Words

counterrevolutionaries · electroencephalographs · electroencephalography
electroencephaloscopes · establishmentarianisms · interdenominationalism

24 Letter Word

electrocardiographically

28 Letter Word

antidisestablishmentarianism

Syllable Written without a Vowel but Pronounced with a Vowel

rhythm (rhyth/m) /r<u>ith</u>-əm/

-asm (as/m) **words:** chasm /<u>ka</u>-zəm/ enthusiasm /in-<u>th</u>o͞o-ze̅-az-əm/ sarcasm /<u>sar</u>-kaz-əm/
spasm /<u>spaz</u>-əm/;   See: Ap. iv-54

-ism (is/m) **words:** capitalism /<u>cap</u>-ə-təl-iz-əm/ communism /<u>com</u>-yə-niz-əm/ dualism
fascism /<u>fash</u>-iz-əm/   idealism /i-<u>de̅l</u>-iz-əm/   socialism /<u>so̅</u>-shəl-iz-əm/;   See: Ap. iv-37, 56

Syllable Written with a Vowel which is not Pronounced

acquittal /ə-<u>kwit</u>-l/ bitten /<u>bit</u>-n/ blatant /<u>bla̅t</u>-nt/ bridal /<u>bri̅d</u>-l/ broaden /<u>brawd</u>-n/ brutal /<u>bro͞ot</u>-l/
cadence /<u>ca̅d</u>-ns/ chattel /<u>chat</u>-l/ combatant /kəm-<u>bat</u>-nt/ committal /kə-<u>mit</u>-l/ deaden /<u>ded</u>-n/
decadent /di-<u>ca̅d</u>-nt/ disputant /dis-<u>pyo͞ot</u>-nt/ eaten /<u>e̅t</u>-n/ Eden /<u>e̅d</u>-n/ enlighten /in-<u>li̅t</u>-n/
fatal /<u>fa̅t</u>-l/ fetal /<u>fe̅t</u>-l/ flatten /<u>flat</u>-n/ forgotten /for-<u>got</u>-n/ frighten /<u>fri̅t</u>-n/ gotten /<u>got</u>-n/
heighten /<u>hi̅t</u>-n/ hidden /<u>hid</u>-n/ impedance /im-<u>ped</u>-ns/ kitten /<u>hid</u>-n/ laden /<u>la̅d</u>-n/ Latin /<u>lat</u>-n/
leaden /<u>led</u>-n/ lighten /<u>li̅t</u>-n/ maiden /<u>ma̅d</u>-n/ Manhattan /man-<u>hat</u>-n/ medal /<u>med</u>-l/ metal
/<u>met</u>-l/ mitten /<u>mit</u>-n/ modal /<u>mod</u>-l/ model /<u>mod</u>-l/ mutant /<u>myo͞ot</u>-nt/ natal /<u>na̅t</u>-l/ patent
/<u>pat</u>-nt/ pedal /<u>ped</u>-l/ pedant /<u>ped</u>-nt/ petal /<u>pet</u>-l/ platen /<u>plat</u>-n/ pollutant /pə-<u>lo͞ot</u>-nt/
prudence /<u>pro͞od</u>-ns/ rebuttal /ri-<u>but</u>-l/ recital /ri-<u>ci̅t</u>-l/ remittance /ri-<u>mit</u>-ns/ remodel /re̅-<u>mod</u>-l/
rodent /<u>rod</u>-nt/ rotten /<u>rot</u>-n/ sadden /<u>sad</u>-n/ Satan /<u>sa̅t</u>-n/ Staten /<u>stat</u>-n/ straighten /<u>stra̅t</u>-n/
strident /<u>strid</u>-nt/ strudel /<u>stro͞od</u>-l/ sudden /<u>sud</u>-n/ Sweden /<u>swe̅d</u>-n/ threaten /<u>thret</u>-n/
Tibetan /ti-<u>bet</u>-n/ tidal /<u>ti̅d</u>-l/ tighten /<u>ti̅t</u>-n/ total /<u>to̅t</u>-l/ vital /<u>vi̅t</u>-l/ widen /<u>wi̅d</u>-n/ written
/<u>rit</u>-n/ yodel /<u>yo̅d</u>-l/;   Note: This vowel dropping occurs most often when an accented syllable
ending with a **t** or **d** is followed by a *vowel-l* or *vowel-n* syllable. This is because /t/, /d/, /l/, and
/n/ are all pronounced with the tongue in approximately the same position.

Old English Prefixes

a-, after-, al(l)-, be-, by-, for-, fore-, in-, ... Ap.iii- 2

mid-, mis-, off-, out-, over-, step-, ... Ap.iii- 3

twi-, un- (not), ... Ap.iii- 4

un- (back), **under-, up-, with-, yester-,** . . . . Ap.iii- 5

Latin Prefixes

ab-, ad- *[ac-, af-, ag-, al-, an-, ap-, ar-, as-, at-],* . . . . . . Ap.iii- 6

ambi-, ante-, bi-, centi- (100), **circum-, cis-,** . . . . . . Ap.iii- 7

com- *[co-, col-, con-, cor-],* . . . . Ap.iii- 8

contra-, de-, ... Ap.iii- 9

dec- (10), **deci-, dis-** *[dif-, di-],* Ap.iii-10

duo- (2), **ex-** *[ef-, e-],* Ap.iii-11

extra-, in- (not) *[il-, im-, ir-, i-],* Ap.iii-12

in- (in) *[il-, im-, ir-],* Ap.iii-13

infra-, inter-, intra-, intro-, juxta-, milli-, multi-, non-, nov- (9), Ap.iii-15

ob *[oc-, of-, o-, op-],* **oct-** (8), **per-, post-,** Ap.iii-16

pre-, pro-, ... Ap.iii-17

quad- (4), **quasi-, quint-** (5), **re-,** Ap.iii-18

retro-, se-, semi-, sept- (7), **sex-** (6), **sub-** *[suc-, suf-, sug-, sum-* Ap.iii-20

sup-, sur-, sus-], **super-, supra-, trans-, tri-** (3), ... Ap.iii-21

ultra-, uni- (1), **vice-,** Ap.iii-22

Greek Prefixes

a-, amphi-, ana-, anti-, ... Ap.iii-22

apo- cata-, cath-, deca- (10), **di-** (2), **dia-, dys-,** Ap.iii-23

ecto-, en- *[el-, em-, er-],* **endo-, ennea-** (9), **epi-,** Ap.iii-23

eu-, ex-, hecto- (100), **hemi-, hepta-** (7), **hexa-** (6), ... Ap.iii-24

hyper-, hypo-, kilo- (1,000), **meso-, meta-, mono-** (1), . . . Ap.iii-24

neo-, octo- (8), **para-, penta-** (5), **peri-,** Ap.iii-25

pro-, syn- *[syl-, sym-, sys-],* **tetra-** (4), **tri-** (3), ... Ap.iii-25

Other Prefixes

en- *[em],* **counter-, mis-, sur-** Ap.iii-26

Appendix iii A Good Beginning (Prefixes)

Old English Prefixes

a- /ə/ abeam abide ablaze aboard about abreast abroad adrift afar afield afire aflame afloat afoot afore afoul afresh aghast agleam ago aground ahead akin alight alike alive along amaze amid amiss anew aright arise asea ashamed ashore aside askance askew aslant asleep aslope asleep astern (O.N.) astir asunder athirst atilt atop awake aware awash away aweary aweigh awhile awoke awry

after- afterbirth afterbrain afterburner aftercare afterglow afterlife afternoon aftertaste afterthought afterward afterworld

al(l)- all-fired allheal all-out allover all-star almighty almost already all right *(Alright* is incorrect.*)* also although altho altogether always

be- /bi/ (unaccented) becalm became because becloud become becoming bedazzle bedeck bedevil bedraggle befall befit befitting before befoul befriend beget begird begone begot begotten behalf behave behavior behead beheld behind behold beholden behoove belabor belated beleaguer belie belief believe belong belonging beloved below bemean bemoan bemuse bemused benumb bereave beseech beseem beset beside besides besmear besmirch besot besought bespeak bespread besprinkle bestow bestraddle bestrew bestride bethink betide betimes betoken betook betray betroth between betwixt beware bewilder bewitch beyond

by- /bī/ bygone bylaw by-pass by-path by-play by-product byroad bystander bystreet bytalk byway byword bywork

for- (away; off; very) forbear forbearance forbid forbidden forever forgave forget forgive forgot forsooth forswear forward

fore- (in front of) forearm forebear forebode forebrain foredoom forefather forefinger forefoot foreglimpse forego foregoing foregone foreground forehand forehead foreknowledge foreleg forelock foreman foremast foremost forename forenoon forerunner foresaid foresail foresee foreshadow foresheet foreshorten foreshow foreside foresight foresighted forestall foretell forethought foretooth forewarn foreword; Also applied to words from Latin: foreclose foreclosure forefront

in- (in) inbeing inboard inborn inbound inbreed inbred inbreeding inburst income incoming indeed indent indoor indoors indraft indrawn indwell infield infielder inflow ingoing ingrown inlaid inland in-law inlay inlet inmate inmost innards inner innermost inning input inroad inset insheathe inshore inside insider insight instead instep insure intake into inwall inward inwards;   See: Latin prefix **in-** in Ap. iii-12,13.

mid- (middle point) midbrain midday middle middy mid-field mid-flight midiron midland Midland Midlands midmost midnight midnoon midrib midriff midship midshipman midships midspring midst midsummer midtown midwatch midway midweek Midwest midwife *("With woman.")* midwinter midyear; <u>With words from Latin</u>: midair midautumn mid-January (et al.) mid-ocean midpoint midriver midsentence midstory midterm

mis- (wrong) misbegotten misbehave misbelief misbrand miscall miscast misdeal misdeed misdo misfire misfit misgiving mishandle mishap mishear mislay mislead mislike mismatch mismate misname misplay misread misreckon missay misshape misshapen misspeak misspell misspend misstep mistake mistaken misthink mistime mistrust misunderstand misunderstanding misword miswrite; [Note: *call, cast, hap, take* & *trust* are Old Norse words. *Spell* is Old French.] <u>See</u>: **mis-** in Other Prefixes.

off- offbeat off-color offhand offish offset offshoot offshore offside offspring off-white

out- outback outbid outboard outbreak outbreed outbuilding outburst outcome outcrop outdo outdone outdoor outdoors outfield outfielder outfit outflow outfoot outfox outgo outgoing outgrow outgrowth outguess outgush outhouse outland outlandish outlast outlaw outlay outlet outline outlive outlook outlying outman outplay outpost outpour outpull output outrage outreach outride outrider outright outroot outrun outsell outset outshine outshoot outside outsider outsit outsmart outspeak outspoken outspread outstanding outstretch outstrip outtell outturn outward outwear outweigh outwit outwork outworn; <u>Also applied to words from Latin</u>: outclass outcry outdated outdistance outmoded outnumber outpost

over- overall overalls overarm overbearing overbid overbite overblow overblown overboard overbuild overburden overcloud overcome overcrop overdo overdraft overdrawn overdrive overeat overflight overflow overgrow overgrowth overhand overhang overhead overhear overheat overkill overlade overlain overland overlap overlay overleap overlie overlive overload overlook overlord overman overmatch overmuch overnight overplay overreach override overrun oversanded overscore overseas oversee overseer oversell overset oversew overshade overshadow overshine overshoe overshoot overshot oversight oversleep oversoul overspend overspread overstep overstrung overtake overthrow overtime overturn overwatch overwear overweening overweigh overweight overwhelm overwhelming overwind overword overwork overwrite overwrought; <u>Also applied to words from Latin</u>: overact overage overarch overbalance overcapitalize overcompensate overcompensation overdue overestimate overexpose overissue overpass overpay overpopulate overpower overpowering overprice overprint overprize overproduce overproduction overprotect overrate overrule oversexed oversigned oversize overspend overstay oversupply overtax overtrick overtrump overturn

step- (related by a previous marriage) stepbrother stepchild stepdaughter stepfather stepmother stepsister stepson

twi- (two, double) /twī/ twibil   twice   twice-laid   twice-told   twilight   twine; /twi/ twill *(a weave)* twin   twin bed   twinberry   twinborn   Twin Cities   twinflower   twin-leaf   twist;   Also from **twi-:** twain   two   two-bits   two-by-four   two-cycle   two-edged two-faced twofer (Sl.) two-fisted twofold two-handed twopence twopenny two-phase two-ply twosome two-spot two-step two-stroke two-time two-way

un-[1] (not) [adjectives & nouns]   unaware   unawares   unbacked   unbaked   unbeaten unbecoming unbeknown unbelief unbeliever unbending unbidden unblessed unbloody unblushing   unbodied   unborn   unbound   unbounded   unbowed   unbred   unbridled unbroken uncaged uncalled uncanny uncared-for unchurched unclad unclean uncouth uncut undoing undone undreamed-of undying unearned unearthly uneven unfair unfeeling unfit unforgettable unfriendly ungodly unhallowed unhandy unhappy (O.N.) unhealthy unheard-of unholy unhoped-for unhurried unkempt unkind unknowable unknown unlaid unlawful unleaded unlearned unlike unlikely unlooked-for unlovely unlucky (M.Du.) unmanly unmanned unmarked unmeaning unmindful unreadable unready unrest unrighteous unripe unsaid unseemly unseen unselfish unsettled unshakable unshaken unsightly unskilled (O.N.) unsmiling (M.E.) unsound unsparing unspeakable unspotted unsteady unstopped unstrung unsung untalked-of untaught unthankful unthinking unthought-of untidy untimely untold untoward untrue untrustworthy untruth untruthful unutterable unwearied unwelcome unwell unwholesome unwieldy unwilling unwise unwitting unworldly unworthy unwound unwritten;   Exception: unless [conj., prep.] *("On less.")*

----This prefix was later freely applied to Old & Middle French words coming from Latin: unable unabridged   unaccompanied   unaccountable   unaccounted-for   unaccustomed unaffected   unappealable   unapproachable   unargued   unarmed   unassailable unassisted   unassuming   unattended   unavoidable   unbalanced   unceremonious uncharitable   unchristian (Gk.)   uncircumcised   uncivilized   uncomfortable uncommercial   uncommitted   uncommon   uncommunicative   uncompromising unconcerned   unconditional   unconformity   unconscionable   unconscious unconsolidated   unconstitutional   uncontrollable   unconventional   unconverted uncounted   uncovered   undeceived   undecided   undemonstrative   undeniable undesirable   undirected   undoubted   undressed   uneasy   uneducated   unemployed unequal   unequivocal   uneventful   unexceptional   unexpected   unexpressive unfailing unfaithful unfamiliar unfavorable unfinished unfortunate unfounded unfrequented unfruitful   ungainly   ungenerous   ungovernable   ungracious   ungrammatical ungrateful   unimpeachable   unimportant   unimproved   unintelligent   uninterested unjust   unlabored   unleavened   unlettered   unlimited   unmentionable   unmerciful unmitigated   unmodulated   unnatural   unnecessary   unnumbered   unoccupied unofficial   unorganized (Gk.)   unorthodox (Gk.)   unpaid   unparalleled (Gk.)   unpeopled unperforated unpleasant unpopular unpracticed (Gk.) unprecedented unprejudiced unpremeditated unprepared unprincipled unprintable unproductive unprofessional unprofitable   unpronounceable   unprovided   unqualified   unquestionable   unreal unreason   unreasonable   unrelenting   unreliable   unremitting   unreserved unresponsive unrestrained unrivaled unruly unsanitary unsatisfied unsaturated unscrupulous unseasonable unseasoned unsocial unsophisticated (Gk.) unspecialized unstable unstudied unsuccessful unsuitable unsuspecting untenable untitled untouchable untraveled untried untutored unused unusual unwarranted

un-[2] (back) [verbs] unbelt unbend unbind unbolt unbuild unburden unbutton uncap unchurch unclasp unclench unclothe uncock undo undraw unearth unfasten unfold ungird unhand unhinge unhitch unhook unknit unlade unlatch unlay unlead unlearn unload unlock unmake unmask (Ar.) unmoor unpack unpeg unpin unravel (M.Du.) unreel unsaddle unscramble (Du.) unseat (O.N.) unsettle unshackle unship unsling unsnap (Du.) unsnarl unstop unstrap unstring untangle (Scan.) unteach unthread untie untwine untwist unwind unwrap unwrinkle unyoke; <u>From Latin:</u> unbalance uncouple unclose uncover undouble undress unfurl unharness unlace unleash unnerve unroll unscrew unseal unveil

under- underarm underbelly underbid underbrush underbuy underclothes undercut underdo underdog underdone underdrain underdrive underfeed underfoot undergird undergo underground undergrowth underhand underhanded underlaid underlay underline underlying undermost underneath underpin underpinning underrun underscore undersea undersell undersheriff undershirt undershoot underside understand understanding understood undertake undertaker undertaking undertow underwaist underwater underway underwear underweight underwent underworld underwrite underwriter; <u>This prefix is also applied to Latin based words:</u> undercarriage undercharge underclass undercurrent underemployed underestimate underexpose undergraduate undernourish underpass underpay underprivileged underproduction underrate undersecretary undersigned undersoil understate understudy undertrick undervalue undervest

up- upbeat up-bow upbraid upbringing updraft upend upgrowth upheaval upheld uphill uphold upholster upkeep upland uplift upmost upon upper uppish upright uprise uprising uproar uproot upset upshot upside upstairs upstanding upstart upstream upstretched upstroke upsweep upswell upswing uptake upthrow uptight upto uptown uptrend upturn upward; <u>With Latin:</u> upcountry update upgrade upper-bracket upper-case upperclassman uppermost upriver upstage upstate upsurge

with- withal withdraw withdrawal withdrawn withhold within with-it without withstand

yester- (the period before) yesterday yesterevening yestermorning yesternight yesternoon yesterweek yesteryear

Latin Prefixes

ab- (away, off) abdicate abducent abduct abduction aberrant aberration abfarad abhenry abhor abhorrent abirritant abject abjure ablation ablative ablegate ablution abnegate abnormal abominate abomination aboriginal aborigine abort abortion abound abrade abrasion abrogate abrupt abscess abscissa abscission abscond absence absent absolute absolution absolve absorb absorbent absorption abstain abstemious abstention abstinence abstract abstraction abstruse absurd absurdity abundant abuse abusive; Also from *ab-* : ament amentia amotion

ad- (to, toward, near) A Chameleon Prefix changing to *a-, ac-, af-, ag-, al-, an-, ap-, ar-, as-* & *at-* depending on its environment. **ad/a-** adage adapt adaptable adaptation adaptive; **a/b-** abase abasement abate abatement abeyance abridge abridgment **ab/b-** abbreviate; **ac/c-** accede accelerate accelerator accent accentuate accept acceptable access accessible accident accidental acclaim acclamation acclivity accolade accommodate accommodation accompany accomplish accomplishment accord according accost account accountable accredit accreditation accrescent accretion accrual accrue accumbent accumulate accuracy accurate accusation accuse accustom; **ad/d-** add addendum addict addiction addition address adduce adduct adductor; **ad/e-** adeem adept adequate ad extremum; **af/f-** affable affair affect affection affectionate afferent affiance affidavit affiliate affiliation affined affinity affirm affirmation affirmative affix afflatus afflict affliction affluence affluent afflux afforest affricative affront affusion; **ag/g-** agglomerate agglutinant agglutination aggrade aggrandize aggravate aggravation aggregate aggress aggression aggressive aggrieve; **a/g-** agist agnomen agree agreeable agreement; **ad/h-** adhere adherent adhesion adhesive adhibit ad hoc ad hominem; **ad/i** adit ad infinitum ad initium ad interim; **ad/j-** adjacent adjective adjoin adjoining adjourn adjudge adjudicate adjunct adjure adjust adjustment adjutant adjuvant; **al/l-** allegation allege allegedly alleviate alliance allied alliteration allocate allocation allow allowance alloy allude allusion alluvial ally; **a/l-** align alignment; **ad/l-** ad-lib ad libitum; **ad/m-** admeasure adminicle administer administration admirable admiration admire admission admit admittance admix admixture admonish admonition; **a/m-** amass ameliorate amenable amoritize amount amuse amusement; **an/n-** annex annexation annihilate annihilation annotate announce announcement annul annulment annunciation Annunciation; **ad/n-** adnate ad nauseam adnoun; **ad/o-** adolescence adolescent adopt adoption adorable adoration adore adorn adornment; **ap/p-** appall appalling appanage apparatus apparel apparent apparently apparition appeal appear appearance appease appeasement appellant appellate appellation appellee appellor append appendage appendix apperceive appertain appetite appetizer appetizing applaud applause appliance applicable application applied apply appoint appointee appointment apportion apportionment apposable appose apposition appositive appraisal appraise appreciate appreciation apprehend apprehension apprentice apprise approach approbation appropriate approval approve approximate appurtenance; **ac/q-** acquaint acquaintance acquiesce acquiescence acquire acquisition acquit acquittal;

ar/r- arraign arraignment arrange (Ger.) arrangement array (Ger.) arrest arrears arrival arrive arrogance arrogant arrogate; **ad/r-** ad rem adrenal adroit; **as/s-** assail assailant assault assemble assembly assent assert assertion assertive assess assessment assets assiduous assign assignment assimilate assimilation assist assistance assistant assize associate association assonance assort assortment assuage assume assumption assurance assure assured assurgent; **ad/s-** adsorb adsorption adsum; **a/sc-** ascend ascension ascent ascertain ascribe ascription; **a/sp-** aspect asperse aspersion aspirant aspirator aspire; **a/st-** astrictive astringe astringent; **at/t** attach (Ger.) attachment attack (Ger.) attain attainment attaint attempt attend attendance attention attentive attenuate attenuation attest attestation attire (O.F.) attitude (From *aptitude*.) attorney attract attraction attractive attribute attribution attrition attune; **ad/u-** adult adulate adulation adulterate adulterer adulteress adumbrate adunc adust; **ad/v-** advection advent Advent adventitious adventure adventurous adverb adversary adverse adversity advert advertise advertisement advice advisable advise adviser advisory advocacy advocate; **a/v-** avail available avalanche avaunt avenge avenue aver averse aversion avert avouch avow avowal avulsion

ambi- (both) ambidextrous ambience ambiance (F) ambient ambiguity ambiguous ambition ambitious ambivalent amputate amputee

ante- (before) ante-bellum antecedent antechamber antedate antediluvian ante meridian (A.M.) ante mortem antenatal antepast antepenult anterior anteroom; Also from *ante-* : ancestor ancient antiquarian antiquate antiquated antique

bi- /bī/ (two) biangular biannual *(Two times a year.)* biauricular biaxial bicameral bicapsular bicarbonate bicentennial biceps bicipital bicolor biconcave biconvex bicorn bicorporal bicultural bicuspid bidentate biennial *(Every two years.)* bifacial bifid bifilar biflex bifocal bifocals bifold bifoliate biform bifurcate bihourly bijugate bilabial bilateral bilinear bilingual biliteral bilobate bilocular bimanous bimanual bimensal bimestrial bimolecular bimonthly (O.E.) bimotored binal binary binate binaural *(bin- variation of bi-)* binocular binomial binucleate biocellate biparietal biparous bipartisan bipartite biped bipinnate biplane bipolar bipropellant biquadrate biquarterly biradial bireme biscuit *(bis- variation of bi-)* bisect bisector biserrate bisexual bissextile bisulcate bisulfate bivalent bivalve biweekly (O.E.) biyearly (O.E.); Base word from Greek: bicephalous bichloride bicycle bigamist bimetalism bipod bisymmetrical bitartrate

centi- (one hundred) centigrade centimo centipede; Base word from Greek: centigram centiliter centimeter centimeter-gram-second centistere; See: **centum** Ap. vii-6.

circum- (around) circumambient circumambulate circumcise circumference circumflex circumfluous circumlocution circumnavigate circumrotate circumscribe circumspect circumstance circumstantial circumvent

cis- (on this side of) cisalpine Cisalpine Gaul cisatlantic cislunar cismontane cispadane

com- (with, together) A <u>Chameleon Prefix</u> changing to *co-, col-, con-* or *cor-* depending on its environment. **co/a-** coadjutant coadjutor coadunate coagulable coagulant coagulate coalesce coalition coarctate coaxial cobelligerent; **com/b-** combat combatant combination combine combo combustion; **con/c-** concatenate concave conceal concealment concede conceit conceited conceive concentrate concentration concentric concept conception conceptual concern concerned concert concession concise conclave conclude conclusion concoct concoction concomitant concord concordance concourse concrete concubine concur concurrent concussion; **co/c-** coconscious; **con/d-** condemn condemnation condensation condense condescend condescending condition conditional condolence condominium condone conducive conduct conduction conductor conduit; **co/e-** coed coeducation coefficient coempt coemption coequal coerce coercion coercive coessential coetaneous coeternal coeternity coeval coexist coexistence coextend coextensive; **con/f-** confab confabulate confection confectionery confederacy Confederacy confer conference confess confession confidant confide confidence confidential configuration confine confinement confirm confirmation confiscate conflagration conflation conflict confluence conform conformation conformity confound confounded confraternity confront confrontation confuse confusion confutation confute; **com/f-** comfort comfortable; **con/g-** congeal congenial congenital congest congestion conglomerate conglomeration conglutinate congratulate congratulations congregate congregation congress Congress congressional congruence congruent; **co/g-** cogitate cogitation; **co/gn-** cognate cognation cognition cognitive cognizable cognizance cognize cognomen cognoscente cognoscible cognovit; **co/h-** cohabit cohere coherence coherent cohere cohesion cohesive; **co/i-** coincide coincidence coition; **com/i-** comitia; **con/j-** conjecture conjoin conjoint conjugal conjugate conjunction conjunctivitis conjuncture conjuration conjure; **col/l-** collaborate collapse collate collateral collation colleague collect collection collective college collegian collide colligate collimate collinear collision collocate collogue colloquial colloquialism collude collusion; **co/l-** colatitude; **com/m-** command commander commando commemorate commemoration commence commend commendation commensal commensurate comment commentary commerce commercial commination commingle (O.E.) commiserate commissar (Rus.) commissary commission commissure commit commitment committee commixture commode commodious commodity commodore (Du.) <u>common</u> (commonality, commoner, commonly, commonplace, commons, communal, commune, communicable, communicate, communication, communicative, communion, communiqué, communism, communist community) commotion commutation commutative commute commuter; **con/n-** connate connatural connect connection connivance connive connoisseur (F.) connotation connote connubial; **co/o-** cooperate cooperation co-opt coordinate copartner coordination; **com/p-** compact companion company comparative compare comparison compartment compass compassion compassionate compatible compatriot compeer compel compendium compensate compensation compete competence competent competition competitive compilation compile complacent complain complaint complaisant complected complement complete completion complex complexion complexity compliance complicate complicated complication complicity compliment comply component comportment compose composer composite composition compost composure compote compound comprehend comprehension compress comprise compromise compulsion compulsive compunction computation compute computer; **con/qu-** conquer conqueror conquest conquistador (Sp.); **cor/r-** corrade correct correction correlate correlation correspond correspondence correspondent corridor corrigendum corrigible corroborate corroboration corrode corrosion corrosive corrugate corrupt corruptible corruption; **con/s-** consanguinity conscience conscientious conscious consciousness conscript conscription consecrate consecration consecutive consensual consensus consent consequence conservation conservatory conserve consider consignment consist consolation console consolidate consonance consonant consortium conspicuous conspiracy conspire constable constant constellation consternation constipation constitute constitution constraint constrict constriction construct construction construe consubstantial consuetude consume consumer consummate consumption; **co/s-** cosecant cosign costar (O.E.); **con/t-** contact contagious contain container contaminate contamination contemplate contemplation contemporaneous contemporary contempt contemptible contend content contention contentment contest contestant context contiguity contiguous continence continent continental contingency contingent continual continuation continue continuity continuous continuum contortion contortionist contour contract contraction contractor contractual contribute contribution contrite contrition contrivance contrive contusion; **co/t-** cotangent cotenant; **con/v-** convalesce convalescent convection convene convenience convenient convent convention conventional converge convergence conversant conversation converse conversion convert convertible convex convey conveyance conveyer convict conviction convince convincing convivial convocation convoke convolution convoy convulse convulsion convulsive; **co/v-** covalence covenant cover; **co/w-** co-worker (O.E.)

contra- (against, opposite, contrary) contraband contrabass contrabassoon contraception contraclockwise contradict contradiction contradistinction contraindicate contralto contraposition contrapuntal contrariety contrary contrast contravene; Also from *contra*- : control controversial controversy counter

de- /di/, /de/, /dē/ listed separately (off; down; completely) /di/ debase debate decapitate decay decease deceased deceit deceive deception decide deciduous decision decisive declaim declare declension decline declivity decoct decrease decree decrepit deduct deduction deface defame default defeasance defeat defect defection defective defector defend defense defensive defer deferred defiance defiant deficiency deficient define definitive deflate deflation deflect deflection deflower defoliate deform deformation defraud defunct defy degenerate degrade degree dejected dejection delectable delete deletion deliberate deliberation delight delimit delineate delinquent delirious delirium deliver delivery delude delusion demand demented demerit demise demit demolish demoralize demote deniable denial denominate denominational denote denounce denude denunciation deny depart department departure depend dependence dependency deplete depletion deplorable deplore deploy deponent deport deportment depose deposit depository depraved depreciate depreciation depress depressed depression deprivation deprive deride derision derisive derivative derive derogatory descend descendant descent describe description descriptive desert (v) /di-zert/ deserter deserve desideratum design designate designer desirable desire desirous desist despair despicable despise despite despoil despondent destroy destroyer destruct destruction destructive detain detect detective detector detention deter detergent deteriorate determinant determination determine determinism deterrent detest detestable detract detractor detruncate devest device devise devote devotion devour devout; /de/ decadence declamation declaration dedicate dedication defecate deference deficit definite definition degradation delegate delegation delicacy delicate deluge demolition demonstrate demonstration denigrate depravation deprecate depredation deputation deputize deputy descant desecrate desecration desert (n) /dez-ert/ designation desolate desolation desperado desperate desperation destination destine destined destiny destitute desultory detonation detriment detrimental devastate devastation devolution; /dē/ debrief decarbonate decelerate decenter decode decolor decompose decomposition decompress decompression decontrol dehumanize dehumidifier demilitarize demobilize demount denationalize denature denotation deodorant departmental deplane depolarize depopulate deportation depot /dē-pō/ desalinization desegregate desegregation desensitize dethrone detour detumescence devaluate devein deviate deviation devious devitalize devocalize devoiced; And: derelict /dair-ə-lict/

dec- (ten) December decillion decemvir decennial decennium; See Gk. prefix **deca-**.

deci- (one tenth) decibel decigram (Gk.) decile deciliter (Gk.) decimal decimate decimeter (Gk.)

dis- (apart, reverse, not) A Chameleon Prefix changing to *dif-* or *di-* depending on its environment. **dis/a-** disability disable disabuse disaccord disadvantage disarmament disarrange disarray disassemble disaster disavow; **dis/b-** disband disbar disbelief disburden disburse; **dis/c-** discard discern discernible discharge disclaim discount discourage discourse discover discreet discrepancy discretion discriminate discuss discussion; **dis/d-** disdainful; **dis/e-** disease disembark disenchant disengage; **dis/f-** disfavor disfigure disfrock; **dif/f-** differ difference different differential differentiate difficult difficulty diffident diffraction diffuse **dis/g-** disgorge disgrace disguise disgust; **di/g-** digest digression; **dis/h-** disharmony dishearten dishonest dishonor; **dis/i-** disincline disinfect disinherit disintegrate disinterest; **dis/j-** disjointed; **dis/l-** dislike dislocate dislodge disloyal; **di/l-** dilapidated dilate dilute; **dis/m-** dismantle dismember dismiss dismount; **di/m-** dimension **dis/o-** disobedient disorder disorient disown; **dis/p-** disparage disparaging disparity dispensable dispensation dispense disperse displace display displease dispose disproportionate disprove disputable dispute; **dis/qu-** disqualify; **dis/r-** disregard disrepute disrespectable disrupt; **di/r-** direct direction dirigible; **dis/s-** dissatisfied dissatisfaction dissection dissent dissertation dissident dissipate dissolute dissolve dissonance dissuade; **dis/t-** distance distemper distill distortion distract distraction distraught distress distribute district distrust disturb; **dis/u-** disunion disuse

duo- (two) duo duotone duologue duodecimal *(Twelve.)* duodecimo duodecuple duodecuplicate duodenal duodenary duodenum *(Part of small intestine--"twelve" fingers long.)* <u>See</u>: **duo** in Ap. vii-12.

ex- /iks/ /igz/ (When unaccented.) (out of) A <u>Chameleon Prefix</u> changing to *ef-* or *e-* depending on its environment. **ex/a-** exacerbate exact exactly exaggerate exaggeration exalt exaltation examination examine example exasperate exasperating; **ex/c-** excavate excavation exceed exceedingly excel excellence excellent except exception exceptional excerpt excess excessive exchange excide excise excitable excite excitement exclaim exclamation exclamatory exclave exclude exclusion exclusive excommunicate excommunication excoriate excrement excrescence excrete excretion excruciating exculpate exculpatory excursion excusable excuse; **e/d-** edentulous edict edit edition editor editorial educate educated education educe edulcorate; **ex/e-** execrable execute execution executioner executive executor exegesis exemplar exemplary exemplification exemplify exempt exemption exercise exert exertion exeunt; **ef/f-** efface effect effective effeminate efferent effervesce effervescence effervescent effete efficacious efficacy efficiency efficient effigy efflorescence efflorescent effluent effluvium efflux effort effortless effrontery effulgence effusion effusive; **ex/f-** exfoliate exfoliation; **e/g-** egest egregious egress; **ex/h-** exhalant exhale exhaust exhaustion exhibit exhibition exhibitor exhilarate exhilarating exhort exhortation exhume; **ex/i-** exigency exiguous exile exist existence existentialism exit; **e/j-** ejaculate ejaculation eject ejecta ejection ejector; **e/l-** elaborate elaboration elapse elated elation elect election elective electorate elegance elegant elevate elevation elevator elicit elide eligibility eligible eliminate elimination elision elite elocution eloign elongate elongation eloquence eloquent elucidate elude elusion elusive; **e/m-** emaciate emaciated emanate emanation emancipate emancipation emasculate emend emerge emergence emergency emergent emeritus emigrant emigrate emigration émigré eminence eminent emissary emission emit emollient emote emotion emotional emotive emulsion emunctory; **e/n-** enate enervate enormous enucleate enumerate enumeration enunciate enunciation; **ex/o-** exonerate exorable exorbitant; **ex/p-** expand expanse expansion expatiate expatriate expect expectant expectation expectorant expediency expedient expedite expedition expeditious expel expend expendable expenditure expense expensive experience experiment experimentation expert expertise expiate expiation expiration expire explain explanation explant expletive explicate explicit explode exploit exploitation exploration explore explorer explosion explosive exponent exponential export exportation expose exposé exposition expostulate exposure expound express expression expressionism expressive expressly expropriate expulsion expunction expunge expurgate expurgatory; **ex/qu-** exquisite; **e/r-** eradicate erase eraser erasure erect erection erode erosion eruct erudite erupt eruption **e/s-** escapade escape escort; **es/s-** essay; **ex/s-** exsanquine exscind exsecant exsect exsert exsiccate; **ex/t-** extant extemporaneous extemporize extend extended extension extensive extent extenuating exterminate extermination exterminator extinct extinction extinguish extinguisher extirpate extol extort extortion extract extraction extradition extricate; **ex/u-** exuberance exuberant exude exult exultation exurbia exuviate; **e/v-** evacuate evacuation evacuee evade evaluate evanesce evanescent evaporate evaporation evasion evasive evection event eventful (*ful = full, O.E.*) eventual eventuality eversion evert evict eviction evidently evidence evident evince eviscerate evocation evoke evolution evolutionary evolve; <u>See</u>: Gk. **ex-**, Ap. iii-24.

extra- (outside, beyond) extrabold extracanonical extracurricular extrados extragalactic extrajudicial extramarital extramundane extramural extraneous extraordinary extraphysical extrapolate extraprofessional extrasensory extraterritorial extraterritoriality extrauterine extravagance extravagant extravagate extravasate extravasation extravascular

in- (not, without) A <u>Chameleon Prefix</u> changing to *il-, im-, ir-* or *i-* depending on its environment. **in/a-** inability inaccessible inaccuracy inaccurate inaction inactive inadaptable inadequacy inadequate inadmissible inadvertent inadvisable inaffable inalienable inalterable inanimate inappeasable inapplicable inappreciable inappreciative inapprehensible inapproachable inappropriate inapt inaptitude inarticulate inartistic inattention inaudible inattentive inauspicious; **im/b-** imbalance; **in/c-** incalculable incapable incapacitate incapacity incautious incertitude incessant incest incestuous inchoate incivility inclement incoercible incognito incognizant incoherence incoherent incombustible incommensurable incommensurate incommodious incommunicable incommunicado (sp.) incommunicative incommutable incomparable incompatible incompetence incompetent incomplete incomprehensible incomprehensive incompressible incomputable inconceivable inconclusive incondensable inconformity incongruent incongruity incongruous inconsequential inconsiderate inconsistency inconsistent inconsolable inconspicuous inconstancy inconstant inconsumable incontaminable incontestable incontinence incontinent incontinuity incontinuous incontrollable incontrovertible inconvenience inconvenient inconversant inconvertible inconvincible incoordination incorporeal incorrect incorrigible incorruptible incredible incredulity incredulous incurable; **in/d-** indecency indecent indecipherable (*cipher, Ar.*) indecision indecisive indeclinable indecomposable indecorous indecorum indefatigable indefeasible indefectible indefensible indefinable indefinite indelible indelicacy indelicate independence independent indemnity indemonstrable indescribable indestructible indeterminable indeterminate indifference indifferent indigestion indignant indignation indirect indiscernible indiscreet indiscretion indiscriminate indispensable indisposed indisputable indissoluble indistinct individual individuality indivisible indocile indolence indolent indomitable indubitable; **in/e-** inedible ineffable ineffective inefficacious inefficiency inefficient inelegance ineligible ineloquent ineluctable ineludible inept ineptitude inequality inequity ineradicable inerasable inerrant inert inertia inescapable inessential inestimable inevitable inexact inexcusable inexorable inexhaustible inexistent inexorable inexpedient inexpensive inexperienced inexpert inexplicable inexplicit inexpressible inexpressive inexpugnable inextinguishable inextricable; **in/f-** infallible infamous infamy infancy infant infantile infantry infecund infelicity infidel infidelity infinite infinitesimal infinitive infinity infirm infirmary infirmity inflexible infrangible infrequent; **in/g-** inglorious ingrate ingratitude; **i/gn** ignoble ignominious ignorance ignorant ignore; **in/h-** inharmonious inhospitable inhuman inhumane inhumanity; **in/i-** inimical inimitable iniquitous iniquity; **in/j-** injure injurious injury injustice; **il/l-** illegal illegality illegible illegitimate illiberal illiberality illicit illimitable illiteracy illiterate illogical illusory; **im/m-** immaculate immaterial immature immaturity immeasurable immediacy immediate immediately immemorial immense immensity immensurable immiscible immobile immobility immobilize immoderate immodest immoral immorality immortal immortality immortalize immovable immune immunity immunize immutable; **in/n-** innocence innocent innocuous innominate innoxious innumerable; **in/o-** inoffensive inofficious inoperable inoperative inopportune inordinate inorganic; **im/p-** impalpable imparity impartial impartiality impartible impassable impasse (F) impassible impassive impatience impatiens impatient impavid impeccable impecunious impenetrability impenetrable impenitent imperceptible imperceptive imperfect imperfection imperishable impermanent impermeable impermissible impersonal impertinence impertinent imperturbable impervious impiety impious implacable impolicy impolite impolitic imponderable impossibility impossible impotence impotent impractical imprecise impregnable imprescriptible improbability improbable improbity impromptu (F) improper improvident improvisation improvise imprudent impudence impudent impunity impure impurity; **in/qu-** inquietude; **ir/r-** irrational irrationality irreconcilable irrecoverable irrecusable irredeemable irreducible irrefrangible irrefutable irregular irregularity irrelevant irreligious irremediable irremissible irremovable irreparable irrepealable irreplaceable irrepressible irreproachable (O.F.) irresistible irresoluble irresolute irresolvable irrespective irresponsible irresponsive irretraceable irretrievable (O.F.) irreverence irreverent irreversible irrevocable; **in/s-** insane insanitary insanity insatiable inscrutable insecure insecurity insensate insensible insensitive insentient inseparable insignificant insincere insipid insipience insobriety insolence insolent insoluble insolvable insolvency insolvent insomnia insomniac instability insubordinate insubordination insubstantial insufferable insufficient insuperable insupportable insuppressible insurmountable insusceptible; **in/t-** intact intangible integer integral integrate integration integrity intemperance intemperate intestate intolerable intolerance intolerant intractable intransigent intransitive; **in/u-** inurbane inutile; **in/v-** invalid inv̲alid invalidate invaluable (*Priceless.*) invariably inveracity invertebrate inviable invincible inviolable invisible invitation invite invocation invoke involuntary invulnerable; <u>Also from **in-**</u>: enemy enmity

in- (in, into, on, within, toward, very, thoroughly)   A <u>Chameleon Prefix</u> changing to *il-, im-,* or *ir-* depending on its environment.   **in/a-** inaugurate inauguration inamorata (It.) inamorato; **im/b** imbibe; **in/b-** inborn inbound; **in/c-** incalescent incandescence incandescent incantation incapsulate incarcerate incarnate incarnation incase incasement incavation incendiary incense incentive inception incidence incident incidental incidentally incinerate incinerator incipient incision incisive incisor incite incitement inclination incline include included inclusion inclusive incorporate incorporated incorporation increase increment incriminate incrust incrustation incubate incubation inculcate incumbent incur incursion incurvate incuse; **in/d-** indebted indent indentation indentured index (Pl. indices.) indicate indication indicative indicator indicia indict indictment indoctrinate induce inducement induct inductance inductee inductile induction inductive inductor indulge indulgence indurate; **in/e-** inebriated; **in/f-** infarct infarction infatuate infatuated infect infection infectious infer inference infix inflame inflammable inflammation inflatable inflate inflated inflation inflect inflection inflict influence influential influenza influx inform informal informality informant information informed informer infraction infringe infringement infuriate infuse infusion; **in/g-** ingeminate ingenious ingenuity ingenuous ingest ingrain ingrained ingratiate ingredient ingress ingurgitate; **in/h-** inhabit inhabitant inhabited inhalant inhalator inhale inhaler inhere inherent inherit inheritance inhibit inhibition inhume; **in/i-** initial initiate initiation initiative; **in/j-** inject injection injunction; **il/l-** illation illuminance illuminate illuminati illumination illusion illusionary illusive illusory illustrate illustration illustrator illustrious; **im/m-** immanence immanent immerge immerse immersion immigrant immolate immolation immigrate immigration imminent immure; **in/n-** innate innerve innovate innovation innuendo; **in/o-** inoculate inoculation; **im/p-** impact impacted impair impairment impale impanel impart impassion impassioned impeach impeachment impedance impede impediment impel impellent impending imperative imperial imperialist imperious impersonate impetigo impetuous impetus impinge implant implantation implausible implement implementation implicate implication implicit implied implode implore implosion imply import importance important importation importer importunate importune impose imposing imposition impost impostor imposture impoverish imprecate impregnate impregnation impress impression impressionable impressionism impressive impressment imprint imprison improve (O.F.) improvement impugn impulse impulsive imputation impute; **in/p-** inpatient; **in/qu-** inquire inquiry inquisition Inquisition inquisitive inquisitor; **ir/r-** irradiate irradiation irrigate irrigation irritability irritable irritant irritate irritating irritation irruption; **in/s-** inscribe inscription insect insecticide inseminate insemination insert insertion insignia insinuate insinuation insist insistent insole inspect inspection inspector inspiration inspire inspissate install (M.F.) installation installment instance instant instantaneous instantly instigate (*in-* = against) instigation instill instinct instinctive institute institution institutional instruct instruction instructive instructor instrument instrumental instrumentation insult (*in-* = on) insulting insurance insure insured insurgence (*in-* = against) insurgency insurgent insurrection; **in/t-** intend intense intensity intent intention intentional inter intestine (*intus* = within < *in-*) intimacy intimate intimation intimidate (*in-* = very) intimidation intinction intonation intoxicant intoxicate intoxicated intoxication intricacy intricate intrigue intrude intrusion intrusive intubation intuit intuition intuitional intuitive; **in/u-** inundate inundation inure inurn; **in/v-** invade invaginate invasion invective inveigh invent invention inventive inventor inventory inverse inversion invert invest investigate investigation investigator investment inveterate invidious invigorate invoice involution involve involved;   <u>See also</u>: Greek prefix **en-** Ap. iii-23.

infra- (below, beneath) infracostal   infra dignitatem *(Beneath one's dignity.)* infralapsarianism   infrared   infrasonic

inter- (together; between)   interact   interaction   intercede   intercept   interception   intercession   intercollegiate   intercom   intercommunication   interconnect   intercontinental   intercostal   intercourse   intercurrent   interdenominational   interdependent   interdict   interdiction   interdisciplinary   interest   interested   interfere   interference   interfuse   intergrade   interim   interior   interject   interjection   interlace   interline   interlocutor   interlude   interlunar   intermarry   intermediary   intermezzo   interminable   intermission   intermittent   intermix   intern   internal   international   internecine   internist   internment   interpenetrate   interpolate   interpose   interpret   interpretation   interregnum   interrelate   interrelation   interrogate   interrogation   interrupt   interruption   intersect   intersection   intersession   intersperse   interstate   interstellar   interstice   intertribal   interurban   interval   intervene   intervention   interview; <u>Also:</u> enterprise   entertain   entertaining   entertainment   entrails   entrepreneur (F)   intellect *(inter- = intel- as chameleon prefix.)* intellectual   intelligence   intelligent   intelligentsia   intelligibility   intelligible

intra- (within)   intracellular   intracostal   intracranial   intramolecular   intramural   intramuscular   intranuclear   intrastate   intravenous; <u>Also:</u> enter   entrance   entrant   entrée (F)   entry   entryway *(way O.E.)*

intro- (in; into; within)   introduce   introduction   introductory   introit   introjection   intromission   introspection   introspective   introversion   introvert

juxta- (near, next to)   juxtapose   juxtaposed   juxtaposit   juxtaposition

milli- (one thousand)   milliampere   millibar   millifarad   milligram   millihenry   milliliter   millimeter   millimicron   million   millionaire   millionth   millipede   millivolt   milliwatt

multi- (many)   multicolored   multiengined   multifarious   multifold   multifoliate   multiform   multilateral   multilingual   multimillionaire   multimotored   multinational   multipartite   multiped   multiphase   multiple   multiplex   multiplicand   multiplication   multiplicity   multiplier   multiply   multipropellant   multipurpose   multisection   multistage   multisyllable   multitude   multitudinous   multivalent   multivalve

non- (not)   nonage   nonappearance   nonchalance (F)   nonchalant   noncom   noncombatant   noncommissioned   noncommittal   noncompliance   nonconductor   nonconformist   nonconformity   noncooperation   nondescript   nondistinctive   noneffective   nonego   nonentity   nonexistence   nonfeasance   nonfiction   nonflammable   nonintervention   nonjoinder   nonmetal   nonobjective   nonpareil   nonparticipating   nonpartisan   nonplus   nonproductive   nonprofit   nonrepresentational   nonresident   nonresistant   nonrestrictive   nonrigid   nonsectarian   nonsense   non sequitur   nonskid (O.N.)   nonstandard (O.F.)   nonstop (O.E.)   nonsupport   nonunion   nonwhite (O.E.)

nov-, non- (nine, ninth)   November   nonillion   nonuple   nonagon   nonuplicate   nones *(Ninth day before the ides.)*

ob- (toward; against; over) A <u>Chameleon Prefix</u> changing to *oc-, of-, o-* or *op-* depending on its environment. **ob/b-** obbligato; **oc/c-** occasion occasional occasionally occident Occident occidental occipital occiput occlude occult occupancy occupant occupation occupational occupy occur occurrence; **ob/d-** obdurate; **ob/e-** obese obesity obedience obedient obey; **ob/f-** obfuscate; **of/f-** offend offense offensive offer offering offertory; **ob/i-** obituary; **ob/j-** object objection objectionable objective objectivity objurgate; **ob/l-** oblate oblation oblige obligate obligation obligatory oblige obliging oblique obliterate oblivion oblivious oblong; **o/m-** omission omit; **ob/n-** obnoxious; **op/p-** opponent opportune opportunity opposable oppose opposite opposition oppositive oppress oppression oppressive opprobrious opprobrium oppugn oppugnant; **ob/s-** obscene obscenity obscure obscurity obsequious observant observation observatory observe obsess obsession obsolescent obsolete obstacle obstetrician obstetrics obstinate obstreperous obstruct obstruction obstruent; **ob/t-** obtain obtrude obtrusive obtuse; **ob/v-** obverse obvert obvious; <u>Note</u>: *office, officer, official, officiate, officious* < *opus* work + *facere* to make.

oct- (eight) octangle octant octave octavo octennial octet octillion octillionth October octodecimo octogenarian *(An 80 year old.)* octogenary octonary octopod octuple octuplicate Octavia *(The eighth born.)* Octavius; <u>See</u>: Gk. prefix **octo-** Ap. iii-25.

per- (through; completely; very) peracidity perambulate perambulation perambulator perceive percept perceptible perception perceptive perceptual percipient percolate percolator percuss percussion perdition perdu perdurable peregrinate peregrine peremptory perennial perfect perfectible perfection perfectionist perfectly perfecto (Sp.) perfervid perfidious perfidy perforate perforated perforation perforce perform performance performer perfume perfumery perfunctory perfuse pergola perhaps (O.N. *happ* = chance, luck) perish perishable perjure perjury permanence permanent permeable permeate permissible permission permissive permit permutable permutation pernicious perorate peroration perpendicular perpetrate perpetual perpetuate perpetuity perplex perplexed perplexing perplexity perquisites (perks) persecute persecution perseverance persevere persiflage persist persistence persistent persnickety perspective perspicacious perspicacity perspicuous perspiration perspire persuade persuasion persuasive pertain pertinacious pertinacity pertinent perturb perturbation pertussis pervade pervasive perverse perversion perversity pervert perverted pervious; <u>Note</u>: **per** as preposition meaning *by the*: per annum   per capita percent (*Per centum,* by the hundred.) percentage percentile   per diem   per interim per mensem   per mill   permillage   per se /sā/ (By itself.); <u>Also</u>: person, persona, personable, personal, personality, personally, personification, personnel < *persona* mask.

post- (after) postaxial post-bellum postdate postdiluvian posterior posterity postern postexilian postfix postglacial postgraduate posthumous postimpressionism postliminium postlude postmeridian post meridiem (P.M.) postmillennial post-mortem postnatal postnuptial post-obit postoperative postorbital postpartum postpone postposition postpositive postprandial postscript (P.S.) postwar; <u>Note</u>:   the **post-** in *postal, postman, postmark, etc.* are from the Latin *posita*, (placed).

pre- (before) preamble preamplifier Pre-Cambrian precancel precaution precautionary precautious precede precedence precedent preceding precept preceptor precession precessional precinct precipice precipitate precipitation precipitous precise precisely precision preclude precocious precognition preconceive preconception precondition preconscious precook precursor precursory predate predecease predesignate predestination predestine predetermine predicable predicament predicate predication predict prediction predigest predilection predispose predisposition predominance predominant predominate preeminent preempt preemption preexilian preexist prefab prefabrication preface prefatory prefect prefer preferable preference preferential preferred prefigure prefix preflight pregnancy pregnant prehension prehistoric preignition prejudge prejudice prejudicial prelate prelim preliminary preliterate prelude premature premedical premeditate premeditation premillennial premise premium premolar premonition prenatal preoccupation preoccupied preordain prepackage (*pack* M.E.) preparation preparatory prepare prepay preponderance preposition prepositional prepositive prepossess preposterous prepotent prepuce prerequisite prerogative presage preschool prescience prescind prescribe prescript prescription prescriptive presence present presentable presentation presentiment presently presentment preserve pre-shrunk (O.E.) preside president presidio (Sp.) presidium (Rus.) presignify prestige prestigious presumable presume presumption presumptuous presuppose pretend pretender pretense pretension pretentious pretext prevail prevailing prevalent prevaricate prevarication prevent prevention preventive preview previous prevision prevocational prewar prexy (president)

pro- (forward, forth; on behalf of; in place of; in favor of) procedure proceed proceeding proceeds process procession processional proclaim proclamation proconsul procrastinate procrastination procreant procreate proctor procurance procurator procure procurement prodigal prodigious prodigy produce producer product production productive profane profanity profess profession professional professor professorial proficiency proficient profile profit profitable profiteer profligate profound profundity profuse profusion progenitor progeny progress progression progressive prohibit prohibition prohibitive project projectile projection projectionist projector prolapse proletarian proletariat proliferate prolific prolix prolocutor prolong prominence prominent promiscuous promise promising promissory promote promotion prompt promptly promulgate pronoun pronounce pronouncement pronunciation propaganda propagate propagation propel propellant propeller propensity propitious proponent proportion proportional proportionment proposal propose proposition propound propulsion prorate prorogation proscribe proscription prosect prosecute prosecution prosecutor prosimian proslavery prospect prospective prospector prospectus prosper prosperity prosperous prostitute prostitution prostrate prostration protect protection protective protector protectorate protégé (F) protest protestant Protestant protestation protract protraction protractor protrude protrusion protuberance protuberant provection provenience proverb proverbial provide providence Providence provident providential provider provision provisional proviso provocation provocative provoke;   <u>Related to **pro-** more distantly</u>: probability probable probably probate probation probe probity proof prosaic prose proud prove; <u>From **proprius**, *one's own*</u>: proper   property   proprietary   proprietor   propriety

quad- (four) quad quadragenarian (40's) quadrangle quadrant quadratic quadrennial quadrennium quadricentennial quadriceps quadrifid quadrilateral quadrilingual quadrille (F) quadrillion quadripartite quadrisyllable quadrivalent quadrivial quadrivium quadrumanous   quadruped   quadruple   quadruplets   quadruplex   quadruplicate

quasi- (as if, nearly)   quasi-devoted quasi-equal quasi-humorous quasi-illness quasi-liberal quasi-luxury quasi-official quasi-protection quasi-scholar quasi-scientific quasi-willing   quasi-victory   quasi-zeal, *etc.*

quint- (five) quint quintet quintuple quintuplet quintessence quintillion quintillionth quintuplicate   quinquennial *(Every five years.)*   quinquennium

re- /ri/, /re/, /rē/ listed separately. (back; again; anew) [Often **red-** before a vowel.] /ri/ rebel (v) rebellion rebellious rebuff (M.F.) rebuke (O.F.) rebuttal (O.F.) recalcitrant recant recede receipt receiptor receivable receive receiver recension receptacle reception receptionist receptive receptor recess (v) recession recessional recessive recidivism recipient reciprocal reciprocate recision recital recite reclaim recline reclusion recognizance recoil (v) reconnaissance record (v) recorder recording recount recoup recover recovery recriminate recrimination recruit recumbent recuperate recur recurrence recurrent redact redaction redecorate redeem redeemer redeeming redemption redemptive redintegrate redintegration redoubt redoubtable redound redress reduce reducer reduction redundancy redundant reduplicate reduplication reecho (Gk.) refection refer refine refined refinement refinery reflect reflection reflective reflector reflexive reform reformatory reformed refraction refractor refrain refresh (O.E.) refresher refreshing refreshment refrigerant refrigerate refrigerator refulgence refund refurbish (O.F.) refusal refuse refute regard (O.F.) regenerate regeneration regenerator regorge regress (v) regression regressive regurgitate regurgitation rehearsal rehearse reheat (O.E.) reject (v) rejection rejoice rejoicing rejoin rejoinder (F) rejuvenate relapse (v) relate related relation relationship relax release relent relentless reliable reliance reliant relief relieve religion religious relinquish reluctance reluctant rely remain remainder remains remand remark (Ger.) remarkable remedial remember remembrance remind (O.E.) remiss remission remit remittance remittent remonstrance remorse remote removable removal remove removed remunerate remuneration remunerative renascence renege renewal renitent renounce renown renowned renunciation repair repast repay repeal repeat repeater repel repent repentance repentant repetitive replace replacement replenish replete repletion reply report reporter repose repository repress repression repressive reprieve reprisal reprise reproach (F) reproof reprove repudiate repugnance repugnant repulse repulsion repulsive repute request require requirement requital rescind research resection resemblance resemble resent resentful resentment reserve reserved reservoir (F) reside residual resign resigned resilience resilient resist resistance resistible resistive resistor resolve resolved resorb resorption resort resound resource resourceful respect respectable respecting resplendent respond respondent response responsibility responsible responsive restore restrain restraint restrict restricted restriction result resultant resume resumption resurge resurgence resurgent resuscitate resuscitation retail (v) retailer retain retainer retaliate retaliation retaliatory retard retardant retardation retarded retention retentive retire (M.F.) retired retirement retiring retort retrace retract retraction retractor retreat retrenchment retrieve (O.F.) retriever return reveal revenge revengeful reverberant reverberate reverberation revere reversal reverse reversible reversion revert review reviewer revile revise revision revival revivalist revive revoice revoke revolt revolting revolutionary revolve revolver revue (F) revulsion reward (O.F.) rewarding; /re/ rebel (n) recipe reciprocity recitation recitative reclamation recluse recognition recognize recollect recollection recommendation recompense reconcilable reconcile reconciliation recondite record (n) recreant recreate recreation recusant redolent referee reference referendum referent refluent reformation Reformation refuge refugee refutation register registrant registrar registration registry relative relativity relegate relevant relic relish remedy reminiscent remnant renaissance (F) Renaissance render rendition renegade renovate renovation reparable reparation repartee repertoire (F) repertory repetend repetition repetitious replica replicate reprehend reprehensible represent representation representative reprimand reprobate reputable reputation requisite requisition reservation residence residency resident residential residue reservation residence residency resident residential residue resignation resolute resolution resonance resonant resonate resonator respiration respirator respite rest *(Remainder.)* restaurant (F) restitution restive restoration résumé (F) resurrect resurrection reticence reticent retinue (F) retribution reveille revel revelation Revelations revelry revenue reverence reverent revocable revocation revolution; /rē/ react reactance reaction reactionary reactivate reactor readjust readjustment readmit reaffirm reanimate rearm rearmament rearrange reassure rebate rebirth reborn (O.E.) rebound (O.F.) (n) recalesce recap recapitulate recapitulation recapture recess (n) recoil (n) recombination recomment recommit reconnoiter reconsider reconsign reconstitute reconstruct reconstruction reconvert recourse recrudesce recycle (Gk.) redeliver redevelop (O.F.) redirect redistrict redouble redraft (O.E.) reenforce reenter reentry reevaluate reexamine refill (O.E.) refit (M.E.) reflex (n) reforest refuel regress (n) rehabilitate rehash (O.F.) reimburse reimport reimpression reincarnate reincarnation reinforce reinforcement reinstall (M.F.) reinstate reinsure (M.E.) reinvest reissue reiterate reject relapse (n) relaxation relay relive (O.E.) relocate reman (O.E.) remarry rematch (O.E.) remodel remount renew (O.E.) reopen (O.E.) reorder reorganize (Gk.) reorient repatriate repercussion rephrase (Gk.) repossess reprint reproduce reproduction reproductive rerun (O.E.) reseat (O.N.) reship (O.E.) reshipment resole resurface retail (n) retake (O.E.) retell (O.E.) retouch (O.F.) retread retrial retry reunify reunion reunite revaluate revamp (O.F.) revest revisit revitalize rewind (O.E.) rewire (O.E.) reword (O.E.) rewrite (O.E.); **From regere, *to rule:*** regent regime regimen regiment regimentation region regional regular regularity regularly regulate regulation regulator rule ruler

retro- (back; behind) retroact retroactive retrocede retrocession retrochoir retrofire retroflex retroflexion retrograde retrogress retrogression retrogressive retrorocket (It.) retrorse retrospect retrospection retrospective retroversion

se- (apart; without) secede secern secession seclude secluded seclusion seclusive secrecy secret secretary secrete secretion secretive secure security sedition seduce seduction seductive segregate segregation select selection selective separable separate separation separatist separator; From **secare**, *to cut*: secant sectile section sectional sectionalism sectionalize sector segment segmental segmentation; From **sentire**, *to feel*: sensate sensation sensational sense senseless sensibility sensible sensitive sensitivity sensitize sensor sensory sensual sensualism sensuality sensuous sentient sentiment sentimental sentimentality sentimentalize sentinel sentry

semi- (partly; half; twice a period) semi (semitrailer) semiannual semiautomatic (Gk.) semibreve semicentennial semicircle semicivilized semicolon (Gk.) semiconductor semiconscious semidiurnal semidome semifinal semifluid semiformal semiliquid semimonthly (O.E.) semiofficial semipermeable semiporcelain semiprecious semiprivate semiprofessional semiquaver semirigid semiskilled (O.N.) semisolid semitone semitrailer semiweekly (O.E.) semiyearly (O.E.)

sept- (seven) September septenary septenial septet septilateral septillion septime septuagenarian (70's) septuple septuplicate

sex- (six) sextet sextan sextant sextile sextuple sextuplet sextuplicate sexennial sext sexagenarian (60's) sexagesimal sexcentenary sextillion sextodecimo

sub- (under; secondary) A Chameleon Prefix changing to *suc-, suf-, sug-, sup-, sus-* & *sur-* depending on its environment. **sub/a-** subagent subalpine subaltern subantarctic subaquatic subarctic subassembly subatomic (Gk.); **sub/b-** subbasement subbass; **sub/c-** subcaliber (Ar.) subcelestial subcellar subcentral subclinical (Gk.) subcommittee subconscious subcontinent subcontract subcontractor subcortex subculture subcutaneous; **suc/c-** succeed success successful succession successive successor succinct succor succubus succumb succussion; **sus/c-** susceptible; **sub/d-** subdeacon (Gk.) subdelegate subdivide subdivision subdominant subdue; **sud/d-** sudden; **sub/e-** subequatorial; **sub/f-** subfamily subfloor (O.E.); **suf/f-** suffer sufferance suffering suffice sufficiency sufficient suffix suffocate suffocation suffrage suffragette suffumigate suffuse suffusion; **sub/g-** subgenus subglacial subgroup (F); **sug/g-** suggest suggestible suggestion suggestive; **sub/h-** subhead (O.E.) subheading subhuman; **sub/i-** subindex subirrigate; **sub/j-** subjacent subject subjection subjective subjoin subjoinder subjugate subjunctive; **sub/k-** subkingdom; **sub/l-** sublease sublimate sublimation sublime subliminal sublunary; **sub/m-** submachine gun (Gk./O.N.) submarginal submarine submediant submerge submersion submicroscopic (Gk.) submission submissive submit submultiple; **sum/m-** summon summoner summons; **sub/n-** subnormal; **sub/o-** suboceanic (Gk.) suborbital suborder subordinary subordinate suborn; **sub/p-** subphylum (Gk.) subplot (O.E.) subpoena subprincipal; **sup/p-** supplant supple supplement supplemental supplementary suppliant supplicant supplication supply support supporter supportive suppose supposed supposition suppository suppress suppression suppuration; **sus/p** suspect suspend suspense suspension suspicion suspicious suspire; **sub/r-** subregion subreption subrogate subrogation sub rosa; **sur/r-** surrogate surreptitious; **sub/s-** subscribe subscript subscription subsequence subsequent subserve subservient subside subsidence subsidiary subsidize subsidy subsist subsistence subsoil subsolar subsonic subspecies substance substandard (O.F.) substantial substantiate substantive substation substitute substitution substratum substructure subsume; **sub/t-** subtangent subtemperate subtenant subtend subterfuge (subter-, *below*) subternatural subterrane subterranean subterrestrial subtile subtitle subtle subtlety subtonic (Gk.) subtorrid subtract subtraction subtrahend subtranslucent subtreasury (Gk.) subtropical (Gk.) subtropics; **sus/t-** sustain sustenance; **sub/u-** suburb suburban suburbanite suburbia; **sub/v-** subvene subvention subversion subversive subvert subvitreous; **sub/w-** subway (O.E.); <u>Note:</u> succulent (From succus, *juice* .); suction (From sugere, *to suck*.)

super- (above; greater than) superable superabound superabundant superannuate superb superbomb supercargo supercarrier supercharge supercharger supercilious superfamily superfemale superficial superfine superfluidity superfluous superheat (O.E.) superhighway (O.E.) superhuman superimpose superintendent superior superjacent superlative supermale superman (O.E.) supermarket supernal supernational supernatural supernormal supernumerary superorder superphysical (Gk.) superpower supersaturate superscribe superscript supersede supersensible supersensual supersex supersonic supersonics superstate superstition superstitious superstratum superstructure supersubtle supertax supertonic (Gk.) supervene supervise supervision supervisor supervisory supreme

supra- (above; beyond) (Akin to super-) supraconductivity supraconscious supraglacial suprahuman supralapsarianism supralateral supraliminal supralittoral supramolecular supramundane supranational supranatural supranormal supraorbital supraordinate supraorganism suprapersonal supraprotest suprarational suprasegmental

trans- (across; beyond; through) transact transaction transatlantic (Gk.) transcalent transceiver transcend transcendent transcendental transcontinental transcribe transcript transcription transect transept transeunt transfer transference Transfiguration transfigure transfix transform transformation transformer transfusion transgress transgression transient transilient transistor transit transition transitive transitory translate translation translator translucent transmigration transmissible transmission transmit transmitter transmutation transoceanic (Gk.) transom transpacific transparency transparent transpiration transpire transplant transponder transport transportation transpose transposition transubstantiation transude transversal transverse transvestite

tri- (three) triad triangle triangular triangulation triaxial tribe tribune tricentennial triceps triceratops tricolor tricorn tricornered tricuspid trident tridimensional triennial triennium trifid trifocals trifold (O.E.) trifoliate triformed trifurcate trigeminal trijugate trilateral trilinear trilingual triliteral trillion trillium trimester trimolecular trimonthly (O.E.) trinal trinary trine trinity Trinity trinomial trio (It.) tripartite tripedal triple triplet triplex triplicate tripody tripos triradiate trireme trisect triserial triskelion trisoctahedron triune trivalent trivalve trivet trivia trivial triviality trivium triweekly (O.E.); <u>See</u>: Greek prefix **tri-**, Ap. iii-25.

ultra- (On the other side of; beyond. Opposite of **cis-**.) ultraconservative ultracritical (Gk.) ultrafilter ultrahigh frequency (UHF) ultraism ultralunar ultramarine ultramicrometer (Gk.) ultramicroscope (Gk.) ultramodern ultramontane ultramundane ultranationalism ultrared ultrasonic ultratropical (Gk.) ultraviolet ultra vires *(Beyond the power of.)*

uni- (one) uniaxial unicameral unicellular unicolor unicorn unicycle (Gk.) unidirectional unifiable unification unified unifilar uniform uniformed uniformity unify unilateral union unionism unionist unionize uniplanar unipolar unique (F) unisexual unison unit Unitarian Unitarianism unitary Unitas Fratrum *("Unity of brothers," The Moravian Church.)* unite united United Nations United States unity univalent univalve universal universalism universality universe university univocal

vice- (substitute, instead of) vice admiral (Ar.) vice-chairman vice-chancellor vice-consul vice-dean vice-director vicegerent vice-president vice-principal vice-regent viceroy vice versa *(conversely)*

Greek Prefixes

a- (without; not; apart) **an-** (before vowels) /ā/ acentric agraphia amoral asexual (L) asocial (L) asymmetric atemporal (L) atheism atheist atheistic atonal atypical avitaminosis (L); /a/ abysmal abyss achromatic adamant adynamia agnostic agnosticism Amazon amethyst amnesia amnesty amorphous analgesic anarchist anarchy anecdotal anecdote anhidrosis anhydrous anomie anorexia apathetic apathy aphorism asbestos asbestosis asphyxia asphyxiate atom atomizer atonality atrophied atrophy; /ə/ alexia anemia anemic anonymous aphagia aphasia aplasia apraxia arrhythmia astigmatic astigmatism asylum ataxia atomic

amphi- (both; around) amphibian amphibious amphigory amphitheater amphora

ana- (up; back; anew; thorough) Anabaptist anachorism anachronism anaclisis anaglyph anagoge anagram analeptic analogous analogue analogy analysis analyst analytic analyze anaplastic anathema anatomy anode; <u>Also</u>: aneurysm

anti- (against) antiaircraft antibiotic antibody (O.E.) anticatalyst antichrist anticlimactic anticlimax antidote antifreeze (O.E.) antigen antihistamine antiknock (O.E.) antimatter (L) antineutron antiparticle (L) antipathy antipersonnel (L) antiperspirant (L) antiphonal antiphony antipope (L) antiproton anti-Semitism antiseptic antislavery (Slavic) antisocial antitank (L) antithesis antithetical antitoxic antitoxin antitrust (O.N.) antivenin (L) antiviral; <u>Also</u>: antagonism antagonist antagonize Antarctic Antarctica anthem antonym

apo- (off; from; away) apocalypse apocalyptic Apocrypha apocryphal apogee apologetic apologist apologize apology apoplexy apostle apostolate apostolic apostrophe apothecary

cata- (down; against; back) catachresis cataclysm catacomb catalepsy catalogue catalyst catalytic catapult cataract catarrh catastrophe catastrophic catatonia; <u>Also</u>: categorize category

cath- (Variation of **cata-**) cathedral catheter catheterize cathode catholic Catholic

deca- (ten) decade decagon *decagram decahedron *decaliter Decalogue Decameron *decameter Decapolis *decare *decastere decathlon; (*May also be **deka-**.) <u>See</u>: Latin prefix **deci-**, Ap. iii-10.

di- (two) diarchy diatomic dicephalous dichlorodiphenyltrichloroethane (DDT) dicrotic digraph dilemma dimorphic dioxide diphase diphthong dipole diptych; <u>Note</u>: dichotomy (*dicho-*, in two; *temnein*, to cut.) dinosaur (*dino-*, terrible; *sauros*, lizard.) diphtheria (*diphthera*, membrane.) diploma (*diploma*, paper folded double.) diplomacy, diplomat, diplomatic dipsomania (*dipsa*, thirst; *-mania*, irrational craving.) discobolus (*diskos*, a discus; *ballein*, to throw.)

dia- (across; apart; completely), **di-** before vowels. diabetes diabetic diachronic diacritical diadem diagnose diagnosis diagnostic diagnostician diagonal diagram dialect dialectical dialectics dialogue dialysis diameter diametrically diapason diaper diaphragm diaphragmatic diarrhea Diaspora diatonic diatribe; <u>Also</u>: dieresis diesis diocese diode diorama diuresis diuretic

dys- (defective; difficult; hard) dysentery dysfunction dysgraphia dyslexia dysmenorrhea dyspepsia dysphagia dysphasia dysphoria dysrhythmia dystaxia dysuria

ecto- (outside, external) ectoderm ectogenous ectomorph ectomorphic ectoplasm

en- (in, into) A <u>Chameleon Prefix</u> changing to *el-*, *em-* or *er-* depending on its environment. ellipse emblem emblematic embolism embryo empathize empathy emphasis emphasize emphatic emphysema empirical empiricism emporium encephalitis encyclical encyclopedia endemic enema energetic energize energy engraft engrave engraving enharmonic enthuse enthusiasm enthusiast enthusiastic entropy enzyme errhine

endo- (within, inside) endocardial endocardium endocrine gland endocrinology endogamy endomorph endomorphic endoparasite endoscope endoskeleton

ennea- (nine) ennead enneagon enneahedron

epi- (upon; among; beside; in addition); **ep-** before vowels; **eph-** before Greek root with /h/ sound. ephemeral ephor epicanthus epicenter epicrisis epicycle epidemic

Ap. iii-23

epidemiology epidermis epiglottis epigram epigraph epilepsy epileptic epilogue epiphany Epiphany episode episodic epistaxis epistemology epistle epithet epitome epitomize epoch epoxy

eu- (good; well) eucalyptus Eucharist eugenicist eugenics Eugene eulogist eulogize eulogy Eunice euphemism euphemistic euphemize euphonic euphonium euphony euphoria euphoric eurhythmics euthanasia euthenics

ex- (out of; from; forth) **ec-** (Before consonants.) eccentric eccentricity Ecclesiastes eclectic eclecticism eclipse ecstasy ecstatic eczema exegesis exodus exorcise exorcism; Note: ecology (*oikos*, home; *-logy*, the study of.) economy (*oikos*, home; *nemein*, to manage.) exotic (*exotikos*, foreign.)

hecto- (one hundred) hectogram hectograph hectoliter hectometer hectostere

hemi- (half) hemialgia hemicrania hemicycle hemiplegia hemisphere hemispheroid

hepta- (seven) heptad heptagon heptahedron heptangular (L) heptarchy Heptateuch

hexa- (six) hexad hexagon hexagonal hexameter hexarchy hexastich Hexateuch

hyper- (above, over) hyperacidity (L) hyperactive hyperalgesia hyperbola hyperbole hyperbolic hypercorrection (L) hypercritical hyperemia hyperesthesia hyperkinesia hypersensitive (L) hyperspace (L) hypertension (L) hyperthermia hyperthyroidism hyperventilation (L) hypervitaminosis (L)

hypo- (under, beneath) **hyph-** before vowels. hyphemia hyphen hyphenate hypoactive hypocenter hypochondria hypochondriac hypocoristic hypocrisy hypocrite hypodermic hypomania hypopituitarism hypostyle hypotenuse hypothalamus hypothermia hypothesis (Pl. hypotheses) hypothesize hypothetical hypothyroidism; hypoxia *(Deficiency of oxygen.)*; Note: hypnosis (From *hypnos*, sleep.)

kilo- (one thousand) kilo kilocalorie kilocycle kilogram kiloliter kilometer kilowatt

meso- (in the middle) mesocephalic mesoderm Mesolithic Era mesomorph mesomorphic meson Mesopotamia mesosphere Mesozoic Era

meta- (after, beyond) metabolic metabolism metabolize metacarpal metacarpus metamorphic metamorphism metamorphosis metaphor metaphysical metaphysics metapsychology metastasis metastasize metatarsal metatarsus metathesis

mono- (one) monocle (L) monocycle monogamous monogamy monogram monograph monolith monologue monomania mononucleosis (L) monophonic monoplane (L) monoplegia monopolize monopoly monorail (O.F.) monosyllabic monotheism monotone monotony monotype monoxide

neo- (new, recent) Neocene neoclassic (L) Neo-Darwinism neoimpressionism (L) Neo-Latin Neolithic Era neologism neomycin neon neophyte neoplasm neoplasty

octo-, octa- (eight) octad octagon octagonal octameter octarchy octopus; See: L. oct- Ap. iii-16.

para- (beside; beyond) parable parabola parabolic paradigm paradox paragon paragraph parallel parallelogram paralysis paralytic paralyze paramecium parameter paramilitary (L) paranoia paranoid paraphernalia paraphrase paraplegia parapsychology parasite parasitic; From other sources: parachute parade paradise paraffin parakeet paramount paramour parapet paratrooper

penta- (five) pentagon pentameter pentarchy Pentateuch pentathlon pentatonic

peri- (around; near) pericarditis pericardium perigee perihelion perimeter period periodic periodical periodontics peripatetic peripheral periphery periphrastic periscope peristalsis peristyle peritonitis

pro- (before; forward) problem proclivity prognosis prognostic prognosticate prognostication program programmer prolegomenon (Pl. prolegomena) prologue propaedeutic prophecy prophesy prophet prophetic prophylactic prophylaxis proptosis propylaeum propylon proscenium proselyte proselytize prosodic prosody prostate prostatectomy prostyle; Note: from protos, first: protocol proton protoplasm prototype protozoa; See: Latin Prefix **pro-** Ap. iii-17.

syn- (with, together) A Chameleon Prefix changing to *syl-, sym-* or *sys-* depending on its environment. syllable syllabicate syllabus syllogism symbiosis symbol symbolic symbolism symbolize symmetrical symmetry sympathetic sympathize sympathy symphonic symphony symposium symptom symptomatic synagogue synapse synchronism synchronize syncopate syncopation syncretism syncretize synergism synod synonym synonymous synopsis syntax synthesis synthesize synthetic systaltic system systematic systematize systemic systole systolic

tetra- (four) tetrachord tetracycline tetrad tetragon tetragram tetrarcy

tri- (three) Triasic tricycle triglyph trigonometry trigraph trihedron trilobite trilogy trimerous triode trioxide tripod triphase triphthong triptych tritone; See: L. prefix **tri-** Ap. iii-21.

NOTE: For references to the following, see Ap. ix at the indicated pages: **hetero-** (9), **homo-** (9), **iso-** (10), **mega-** (12), **micro-** (12), **pan-** (14), **poly-** (15).

Other Prefixes

en- /in/ (unaccented) (Old French, Latin *in-*); **em-** before *b* & *p*.; [Often verb forming.] embalm embankment embargo embark embarkation embarrass embarrassing embarrassment embassy embattle embay embellish embellishment embezzle embitter emblaze emblazon embody (O.E.) embolden (O.E.) embouchure embrace embrasure (F) embroider (M.F.) embroil (F) employ employee employer employment enable enact enactment enamor encamp encampment encase enchain enchant enchanting enchantment enchantress enchase encircle enclave enclose enclosure encode encompass encounter encourage encouragement encouraging enculturation encumber encumbrance endorse endorsement endow endowment endue endurable endurance endure enduring enface enfeeble enfilade (F) enforce enfranchise engage (F) engagement engaging engender engine engineer engineering engorge (F) engrain engrave (O.E.) engraving engross engrossing engulf enhance enjoin enjoy enjoyable enjoyment enlarge enlargement enlist enlistment enliven (O.E.) enmasse (F) enmesh (M.Du.) ennoble enrage enrapt enrapture enrich enrichment enroll enrollment en route (F) ensanguine ensconce (Du.) ensemble enshrine (O.E.) ensign enslave (Slav) ensnare (O.E.) ensnarl (O.E.) ensphere ensue ensure (O.F.) entablature entail enthrone entice enticement entire entirely entitle entrain entrance entreat entreaty entrench entrenchment entrust (O.N.) entwine (O.E.) envelop envelope envelopment enviable envious environment envisage envision envoy envy entomb (O.E.); <u>See</u>: Gk. prefix **en-** Ap. iii-23.

counter- (From French *contre* from Latin *contra*.) counter counteract counterargument counterattack counterbalance countercharge countercheck counterclaim counterclockwise (M.Du.) counterespionage counterfeit counterinsurgency counterintelligence countermand countermarch countermeasure countermove counteroffensive counteroffer counterpart counterpoint counterpoise counterpropaganda counterproposal counterreformation Counter Reformation counterrevolution countersign countersink (O.E.) counterspy counterstroke (M.E.) countertenor countertype countervail counterweight (O.E.)

mis- (From Old French *mes-* from Latin *minus*.) misadventure misadvise misalliance misally misapply misapprehend misapprehension misappropriate miscarriage mischief mischievous miscolor misconceive misconception misconduct misconstruction misconstrue miscount miscreant miscreate miscue misdate misdemeanor misdirect misdirection misdoubt misemploy misfeasance misfortune misgovern misinform misinterpret misjoinder misjudge mismanage mismarriage misnomer misplace misplead misprint misprision misprize mispronounce misquote misremember misreport misrepresent misrule misstate mistranslate mistreat mistrial misusage misuse misvalue misventure; <u>See</u>: Old English prefix **mis-** Ap. iii-3.

sur- (above; beyond; over) (Old French from Latin *super* or *sursum*, upwards) surcharge surcingle surface surfeit surmise surmount surname surpass surpassing surplice surplus surprise surrealism surrender surreptitious surround surrounding surtax surveillance survey surveyor survival survive survivor

Old & Middle English Suffixes

-**burg**, (-berg), (-borough), (-bourg), (-burgh), (-bury), ... Ap. iv- 4

-**cester**, -**dom**, -**ed**, ... Ap. iv- 4

-**edly**, -**en**, -**enly**, -**er** (noun), ... Ap. iv- 5

-**er** (verb), ... Ap. iv- 6

-**er** (adj.), -**er** (Comp. adj.), (-ier), -**er** (adv.), ... Ap. iv- 7

-**er** (prep.), -**erly**, -**ern**, -**est** (Super. adj.), ... Ap. iv- 7

(-iest), -**field**, -**fold**, -**for**, -**fold**, -**ful**, -**fully**, ... Ap. iv- 8

-**hood**, -**ing** (adj.), -**ing** (noun), ... Ap. iv- 9

-**ing** (prep., conj., p.p.)-**ingly**, -**ish**, -**ishly**, -**land**, -**le**, -**less**, -**lessly**, Ap. iv-10

-**like**, -**ling**, -**ly**, ... Ap. iv-11

-**man**, -**manly**, -**most**, -**ness**, ... Ap. iv-12

-**ock**, -**of**, -**ship**, -**shire**, -**some**, ... Ap. iv-13

-**somely**, -**son**, -**ster**, -**teen**, -**th**, ... Ap. iv-13

-**the**, -**thorp**, -**ton**, -**town**, .-**ty**, -**ward**, ... Ap. iv-14

-**wardly**, -**ware**, -**way**, -**ways**, -**wise**, -**woman**, ... Ap. iv-14

-**work**, -**worthy**, -**worthily**, -**wright**, -**y** . . . . Ap. iv-15

Latin Suffixes

-**a**, (-ia), ... Ap. iv-16

-**ability**, -**able**, ... Ap. iv-17

-**ableness**, -**ably**, -**ace**, ... Ap. iv-18

-**aceous**, -**ade**, ... Ap. iv-18

-**age**, al^1, ... Ap. iv-19

(-ial^1), -**al**^{2}, ... Ap. iv-19

(-eal^2), (-ial^2), (-ual^2), ... Ap. iv-20

-**ally**, -**amine**, -**an**, ... Ap. iv-20

(-ean), (-ian), -**ana**, -**ance**, ... Ap. iv-21

(-eance), (-iance), (-uance), ... Ap. iv-22

-**ancy**, -**ane**, -**anely**, -**ant**^{1} . . . . Ap. iv-22

(-iant^1), (-uant^1), -**ant**^{2}, ... Ap. iv-22

(-eant^2), (-iant^2), (-uant^2), -**antly**, -**ar**^{1}, (-iar), ... Ap. iv-23

-**ar**^{2}, -**arily**, -**arity**, -**arium**, -**arly**, ... Ap. iv-23

-ary[1], (-iary[1]), -ary[2], (-iary[2]), -as, -ate[1], ... Ap. iv-24

(-iate[1]), -ate[2], ... Ap. iv-25

(-iate[2]), -ate[3], (-iate[3]), -ately, ... Ap. iv-26

-ator, -atory, -cia, -cial, -cially, ... Ap. iv-26

-cian, -ciate, -ciency, -cient, -ciently, ... Ap. iv-27

-cion, -cious, -ciously, -cise, ... Ap. iv-27

-cisely, -cle, -cule, -cy, (-acy), ... Ap. iv-27

-e (Non-silent final *e*), -el, ... Ap. iv-28

-ella, -em, -en, -ence . . . . Ap. iv-28

(-ience), (-cience), (-tience), -ency, -end, -ent, ... Ap. iv-29

(-ient), (-uent), -ental, -entally, -ently, -ery, -esce, ... Ap. iv-30

-escence, -escent, -escently, -ese, ... Ap. iv-31

-ete, -etely, -ey, -facient, ... Ap. iv-31

-faction, -factor, -ferous, ... Ap. iv-31

-fic, -fically, -fication, -ficator, -fice, -ficent, ... Ap. iv-32

-ficently, -fy, (-ify), -fier (-ifier) -geous, ... Ap. iv-32

-geously, -geousness, -gious -giously, ... Ap. iv-33

-giousness, -ibility, -ible, -ibly, -ic, ... Ap. iv-33

-ical, -ically, -icalness, -ice, -id, -ide, -idly, ... Ap. iv-34

-il, -ile, -ilely, -ility, ... Ap. iv-35

-ily, -in, -ine, -inely, ... Ap. iv-35

-ineness, -ion, -ior, -iorly, -is, ... Ap. iv-36

-ise, -isely, -ish, -ism, ... Ap. iv-36

-ist, -istic, ... Ap. iv-37

-istically, -it, -ite, ... Ap. iv-38

-itely, -ive, -ment, ... Ap. iv-38

-mental, -mentally, -mony, ... Ap. iv-39

-ol, -ole, -or, ... Ap. iv-39

-orily, -oriness, -ory, -ose, ... Ap. iv-40

-osely, -oseness, -osity, -ous, (-eous), (-ious), ... Ap. iv-41

(-uous), -ously, -ousness, -ry, -sia, -sion, (-asion), ... Ap. iv-42

(-esion), (-ision), (-osion), (-usion), -sional, -sionally, -sive, . Ap. iv-43

(-asive), (-esive), (-isive), (-osive), (-usive), ... Ap. iv-43

-sively, -siveness, -sivity, ... Ap. iv-43

-sure, -tain, -tia, -tial, -tially . . . . Ap. iv-44

Ap. iv CONTENTS . **Latin Suffixes** continued

-**tian**, -**tiate**, -**tient**, -**tiently**, -**tion**[1], ... Ap. iv-44
(-ation), ... Ap. iv-45
(-etion), ... Ap. iv-46
(-ition), (-otion), (-ution), -**tion**[2], -**tional**, ... Ap. iv-47
-**tionally**, -**tionary**, -**tious**, -**tiously**, -**tive**, ... Ap. iv-47
(-ative), (-etive), (-itive), (-otive), (-utive), ... Ap. iv-48
-**tively**, -**tiveness** -**tivity**, ... Ap. iv-48
-**trix**, -**tual**, -**tually**, -**tuary**, -**tude**, ... Ap. iv-49
-**tural**, -**turally**, -**ture**, -**ty**, (-ety), (-ity), ... Ap. iv-49
-**ude**, -**ule**, -**ulence**, -**ulent**, ... Ap. iv-50
-**ulently**, -**ulosity**, -**ulous**, ... Ap. iv-51
-**ulously**, -**ulousness**, -**um**, (-ium), ... Ap. iv-51
-**ure**, -**us**, (-ius), ... Ap. iv-52
-**use**, -**ute**, -**utely**, -**xion**, -**xious**, ... Ap. iv-53
-**xiously**, -**xiousness** -**y** . . . . Ap. iv-53

GREEK SUFFIXES

-**a**, -**ad**, -**asm**, -**ast**, -**ene**, -**es**, ... Ap. iv-54
-**eum**, -**gen**, -**ia**, -**iac**, -**ic**, ... Ap. iv-54
-**ical**, -**ically**, ... Ap. iv-55
-**is**, -**ism**, -**ist**, -**ite**, -**ize**, ... Ap. iv-56
-**ization**, -**lyze**, -**ode**, -**oid**, -**om**, ... Ap. iv-57
-**on**, -**os**, -**ose**, -**osis**, ... Ap. iv-58
-**ous**, -**ously**, -**sis**, -**tery**, -**tic**, ... Ap. iv-59
-**tron**, -**um**, -**y** . . . . Ap. iv-60

OTHER SUFFIXES

-**ac**, -**ah**, -**ain**, -**aire**, ... Ap. iv-61
-**ard**, -**ardly**, -**art**, ... Ap. iv-61
-**eer**, -**el**, -**esque**, ... Ap. iv-62
-**esquely**, -**ess**, -**et**, ... Ap. iv-62
-**ette**, -**eur**, -**grad**, -**kin**, -**let**, -**nik**, ... Ap. iv-63
-**o**, -**ot**, -**op**, -**que**, (-ique), -**quely**, ... Ap. iv-64
-**ski**, -**sky**, -**ute**, -**ville**, -**y** . . . . Ap. iv-64

Old & Middle English Suffixes

-burg /berg/ (noun) *[Town.]* Fitchburg Hamburg /häm-berg/ Hapsburg Harrisburg Hattiesburg Hindenburg (Name.) Johannesburg Luxemburg (Name.) Marburg Petersburg Salzburg Sandburg (Name.) Sharpsburg St. Petersburg Wilkinsburg Williamsburg Vicksburg Würzburg; **berg** /berg/ (Ger.) Heidelberg Nuremberg Schonberg (Name) Svedberg (Sw. name.) Württemberg; **-borough** /ber-ō/ Marlborough Peterborough Scarborough Yarborough; **-bourg** /boorg/ (F) Luxembourg Strasbourg Cherbourg; **-burgh** /berg/ Edinburgh /-ber-ə/ Pittsburgh Plattsburgh Roxburgh /ber-ə/; **-bury** /ber-ə/ Newbury Waterbury, *etc.*   See: -ville in Other Suffixes.

-cester /ster/ (noun) *[Camp. L. castra.]* Gloucester /glos-ter/ Worcester /woos-ter/

-dom /dəm/ (noun) *[Condition, domain, rank.]* boredom Christendom czardom dukedom earldom freedom heathendom heirdom kingdom martyrdom officialdom popedom rebeldom sheikdom subkingdom thralldom Yankeedom

-ed[1] /id/ (After *t* & *d*.) (Past tense verb, past participle, or adj.) accepted acquainted affected acted added assorted attended blasted commanded conceited concerted consulted contented crowded cultivated dated decided degraded dejected delighted departed devoted disappointed discontented disgusted disinterested disjointed distorted distracted divided dotted drifted dusted educated elated elevated ended excited exhausted expanded extended fated folded frosted gifted granted guarded haunted hinted hunted included indebted inflated inhabited intended interested interrupted insisted invented landed lasted lifted limited loaded melted misguided mounted needed nested operated painted parted planted pointed pretended printed provided punted related repeated restricted rusted salted sanded seated sided sifted sighted slanted spirited spotted stated stilted subtracted superannuated suspended sweated talented tended tented tested tinted truncated waited wanted

-ed[2] /t/ (After all unvoiced letters but *t*.) (Past tense verb, past participle, or adj.) accomplished advanced asked attacked backed blinked blocked bumped camped checked cracked deceased depressed detached discussed distinguished distressed embarrassed experienced expressed finished fixed flunked forced gulped helped honked hoped iced impressed jumped kicked kissed limped marked missed mixed packed passed picked polished practiced puffed risked shaped touched typed

-ed[3] /d/ (After all voiced letters but *d*.) (Past tense verb, past participle, or adj.) abandoned accustomed advised aged agreed allied applied armed ashamed assumed assured authorized banged blamed canned carried called colored compelled composed concerned conditioned confined confirmed considered cornered cried cultured damaged declared deserved destined determined disadvantaged diseased disturbed engaged exposed favored featured figured filled filmed frightened gnarled grilled happened healed hurried hushed implied inclined informed injured insured involved killed learned lettered lived loved mailed mannered married mended misspelled motored muscled pickled principled qualified quizzed raised reasoned refined reformed registered removed reserved resigned resolved retired screamed seemed served signaled skilled smelled spelled spilled starred strained studied summoned tired traveled troubled used valued varied watered weathered yelled

-edly /id-lē/ (adv.) (Adverb forming **-ly** ending added to **-ed** ending adjectives.) absentmindedly admittedly advisedly allegedly assuredly belatedly conceitedly confusedly contentedly decidedly dejectedly delightedly deservedly determinedly devotedly disappointedly disgustedly dispiritedly distractedly elatedly evenhandedly exaggeratedly excitedly guardedly halfheartedly hurriedly kindheartedly learnedly markedly misguidedly notedly opinionatedly perplexedly pointedly premeditatedly presumedly purportedly repeatedly reportedly reputedly sophisticatedly spiritedly supposedly tiredly undoubtedly unexpectedly unitedly unlimitedly unreservedly

-en[1] /ən/ (verb) awaken cheapen dampen darken deafen deepen dishearten enliven fasten glisten happen harden hasten hearten lengthen lessen listen loosen moisten open quicken ripen sharpen shorten sicken slacken smarten smoothen soften steepen stiffen strengthen thicken toughen weaken worsen; /n/ (*d* or *t* after vowel sound. Note that *d, t, & n* all have same tongue position.) broaden deaden enlighten flatten frighten heighten lighten sadden straighten threaten tighten widen

-en[2] /ən/ (verb) (Past participle.) broken chosen driven fallen frozen given mistaken spoken stolen taken; /n/ bitten eaten forgotten gotten hidden written; Note: been /bin/ seen /sēn/

-en[3] /ən/ (adj.) ashen barren brazen cloven craven drunken earthen even flaxen golden graven oaken olden shaven silken sullen waxen wooden; /n/ laden leaden rotten sudden

-en[4] /ən/ (noun) aspen burden chicken children (pl.) delicatessen eleven garden haven heaven kitchen linen oven oxen (pl.) raven seven siren token warden women (pl.); /n/ Eden kitten maiden sauerbraten; Names: Arden Helen Reuben Tutankhamen Warren Yemen; /n/ Staten Island Sweden See: Latin Suffix **-en**, Ap. iv-28.

-enly /ən-lē/ (adv.) (Adverb forming **-ly** added to **-en** adjective.) brazenly brokenly cravenly drunkenly evenly misshapenly mistakenly outspokenly suddenly

-er[1] /er/ (noun) accuser adventurer adviser airliner anger angler announcer answer appetizer backer badger baker banker banner banter barber barker barter batter beater beaver biker binder biographer bladder blazer bleacher blender blinker blister blocker blotter blunder boiler bomber booster border bother boulder bouncer boxer broker brother bubbler bumper burger burner butcher butler butter buyer buzzer caller camper cancer canner carpenter carrier catcher center chapter charter character chatter checker chowder cider cinder cipher clatter cleaner cleanser climber clincher clinker clipper cluster clutter coaster cobbler commander composer computer consumer container controller cooker cooler copper corner counter coupler cover cracker crater creamer crier cruiser cucumber customer cycler cylinder dagger damper dancer danger daughter dealer defroster deserter designer destroyer developer diaper diner dinner dipper disclaimer disorder dispatcher dispenser divider dodger doer drawer dreamer driller drinker driver drummer eater elder ember employer encounter eraser explorer extinguisher farmer father feather feeder fertilizer fever fiber fibber fielder fighter filibuster filler filter financier finger flicker flier flower folder follower forecaster foreigner forester founder freezer freighter fritter gardener gender geyser ginger girder giver glacier glider glimmer golfer goner gopher grinder grocer grounder grower gunner gutter hacker hamburger hammer hanger handler hauler healer heater helper hiker hitter hunger hunter importer informer insider insurer interpreter jailer jester jeweler jogger joker juggler juicer jumper kicker killer kindergartner ladder laughter lawyer layer leader lecturer letter lever liner liver lobster locker lodger logger loser lover lumber maker manager manner marker master matter member merger messenger meter miner minister mister mixer monster mother murder neither nerve November number offer officer opener order other otter ouster oyster owner paper partner passenger passer pepper philosopher pitcher planer planner planter plaster plater platter player pledger plumber pointer poster powder power prayer preacher printer prisoner producer programmer promoter prompter propeller provider publisher punter quarter racer rafter raider rancher ranger reader receiver refresher register remainder renter reporter retailer reviewer revolver rider river robber rocker roller roofer roomer rooster rower rubber rudder ruler runner saucer saver scavenger scepter semester sender September settler shelter shiver shooter shopper shower shudder shutter silver singer sister sitter skater skier skipper slander‿ slaughter slayer sledder sleeper slipper sliver slumber smoker smuggler sneaker soccer sparkler speaker speeder speller spider splinter sprinkler stapler starter steamer sticker stinger stopper stranger streamer stretcher stutter summer super supper supporter surfer surrender suspender sweater sweetener talker tanker teacher teenager temper thinker thriller thunder tiger timber timer tinder toaster tower trader trailer trainer tranquilizer transfer transformer transmitter traveler treasurer trigger trucker trumpeter tumbler twister usher viewer voter voucher wager waiter walker watcher water waver wearer whaler whimper whisker whisper whistler whopper widower winner winter wiper wonder worker wrapper wrecker wrestler writer zipper;   (pronoun) her

-er[2] /er/ (verb) administer alter answer blunder bolster bother clobber cluster clutter confer conquer consider cover decipher defer deliver desert /di-<u>zert</u>/ deter differ discover encounter enter fester filter flatter flounder flower flutter foster founder fritter gather glimmer glitter hammer hamper hinder linger litter lower maneuver master matter minister murder muster mutter number offer order pamper plaster plunder ponder powder prefer recover refer register remember scatter shatter shelter shiver shower shudder simper slander slaughter slobber slumber smolder smother snicker spatter splatter splutter squander stagger stammer stutter suffer surrender swagger swelter tamper taper tether tinker titter totter transfer trigger twitter uncover unlimber upholster usher wander waver whisper wonder

-er³ (adj.) aflutter amber bitter dapper clever elder either former improper inner proper sober somber subcaliber other slender sinister tender upper utter yonder

-er⁴ (Comparative form of adj.) better blacker bluer blunter braver brighter broader browner calmer cleaner closer cooler crisper damper darker dimmer duller elder farther faster fatter firmer fitter greater greener harder higher hotter later lesser lighter longer louder lower madder meaner milder moister narrower nearer nicer older quicker rapider redder riper rougher sadder sharper shorter sicker slicker slimmer slower smarter softer sooner sounder stronger stupider swifter tamer tanner tenderer thinner tighter timider tireder tougher trimmer vivider weaker wetter whiter wider yellower younger; *Better worse more less* are also comparatives.

(-ier) /ē-er/ (Comparative of adj. ending in *y*. Change **y** to **i** and add **-er,** e.g., *happy* to *happier.*) angrier bossier brawnier breezier bulkier bumpier bushier busier cheerier chewier chillier choosier choppier cloudier clumsier cozier crabbier craftier crankier crazier creakier creepier curlier daintier dewier dingier dirtier dizzier dreamier drearier drowsier dustier easier emptier filthier flimsier fluffier foggier friskier frostier funnier fussier gaudier glassier gloomier goofier greasier greedier grimier grouchier grumpier happier hardier healthier huskier icier juicier lazier luckier lumpier merrier mightier mistier moodier muddier murkier nastier naughtier needier nosier nuttier perkier prettier punier rainier riskier ritzier roomier rustier saltier sexier shabbier shaggier sillier skimpier skinnier sleazier sleepier slimier sloppier smellier smokier sneakier snootier snowier soapier soggier spookier squeakier steadier stickier stingier stormier stringier sturdier sunnier tardier tastier teenier thirstier thriftier tidier trickier uglier unrulier wackier wearier worthier zanier; <u>See</u>: **-y** in Ap. iv-15.

-er⁵ (adv.) hither later rather sooner;   **-er⁶** (prep.) after

-erly¹ /er-lē/ (adj., adv.) *[In the direction of.]* easterly northeasterly northerly northwesterly southeasterly southerly southwesterly westerly

-erly² /er-lē/ (adv.) *[Characteristic of.]* bitterly brotherly (+adj.) cleverly disorderly elderly fatherly (+adj.) formerly improperly motherly (+adj.) properly sinisterly sisterly (+adj.) slenderly soberly somberly tenderly unmannerly utterly

-ern /ern/ (adj.) *[To, toward.]* eastern midwestern northeastern northern northwestern southeastern southern southwestern western; <u>Unrelated</u>: cavern (L) concern (L) fern (O.E.) govern (O.F.) lectern (L) modern (L) pattern (L) stern (O.E.) tavern (L)

-est /est/ (Superlative form of adj.) blackest bluest boldest bravest brightest broadest brownest calmest cleanest closest coolest dampest darkest dimmest dullest dumbest eldest farthest fastest fattest firmest fittest flattest furthest greatest hardest highest

Ap. iv-7

horridest hottest kindest latest lightest longest loudest lowest maddest meanest mildest moistest narrowest nearest nicest oldest quickest reddest ripest roughest saddest sharpest shortest sickest slowest smartest softest soonest soundest strongest stupidest swiftest tamest thinnest tightest timidest tiredest toughest trimmest vividest weakest wettest whitest widest yellowest youngest;
Best worst least most are also superlatives.

<u>Note</u>: Other words, mainly from Latin, happen to end in **-est**. acquest arrest attest bequest congest conquest contest detest digest divest forest harvest honest immodest infest ingest inquest interest invest jest lest manifest modest molest nest pest protest quest rest suggest tempest test vest west

(-iest) /ē-est/ (Superlative form of adj. ending in –y.)   [Change **y** to **i** and add **-est**, e.g., *happy* to *happiest*.] angriest balmiest billowiest bossiest bounciest brainiest breeziest bulkiest bumpiest bushiest busiest catchiest cheeriest chewiest chilliest chintziest choosiest cloudiest clumsiest cockiest coziest crabbiest crankiest craziest creepiest crispiest crumbiest dingiest dinkiest dirtiest dizziest dreamiest dreariest dressiest drowsiest dustiest easiest fanciest filthiest flakiest flashiest foggiest funniest fussiest giddiest glassiest gloomiest goofiest greediest grouchiest grumpiest guiltiest happiest healthiest holiest huskiest itchiest luckiest lumpiest lustiest mightiest moodiest muggiest murkiest nastiest naughtiest neediest niftiest noisiest nuttiest prettiest pudgiest rainiest riskiest ritziest saltiest sandiest sassiest sexiest shabbiest skinniest sleepiest slimiest sloppiest smelliest smokiest sneakiest soapiest soggiest sorriest spunkiest steadiest stickiest stingiest stormiest sunniest tardiest tastiest thirstiest touchiest ugliest

-field /fēld/ Chesterfield Garfield Sheffield Springfield

-fold *[Number of parts or times.]* eightfold fivefold fourfold hundredfold manifold multifold (L) ninefold onefold sevenfold sixfold tenfold thousandfold threefold trifold twofold;   <u>Also</u>: billfold blindfold centerfold infold sheepfold unfold

-for unaccounted-for uncalled-for uncared-for unhoped-for unlooked-for

-ford Bradford Hartford Haverford Medford Strafford Waterford Wexford

-ful /fəl/ (adj.) *[Full of.]* awful bashful beautiful careful cheerful colorful deceitful delightful disgraceful doubtful dreadful faithful fearful flavorful forceful forgetful frightful fruitful graceful grateful harmful hateful helpful hopeful joyful meaningful mindful mouthful needful pitiful playful powerful resentful resourceful respectful restful rightful roomful shameful sinful skillful sorrowful spiteful successful tactful tankful tasteful tearful thankful thoughtful trustful truthful tuneful uneventful unfaithful unfruitful ungrateful unsuccessful useful vengeful wasteful willful zestful

-fully /fəl-ē/ (adv.) (Adverb forming **-ly** added to **-ful** adjective.) awfully beautifully carefully doubtfully faithfully forcefully frightfully gracefully hopefully peacefully powerfully respectfully successfully thoughtfully truthfully usefully willfully, *etc.*

-hood /hŏŏd/ (noun) *[Condition of; class of.]* adulthood childhood falsehood knighthood livelihood manhood neighborhood parenthood priesthood sainthood

-ing[1] /ing/ (adj.) accepting adoring agonizing ailing alarming alluring amazing amusing annoying appalling appealing appetizing approving astonishing astounding bewildering blinding blushing boring bouncing brooding burning charming chattering chilling clinging coming commanding compelling complaining condescending conflicting confusing continuing convincing damaging daring dashing deadening deafening deceiving demanding depressing despairing detracting disappointing discouraging discriminating disgusting distracting disturbing domineering doting doubting dying embarrassing enchanting encouraging endearing enduring enterprising entertaining enticing everlasting exasperating exciting excruciating exhausting exhilarating extenuating fascinating fighting flickering flowering foreboding forgiving forthcoming frightening frustrating glowing gratifying halting hanging haunting hesitating horrifying humiliating impending imposing incoming increasing indiscriminating infuriating inquiring insulting interesting intriguing invigorating inviting irritating lasting limiting living longing losing loving maddening menacing misleading missing moaning moving mystifying nauseating neighboring outstanding overbearing participating perplexing pleasing preceding pressing prevailing promising provoking puzzling rambling reassuring refreshing resounding retiring revealing revolting rewarding rousing satisfying searching sickening singing smiling snarling sparkling speeding standing startling stunning surprising surrounding sweltering swinging talking tantalizing taunting taxing teasing tempting terrifying threatening thrilling touching unbecoming unceasing uncompromising unrelenting unwilling varying waiting warning weeping whining whispering willing winding winning

-ing[2] /ing/ (noun) acting accounting advertising aging backing banking being billing bowling boxing breaking brewing briefing building calling camping canning ceiling clearing clothing coloring consulting covering craving crossing crying curbing cutting dairying darling dealing drawing drilling driving dwelling dying eating engineering engraving etching farming feeling fencing filling fishing flavoring flooring footing frosting gathering greeting happening hardening heading hearing helping hiding housekeeping housing humming hunting ironing icing jesting juggling keeping killing kindling knitting landing laughing launching leaning learning lettering lightning liking lining lodging logging losing lying making meaning meeting mining misunderstanding molding moonlighting morning nursing opening outing packing padding paddling paving peeling plumbing printing railing rating reasoning ruling running saving scaffolding seasoning seating seeing serving setting sewing shaving showing siding singing sitting skiing sledding spacing spanking speaking speeding spelling spelunking sprinkling stabbing staging standing stocking stuffing suffering surfing surveying sweeping sweetening swelling swimming tackling tailoring taking talking teaching Thanksgiving thinking timing topping training turning understanding upbringing waiting warning washing watering wedding weightlifting whipping whispering winning wiring woodcarving wording wrapping wrestling writing yachting

Ap. iv-9

-ing³ /ing/ (prep.) barring concerning considering during excepting failing regarding respecting saving touching

-ing⁴ /ing/ (conj.) providing seeing

-ing⁵ /ing/ (present participle) acting crying hunting seeing sewing training winning, *etc.*

-ingly /ing-lē/ (adv.) (Adverb forming **-ly** added to **-ing** adjective.) accordingly amazingly chillingly convincingly depressingly disapprovingly encouragingly increasingly invitingly pleasingly refreshingly surprisingly trustingly willingly, *etc* <u>See</u>: **-ing¹** Ap. iv-9.

-ish¹ /ish/ (noun, adj.) *[Belonging to a national or other group.]* Amish British Cornish Danish English Finnish Flemish Frankish Gaulish Irish Jewish Kurdish Lettish Moorish Pictish Polish Rhenish Scottish Spanish Swedish Turkish Wendish Yiddish

-ish² /ish/ (adj.) *[Like; somewhat.]* amateurish babyish bookish boorish boyish childish coolish devilish feverish fiendish foolish freakish girlish goodish grayish impish kittenish knavish latish mannish modish oddish oldish old-womanish outlandish peevish piggish prudish reddish roguish roundish rowdyish selfish sheepish sickish sluggish smallish snobbish squeamish standoffish stylish sweetish tallish ticklish tigerish unselfish uppish weakish;   <u>See</u>: Latin Suffix **-ish** Ap. iv-36.

-ishly /ish-lē/ (adv) (Adverb forming **-ly** added to **-ish²** adjective. A few examples are given here.) boorishly boyishly fiendishly foolishly peevishly selfishly, *etc.*

-land /lənd/ (noun) *[Name, place.]* Cleveland Cumberland England Falkland Finland Holland Iceland Ireland Maryland Midland Portland Scotland Shetland Switzerland; /land/ dreamland fatherland Lapland motherland Somaliland Sudetenland tableland

-le /əl/ (verb) (Verb frequentative, e.g., *spark* > *sparkle*.) chuckle crackle crumple curdle dabble dazzle draggle dribble dwindle fizzle fondle jiggle joggle jostle ramble ramshackle scuffle scuttle sniffle snuffle snuggle sparkle straggle topple trample

-less /lis/ (adj.) *[Lacking the preceding concept.]* aimless blameless bottomless boundless brainless careless changeless cheerless colorless dauntless deathless doubtless effortless endless expressionless faithless fatherless fathomless faultless fearless featureless flawless flightless formless friendless fruitless gainless graceless groundless guiltless hapless harmless heartless heedless helpless hopeless jobless joyless landless lawless lifeless lightless limitless listless loveless luckless matchless meaningless mindless needless penniless reckless relentless pitiless powerless priceless profitless quenchless regardless relentless remorseless restless ruthless selfless senseless shameless speechless spineless spiritless spotless stateless tactless tasteless thankless timeless tireless useless wordless;   <u>Exceptions</u>: /les/ less unless

-lessly /lis-lē/ (adv.) (Adverb forming **-ly** added to **-less** adjective.) breathlessly carelessly endlessly fearlessly flawlessly helplessly recklessly relentlessly ruthlessly selflessly shamelessly thoughtlessly tirelessly uselessly, *etc.*   <u>See</u>: **-less** above.

Ap. iv-10

-like /līk/ (adj.) *[Similar to first word in compound.]* birdlike boxlike catlike childlike deathlike doglike domelike dreamlike flowerlike flutelike ghostlike godlike hairlike homelike humanlike jellylike jewellike ladylike lifelike manlike mirrorlike puppylike ratlike ringlike rocklike rubberlike sportsmanlike threadlike tigerlike toothlike toylike tublike warlike waxlike weblike winglike workmanlike, *etc.*   And: dislike unlike

-ling /ling/ (noun)   *[Little; young; minor; related to.]* changeling darling duckling dumpling earthling fatling firstling foundling godling gosling nestling nursling sapling seedling sibling sproutling starling sterling stripling weakling weanling yearling

-ly¹ /lē/ (adj.) *[Like, pertaining to.]* beastly bristly brotherly bubbly burly chilly comely comradely costly courtly crackly crinkly crumbly cuddly curly deadly deathly drizzly early earthly elderly fatherly friendly frilly ghastly ghostly godly goodly grumbly heavenly hilly holy homely jolly likely lively lonely lovely lowly manly motherly nightly oily only orderly richly saintly scholarly scribbly seemly shapely sickly silly sisterly smelly stately surly timely tingly ugly unearthly unfriendly ungainly unlikely unseemly unsightly untimely unholy unruly unsightly wobbly; *[At a certain interval.]* annually bimonthly biweekly daily half-hourly hourly momently monthly quarterly semimonthly semiweekly weekly yearly

-ly² /lē/ (adv.) ably abruptly absolutely absurdly abundantly adeptly adroitly adversely amiably amply aptly aversely badly barely blatantly brusquely blindly bluntly boldly bravely briefly brightly briskly broadly calmly capably certainly chiefly clearly cleverly closely coldly commonly completely concisely conversely coolly correctly costly covertly cowardly coyly crudely cruelly daily deadly dearly deathly deeply defiantly devoutly directly difficultly dimly directly distinctly dryly dumbly eagerly earnestly elegantly elusively eminently entirely equally evasively evenly evidently exactly explicitly expressly extremely fairly falsely fatally feebly fervently fiercely finely firmly flatly fondly frankly franticly freely frequently friendly fully futilely gently gladly glibly glumly grandly gravely greatly grimly hardly harshly highly honestly hotly ideally immodestly imprecisely inaptly indirectly insanely insincerely insipidly instantly intensely invalidly jointly justly keenly kindly largely lastly lately legally legibly leisurely leniently lewdly lightly likely locally lonely loosely loudly lovably loyally madly mainly manifestly meekly merely mildly minutely modestly morally morosely mostly namely narrowly nearly neatly neighborly newly nicely nightly notably obscurely oddly only openly orally orderly outwardly overly overtly partly perfectly perversely plainly poorly precisely presently privately probably profoundly promptly properly prudently publicly purely purposely quaintly quickly quietly randomly rarely rashly really remotely richly rightly roughly roundly routinely royally rudely sadly safely savagely scarcely secretly securely serenely severely sharply shortly shrewdly shyly sickly silently simply sincerely slightly slowly slyly smartly smoothly smugly soberly softly solely solemnly sorely soundly splendidly squarely steadfastly sternly strangely strictly strongly stubbornly succinctly suddenly supremely surely sweetly swiftly tacitly tamely tensely thickly thinly thoroughly thusly tightly timely tiredly tonally totally truly uncertainly unduly unequally unevenly unfairly unfriendly uniformly unjustly unlikely unseemly untimely unwisely uselessly usually utterly vaguely vainly vastly venally verbosely visibly warmly weakly weedily weirdly wholly widely wildly wisely wrongly; <u>See also</u>: O.E. suffixes **-edly, -enly, -erly, -fully, -ingly, -ishly, -lessly, -manly, -somely, -wardly, -worthily;** Latin suffixes **-ably, -ally, -anely, -antly, -arily, -arly, -ately, -cially, -ciently, -ciously, -cisely, -entally, -ently, -escently, -etely, -fically, -ficently, -geously, -giously, -ibly, -ically, -idly, -ilely, -ily, -inely, -iorly, -isely, -istically, -itely, -mentally, -orily, -osely, -ously, -sionally, -sively, -tially, -tiently, -tionally, -tiously, -tively, -tually, -turally, -ulently, -ulously, -utely, -xiously;** Gk. suffixes **-ically, -ously;** Other Suffixes **-esquely.**

-man /mən/ (noun) *[Activity, interest, or status of a particular man.]* (Forms a compound word.) airman alderman artilleryman assemblyman bondsman brushman cattleman chairman churchman clansman clergyman committeeman congressman councilman craftsman dairyman draftsman Dutchman Englishman fisherman flagman foreman freshman frogman frontiersman gentleman guardsman guildsman gunman hangman helmsman henchman herdsman highwayman horseman infantryman Irishman journeyman juryman kinsman Klansman laundryman layman lineman longshoreman lumberman Manxman merchantman midshipman militiaman motorman nobleman Norman Norseman nurseryman oarsman Orangeman packman patrolman pitchman plainsman plowman policeman postman pressman raftsman ranchman rifleman salesman Scotsman seaman selectman shopman showman signalman spaceman spokesman sportsman statesman stockman switchman swordsman townsman trackman tradesman trainman tribesman truckman underclassman upperclassman warehouseman watchman waterman Welshman wheelman woodsman yachtsman yardman yeoman; /man/ anchor man ape man ashman best man black man bogeyman businessman cameraman cave man chessman common man confidence man doorman end man enlisted man gag man gasman handyman he-man hired man iceman Java man junkman letterman madman medicine man milkman minuteman Neanderthal man newsman newspaperman overman Paleolithic man Peking man Piltdown man plainclothes man pointman ragman red man repairman rewrite man sandman secondstory man serviceman snowman straight man straw man strongman stunt man superman track man trigger man trolleyman utility man weatherman white man workingman yes man

-manly /man-lē/ (adj.) gentlemanly sportsmanly statesmanly, *etc.*

-most /mōst/ (adj.) (Forms superlative from adjective.) almost easternmost endmost farthermost foremost furthermost hindmost inmost innermost lowermost northernmost outermost outmost southernmost topmost uppermost utmost uttermost westernmost

-ness /nis/ (noun) *[state of being]* (**-ness** added to adj. to form noun. Adj. ending in *y* changes to *i*.) baldness bareness blessedness boldness business busyness calmness cleanliness clearness cleverness closeness conciseness consciousness coziness dampness darkness deafness drunkenness dullness earthiness easiness exactness fairness firmness fondness foolhardiness forgiveness frankness forwardness fullness gladness goodness happiness hardiness hardness heaviness highness holiness iciness idleness illness indebtedness kindness lateness laziness likeness loudness madness nearness neatness neediness openness preparedness readiness recklessness righteousness rudeness selfishness sickness slowness smugness softness soreness spotlessness sweetness tameness thickness thoughtlessness togetherness ugliness unconsciousness unpleasantness vastness weakness wickedness wilderness, *etc.*

-ock /ok/ (noun) (Common ending, but may mean *small.) aftershock alpenstock antiknock bitstock *bullock *buttock deadlock feedstock flintlock forelock gamecock *hillock hollyhock interlock livestock *mullock overstock poppycock roadblock rootstock shamrock shuttlecock stopcock weathercock woodcock

-of /əv/ (adj.) undreamed-of unheard-of untalked-of unthought-of well-thought-of

-ship /ship/ (noun) *[Condition; rank; skill.]* brinkmanship censorship championship citizenship companionship courtship dictatorship fellowship friendship governorship hardship horsemanship internship interrelationship kingship kinship leadership lordship oarsmanship ownership partnership relationship salesmanship scholarship seamanship sportsmanship township trusteeship tutorship workmanship yachtsmanship

-shire /shear/ or /sher/ (noun) *[Territorial division in Britain.]* Berkshire Gloucestershire Hampshire Lancashire Lincolnshire New Hampshire Wiltshire Yorkshire

-some /səm/ (adj.) *[Tending to be.]* awesome bothersome burdensome cumbersome fearsome foursome frolicsome gruesome handsome lonesome quarrelsome threesome tiresome troublesome twosome unwholesome wholesome winsome

-somely /səm-lē/ (adv.) (Adverb forming **-ly** added to **-some** adjective.) awesomely fearsomely gruesomely handsomely lonesomely quarrelsomely, *etc.* Ṣee: **-some**.

-son /sən/ (name) *[Son of.]* Emerson Ericson Gibson Harrison Jackson Janson Jefferson Johnson McPherson Neilson, *etc.*

-ster /ster/ (noun) *[One who makes; one who belongs to.]* gangster huckster pollster prankster punster roadster songster speedster spinster teamster trickster youngster

-teen /tēn/ (noun, adj.) *[Plus ten.]* thirteen fourteen fifteen sixteen seventeen eighteen nineteen

-th /th/ (adj.) (Used with ordinal numbers.) **-eth** (After vowels.) fourth fifth sixth seventh eighth ninth tenth eleventh twelfth thirteenth fourteenth fifteenth sixteenth seventeenth eighteenth nineteenth twentieth thirtieth fortieth fiftieth sixtieth seventieth eightieth ninetieth hundredth thousandth millionth billionth trillionth umpteenth, *etc.* Also with many Old & Middle English nouns:--berth betroth breadth broth dearth hearth heath Kenneth kith loath pith Ruth sheath sloth stealth swath troth uncouth worth wraith wrath wreath; Ṣee: **th** Ap.i-39 for initial and medial positions.

<u>Others</u>: froth (O.N.)   girth (O.N.)   hyacinth (Gk.)   labyrinth (Gk.)   megalith (Gk.) monolith (Gk.)   osteopath (Gk.)   sleuth (O.N.)   sociopath (L/Gk.)   vermouth (Ger.) zenith (Ar.)

-the (voiced <u>th</u>) (verb) (**-th** /th/ unvoiced = **noun**)   bath ba<u>the</u> /bā<u>th</u>/   breath brea<u>the</u> /bre<u>th</u>/ loath (adj.) loa<u>the</u>   sheath shea<u>the</u>   sooth soo<u>the</u>   swath swa<u>the</u>   teeth tee<u>the</u> wreath wrea<u>the</u>;   And: blithe /blī<u>th</u>/ or /blī<u>th</u>/ (adj.)   ti<u>the</u> (n,v)   wi<u>the</u> (n)   wri<u>the</u> (v)

-thorp(e) (noun) *[Village, hamlet.]* Linthorp Oglethorpe, *etc.*

-ton /tən/ (noun) *[Town.]* Appleton Arlington Boston Brockton Burlington Charleston Chesterton Edmonton Galveston Hamilton Hampton Lewiston Princeton Scranton Washington;   <u>Also</u>: singleton simpleton

-town /town/ (noun) Georgetown Levittown Provincetown Yorktown Youngstown

-ty /tē/-(noun) *[Ten times.]* twenty thirty forty fifty sixty seventy eighty ninety <u>See</u>: Latin suffix **-ty** Ap. iv-49.

-ward /werd/ (adj.) *[Directed toward.]* afterward awkward (O.N.) backward cityward downward earthward eastward forward heavenward homeward inward landward leeward northward onward outward seaward shoreward sideward southward toward untoward upward wayward westward windward; <u>See</u>: Old French suffix **-ard** Ap. iv-61.

-wardly /werd-lē/ (adv.)   (Adverb forming **-ly** added to **-ward** adjective.) awkwardly backwardly   forwardly   westwardly, *etc.*   <u>See</u>: **-ward** above.

-ware /wair/ (noun) agateware glassware hardware kitchenware software stemware stoneware   tableware   tinware   warehouse   wareroom   woodenware

-way /wā/ airway alleyway archway areaway breezeway causeway companionway doorway driveway expressway fairway freeway gangway gateway guideway hallway hatchway highway keyway midway passageway railway roadway runway shipway skyway sluiceway speedway spillway stairway steerageway sternway straightway subway   superhighway   thruway   tramway   underway   walkway   waterway; **(-away)** castaway cutaway faraway flyaway foldaway getaway giveaway hideaway layaway runaway stowaway straightaway throwaway walkaway

-ways /wāz/ edgeways endways folkways noways sideways

-wise /wīz/ (adj., adv.) clockwise (M.D.) crosswise counterclockwise contrariwise (L) cornerwise crosswise edgewise endwise leastwise lengthwise likewise longwise moneywise (L) nowise otherwise sidewise slantwise (Scan.) stepwise weather-wise

-woman /woom-ən/ (May be substituted for many of the **-man** entries.) chairwoman congresswoman clubwoman Englishwoman gentlewoman horsewoman laundrywoman laywoman noblewoman policewoman sportswoman townswoman workingwoman, *etc.*

-work /werk/ (noun) basketwork brickwork bridgework brushwork cabinetwork clockwork cutwork fieldwork glasswork handiwork housework ironwork lifework metalwork network piecework presswork rackwork roadwork scrollwork shopwork spadework steelwork stonework timberwork tinwork waxwork woodwork

-worthy /wer-$\underline{th}$ē/ (adj.) *[Meriting; valuable as.]* airworthy blameworthy newsworthy noteworthy praiseworthy seaworthy thankworthy trustworthy untrustworthy

-worthily /wer-$\underline{th}$ə-lē/ (adv.) newsworthily praiseworthily trustworthily, *etc.*

-wright /rīt/ (noun) *[One who constructs.]* millwright playwright shipwright wheelwright

-y /ē/ (adj.) (Remember the 1-1-1-V Rule: *bag + y = baggy.* Note that some of these adjectives come from nouns ending in *e*. The *e* is simply changed to *y*, thus *juice = juicy, stone = stony*, etc.) airy almighty angry any arty baggy balmy batty bawdy beefy billowy bony bossy bouncy brainy brassy brawny breathy breezy buggy bulky bumpy burly bushy busy catchy chancy chatty cheery cheesy chewy chilly choosy choppy chubby chummy chunky clammy classy cloudy clumsy cocky colicky corny cozy crabby crafty craggy cranky crazy creaky creamy creepy crispy crumby crummy crusty curly dainty dewy dingy dinky dirty dizzy doughy drafty dreamy dreary dressy drippy droopy drowsy dumpy dusky dusty earthy easy edgy empty every fancy fatty faulty feathery feisty fidgety filthy finicky flaky flashy fleecy fleshy flighty flimsy floppy flowery fluffy foamy foggy foolhardy foxy frilly frisky frosty funny fussy fuzzy gaudy giddy giggly glassy glittery gloomy glossy goofy gory gossipy grassy greasy greedy grimy gritty grouchy grubby grumpy guilty gummy gusty hairy happy hardy hasty haughty hazy healthy hearty hefty hilly holy huffy husky icy iffy itchy jaunty jazzy jerky jolly juicy jumpy kinky knotty lanky lazy leafy leery lengthy lofty loony lucky lumpy lusty many marshy merry mighty milky misty moldy moody muddy muggy murky mushy musty nasty naughty needy nervy newsy nifty nippy nosy nutty peppy perky pesky petty phony piggy plucky porky pretty pudgy puffy puny rainy raspy risky ritzy rocky roomy rosy rowdy rubbery ruby ruddy rusty salty sandy sassy saucy scanty scraggy scrubby scrappy seamy seedy sexy shabby shady shaggy shaky shiny shoddy showy silly silky sketchy skimpy skinny sleazy sleepy slimy slippery sloppy smelly smoky smudgy smutty snappy sneaky snippy snoopy snotty snowy soapy soggy sorry sooty soupy speedy spicy spongy spooky spotty spunky squeaky starchy starry steady stealthy steamy sticky stingy stocky stony stormy streaky stringy sturdy sugary sulky sunny swanky tacky tardy tasty teeny thirsty thorny thrifty tidy tiny touchy trashy tricky trusty ugly uncanny uneasy unlucky unruly unsavory unsteady unworthy wacky watery wavy waxy weary weedy wiry woody wordy worthy zany zippy;

Note: Most of these words may be made into the **comparative** form of the adjective by *"Changing **y** to **i** and adding **er**."* *Hasty* becomes *hastier*. The **superlative** form of the adjective is formed by *"Changing **y** to **i** and adding **-est**."* *Hasty* becomes *hastiest*. The adjective becomes an **adverb** by *"Changing **y** to **i** and adding **-ly**."* *Hasty* becomes *hastily*.
<u>See:</u> **-ier** Ap. iv-7, **-iest** Ap. iv-8, **-ily** Ap. iv-35.

Latin Suffixes

-a /ə/ (noun) (**-a** is L fem. sing. Its pl. is **-ae.** Neut. sing. **-um** has a pl. of **-a.**) abscissa alga *(algae)* alumna *(alumnae)* amphora *(amphorae)* angina antenna *(antennae)* aorta *(aortae)* aqua area arena armada aurora basilica boa bursa camera cantata cicada conjunctiva copula corona curiosa (pl.) dejecta (pl.) diva (It.) fibula fistula flora formula fossa gladiola harmonica impedimenta (pl.) ingesta (pl.) larva Libra Luna macula mamma mammilla maxilla mensa minutia *(minutiae)* mesa (Sp.) militia miscellanea mozzarella (It.) nebula *(nebulae)* nova *(novae)* novena novella opera patella peninsula penumbra persona placenta propaganda pupa retina rotunda saliva siesta (Sp.) sierra (Sp.) spatula stamina stanza tarantula (It.) tela tempera tenebra terra tibia toga trachea tuba ulna ultima umbra urethra Ursa uvea uvula vagina vertebra *(vertebrae)* via vibrissa visa vista vita vulva; **Geographic Names:** Africa Alabama Alaska Albania Alberta Argentina Arizona Aurora Botswana Herzegovina Montana Montezuma Mt. Etna Panama Rumania Venezuela; **Personal Names:** Agatha Aida /ä-ē-də/ Alexandra Anastasia Angela Angelica Anita Anna Athena Augusta Ava Barbara Bathsheba Bertha Brenda Carla Christina Clara Cleopatra Diana Donna Dora Edna Ella Elsa Emma Erica Erma Esmeralda Eva Evita Felicia Flora Frieda Georgiana Greta Hedda Helena Henrietta Hilda Ida Ilona Irma Johanna Juanita /hwä-nē-tä/ Juliana Katrina Klara Laura Pamala Pandora Susanna Lenora Lila Linda Lisa Lola Loretta Louella Marcella Marsha Martha Matilda Melinda Melissa Miranda Moira Mona Monica Myra Nora Norma Olga Pamela Paula Priscilla Ramona Rebecca Rhoda Rita Roberta Rosa Sandra Selma Sheila Stella Teresa Thelma Theresa Tina Trina Ursula Vanessa Vera Veronica Viola Wanda Wilhelmina Willa Wilma Yolanda

(-ia) /ē-ə/ (noun) alluvia (pl.) aria bacchanalia (pl.) bignonia (Name) cafeteria (Am.Sp.) claustrophobia (L/Gk.) cornucopia curia egomania (L/Gk.) forsythia (Name) genitalia (pl.) gloria Gloria gloxinia (name) hernia in absentia insignia insomnia intelligentsia juvenilia (pl.) mafia (It.) malaria (It.) media (pl.) memorabilia millennia (pl.) quadriplegia (L/Gk.) regalia (pl.) saturnalia (pl.) sinfonia (It.) suburbia tibia trivia zinnia; /yə/ alleluia begonia camellia dahlia gardenia magnolia pogonia passacaglia petunia pneumonia; **Geographic Names:** /ē-ə/ Albania Alexandria Algeria Arabia Armenia Assyria Austria Babylonia Bavaria Bohemia Bolivia Bosnia Britannia Bulgaria Caledonia Cambodia Colombia Czechoslovakia Estonia Ethiopia Gambia India Latvia Liberia Lithuania Macedonia Manchuria Mauritania Mesopotamia Moldavia Mongolia Moravia Nigeria Olympia Peoria Philadelphia Pretoria Romania Sardinia Scandinavia Serbia Siberia Slovakia Slovenia Syria Tanzania Tasmania Transylvania Victoria Yugoslavia Zambia; /yə/ Australia California Georgia /jor-jə/ Pennsylvania Somalia Virginia; /shə/ Croatia Phoenicia Silesia; /zhə/ Asia Melanesia Rhodesia Tunisia; /shē-ə/ Venetia; **And:** Prussia /prush-ə/ Russia /rush-ə/; Note: usually adding an *n* shows a person from this area; an *Albanian* is from *Albania*. See: **-ian** Ap. iv-21. **Personal Names:** /ē-ə/ Antonia Cecilia Claudia Cynthia Delphinia Eugenia Gloria Iphigenia LaGuardia Lavinia Lusitania Lydia Maria Octavia Olivia Olympia Sophia Sylvia Valeria Victoria Zenobia; /yə/ Camellia Cordelia Cornelia Delia Julia Ophelia Segovia Sonia Virginia

-ability /ə-bil-ə-tē/ (noun) (Formed from **-able** adjective.) accountability adaptability advisability applicability availability believability capability conceivability creditability culpability demonstrability dependability desirability disability durability educability employability enforceability excitability habitability heritability immovability impassability impenetrability imperishability impracticability impressionability improbability inability incapability inconceivability indispensability indistinguishability inevitability inexcusability inheritability insatiability inseparability instability insurability interchangeability intolerability intractability invariability invulnerability irreconcilability irrefutability irremovability irreplaceability irretrievability irrevocability irritability justifiability liability likability livability lovability malleability manageability maneuverability marketability measurability modifiability movability mutability navigability negotiability operability palatability penetrability perishability pliability portability practicability predictability preferability preventability probability punishability readability reasonability recognizability reconcilability reliability reparability respectability serviceability sociability stability suitability supportability survivability tenability transportability trustability unaccountability unavailability unsociability unsuitability usability variability venerability verifiability viability vulnerability washability wearability workability

-able /ə-bəl/ (adj.) abominable acceptable accountable adaptable admirable adorable advisable affable agreeable allowable alterable amenable amicable applicable appreciable approachable attainable available bearable breakable changeable charitable comfortable commensurable comparable compliable conformable creditable culpable cultivable curable debatable delectable demonstrable deniable dependable deplorable desirable despicable detestable differentiable disagreeable discreditable dishonorable dispensable disposable disputable doable drinkable durable educable endurable enjoyable enviable equitable exchangeable excitable excusable expendable fashionable favorable flammable formidable habitable honorable hospitable imaginable immeasurable immedicable immovable immutable impassable impeachable impeccable impenetrable imperturbable implacable imponderable impressionable improbable inadvisable inalienable inalterable inapplicable inapproachable incalculable incapable incommunicable incomparable inconceivable inconsiderable inconsolable incontestable incontrollable incurable indefinable indescribable indeterminable indispensable indisputable indistinguishable indubitable inescapable inestimable inevitable inexcusable inexplicable inheritable inhospitable inimitable innumerable inoperable insatiable inscrutable inseparable insolvable insufferable insupportable insurmountable interchangeable interminable intolerable intractable invaluable invariable inviable inviolable invulnerable irreconcilable irredeemable irrefutable irremediable irremovable irreparable irreplaceable irreproachable irretrievable irrevocable irritable judicable justifiable knowledgeable laughable liable likable malleable manageable marketable marriageable measurable medicable memorable mistakable movable mutable miserable navigable negotiable nonflammable numerable objectionable observable operable opposable palatable passable payable peaceable penetrable perishable personable pitiable placable pleasurable pliable ponderable portable practicable predictable preferable pregnable presentable presumable probable procurable profitable punishable questionable quotable readable reasonable receivable reconcilable rectifiable redeemable reliable remarkable remediable removable reputable respectable returnable revocable seasonable separable serviceable shipable sociable specifiable suable sufferable suitable supportable taxable teachable tenable terminable tolerable tractable transportable treasonable unaccountable unapproachable unassailable unavoidable unbearable unbelievable uncharitable uncomfortable unconscionable uncontrollable undeniable undesirable unemployable unfavorable unflappable ungovernable unimaginable unmentionable unmistakable unprintable unprofitable unpronounceable unquestionable unreadable unreasonable unreliable unseasonable unshakable unsociable unspeakable unsuitable untouchable unwarrantable usable valuable variable venerable verifiable veritable viable violable vulnerable washable wearable workable; /ā-bəl/ disable enable unable; <u>Note the nouns</u>: constable parable

-ableness /ə-bəl-nis/ (adv.) (Noun forming **-ness** may be added to some **-able** adjectives.) abominableness allowableness alterableness notableness, *etc.* (However, **-ability** is the more common noun ending, e.g. *accountability.* Many **-able** adjectives may have either **-ness** or **-ability** noun endings.) acceptableness, *acceptability* adaptableness, *adaptability* admirableness, *admirability* adorableness, *adorability* advisableness, *advisability* affableness, *affability* agreeableness, *agreeability* separable, *separability,* *etc.* Dictionaries usually list the most common form first. <u>See</u>: **-able** and **-ability** on previous page.

-ably /ə-blē/ (adv.) (Most **-able** adjectives may become **-ably** adverbs.) admirably adorably agreeably arguably believably capably certifiably comfortably conceivably considerably creditably deplorably enjoyably favorably improbably inappreciably incapably intolerably justifiably knowledgeably notably peaceably pleasurably predictably preferably presumably probably profitably questionably reasonably remarkably respectably tolerably unavoidably unbearably undeniably understandably unfavorably unquestionably unreasonably valuably, *etc.* <u>See</u>: **-able** on previous page.

-ace /is/ (noun) furnace grimace Horace menace necklace palace pinnace pomace populace preface resurface solace surface terrace Wallace
-ace /ās/ (verb) apace (adv.) deface disgrace displace face (+n) efface embrace enlace grace (+n) Grace (n) lace (+n) mace (+n) outface outpace pace (+n) place (+n) race (+n) replace retrace space (+n) trace (+n)

-aceous /ā-shəs/ (adj.) *[Of the nature of.]* carbonaceous cretaceous crustaceous curvaceous farinaceous herbaceous olivaceous pomaceous predaceous saponaceous sebaceous testaceous; <u>See</u>: -cious Ap. iv-27, **-ferous** Ap. iv-31, **-ous -eous**, and **-ious**, Ap. iv-41, **-tious** Ap. iv-47, and **-ulous** Ap. iv-51.

-ade /ād/ (noun) accolade aquacade arcade balustrade barricade blockade brigade cannonade cascade cavalcade charade colonnade crusade decade escapade esplanade (or /äd/) grenade lemonade marinade marmalade masquerade orangeade palisade parade promenade renegade serenade stockade; /ad/ comrade; (verb) /ād/ abrade brocade degrade dissuade evade invade persuade pervade promenade retrograde serenade

-age¹ /-ij / (noun) *[Collection, condition, relation of.]* acreage adage advantage amperage anchorage appendage assemblage average baggage bandage beverage blockage bondage breakage brokerage cabbage carnage carriage Carthage cartilage cleavage coinage cottage courage coverage cribbage damage disadvantage discourage (n) disparage (n) dockage dosage dotage drainage encourage (n) envisage (n) flowage foliage footage forage freightage frontage garbage heritage hermitage homage hostage image language leakage leverage lineage linkage luggage manage (n) marriage message mileage miscarriage mismanage (n) misusage moorage mortgage mucilage ohmage orphanage outage package parentage parsonage passage patronage percentage personage pilferage pilgrimage pillage plumage portage postage poundage presage ravage (n) roughage rummage salvage sausage savage scrimmage seepage sewage shortage shrinkage silage slippage spoilage steerage storage stowage suffrage tillage tonnage truckage tutelage umbrage usage vantage verbiage village vintage visage voltage voyage wastage wattage wordage wreckage yardage;
-age² /äzh/ (noun) **(French)** barrage bon voyage collage corsage décolletage espionage fuselage garage gavage massage menage mirage montage moulage persiflage potage sabotage triage;
-age³ /āj/ assuage cage engage outrage page rage rampage sage teenage iceage, etc

-al¹ /əl/ (noun) admiral animal annal appraisal approval arrival avowal betrayal betrothal cannibal capital carnival carousal corporal crystal cymbal decimal deposal diagonal disapproval disavowal dismissal dispersal disposal espousal festival funeral hospital hymnal interval journal madrigal mammal marshal mescal mineral missal mural oval pedestal periodical perusal plural portal portrayal principal prodigal processional proposal radical rascal recessional reciprocal refusal rehearsal removal renewal rental reprisal reversal revival rival sabbatical sandal scandal signal spiral survival tribunal urinal vandal vassal withdrawal; /l/ acquittal committal medal metal pedal petal rebuttal recital total; Note: /t/, /d/, & /l/ have same tongue position.

(-ial¹) /ē-əl/ marsupial serial; /ī-əl/ (*i* is in accented syllable.) decrial denial dial vial

-al² /əl/ (adj.) abdominal abnormal aboriginal abysmal accidental adrenal agonal amoral anal ancestral anecdotal annual antidotal antiphonal antiviral apocryphal astral atonal aural autumnal axial banal baptismal basal behavioral bicameral bicultural bifocal bilateral binal botanical capital cardinal carnal carpal causal central centrifugal centripetal cerebral choral coastal coincidental collateral colloquial colossal communal conditional confessional congenital congressional conjugal consensual continental continual contrapuntal corporal criminal dental dermal diagonal dialectal digital disloyal dismal doctrinal dorsal dual electoral elemental emotional ephemeral Episcopal epochal equal equivocal eternal external extramural farcical fecal federal festal feudal final fiscal floral focal formal fraternal frugal fugal fungal gastrointestinal general genital germinal global guttural herbal hexagonal homicidal horizontal identical illegal illiberal illogical immoral immortal impersonal inaugural incidental infernal infinitesimal informal integral intercontinental internal interpersonal intertribal intestinal intramural isothermal lateral latitudinal legal lethal liberal lingual literal local longitudinal loyal marginal marital marshal maternal maximal mayoral medicinal medieval mental metacarpal metatarsal minimal monaural monumental moral mortal multilateral municipal nasal nautical naval Neanderthal neural neutral nocturnal nominal noncommittal nonmoral normal numeral occasional occidental octagonal optimal oral orchestral ordinal oriental original oval palatal papal pastoral paternal patriarchal pectoral penal Pentecostal peripheral personal phenomenal pivotal plural political polygonal polyhedral postal postnatal prenatal primeval primal principal prodigal puritanical pyramidal quizzical reciprocal rectal regal regional renal rhinal royal rural seasonal semifinal semiformal seminal several signal sinistral skeletal societal spectral spinal spheroidal spiral spousal statistical subliminal submarginal subnormal suborbital suicidal temporal terminal thermal tonal transcendental transversal triagonal tribal trifocal trilateral triumphal unequal unequivocal unicameral unilateral universal vaginal vegetal verbal vernal vertebral vertical vesperal vestal vicinal vigesimal viral virginal visceral vocal withdrawal (O.E.) zonal; /l/ bridal brutal fatal fetal modal natal tidal vital; See: **-cial** Ap. iv-26, **-mental** Ap. iv-39, **-tial** Ap. iv-44, **-tional** Ap. iv-47, **-tual** Ap. iv-49.

(-eal²) /ē-əl/ arboreal cereal (n) corporeal ethereal funereal ideal lineal venereal

(-ial²) /ē-əl/ adverbial aerial alluvial arterial axial bacterial bicentennial biennial bilabial binomial bronchial burial centennial ceremonial colonial congenial conspiratorial convivial custodial dictatorial directorial editorial equatorial extraterritorial factorial filial genial gladiatorial gubernatorial immaterial immemorial imperial industrial janitorial jovial malarial managerial marsupial material medial memorial menial mercurial millennial ministerial monomial parochial perennial pictorial polynomial primordial professorial proverbial quadrinomial radial remedial sectorial serial terrestrial territorial testimonial triennial trinomial trivial tutorial venial vestigial; /ī-əl/ trial; /yəl/ familial; /jəl/ cordial; /shəl/ controversial; /zhəl/ ambrosial

(-ual²) /yōō-əl/ (adj.) biannual manual semiannual; /ōō-əl/ menstrual; /shōō-əl/ asexual bisexual sensual sexual supersensual; /zhōō-əl/ casual unusual usual visual; /gwəl/ bilingual multilingual trilingual

-ally /əl-ē/ (adv.) (Adverb forming **-ly** added to **-al** adjective.) accidentally actually annually basically continually diagonally editorially equally finally generally gradually ideally legally nationally naturally normally occasionally orally originally personally practically remedially specifically usually vertically virtually, *etc.*

-amine /ə-mēn/ (noun) *[Ammonia derivative.]* amphetamine antihistamine histamine prolamine thiamine; Other: jessamine /jes-ə-min/

-an¹ /ən/ (noun) Alan artisan Brahman brogan Bunyan charlatan Ethan Ian /ē-ən/ Ivan Jonathan Jordan leviathan MacMillan Morgan Nathan pelican publican sacristan Sullivan sultan Sheboygan shenanigan Tarzan toboggan (+v) turban Urban Vatican Vulcan woman; /an/ Afghanistan Turkestan Yucatan; /n/ Manhattan Satan

-an² /ən/ (adj.)   bipartisan Gargantuan Minoan Mycenaean nonpartisan urban

-an³ /ən/ (both noun & adj.) American Anglican Augustan Chinookan cosmopolitan Dominican Franciscan Genevan German human Incan interurban Jamaican Libyan Lutheran metropolitan Mexican Nicaraguan orphan Ottoman pagan partisan puritan Puritan quartan republican Republican Roman sylvan Trojan veteran; /n/ Tibetan

(-ean) /ē-ən/ (both noun & adj.) *[Connected with country, person, group or doctrine.]* cesarean Epicurean European Galilean Indo-European Judean Korean Mediterranean Shakespearean Tennessean; /shən/ crustacean;   (adj. only) Aegean Archimedean Euclidean Herculean Linnean Periclean protean Procrustean subterranean

(-ian) /ē-ən/ (noun, adj.) agrarian Algonquian Amazonian amphibian Appian Appalachian Aristotelian authoritarian barbarian callipygian Cartesian collegian comedian custodian Darwinian Dionysian disciplinarian doctrinarian Draconian egalitarian Elysian Episcopalian equalitarian equestrian Estonian Ethiopian Freudian Gregorian guardian Hadrian historian humanitarian Jeffersonian Kiwanian lesbian libertarian librarian Machiavellian Malthusian median meridian Merovingian millenarian Mousterian obsidian octogenarian Olympian parliamentarian pedestrian Pre-Cambrian Presbyterian proletarian radian reptilian Rotarian ruffian sectarian seminarian septuagenarian simian stentorian theologian Thespian totalitarian tragedian Trinitarian Unitarian utilitarian utopian valedictorian vegetarian veterinarian Victorian Vivian Wagnerian /väg-nair-ē-ən/; /yən/ civilian Maximillian vaudevillian; /zhən/ Caucasian;
People from places: /ē-ən/ Alabamian Albanian Algerian Arabian Arizonian Armenian Athenian Austrian Bavarian Bohemian Bolivian Bulgarian Cambodian Canadian Columbian Cyprian Hungarian Indian Iranian Italian Jordanian Macedonian Manchurian Mississippian Mongolian Moravian Nigerian Panamanian Pennsylvanian Peruvian Romanian Salvadorian Sardinian Scandinavian Serbian Siberian Sicilian Slovenian Somalian Sumerian Syrian Thessalonian Ukrainian; /ən/ Hessian Prussian Russian; /jən/ Belgian Norwegian; /yən/ Brazilian Hawaiian

-ana /an-ə/ (noun) Americana banana bandana cabana Havana Indiana Louisiana Montana sultana tympana (Pl. of *tympanum*.); /ä-nə/ Ghana iguana marijuana nirvana

-ance /əns/ (noun) abundance acceptance accordance acquaintance admittance allegiance allowance ambulance annoyance appearance appliance arrogance assistance assonance assurance attendance balance brilliance /bril-yəns/ capacitance clairvoyance clearance cognizance conductance conformance connivance consonance Constance contrivance conveyance countenance deliverance disappearance discordance disinheritance dissemblance dissonance distance disturbance dominance entrance elegance encumbrance endurance exorbitance extravagance exuberance forbearance fragrance governance grievance guidance hindrance ignorance imbalance importance inductance inheritance insignificance instance insurance intemperance intolerance irrelevance maintenance malfeasance nuisance observance ordinance ordnance penance performance perseverance predominance preponderance reconnaissance reluctance remembrance repentance repugnance resemblance resistance resonance semblance severance significance substance surveillance sustenance temperance tolerance utterance valance vigilance; /ans/ advance askance circumstance enhance entrance (v) finance happenstance romance stance; /äns/ nonchalance (F) renaissance (F) Renaissance (F); /ns/ impedance pittance remittance

(-eance) /ē-əns/ (noun) permeance vengeance /ven-jəns/

(-iance) /ē-əns/ (noun) ambiance dalliance deviance insouciance (F) luxuriance radiance suppliance valiance variance; /ī-əns/ alliance compliance reliance

(-uance) /yo͞o-əns/ (noun) continuance discontinuance; /o͞o-əns/ nuance pursuance

-ancy /ən-sē/ (noun) (A variation of **-ance**. From **-ant²** adj.) ascendancy brilliancy buoyancy compliancy consonancy constancy discrepancy dormancy errancy expectancy flippancy infancy malignancy occupancy pliancy pregnancy vacancy

-ane¹ /ān/ (adj.) (To distinguish words with corresponding forms.) germane *(German)* humane *(human)* inhumane *(inhuman)* urbane *(urban)*; Other adjectives: antemundane arcane inane insane montane mundane profane submontane subterrane

-ane² /ān/ (noun) *[Chemical suffix.]* butane methane octane pentane propane urethane; Other nouns: cellophane hurricane membrane

-anely /ān-lē/ (adv.) (Adverb forming **-ly** added to **-ane** adjective.) germanely humanely insanely mundanely, *etc.*

-ant¹ /ənt/ (noun) *[Act or process of doing.]* accountant annuitant antiperspirant appellant applicant aspirant assailant assistant attendant celebrant claimant coagulant communicant complainant concomitant consonant (+adj.) consultant contestant coolant cosecant covenant currant defendant deodorant depressant descendant determinant defendant disinfectant emigrant entrant exhalant expectorant fumigant hydrant immigrant infant informant inhabitant inhalant instant intoxicant irritant itinerant lieutenant litigant lubricant mendicant (+adj.) merchant migrant militant mordant noncombatant occupant pageant peasant penchant pendant pennant pheasant quadrant participant restaurant servant sergeant stimulant subdominant supplicant sycophant tenant tremulant tyrant vagrant warrant (+v); /ant/ chant (+v) commandant descant (+v) enchant (v) gallivant (v) grant (+v) Levant (n) pant (v) plant (+v) rant (v) recant (v) slant (+v) supplant (v); /nt/ combatant disputant mutant pedant pollutant

(-iant¹) /ē-ənt/ (noun) asphyxiant euphoriant inebriant submediant suppliant

(-uant¹) /yo͞o-ənt/ (noun) continuant; /o͞o-ənt/ truant

-ant² /ənt/ (adj.) aberrant abundant adamant appendant arrogant ascendant buoyant clairvoyant cognizant complaisant concomitant consonant constant conversant defiant discordant discrepant dissonant distant dominant dormant elegant errant exorbitant expectant extant extravagant exuberant flagrant flamboyant flippant fragrant gallant hesitant important incessant indignant infant insignificant instant intolerant irrelevant jubilant malignant mendicant militant observant petulant pleasant poignant /poin-yənt/ predominant pregnant preponderant protuberant rampant recalcitrant redundant relevant reliant reluctant repentant repugnant resistant resonant significant stagnant tolerant trenchant triumphant truant unimportant unpleasant vacant verdant vibrant vigilant;   /ant/ aslant   scant;   /änt/ avant-garde (F)   nonchalant (F); /nt/ blatant   mutant

(-eant²) /ē-ənt/ (adj.) procreant

(-iant²) /ē-ənt/ (adj.) asphyxiant brilliant /bril-yənt/ invariant luxuriant radiant suppliant valian   variant;   /ī-ənt/ (When *i* is in an accented syllable.) compliant giant pliant

(-uant²) /yōō-ənt/ (adj.)   attenuant   evacuant;   /ōō-ənt/ pursuant truant

-antly /ənt-lē/ (adv.) (Adverb forming **-ly** added to **-ant** adjective.) abundantly arrogantly blatantly brilliantly constantly distantly fragrantly gallantly hesitantly ignorantly incessantly instantly militantly pleasantly radiantly relevantly tolerantly valiantly, *etc.*

-ar¹ /er/ (adj.) angular bipolar cellular circular curricular curvilinear dissimilar extracurricular globular granular insular irregular jocular jugular linear lunar modular molecular muscular nuclear octangular particular perpendicular polar popular rectangular rectilinear regular secular similar singular solar spectacular stellar triangular tubular vascular vehicular verisimilar vulgar;   /are/ afar (adv.) far (adv.)

(-iar) /yer/ (adj.) familiar   peculiar   unfamiliar

-ar² /er/   (noun) altar beggar burglar bursar Caesar calendar Caspar caterpillar cedar cellar Cheddar collar cougar dollar Edgar exemplar friar Gibraltar grammar Hagar hangar liar molar mortar Nebuchadnezzar nectar Oscar pedlar pillar poplar scholar scimitar sugar tartar templar vernacular vicar vinegar;   /are/ bar bazaar cigar   czar   Dagmar   gar   Ishtar   jaguar   jar   knar   mar (+v)   star

-arily /air-i-lē/ (adv.) (Adverb forming **-ly** added to **-ary** adjectives with *y* to *i* change.) arbitrarily contrarily customarily evolutionarily extraordinarily militarily momentarily necessarily ordinarily primarily secondarily temporarily voluntarily;   See: **-ary¹**. Ap. iv-24.

-arity /air-i-tē/ (noun) (Noun forming **-ity** added to **-ar** adjectives.) circularity irregularity muscularity polarity popularity similarity vulgarity; Plural: **-arities**, similarity, *similarities*.

-arium /air-ē-əm/ (noun) *[A place.]* aquarium herbarium planetarium sanitarium solarium terrarium;   Other: honorarium;   See: **-ium** Ap. iv-51.

-arly /er-lē/ (adv.) (Adverb forming **-ly** added to **-ar** word.) circularly familiarly irregularly jocularly linearly modularly molecularly muscularly particularly peculiarly popularly regularly scholarly secularly similarly singularly spectacularly vulgarly, *etc.*

-ary[1] /air-ē/ (noun) *[Pertaining to.]* adversary apothecary bursary /-er-ē/ capillary commentary commissary concessionary constabulary contemporary contrary corollary coronary customary dictionary dignitary documentary dromedary emissary February functionary itinerary January lapidary library luminary mercenary military millenary missionary ovary /ō-və-rē/ reactionary revolutionary rosary secretary seminary supernumerary Tipperary veterinary visionary vocabulary; /er-ē/ anniversary auxiliary beneficiary boundary or /boun-drē/ burglary bursary Calvary concessionary dispensary glossary granary Hillary Hungary infirmary notary quandary or: /kwon-drē/ rotary summary; Plural: **-aries**, dictionary, *dictionaries.*

(**-iary**[1]) /ē-air-ē/ (noun) apiary aviary breviary ciliary fiduciary incendiary intermediary judiciary laniary stipendiary subsidiary; Plural: **-iaries**, aviary, *aviaries*

-ary[2] /air-ē/ (adj.) *[Pertaining to.]* alimentary arbitrary capillary cautionary concessionary contemporary contrary (+adv.) coronary culinary customary deflationary dietary disciplinary discretionary diversionary evolutionary exclusionary expansionary extraordinary fragmentary funerary hereditary honorary illusionary imaginary incendiary inflationary insurrectionary interdisciplinary intermediary interplanetary involuntary legendary literary military momentary monetary necessary ordinary paramilitary pituitary planetary plenary precautionary preliminary primary probationary provisionary pulmonary reactionary residuary revisionary revolutionary salutary sanitary sanguinary secondary sedentary sedimentary solitary stationary temporary unsanitary urinary visionary voluntary; /er-ē/ auxiliary binary complementary or: /kom-plə-men-trē/ complimentary or: /kom-plə-men-trē/ elementary or: /el-ə-men-trē/ exemplary mammary parliamentary rotary rudimentary supplementary; See: **-iary**[2] below, **-arily** Ap. iv-23, and **-tionary** Ap.iv-47.

(**-iary**[2]) /ē-air-ē/ (adj.) biliary domiciliary pecuniary stipendiary subsidiary superciliary

-as /əs/ (noun) alias Aquinas Atlas Barnabas bias canvas Caracas Christmas Dallas fracas Honduras Judas Kansas Las Vegas Pallas pancreas Protagoras Texas Thomas; /əz/ Carolinas Himalayas Moluccas pampas; /as/ Madras sassafras

-ate[1] /āt/ (verb) abdicate abate accelerate accentuate acclimate accommodate accumulate activate adjudicate administrate adulate adulterate advocate agitate alienate allocate alternate ameliorate automate aggravate amputate annihilate annotate anticipate antiquate approximate arbitrate articulate assassinate assimilate attenuate authenticate calculate calibrate capitulate captivate carbonate castigate castrate celebrate circulate circumambulate circumnavigate clorinate coagulate cogitate collaborate collate commemorate commiserate communicate compensate complicate concentrate confederate confiscate conglomerate conglutinate congratulate congregate conjugate consecrate consolidate constellate constipate consummate contaminate contemplate contraindicate cooperate coordinate copulate correlate corroborate create cremate culminate cultivate date deactivate debate debilitate decapitate decarbonate decimate decorate decontaminate dedicate de-escalate deflate degenerate dehydrate delegate deliberate demarcate demonstrate depopulate deprecate desecrate desegregate desiccate designate deteriorate devaluate devastate dictate dilate discombobulate discriminate disintegrate dislocate disseminate dissipate domesticate dominate donate duplicate educate ejaculate elaborate elate elevate eliminate elongate elucidate emanate emancipate emasculate emigrate emulate enervate enumerate equate equivocate eradicate escalate estimate evacuate evaluate evaporate exacerbate exaggerate exasperate excavate excommunicate exculpate exhilarate exonerate expectorate explicate extenuate exterminate extrapolate extricate fabricate facilitate fascinate federate fixate flagellate fluctuate fluoridate formulate fornicate frustrate fumigate generate germinate gesticulate gradate graduate granulate gravitate gyrate habituate hallucinate hesitate hibernate hyphenate illuminate illustrate imitate immigrate impersonate implicate impregnate inactivate inaugurate incapacitate incapsulate incarcerate incinerate incorporate incriminate incubate inculcate indicate indoctrinate infatuate infiltrate inflate innovate inoculate inseminate insinuate instigate insulate integrate interpolate interrogate intimate intimidate intoxicate inundate invalidate investigate invigorate irrigate irritate isolate lacerate lactate laminate legislate legitimate levitate liberate liquidate litigate locate lubricate machinate marinate masticate masturbate matriculate medicate meditate meliorate menstruate migrate misappropriate miscalculate moderate modulate motivate mutate mutilate narrate nauseate navigate necessitate negate negotiate nominate numerate obligate obliterate officiate orate orchestrate orientate originate oscillate ovulate penetrate percolate perforate permeate perpetrate perpetuate populate postulate precipitate predicate prefabricate prevaricate probate procrastinate prorate palpitate participate placate pollinate pontificate predicate predominate premeditate procreate proliferate promulgate propagate pulsate punctuate recapitulate reciprocate recreate re-create recuperate refrigerate regenerate regulate regurgitate rehabilitate reinstate reiterate rejuvenate relate relegate renovate replicate resonate resuscitate reverberate rotate salivate satiate saturate segregate separate simulate speculate stagnate stimulate stipulate subjugate sublimate subordinate substantiate suffocate syllabicate syncopate syndicate tabulate terminate tolerate translate transliterate ulcerate undulate urinate vacate vaccinate vacillate validate valuate vegetate ventilate vibrate vindicate violate; See: **-ciate** Ap. iv-27 and **-tiate** Ap. iv-44.

(-iate[1]) /ē-āt/ (verb) abbreviate affiliate alleviate appropriate asphyxiate conciliate defoliate deviate disaffiliate expatriate expropriate foliate gladiate (adj.) humiliate inebriate infuriate ingratiate mediate opiate radiate repatriate repudiate retaliate

-ate[2] (noun) /it/ advocate agate alternate baccalaureate barbiturate bicarbonate celibate certificate chocolate climate conglomerate consulate degenerate delegate directorate doctorate duplicate electorate estimate frigate graduate insubordinate intimate invertebrate moderate palate pirate pomegranate postgraduate postulate precipitate predicate private profligate senate sophisticate subordinate surrogate syndicate triumvirate ultimate vertebrate; /āt/ acetate candidate chordate citrate delegate estate hydrate ingrate lactate magistrate magnate mandate nitrate nucleate phosphate potentate primate prostate rabbinate rebate reprobate sensate stylobate sulfate vulgate

(-iate²) /ē-it/ (noun) affiliate associate deviate expatriate inebriate intermediate opiate radiate repatriate variate

-ate³ /it/ (adj.) accurate adequate affectionate aggregate alternate animate appellate approximate articulate celibate commensurate compassionate confederate considerate corporate degenerate deliberate delicate designate desolate desperate determinate discriminate disparate dispassionate disproportionate duplicate effeminate elaborate fortunate graduate illegitimate illiterate immaculate immoderate inaccurate inadequate inanimate inarticulate incarnate incommensurate inconsiderate indelicate indeterminate indiscriminate inordinate insubordinate intemperate intimate intricate inveterate inviolate legitimate literate moderate obdurate obstinate passionate precipitate predeterminate predicate private proportionate separate subordinate temperate ultimate unfortunate; /āt/ capsulate cognate dentate globate insensate intestate irate Latinate laureate lunate nucleate ornate ovate pedate pennate plumate probate prostate prostrate reprobate sedate sensate serrate spinate testate tubate valvate vulgate

(-iate³) /ē-it/ (adj.) appropriate associate collegiate expatriate foliate immediate inappropriate inebriate intercollegiate intermediate mediate opiate radiate

-ately /it-lē/ (adv.) (Adverb forming **-ly** added to **-ate** adjective.) accurately adequately appropriately delicately desperately elaborately fortunately immediately moderately ornately privately separately ultimately, *etc.*   <u>See</u>: **-ate**.

-ator /ā-ter/ (noun) *[One who or that which does.]* (Some from *-ate* verbs.) aviator decorator delineator demonstrator denominator detonator dictator duplicator evocator gladiator illuminator illustrator mediator perambulator radiator, *etc.* <u>See</u>: **ate**.

-atory /ə-tor-ē/ (adj.) *[Pertaining to.]* accusatory anticipatory circulatory compensatory declamatory dedicatory defamatory denunciatory derogatory discriminatory exclamatory explanatory exploratory gustatory hallucinatory improvisatory inflammatory investigatory judicatory laudatory mandatory manipulatory migratory nondiscriminatory obligatory participatory predatory preparatory reciprocatory recriminatory regulatory remuneratory respiratory retaliatory salutatory signatory supplicatory vindicatory; (noun) conservatory crematory laboratory lavatory observatory oratory purgatory reformatory

-cia /shə/ Alicia Marcia Patricia; <u>But</u>: (It.) Lucia /loo-<u>ch</u>ē-ə/ valencia /və-<u>len</u>-shē-ə/ Valencia

-cial /shəl/ (adj.) *[Pertaining to; characterized by.]* antisocial artificial asocial beneficial commercial controversial crucial especial facial fiducial financial glacial interracial judicial official prejudicial provincial racial sacrificial social special superficial

-cially /shəl-ē/ (adv.) (Adverb forming **-ly** added to **-cial** adjective.) artificially commercially crucially especially financially officially socially specially, *etc.* <u>See</u>: **-cial**.

-cian /shən/ (noun) academician arithmetician beautician clinician Confucian cosmetician diagnostician dialectician electrician esthetician geometrician Grecian logician magician mathematician mortician musician obstetrician optician patrician pediatrician Phoenecian physician politician rhetorician statistician tactician technician

-ciate /shē-āt/ (verb) annunciate appreciate associate depreciate dissociate emaciate excruciate glaciate officiate; /sē-āt/ denunciate enunciate

-ciency /shən-sē/ (noun) (Noun form of **cient** adjective.) deficiency efficiency inefficiency insufficiency proficiency sufficiency; <u>See</u>: **-cy** Ap. iv-27.

-cient /shənt/ (adj.) ancient coefficient deficient efficient inefficient insufficient omniscient prescient proficient sufficient; <u>See</u>: **-facient** Ap. iv-31.

-ciently /shənt-lē/ (adv.) (Adverb forming **-ly** added to **-cient** adjective.) deficiently efficiently proficiently sufficiently, *etc.*

-cion /shən/ (noun) coercion suspicion

-cious /shəs/ (adj.) *[Characterized by.]* atrocious audacious auspicious avaricious capricious Confucious (name) delicious efficacious fallacious ferocious gracious judicious loquacious luscious malicious mendacious meretricious officious pernicious perspicacious pertinacious precious precocious pugnacious rapacious sagacious salacious spacious specious suspicious tenacious veracious vicious vivacious voracious; <u>And</u>: conscious preconscious semiconscious subconscious unconscious

-ciously /shəs-lē/ (adv.) (Adverb forming **-ly** added to **-cious** adjective.) deliciously graciously precociously preciously suspiciously viciously, *etc.*

-cise /sīz/ (verb) (From L. *caedere*, to cut.) circumcise excise incise exercise (from L. *ex + arcere*, to enclose) exorcise (from L. *ex + horkos*, oath); /sīs/; (adj.) concise imprecise precise; (noun) excise (From M.Du *excijs* < L. *ad + census*, tax.)

-cisely /sīs/ (adv.) (Adverb forming **-ly** added to **-cise** adjective.) concisely precisely

-cle /kəl/ (noun) *[small]* article canticle carbuncle circle corpuscle /<u>cor</u>-pəs-əl/ cuticle manacle muscle /<u>mus</u>-əl/ particle pinnacle tabernacle testicle tubercle uncle ventricle

-cule /kyo͞ol/ (noun) *[small]* animalcule crepuscule floccule macromolecule majuscule minuscule molecule opuscule reticule; <u>Not diminutives</u>: bascule macule ridicule

-cy /cē/ (noun) *[State, quality, rank.]* bankruptcy mercy normalcy policy prophecy
Note: Plural formed by changing 'y' to 'i' and adding '-es'; e.g., policy, *policies*

(-acy) /ə-sē/ (noun) *[State, quality, rank.]* accuracy adequacy advocacy bureaucracy candidacy celibacy confederacy conspiracy degeneracy delicacy democracy diplomacy effeminacy efficacy fallacy illegitimacy illiteracy immaculacy immediacy immoderacy inaccuracy inadequacy indelicacy inefficacy intimacy intricacy inveteracy legacy legitimacy literacy lunacy magistracy obduracy obstinacy Papacy pharmacy piracy prelacy primacy privacy procuracy profligacy   regeneracy; <u>Plural:</u> **-acies**, fallacy, *fallacies; legacy,* legacies;   <u>See:</u> **-ancy** Ap. iv-22, **-ciency** Ap. iv-27, and **-ency** Ap. iv-29.

-e /ē/ (noun) (Non-silent final *e*.) adobe agape Andromache ante Antiope Apache apagoge Aphrodite Arachne Boise Brontë calliope Calliope Chile Circe Daphne dele epitome facsimile kamikaze karate machete Nike posse recipe reveille sarape schipperke sesame Shoshone simile tamale vigilante; /ā/ dolce (adj.) forte (adj.).

-el /əl/ (noun) (Often a diminutive; *also a verb.) (From Latin *-ellus*.) angel apparel bowel cancel (v) caramel chancel *channel chapel charnel chisel camel carrel *counsel damsel dishevel (v) *duel *fuel *funnel gavel gruel hostel impanel (v) infidel jewel *kennel laurel level (+adj.) *libel lintel mantel *marvel minstrel morsel muscatel mussel newel novel (+adj.) *panel *parcel pari-mutuel *pommel *quarrel rebel *revel satchel scalpel sentinel sequel squirrel *tassel *tinsel *trammel *travel *trowel vessel vowel wastrel; /l/ chattel *model remodel (v); <u>From other sources:</u> babel bagel barrel bevel brothel carousel carpel citadel colonel /<u>ker</u>-nəl/ decibel /<u>des</u>-ə-bel/ diesel dowel drivel duffel easel enamel flannel gospel gravel grovel hazel Israel kernel label mackerel materiel /mə-tear-ē-<u>el</u>/ mongrel navel nickel novel parallel petrel pickerel pretzel ravel (v.) scoundrel shekel shovel shrapnel shrivel snivel snorkel sorrel spaniel streusel swivel towel tunnel weasel yokel; /l/ strudel yodel;   <u>Nouns with accent on last syllable:</u> /el/ hotel motel personnel cartel morel Noël pastel lapel;   <u>Verbs with accent on last syllable:</u> /el/ compel dispel excel expel impel propel rebel repel

-ella /el-ə/ (noun) Cinderella citronella clarabella patella salmonella (Name.) terrella

-em /əm/ (noun) Bethlehem (Heb.) harem (Ar.) Harlem (Du.) Jerusalem (Heb.) Moslem (Ar.) postmeridiem (P.M.)   post-mortem   problem requiem Salem *(Jerusalem)* stratagem system tandem theorem totem; /em/ diadem ibidem /i-<u>bī</u>-dem/ mayhem (O.F.)

-en /ən/ (noun) abdomen acumen albumen alien citizen cyclamen delicatessen dozen foramen hyphen lichen mitten (F) mizzen morgen omen oxygen regimen rumen Saracen sauerbraten (Ger.) siren specimen Tutankhamen warden   Yemen; /n/ platen Staten Island Sweden;   <u>See:</u> Old English Suffix **-en** Ap. iv-5.

-ence /əns/ (noun) *[Action, quality, state, or condition.]* (From **-ent** adjectives.) abhorrence absence abstinence acquiescence adherence adolescence affluence belligerence benevolence coherence coincidence competence concurrence condescendence condolence conference confidence confluence congruence conscience consequence continence convergence correspondence crapulence credence decadence deference difference diffidence diligence dissidence divergence eloquence emergence eminence equivalence essence evidence excellence existence flatulence florescence immanence imminence imprudence impudence incandescence incidence incoherence incompetence incontinence independence indifference indigence indolence indulgence inference influence innocence insolence insurgence intelligence interference iridescence irreverence jurisprudence magnificence negligence occurrence omnipotence omnipresence omniscience opulence penitence permanence persistence pestilence preference presence prominence providence quintessence recurrence reference refulgence reminiscence residence resilience resplendence resurgence reticence reverence science sentence sequence silence somnolence subsistence transference transience truculence tumescence turbulence valence violence virulence; /ns/ cadence prudence;   And: /ens/ commence (verb)

(-ience) /ē-əns/ ambience audience disobedience expedience experience incipience inexpedience inexperience insipience lenience obedience percipience provenience recipience salience sapience; /yəns/ convenience inconvenience prevenience resilience

(-cience) /shəns/   nescience *(Lack of knowledge.)*;   **(-tience)** /shəns/ consentience dissentience impatience patience;   /shē-əns/ sentience *(A conscious state.)*

-ency /ən-sē/ (noun) (Alternate form of **-ence** nouns, from **-ent** adjectives or *nouns.) absorbency adjacency *agency ardency astringency belligerency clemency cogency competency complacency congruency consistency constituency contingency currency decency delinquency despondency emergency equivalency Excellency expediency fervency insurgency leniency nonresidency permanency persistency *presidency *regency *residency resiliency solvency *superintendency tendency transcendency transparency urgency;   Note: plural **-encies**, currency, *currencies*;   See: **-cy** Ap. iv-27.

-end /end/ (verb) amend append apprehend ascend attend coextend commend comprehend depend descend emend extend misapprehend offend portend pretend recommend reprehend suspend transcend; (noun) addend dividend legend repetend stipend subtrahend minuend;   (adj.) reverend

-ent¹ /ənt/ (noun) accent /-ent/ accident adherent adolescent advent agent antecedent ascent assent client coincident comment component consent constituent continent convent correspondent cotangent crescent current delinquent dependent deponent descent detergent deterrent discontent dissident docent equivalent existent exponent incident incumbent independent innocent insurgent intransigent malcontent mordent nonresident occident opponent parent penitent portent precedent present president proponent recipient regent repellent resident respondent serpent solvent superintendent talent tangent torrent transient unguent vice-president; /nt/ rodent; **When accented**: /ěnt/: absent assent circumvent event extent indent lament prevent relent represent resent;   **Note**: Often /-nt/ after accented /t/ or /d/: decedent jurisprudent patent student trident

-ent² /ənt/ (adj.) abhorrent absent absorbent acquiescent adjacent ambivalent antecedent apparent ardent belligerent benevolent clement cogent coherent competent complacent concurrent confident consequent consistent constituent contingent corpulent current decadent decent delinquent dependent despondent different diffident diligent dissident divergent eloquent emergent eminent equivalent

Ap. iv-29

evident excellent existent fervent fluent flatulent fluorescent fraudulent frequent immanent imminent impenitent impermanent impertinent impotent imprudent impudent inadvertent incandescent inclement incoherent incompetent inconsistent incontinent indecent independent indifferent indigent indolent indulgent infrequent inherent innocent insistent insolent insurgent intelligent interdependent intermittent intransigent iridescent irreverent latent magnificent malcontent malevolent munificent nascent negligent nonviolent obsolescent opponent penitent permanent persistent pertinent pestilent preeminent present prevalent prominent prudent pungent putrescent recent recurrent relucent reminiscent resident resilient resplendent resurgent reticent reverent sentient silent somnolent stringent subsequent subsistent succulent tangent transcendent translucent transparent tumescent unintelligent urgent vehement violent virulent; /-nt/ patent potent strident;
<u>See</u>: **-cient** Ap. iv-27 and **-tient** Ap. iv-44.

(-ient²) /ē-ənt/ (adj.) ambient disobedient disorient (v) expedient (+n) gradient (+n) impedient (+n) incipient inexpedient ingredient (n) lenient nutrient (+n) obedient orient (+n, v) percipient (+n) prescient prurient recipient (+n) salient sapient subservient transient transilient; /yənt/ convenient ebullient emolient (+n) inconvenient resilient

(-uent²) /ōō-ənt/ (adj.) abluent affluent congruent incongruent

-ental /ent-əl/ (adj.) (Adjective forming **-al** added to some **-ent** noun.) accidental coincidental continental incidental parental transcendental

-entally /ent-əl-ē/ (adv.) (Adverb forming **-ly** added to **-ental** adjective.) accidentally coincidentally continentally incidentally parentally transcendentally

-ently /ənt-lē/ (adv.) (Adverb forming **-ly** added to **-ent²** adjective.) apparently confidently currently decently differently evidently expediently frequently inadvertently independently intelligently obediently presently recently violently, *etc.*

-ery /er-ē/ (noun) *[Place; collection; trade.]* adultery archery artillery bakery baptistery battery bookbindery bowery bravery (Or: /brāv-rē/) brewery bribery cajolery chancery chicanery cookery creamery cutlery deanery debauchery delivery demagoguery discovery distillery drapery drudgery effrontery embroidery finery fishery flattery forgery greenery grocery gunnery haberdashery hatchery hosiery knavery machinery millinery mockery Montgomery nondelivery nunnery nursery ornery (adj.) perfumery periphery pottery prudery quackery recovery refinery robbery scenery scullery shrubbery skulduggery slavery (Or: /slāv-rē/) snobbery surgery tannery thievery tomfoolery treachery trickery vinery volery waggery winery witchery; /air-ē/ cemetery confectionery monastery presbytery stationery;
<u>Plural</u>: **-eries**, delivery, *deliveries* surgery, *surgeries*; <u>See</u>: **-ry** Ap. iv-42.

-esce /es/ (verb) *[To become or grow.]* acquiesce coalesce convalesce effervesce effloresce evanesce luminesce phosphoresce recalesce recrudesce
Ap. iv-30

-escence /es-əns/ (noun) *[State or quality of.]* acquiescence adolescence alkalescense calescence coalescence convalescence detumescence effervescence efflorescence evanescence excrescence florescence incandescence iridescence luminescence obsolescence phosphorescence quiescence recalescence recrudescence rejuvenescence

-escent /es-ənt/ (adj.) *[Beginning to be, have, or do.]* acquiescent adolescent alkalescent arborescent calescent coalescent calorescent convalescent crescent effervescent efflorescent evanescent excrescent ignescent incandescent increscent iridescent lactescent latescent luminescent obsolescent phosphorescent quiescent recalescent recrudescent rejuvenescent rubescent tumescent vaporescent vitrescent

-escently /es-ənt-lē/ (adv.) (Adverb forming **-ly** added to **-escent** adjective.) adolescently convalescently effervescently incandescently obsolescently, *etc.*

-ese /ēz/ (adj., noun) *[A native of; the language of.]* Burmese Chinese *computerese* Congolese Japanese Javanese *journalese* Lebanese Maltese Pekingese Portuguese Siamese Taiwanese Viennese Vietnamese, *etc.*

-ete /ēt/ (verb) accrete (*ad + crescere* to grow.) aesthete (n. Gk.) compete (L. *com + petere*, to seek.) complete (+adj.) (*com + plere*, to fill.) concrete (+n, adj.) (*com + crescere*, to grow.) delete (*delere*, erase.) deplete (*de + plere*, to fill.) effete (adj.) esthete incomplete (adj.) obsolete (adj.) paraclete (n. Gk.)

-etely /ēt-lē/ (adv.) (Adverb forming **-ly** added to **-ete** adjective.) completely concretely, *etc.*

-ey /ē/ (noun) attorney donkey medley; /ā/ obey they, *etc.* <u>See:</u> **-ey** in Ap. i-23.

-facient /fā-shənt/ (adj.) *[Causing.]* abortifacient absorbefacient calefacient febrifacient parturifacient rubefacient tumefacient

-faction /fak-shən/ benefaction calefaction dissatisfaction liquefaction olfaction petrifaction putrefaction rarefaction satisfaction stupefaction tumefaction

-factor /fak-ter/ (noun) *[One who makes.]* (From Latin verb *facere*, to make.) benefactor factor malefactor

-ferous /fer-əs/ (adj.) *[Bearing or producing.]* (From Latin verb *ferre*, to bear.) aeriferous *(air)* aluminiferous *(aluminum)* aquiferous *(water)* argentiferous *(silver)* auriferous *(gold)* bacciferous *(berries)* bulbiferous *(bulbs)* calciferous *(calcium carbonate)* carboniferous *(carbon)* conchiferous *(shells)* coniferous *(cones)* cruciferous *(cross)* crystalliferous *(crystals)* cupriferous *(carbon)* floriferous *(flowers)* fossiliferous *(fossils)* fructiferous *(fruit)* glandiferous *(acorn)* graniferous *(grain)* herbiferous *(herbs)* lactiferous *(milk)* laniferous *(wool)* laticiferous *(latex)* luminiferous *(light)* mammiferous *(breasts)* melliferous *(honey)* metalliferous *(metal)* nickeliferous *(nickel)* odoriferous *(an odor)* ossiferous *(bones)* oviferous *(eggs)* petaliferous *(petals)* piliferous *(hair)* platiniferous *(platinum)* plumbiferous *(lead)* polliniferous *(pollen)* poriferous *(pores)* quartziferous *(quartz)* resiniferous *(resin)* saliferous *(salt)* sanguiferous *(blood)* sebiferous *(fat)* seminiferous *(semen)* setiferous *(bristles)* siliciferous *(silica)* somniferous *(sleep)* soniferous *(sound)* sporiferous *(spores)* stanniferous *(tin)* stelliferous *(stars)* sudoriferous *(sweat)* thuriferous *(incense)* umbriferous *(shade)* uriniferous *(urine)* viniferous *(wine)* vociferous *(loud voice)* zinciferous *(zinc)*

-fic /fik/ (adj.) *[Making.]* (From Latin verb *facere*, to make.) beatific benefic calorific deific frigorific honorific horrific malefic nonspecific pacific Pacific prolific scientific soporific specific sudorific tenebrific terrific torporific transpacific unscientific unspecific vaporific; Other: traffic (n, v) See: **-ic** Ap. iv-33, 54, **-istic** Ap. iv-37, **-tic** Ap. iv-59.

-fically /fik-lē/ (adv.) (Adverb producing **-ly** added to some **-fic** adjectives.) beatifically honorifically horrifically pacifically prolifically scientifically specifically terrifically

-fication /fə-ka-shən/ (noun) *[Causing to be.]* (From Latin verb *facere*, to make.) aerification ammonification amplification calorification clarification classification deification edification exemplification glorification gratification identification intensification justification magnification modification mortification mystification nitrification nullification pacification personification purification ramification ratification rectification signification solidification specification unification verification vilification

-ficator /fə-cā-ter/ (noun) pacificator (pacificatory, adv.) vinificator

-fice /is/ (noun) (From *facere,* to make.) artifice benefice edifice interoffice office orifice; /īs/ suffice (v) sacrifice (+v)

-ficent /fə-sənt/ (adj.) beneficent magnificent munificent

-ficently /fə-sənt-lē/ (adv.) (Adverb forming **-ly** added to **-ficent** adjective ending.) beneficently magnificently munificently

-fy /fī/ (verb) *[To do or make.]* (From Latin verb *facere*, to make.) casefy cockneyfy liquefy putrefy rarefy stupefy tepefy tumefy torrefy;
Third person singular: **-fies,** liquefy *liquefies*

(-ify) /ə-fī/ (verb) *[To do or make.]* (From Latin verb *facere*, to make.) amplify beautify certify clarify classify codify crucify dehumidify deify dignify disqualify dissatisfy diversify edify electrify falsify fortify glorify gratify horrify humidify identify intensify justify magnify modify mortify mummify mystify notify nullify objectify pacify personify petrify purify qualify quantify ratify rectify sanctify satisfy signify simplify solidify specify stratify terrify testify typify unify verify vilify; See: **-fy**.

-fier /ə-fī-er/ (noun) (Noun form of **-fy** verbs.) liquefier putrefier rarefier stupefier

(-ifier) /ə-fī-er/ (noun) (Noun form of **-ify** verbs.) amplifier classifier dehumidifier justifier magnifier modifier purifier qualifier simplifier unifier verifier, *etc.* See: **-ify**.

-geous /jəs/ (adj.) advantageous courageous disadvantageous gorgeous outrageous rampageous umbrageous; See: **-gious** Ap. iv-33, **-ous** Ap. iv-41.

-geously /jəs-lē/ (adv.) (Adverb form **-ly** added to **-geous** adjective.) advantageously courageously disadvantageously gorgeously outrageously rampageously; See: **-geous**.

-geousness /jəs-nis/ (noun) (Noun forming **-ness** added to **-geous** adjective.) advantageousness courageousness disadvantageousness gorgeousness rampageousness

-gious /jəs/ (adj.) ambagious contagious egregious irreligious litigious prestigious prodigious religious sacrilegious; See: **-geous** on previous page and **-ous** Ap. iv-41.

-giously /jəs-lē/ (adv.) (Adverb form **-ly** added to **-gious** adjective.) contagiously egregiously irreligiously litigiously prestigiously prodigiously religiously sacrilegiously

-giousness /jəs-nis/ (noun) (Noun forming **-ness** added to **-gious** adjective.) ambagiousness contagiousness egregiousness litigiousnesss prestigiousness prodigiousness religiousness sacrilegiousness; See: **-gious** above.

-ibility /ə-bil-ə-tē/ (noun) (Variation of **-ability**.) accessibility admissibility combustibility compatibility corruptibility credibility digestibility divisibility eligibility exhaustibility fallibility feasibility flexibility fusibility gullibility illegibility implausibility impossibility inadmissibility incompatibility inconvertibility incredibility indivisibility ineligibility inexpressibility infallibility infeasibility inflexibility intelligibility invincibility invisibility irascibility irresponsibility irreversibility legibility perfectibility permissibility plausibility possibility reducibility reproducibility resistibility responsibility sensibility suggestibility susceptibility visibility; Plural: **-ibilities**

-ible /ə-bəl/ (adj.) accessible admissible audible compatible contemptible corruptible credible digestible dirigible discernible divisible edible eligible fallible feasible flexible forcible gullible horrible illegible imperceptible impermissible implausible impossible inadmissible inaudible incompatible incomprehensible incorrigible incorruptible incredible indefensible indelible indestructible indiscernible indivisible ineligible inexpressible infallible inflexible insensible intangible intelligible invincible invisible irascible irresponsible irreversible negligible perceptible perfectible permissible plausible possible reprehensible responsible reversible sensible suggestible susceptible tangible terrible visible; (noun) crucible dirigible mandible

-ibly /ə-blē/ (adv.) (Any **-ible** adjective may become an **ibly** adverb.) audibly horribly incredibly invisibly negligibly perceptibly possibly responsibly sensibly terribly visibly, *etc.*

-ic /ik/ (adj.) (From Latin **-icus**.) Adriatic angelic aquatic alcoholic algebraic Arabic artistic Atlantic Baltic bureaucratic caloric Celtic centric civic classic concentric dietetic domestic egocentric egotistic erratic Gaelic Hispanic Icelandic inorganic intrinsic Islamic jingoistic Jurassic lunatic majestic masonic Nordic operatic Pacific patristic platonic prosaic pubic public Punic quadratic quixotic Rabbinic robotic romantic rustic satanic scenic Slavic sonic supersonic sylvatic Teutonic transatlantic transoceanic ultrasonic vitric vocalic volcanic vitriolic; Many acid types: acetic, ascorbic, boric, carbolic, citric, lactic, malic, oleic, quinic, suberic, sulfuric, tannic, telluric, vanillic, *etc.* (noun) arsenic aspic attic fabric fanatic frolic garlic lunatic picnic relic republic traffic tunic;   <u>Often -ics as singular noun</u>: antics dietetics histrionics obstetrics statistics supersonics; <u>See</u>: **-fic** Ap. iv-32, **-istic** Ap. iv-37, & Gk. **-ic** Ap. iv-54, **-tic** Ap. iv-59.

-ical /i-kəl/ (adj.) chemical classical fanatical identical lackadaisical medical numerical oratorical radical satirical statistical whimsical;   <u>See</u>: Gk. **-ical** Ap. iv-55.

-ically /ik-lē/ [Note dropped syllable: /ik-ə-lē/] (adv.) (L -ic-al + O.E. -ly.) aquatically artistically chauvinistically communistically concentrically domestically dualistically economically egoistically erratically extrinsically fatalistically generically humanistically idealistically imperialistically individualistically intrinsically jingoistically journalistically legalistically linguistically majestically masochistically materialistically mechanistically militaristically moralistically operatically opportunistically optimistically paternalistically pessimistically pluralistically prolifically puritanically quixotically quizzically rationalistically realistically romantically rustically sadistically satanically scientifically simplistically socialistically sociologically specifically stylistically surrealistically terrifically;   However, if the word has an **-al** form (see **-ical**) , the extra syllable may be pronounced: /ik-ə-lē/: chemically classically fanatically identically lackadaisically medically numerically oratorically radically satirically statistically vertically whimsically;   <u>Exception</u>: publicly;   <u>See</u>: Gk. suf. **-ically** Ap. iv-55.

-icalness /i-kəl-nis/ (noun) identicalness lackadaisicalness radicalness satiricalness

-ice /is/ (noun) *[Condition, quality, or act.]* accomplice apprentice armistice artifice auspice avarice bodice chalice cornice cowardice crevice dentifrice disservice edifice hospice injustice jaundice justice lattice malice malpractice notice novice office orifice poultice practice precipice prejudice service solstice; /īs/. advice device entice sacrifice suffice; <u>Plus one syllable words</u>: dice ice lice mice nice rice vice price slice splice twice;   /ēs/ caprice police;   /ish/ licorice

-id /id/ (adj.) (Most from Latin with masc. ending dropped, e. g. *humidus* becomes *humid.*) acid arid avid candid fervid fetid flaccid florid frigid fluid horrid humid insipid intrepid invalid languid limpid lipid liquid livid lucid lurid morbid pallid placid putrid rancid rapid rigid solid sordid splendid squalid stolid stupid tepid timid torrid tumid valid vivid; (noun) aphid cuspid druid hominid katydid orchid pyramid

-ide /īd/ (noun) (Used in names of chemical compounds.) boride bromide carbide chloride cyanide dioxide fluoride glyceride halide hydroxide iodide monoxide nitride nuclide (an atom) oxide peroxide sulfide telluride thalidomide; <u>Others</u>: coincide collide confide decide deride divide elide guide hide preside pride side subside, *etc.*   <u>And</u>: Candide /kan-dēd/;   <u>See</u>: suicide, *etc.* under **caedo** in Ap. vii-5.

-idly /id-lē/ (adv.) (Adverb forming **-ly** added to **-id** adjective.) candidly humidly lucidly morbidly rapidly rigidly solidly splendidly stupidly timidly validly vividly, *etc.*

-il /əl/ (noun) anvil April basil civil codicil council devil evil fossil nostril pencil peril pupil stencil tonsil utensil vigil; /il/ Brazil daffodil gerbil tranquil (adj.) until (prep.)

-ile /əl/ (adj.) agile contractile docile domicile (n) ductile facile febrile fertile fragile futile hostile juvenile (+n) missile (+n) mobile projectile (+n) virile volatile; /il/ extensile imbecile (+n) labile mercantile prehensile puerile retractile sterile tactile tensile textile (+n) tractile versatile; /īl/ beguile (v) bile (n) camomile (n) compile (v) crocodile (n) defile (v) Gentile (n) infantile percentile quartile (+n) reconcile (v) reptile (n) senile servile revile (v) turnstile (n); /ēl/ automobile (n) Castile mobile Mobile;

-ilely /ə-lē/ (adv.) (Adverb forming **-ly** added to **-ile** adjective.) agilely docilely facilely fertilely fragilely futilely hostilely juvenilely sterilely versatilely

-ility /il-ə-tē/ (noun) (Formed from **-ile** adjectives.) agility facility fertility fragility futility hostility imbecility mobility senility stability versatility virility volatility

-ily /ə-lē/ (adv.) (**-y** ending of adjective changed to **-i-** and adverb forming **-ly** added.) angrily busily crazily daintily dizzily easily greedily happily hardily lazily merrily momentarily naughtily snappily thriftily wearily, *etc*. See: OE suf. **-y** for orig. adj. Ap. iv-15.

-in /in/ (noun) (Common ending from various sources.) assassin begin Berlin bobbin bulletin Darwin Dublin dolphin basin bulletin cabin chagrin cousin gelatin gherkin gremlin griffin javelin Kremlin Lenin mandarin margin marlin martin maudlin Merlin moccasin muffin muslin napkin origin penguin pumpkin Rasputin resin robin rosin Saladin Sanhedrin satin sequin Stalin tarpaulin toxin twin urchin vermin violin virgin vitamin Wisconsin zeppelin; /n/ Latin; As chemical ending: aspirin casein globulin heroin insulin lanolin lecithin melanin neomycin pectin penicillin pepsin tuberculin

-ine /īn/ (adj., noun, verb) alkaline alpine bovine calamine canine carbine Caroline columbine combine concubine confine cosine decline define divine intertwine iodine Palestine porcupine quinine recline refine sine turbine turpentine twine valentine; /in/ Benedictine Catherine citrine clandestine crinoline crystalline destine determine discipline doctrine endocrine engine ermine examine famine feminine genuine heroine illumine imagine intestine jasmine margarine masculine medicine predestine predetermine rapine sanguine strychnine turbine urine; /ēn/ amphetamine antihistamine aquamarine Argentine Augustine beguine bromine Byzantine caffeine chlorine codeine Constantine cuisine dentine figurine Florentine fluorine gabardine guillotine histamine Josephine latrine libertine machine magazine marine mezzanine morphine nectarine nicotine Philippine Philistine praline pristine quarantine ravine routine saline saltine sardine serpentine Sistine sordine submarine tambourine tangerine trampoline vaccine Vaseline wolverine

-inely /in-lē/ (adv.) (Adverb ending **-ly** added to **-ine** adjective ending.) clandestinely femininely genuinely masculinely sanguinely; See: **-ine** above.

-ineness /i-nis/ (noun) (Noun ending **-ness** added to **-ine** adjective.) clandestineness feminineness (femininity) genuineness masculineness (masculinity) sanguineness; <u>See</u>: **-ine**

-ion /yən/ battalion billion bullion bunion champion clarion communion companion cotillion dominion grunion hellion medallion million minion onion opinion pavilion pinion Pygmalion rapscallion rebellion reunion scallion scullion stallion trillion union vermilion; /ən/ cushion fashion; /ē-ən/ accordion alluvion carrion centurion criterion enchiridion oblivion perihelion prothalamion scorpion; /jən/ contagion legion religion; /shən/ stanchion; /ī-ən/ ion Orion scion Zion

-ior /ē-er/ (adj.) (From Latin comparative form.) anterior exterior (+n) inferior interior (+n) posterior superior ulterior; /ī-ər/ prior; (noun) /yər/ behavior junior misbehavior pavior savior Savior (Saviour) seignior senior warrior

-iorly /ē-er-lē/ (adv.) (Adverb forming **-ly** added to **-ior** adjective.) anteriorly exteriorly inferiorly interiorly posteriorly superiorly ulteriorly; <u>See</u>: **-ior** above.

-is /is/ (noun) apsis *(Pl. apsides)* auris classis cuspis *(cuspides)* digitalis finis gratis (adj.) ibis parvis pelvis penis portcullis proboscis *(proboscides)* tennis torticollis trellis tussis unguis *(ungues);* <u>From other sources</u>: abatis (F) brewis (M.E.) chassis /<u>shas</u>-ē/ (F) clevis (O.E.) Davis Dennis Elis Ellis Francis haggis (M.E.) Isis (Egy.) Kiwanis (Am.Ind.) Lewis Memphis (Egy.) morris (Moorish) précis /<u>prā</u>-sē/ (Fr.) syphilis (Name: Syphilis, character in 16th cent. poem.) tamis (F) Sardis Tigris Tunis; <u>See</u>: **-is** Ap. iv-56 **-sis** Ap. iv-59.

-ise /īz/ (verb) (Var. of Gk. **-ize**.) advertise advise apprise arise chastise circumcise comprise compromise (+n) demise (n) despise devise disenfranchise disguise (+n) enterprise (n) excise (+n) exercise (+n) exorcise franchise (n) guise improvise incise merchandise (+n) reprise (n) revise rise supervise surmise surprise (+n) televise uprise; /is/ (noun) anise mortise premise promise treatise; /īs/ (adj.) concise imprecise paradise (n) precise; /ēz/ (noun) chemise expertise vocalise; /ēs/ (noun) camise (Ar.) valise; And: marquise (F) /mar-<u>kē</u>/; <u>See</u>: O.E. **-wise** Ap. iv-14 and Gk. **-ize** Ap. iv-56.

-isely /īs-lē/ (adv.) (Adverb forming **-ly** added to **-ise** adjective.) concisely precisely

-ish /ish/ (verb) abolish accomplish admonish anguish banish brandish burnish cherish demolish diminish distinguish embellish establish extinguish famish finish flourish furbish furnish garnish impoverish languish perish polish publish punish ravish refurbish relinquish relish replenish skirmish tarnish vanish vanquish varnish; (noun) anguish dervish hashish Kaddish parish radish relish rubbish skirmish varnish

-ism /iz-əm/ (noun) *[A theory, doctrine or condition.]* (From Latin **-ismus**.) absenteeism absolutism activism altruism animalism botulism capitalism centralism classicism collectivism colloquialism colonialism commercialism communism conservatism constitutionalism conventionalism defeatism deism denominationalism departmentalism determinism deviationism dualism egoism egotism emotionalism escapism exhibitionism existentialism expansionism expressionism extremism factionalism

fanaticism fascism fatalism favoritism federalism feminism feudalism formalism fraternalism functionalism fundamentalism gradualism humanism humanitarianism idealism imperialism impressionism individualism industrialism infantilism institutionalism instrumentalism intellectualism internationalism intuitionism invalidism irrationalism isolationism journalism legalism liberalism literalism mannerism materialism mercantilism militarism modernism moralism nationalism naturalism negativism nepotism neutralism nihilism nudism objectivism paternalism perfectionism pessimism pluralism pointillism positivism professionalism protectionism Protestantism provincialism puritanism radicalism rationalism realism recidivism relativism romanticism sectarianism secessionism sectionalism secularism sensationalism sensualism socialism solipsism specialism spiritualism statism subjectivism supernaturalism surrealism territorialism terrorism tourism traditionalism transcendentalism transvestitism tribalism unionism Unitarianism Universalism urbanism utilitarianism vegetarianism ventriloquism voluntarism vulgarism;
Other sources: alcoholism Americanism behaviorism Bolshevism bossism Buddhism Calvinism cannibalism chauvinism Confucianism cretinism czarism Darwinism Hinduism Judaism Maoism Marxism masochism McCarthyism mesmerism momism Mongolism sadism Satanism Semitism Shiism Shamanism Sikhism spoonerism Stalinism Sufism Taoism /dow-iz-əm/ truism vandalism voodooism witticism Zionism Zoroastrianism;   See: Greek suffix -ism Ap. iv-56.

-ist /ist/ (noun) *[A person who does, is, or believes something.]*   (From Latin **ista**.) abortionist accompanist activist Adventist aerialist agriculturist alpinist altruist arsonist artist capitalist careerist centrist classicist collaborationist colonist columnist communist conformist conservationist contortionist conversationalist copyist cornettist defeatist deist dentist educationalist egoist egotist escapist essayist evolutionist exhibitionist extortionist extremist fascist fatalist federalist feminist finalist florist humanist humorist idealist imperialist impressionist individualist industrialist instrumentalist internist interventionist isolationist journalist jurist librettist liturgist loyalist manicurist materialist medalist militarist minimalist modernist moralist motorist nationalist naturalist nonconformist novelist nudist nutritionist oculist opportunist panelist perfectionist pessimist pluralist precisionist prohibitionist projectionist propagandist publicist pugilist purist rapist realist receptionist reservist revisionist revolutionist ritualist royalist satirist scientist secularist segregationist separatist socialist soloist specialist stylist suffragist terrorist tourist traditionalist unionist vacationist vocalist; From other sources: alarmist Bolshevist cellist druggist faddist flutist harpist Marxist parachutist pianist rightist Trappist violinist violist violoncellist; Coincidental ending from verb *sistere* (to stand): assist consist desist exist persist resist subsist;   A non-person noun: Eucharist;   See: Gk. Suf. -ist Ap. iv-56.

-istic /is-tik/ (adj.) *[Having the qualities of.]* (From Latin **-isticus**.) altruistic animalistic antagonistic artistic capitalistic characteristic collectivistic commercialistic communistic deterministic dualistic egoistic egotistic emotionalistic exhibitionistic expressionistic fascistic fatalistic feministic fetishistic feudalistic floristic formalistic futuristic humanistic idealistic imperialistic impressionistic individualistic intellectualistic

Ap. iv-37

irrationalistic journalistic legalistic liberalistic linguistic manneristic materialistic militaristic modernistic moralistic nationalistic naturalistic negativistic nihilistic objectivistic obstructionistic opportunistic optimistic paternalistic pessimistic positivistic primitivistic propagandistic ritualistic secularistic simplistic socialistic spiritualistic statistic (+n) surrealistic terroristic unrealistic; <u>Often a plural form used as singular</u>: linguistics patristics statistics; <u>From other sources</u>: behavioristic Buddhistic Calvanistic cannibalistic chauvinistic jingoistic masochistic sadistic truistic; <u>See</u>: Latin suffixes **-fic** Ap. iv-32 **-ic** Ap. iv-33 and Greek suffixes **-ic** Ap. iv-54, **-tic** Ap. iv-59.

-istically /is-tik-lē/ (adv.) (Adverb forming **-ally** added to **-istic** adjective.) artistically egotistically idealistically optimistically pessimistically realistically simplistically, *etc.*

-it /it/ (verb) (Often a result of a dropped Latin inflection, *-us, -um, -are, -ere*.) accredit acquit admit audit commit credit deposit discredit edit elicit emit exit exhibit inhabit inherit inhibit limit intuit merit omit orbit permit posit profit prohibit solicit spirit split submit transmit visit vomit; (noun) affidavit audit bandit conduit credit cubit culprit debit deficit demerit deposit digit gambit habit hermit Jesuit legit (slang) limit merit obit (Short for *obituary*) orbit permit plaudit profit pulpit pundit rabbit Sanskrit spirit split summit transit unit visit vomit; (adj.) decrepit explicit illicit implicit inexplicit legit tacit; (interj.) prosit /<u>prō</u>-zit/

-ite[1] /īt/ (verb) /īt/ cite expedite extradite ignite incite invite recite reunite unite

-ite[2] (noun) /īt/ appetite bauxite calcite Canaanite cosmopolite despite (+ prep.) dolomite geyserite granulite Hussite Israelite Masonite Mennonite Muscovite plebiscite satellite Semite Shiite /<u>shē</u>-īt/ socialite suburbanite sulfite termite vermiculite; /it/ granite perquisite ("perk") respite; <u>See</u>: Greek suffix **-ite** Ap. iv-56.

-ite[3] /it/ (adj.) composite definite explicit exquisite favorite indefinite infinite (+n) opposite (+n) requisite; /īt/ contrite erudite finite polite recondite tripartite

-itely /it-lē/ (adv.) (Adverb forming **-ly** added to **-ite** adjective.) definitely explicitly exquisitely indefinitely infinitely contritely eruditely politely, *etc.* <u>See</u>: **-ite**[3] above.

-ive /iv/ (adj.) (Almost exclusively **-sive** and **-tive**.) coercive conducive gerundive reflexive; /īv/ (verb) arrive contrive deprive derive revive strive survive thrive

-ment[1] /mənt/ (noun) *[The product, result, means, process, quality or state of.]* abatement abolishment abridgment abutment accompaniment accomplishment acknowledgment achievement adjournment adjustment adornment advancement advertisement agreement ailment alignment allotment amazement amendment amusement announcement annulment apartment appeasement appointment apportionment argument armament arraignment arrangement assessment assignment assortment astonishment atonement attainment basement casement commandment commencement commitment compartment complement compliment condiment confinement consignment containment contentment department deportment detachment detriment development disagreement disappointment disarmament disbursement displacement document element embankment embarrassment embellishment embodiment employment enchantment encouragement endearment endorsement endowment enforcement engagement enjoyment enlargement enlightenment enlistment enrichment entertainment entrenchment environment equipment establishment excitement excrement experiment figment filament firmament fragment fulfillment garment government impairment impeachment impediment implement improvement increment indictment /in-dīt-mənt/ inducement infringement installment instrument internment investment judgment ligament liniment management measurement moment monument movement nourishment nutriment ointment ornament parchment parliament pavement payment pediment pigment predicament pronouncement proportionment punishment refinement refreshment regiment replacement requirement resentment retirement rudiment sacrament sediment segment sentiment settlement shipment statement supplement temperament tenement testament tournament treatment; (adj.) vehement; Note: /mənt/ for noun; /ment/ for verb: augment, compliment, implement, torment, etc.

-ment² /män/ (noun) (French)   débridement   dénouement   rapprochement

-mental /men-təl/ (adj.) [Pertaining to.] departmental detrimental experimental fundamental incremental instrumental judgmental sentimental temperamental, etc.

-mentally /men-tə-lē/ (adv.) (Adverb forming -ly added to -mental adjective.) detrimentally experimentally fundamentally incrementally instrumentally, etc.

-mony /mō-nē/ (noun) [Condition, state.] acrimony alimony ceremony hegemony matrimony palimony parsimony patrimony sanctimony testimony; /mə-nē/ harmony

-ol /ōl/ (noun) [Alcohol base.] Ar. aerosol cholesterol glycol methanol naphthol petrol phenol sterol vitriol; /ôl/: alcohol geraniol menthol; Others: /əl/ Bristol capitol idol Mongol pistol symbol viol; /ōl/ control patrol Sevastopol; /ôl/ parasol protocol

-ole /ōl/ (noun) [Small, little.] aureole banderole camisole oriole ostiole petiole; Others: barcarole bole cabriole cajole capriole caracole casserole condole (v) console (n) /kon-sōl/, (v) /kən-sōl/ creole dole escarole hole insole mole Nicole parole pole resole rigmarole role Seminole sole stole variole whole; From Greek: diastole /dī-as-tə-lē/ (Heart relaxation.) dipole hyperbole /hī-per-bə-lē/ systole /sis-tə-lē/ (Heart contraction.)

-or /er/ (noun) [A person or thing that does something.] abductor accelerator actor adductor administrator aggressor agitator alligator alternator ambassador ancestor anchor animator applicator arbitrator arbor armor assessor auditor author bachelor benefactor calculator cantor capacitor captor carburetor censor chancellor cinerator collector commentator compensator competitor compressor conductor confessor conqueror conservator conspirator constrictor contactor contractor counselor creator creditor cultivator curator debtor defector depositor depressor detector detractor dilator director dissector distributor divisor doctor donor editor educator ejector elector elevator emperor equator eradicator escalator excavator executor exhibitor extensor exterminator extractor factor flexor generator governor guarantor impostor incinerator incisor incubator indicator inhalator inheritor injector inquisitor inspector instructor insulator intercessor intermediator interrogator inventor investigator janitor judicator juror lector legislator liberator liquidator lubricator major malefactor mayor mentor meteor minor moderator modulator monitor motor navigator neighbor numerator objector operator oppressor orator oscillator parlor pastor plexor possessor precursor predator predecessor predictor proctor procurator professor projector proprietor prosecutor prospector protector protractor reactor Realtor receptor rector reflector refractor refrigerator regulator resistor resonator respirator retractor rotator rotor rumor sailor scissor sculptor selector senator sensor separator solicitor spectator speculator splendor sponsor successor succor suitor supervisor surveyor survivor tabulator tailor tenor tensor terminator tormentor tractor traitor transgressor transistor translator tutor ventilator vibrator victor visitor;   (Other nouns) *[Quality, state, or condition.]* + ardor camphor + candor +*clamor +*color corridor + demeanor +*dishonor +*endeavor error +*favor + fervor +*flavor furor +*harbor +*honor horror +*humor +*labor languor liquor manor *mirror + misdemeanor + odor pallor + rancor razor + rigor +*rumor +*savor sector sopor squalor stupor terror torpor tremor + tumor + valor + vapor vector + vigor visor;   * Also verbs. (+ British spelling: *ardour, candour, clamour, colour, favour, flavour, harbour, honour humour, labour, odour, rancour, rigour, vigour,* etc.) American spelling exceptions: glamour Saviour;   Pronunciation Exceptions: /or/ abhor Bangor condor conquistador cuspidor for humidor matador metaphor Monsignor picador Salvador Signor Thor;   See: **-our** Ap. i-30 and **-factor** Ap. iv-31.

-orily /or-ē/ (adj.) (**-ory** adjective ending changed to **-ori-** and adverb forming **-ly** is added.) compulsorily contradictorily cursorily illusorily introductorily satisfactorily, *etc.*

-oriness /or-ē-nis/ (noun)   (**-ory** adjective ending changed to **-ori-** and noun forming **-ness** is added.) compulsoriness goriness satisfactoriness savoriness transitoriness, *etc.*

-ory /or-ē/ or /ər-ē/ (adj.) advisory auditory compulsory contradictory cursory desultory dilatory dissatisfactory excretory expository extrasensory gory illusory intercessory introductory ivory monitory olfactory peremptory perfunctory persecutory possessory precursory prohibitory promissory provisory redemptory revisory satisfactory savory sensory statutory supervisory transitory valedictory; (noun) accessory allegory armory category chancellory clerestory consistory depository directory dormitory factory glory Gregory hickory history inventory ivory memory oratory promontory protectory rectory refectory repertory repository story suppository territory theory Tory trajectory valedictory victory; Plural: **-ories**, glory *glories* inventory *inventories* memory *memories*; See: **-atory** Ap. iv-26.

-ose /ōs/ (adj.) *[Full of, like.]* bellicose cellulose (n) comatose diagnose (v) erose grandiose granulose jocose lachrymose morose otiose /ō-shē-ōs/ pilose plumose rugose spinose tumulose varicose ventricose verbose vorticose; /ōz/ (verb) appose compose decompose depose expose oppose predispose primrose repose

-osely /ōs-lē/ (adv.) (Adverb forming **-ly** added to **-ose** adjective.) grandiosely jocosely morosely spinosely verbosely, *etc.*

-oseness /os-nis/ (noun) (Noun forming **-ness** added to a very few **-ose** adjectives.) moroseness operoseness verboseness; <u>Note dual possibility of</u> : adiposeness, *adiposity* jocoseness, *jocosity*

-osity /os-ə-tē/ (noun) (Forming nouns from most adjectives ending in **-ose** and **-ous**.) bellicosity curiosity generosity grandiosity impecuniosity impetuosity luminosity monstrosity nebulosity pomposity religiosity scrupulosity tuberosity verbosity virtuosity viscosity; animosity (From noun, *animus*) <u>Plural</u>: **-osities**, curiosity, *curiosities.*

-ous /əs/ (adj.) *[Of the nature of; full of.]* adulterous adventurous ambidextrous amorous anxious bigamous bituminous boisterous bulbous cadaverous calamitous callous cancerous cantankerous carnivorous cavernous chivalrous circuitous clamorous conterminous covetous dangerous decorous desirous dexterous disastrous dolorous enormous equanimous erogenous fabulous famous felicitous fibrous fortuitous frivolous fatuous fungous gelatinous generous glamorous gluttonous gratuitous grievous hazardous horrendous humorous indecorous indigenous infamous iniquitous intravenous jealous joyous languorous larcenous lecherous libelous libidinous ludicrous luminous lustrous magnanimous marvelous mischievous monstrous mucous multitudinous momentous mountainous murderous murmurous mutinous nebulous nervous numerous obstreperous odorous ominous omnivorous onerous perilous pilous platitudinous poisonous pompous ponderous porous posthumous precipitous preposterous prosperous pulchritudinous rancorous rapturous raucous ravenous rigorous riotous ruinous scandalous scrupulous scurrilous slanderous solicitous sonorous spiritous stupendous thunderous timorous traitorous treacherous treasonous tremendous ubiquitous ulcerous unanimous valorous vaporous venomous vigorous villainous viscous viviparous vociferous voluminous vortiginous wondrous zealous; <u>See</u>: **-aceous** Ap. iv-18, **-ferous** Ap. iv-31 and **-ulous** Ap. iv-51.

(-eous) /ē-əs/ aqueous arboreous beauteous bounteous citreous contemporaneous courteous discourteous duteous erroneous extemporaneous extraneous gaseous heterogeneous hideous homogeneous igneous instantaneous miscellaneous osseous piteous plenteous righteous /rī-chəs/ sanguineous simultaneous spontaneous subaqueous

(-ious) /ē-əs/ abstemious acrimonious amphibious calumnious ceremonious commodious compendious copious curious deleterious delirious devious dubious envious euphonious fastidious felonious furious glorious gregarious harmonious hilarious ignominious illustrious impecunious imperious impervious impious industrious injurious insidious invidious laborious lascivious lugubrious luxurious melodious meritorious multifarious mysterious nefarious notorious oblivious obsequious obvious odious parsimonious penurious perfidious perjurious pervious precarious previous punctilious riparious salubrious sanctimonious serious spurious studious supercilious tedious uproarious usurious vainglorious various vicarious victorious; /yəs/ bilious ingenious rebellious; <u>And</u>: pious /pī-əs/ religious /ri-lij-əs/ <u>See</u>: **-cious** Ap. iv-27 **-tious** -47.

(-uous) /yo͞o-əs/ /o͞o-əs/ (Remember **-du-** /jo͞o/ & **-tu-** /cho͞o/.) ambiguous arduous assiduous celluous congruous conspicuous contemptuous contiguous continuous deciduous discontinuous disingenuous fatuous impetuous incestuous incongruous ingenuous innocuous mellifluous nocuous perspicuous presumptuous promiscuous sensuous superfluous strenuous sumptuous tempestuous tenuous tortuous tumultuous unambiguous unctuous vacuous virtuous voluptuous

-ously /əs-lē/ (adv.) (Adverb forming **-ly** added to **-ous** adjective.) anxiously boisterously conspicuously curiously erroneously jealously nervously obviously seriously simultaneously strenuously tremendously unanimously vigorously, *etc.*

-ousness /əs-nis/ (noun) (Noun forming **-ness** added to som **-ous** adjectives.) adventurousness callousness conspicuousness deviousness nervousness seriousness, *etc.*

-ry /rē/ (noun) (Variation of **-ery**.) ancestry artistry balladry banditry basketry bawdry belfry bigotry carpentry cavalry century chemistry cherry chicory chivalry circuitry citizenry coquetry country Coventry dentistry deviltry dowry entry falconry forestry foundry fury gadgetry gallantry gantry gentry gimmickry glory Harry Henry heraldry history husbandry imagery industry infantry inquiry jewelry laundry masonry Mercury mimicry ministry missilry musketry pageantry palmistry pantry parquetry parry (+v) pastry peasantry pedantry penury perjury pleasantry poetry polyandry poultry puppetry quarry query reentry registry revelry ribaldry rivalry rocketry savagery sentry sophistry story summitry symmetry tapestry theory toiletry usury vestry victory weaponry wizardry zealotry; Plural: **-ies,** entry, *entries;* inquiry, *inquiries;*   (adj.) angry hungry paltry sultry tawdry wintry; (verb) /rī/ (One syllable words.) cry dry fry pry try;   Third person singular of verbs: cry, *cries;* dry, *dries;*   See: **-ary** Ap. iv-24, **-ery** Ap. iv-30 and Greek combining forms **-latry** Ap. ix-11 and **-metry** Ap. ix-12.

-sia /zhə/ (noun) ambrosia Asia euthanasia Indonesia Malaysia Micronesia Persia

-sion[1] /shən/ (noun) accession admission aggression apprehension ascension commission compassion comprehension compression compulsion concession concussion condescension confession convulsion declension decommission decompression depression diapason digression dimension discussion dispersion dissension emission emulsion expansion expression expulsion extension fission hypertension impassion impression impulsion intercession intermission mansion mission obsession omission oppression passion pension permission percussion possession precession pretension procession profession progression propulsion recession regression remission repercussion repression repulsion revulsion secession session submission succession suppression suspension tension torsion transmission

-sion[2] /zhən/ aspersion aversion conversion dispersion diversion emersion excursion extroversion immersion incursion introversion inversion perversion reversion submersion subversion version vision
(-asion[2]) /ā-zhən/ abrasion erasion evasion invasion occasion persuasion

(-esion²) /ē-zhən/ adhesion cohesion lesion

(-ision²) /i-zhən/ collision decision derision division elision envision incision indecision precision provision revision subdivision supervision television vision

(-osion²) /ō-zhən/ corrosion erosion explosion implosion

(-usion²) /ōō-zhən/ allusion collusion conclusion contusion delusion diffusion disillusion elusion exclusion illusion inclusion intrusion malocclusion preclusion protrusion seclusion; /yōō-zhən/ confusion fusion infusion profusion transfusion

-sional /shən-əl/ (adj.) confessional (+n) congressional extensional processional (+n) professional recessional (+n) secessional sessional torsional; /zhən-əl/ delusional diversional divisional illusional occasional provisional

-sionally /shə-nə-lē/ (adv.) congressionally dimensionally extensionally processionally professionally unprofessionally sessionally successionally torsionally; /zhən-lē/ divisionally occasionally provisionally

-sive /siv/ (adj.) *[Tendency to; quality of.]* aggressive apprehensive cohesive collusive comprehensive compressive compulsive convulsive corrosive cursive defensive depressive digressive discursive excessive exclusive expansive expensive expressive extensive impassive impressive impulsive inconclusive inexpensive inoffensive intensive intrusive massive obsessive offensive oppressive passive pensive percussive permissive possessive progressive protrusive recessive regressive repressive repulsive responsive submissive subversive successive unexpressive unresponsive

(-asive) /ā-siv/ abrasive assuasive dissuasive evasive persuasive pervasive

(-esive) /ē-siv/ adhesive

(-isive) /ī-siv/ derisive decisive divisive incisive indecisive

(-osive) /ō-siv/ erosive explosive (+n.) plosive (+n.) purposive /per-pə-siv/

(-usive) /yōō-siv/ abusive amusive diffusive effusive infusive; /ōō-siv/ allusive conclusive delusive elusive extrusive illusive inclusive obtrusive occlusive seclusive

-sively /siv-lē/ (adv.) (Adverb forming **-ly** added to **-sive** adjective.) aggressively comprehensively compulsively expensively extensively impressively inconclusively intrusively offensively persuasively responsively submissively successively, *etc.*

-siveness /siv-nis/ (noun) (Noun forming **-ness** is added to **-sive** adjective.) abusiveness adhesiveness cohesiveness decisiveness elusiveness exclusiveness intrusiveness, *etc.*

-sivity /siv-i-tē/ (noun) (Or noun forming **-sivity** is added to **-sive** adjective.) exclusivity impassivity impulsivity passivity, *etc.*   <u>See</u>: **-sive, -siveness** Ap. iv-43.

-sure /zhər/ (noun) closure composure disclosure displeasure enclosure exposure foreclosure leisure measure pleasure treasure; And: seizure; But: /shoor/ assure cocksure ensure insure reassure unsure;   /sher/ censure erasure fissure pressure

-tain /ān/ (verb) (From L. *tenere, to hold.*) abstain appertain contain detain entertain maintain obtain pertain retain sustain; And from other roots: ascertain attain disdain; (noun) /ən/ Britain captain certain (adj.) chieftain curtain fountain mountain uncertain

-tia /shə/ (noun) absentia consortia Dalmatia dementia inertia Lucretia militia minutia Nova Scotia Portia;   But: differentia /dif-e-ren-shē-ə/ poinsettia /poin-set-ē-ə/

-tial /shəl/ (adj.) *[Pertaining to; characterized by.]* circumstantial confidential consequential credential (+n) deferential differential (+n) essential evidential existential expediential experiential exponential impartial inconsequential inferential influential initial insubstantial jurisprudential martial nuptial palatial partial penitential pestilential postnuptial potential preferential presidential providential prudential referential residential reverential sequential spatial substantial tangential torrential unessential unsubstantial;   /chəl/ bestial celestial

-tially /shəl-ē/ (adv.) (Adverb forming **-ly** added to **-tial** adjective.) beneficially circumstantially confidentially consequentially essentially existentially experientially impartially influentially potentially preferentially sequentially substantially, *etc.*

-tian /shən/ (noun, name) *[Often person or group name.]* Aleutian Christian Dalmatian dietitian Egyptian Galatian Haitian Lilliputian Martian Tahitian Titian Venetian

-tiate /shē-āt/ (verb) circumstantiate consubstantiate differentiate expatiate ingratiate initiate insatiate licentiate negotiate novitiate (n) propitiate satiate vitiate

-tient /shənt/ consentient (adj.) dissentient (n, adj.) impatient (adj.) inpatient (n) insentient (adj.) outpatient (n) patient (n, adj.) quotient (n) sentient (adj.) volitient (adj.)

-tiently /shənt-lē/ (adv.) (Adverb forming **-ly** added to **-tient** adjective.) consentiently dissentiently impatiently insentiently patiently sentiently volitiently

-tion[1] /shən/ (noun) *[Action, process, condition, state, or result of.]* (Note: **-ation, -etion, -ition, -otion, & -ution** follow.) abduction abortion absorption abstention abstraction action addiction adoption affection affliction assertion assumption attention attraction auction benediction caption caution collection combustion compunction conception concoction conduction confection congestion conjunction connection conniption conscription constriction construction consumption contention contortion contraception contraction contradiction contraption convection convention conviction correction corruption deception deduction defection deflection dejection dereliction description desertion destruction detection detention detraction diction diffraction digestion direction disruption dissatisfaction dissection distinction distortion distraction dysfunction ejection election erection eruption exception exemption exertion exhaustion extinction extortion extraction faction fiction fraction friction function genuflection gumption imperception imperfection inception indigestion induction infection inflection infliction infraction injection injunction inscription insertion inspection instruction insurrection interaction interception interjection interruption intersection intervention introduction introjection introspection invention irruption junction jurisdiction malfunction mention misconception nonfiction nonintervention objection obstruction option overproduction perception perfection portion preconception prediction predilection prescription presumption prevention production projection proportion protection reaction reception recollection reconstruction redemption reduction reflection refraction rejection reproduction restriction resumption resurrection retention retraction sanction satisfaction section seduction selection subjection subscription subtraction suction traction transaction transcription unction; See: -faction Ap. iv-31, -fication Ap iv-32.

(-ation) /ā-shən/ (noun) abbreviation aberration abomination acceleration acclamation accommodation accreditation acculturation accumulation activation adaptation adjudication administration admiration adoration adulation adulteration affectation affiliation affirmation aggravation agitation alienation allegation alliteration allocation alteration altercation alternation amalgamation amelioration animation annexation annihilation annotation annunciation anticipation application appreciation appropriation approximation arbitration argumentation articulation asphyxiation aspiration assimilation association attenuation augmentation auscultation automation aviation avocation calculation cancellation capitulation carnation causation celebration certification cessation circulation citation clarification codification coeducation collation coloration combination commemoration commendation commiseration communication commutation compensation compilation complication computation concentration condemnation condensation confederation configuration confirmation confiscation conflagration conflation conformation confrontation conglomeration congratulation congregation conjugation connotation consecration conservation consideration consolation consolidation constellation consternation constipation consultation consummation contamination contemplation continuation conversation convocation cooperation coordination copulation coronation corporation correlation corroboration creation culmination cultivation damnation deceleration declamation declaration decoration dedication defamation deflation deformation degeneration degradation delegation deliberation demarcation demonstration denomination denotation denunciation deportation depravation depreciation depredation deprivation deputation derivation desecration desegregation designation desolation desperation destination deterioration determination detonation devastation deviation dictation dilapidation dilation discoloration discontinuation discrimination disinclination disintegration dispensation disputation disqualification dissertation dissimulation dissipation distillation divination documentation domination donation duplication duration edification education ejaculation elaboration elation electrification elevation elimination elongation emanation emancipation embarkation emigration enumeration enunciation equalization equation equivocation eradication estimation evacuation evaporation exaggeration exaltation examination exasperation excavation exclamation excommunication exhalation exhilaration exhortation expectation expectoration experimentation expiation expiration explanation explication exploitation exploration extermination exultation fabrication fascination federation fermentation fibrillation figuration filtration fixation flirtation fluctuation forestation formation formulation fornication fragmentation frustration gemination generation germination gestation gesticulation gradation graduation gravitation gyration habitation hallucination hesitation hibernation homogenization humiliation hyperventilation illumination illustration imagination imitation immigration immolation implantation implementation implication importation impregnation improvisation inauguration incantation incarnation inclination incorporation incubation indentation indication indignation inflation innovation inoculation insemination insinuation inspiration installation instigation instrumentation insubordination insulation integration interpolation interpretation interrogation intimation intimidation intonation intoxication investigation invitation invocation irrigation irritation isolation jubilation laceration lactation lamentation lamination legation legislation levitation liberation limitation liquidation litigation location lubrication machination malformation manifestation manipulation masturbation maturation mediation medication meditation melioration menstruation migration miscalculation moderation modulation motivation multiplication mutation narration nation navigation negation negotiation nomination notation obligation observation occupation operation oration orchestration ordination orientation ornamentation oscillation ovation ovulation oxidation pagination palpitation participation penetration permutation perspiration perturbation pigmentation plantation pollination population precipitation predestination predication preoccupation preparation presentation preservation prestidigitation prevarication privation probation proclamation procrastination prolongation propagation protestation provocation publication pulsation punctuation qualification quotation radiation recapitulation recitation reclamation recommendation reconciliation recreation reevaluation reformation refutation regeneration regimentation registration regulation regurgitation rehabilitation reincarnation relation relaxation relocation remuneration renunciation reparation repatriation replication representation reputation reservation resignation respiration restoration resuscitation retaliation retardation revelation reverberation revocation rotation ruination salivation salutation salvation sanitation saturation sedation sedimentation segmentation segregation sensation separation simulation situation solicitation sophistication speculation starvation station stipulation strangulation sublimation suffocation summation syncopation syndication taxation telecommunication temptation termination tintinnabulation titillation toleration Transfiguration transformation translation transmigration transportation trepidation triangulation tribulation ulceration undulation vacation vaccination valuation variation vegetation veneration vexation vibration vindication violation visitation vocation

(-etion) /ē-shən/ (noun) completion concretion deletion depletion excretion repletion secretion; /e-shən/ discretion indiscretion

(-ition) /i-shən/ (noun) abolition acquisition addition admonition ambition ammunition apparition attrition audition coalition cognition competition composition condition contrition decomposition definition demolition deposition disposition edition erudition exhibition expedition exposition extradition fruition ignition imposition indisposition inhibition intuition juxtaposition malnutrition nutrition opposition partition petition position predisposition premonition preposition prohibition proposition recognition recondition rendition repetition requisition sedition superstition supposition tradition transition transposition tuition volition

(-otion) /ō-shən/ (noun) commotion devotion locomotion lotion motion notion potion promotion

(-ution) /o͞o-shən/ (noun) constitution convolution devolution dilution diminution dissolution evolution institution pollution prostitution resolution restitution revolution solution substitution; /yo͞o-shən/ (After /b/ and /k/.) attribution circumlocution contribution distribution elocution execution locution persecution prosecution retribution

-tion² /chən/ (After *s*.) (noun) bastion combustion congestion ingestion question suggestion

-tional /shən-əl/ (adj.) *[Pertaining to.]* (Adjective forming **-al** added to **-tion** noun.) additional conditional constitutional conventional educational emotional exceptional functional intentional irrational national optional proportional rational traditional, *etc.*

-tionally /shə-nə-lē/ (adv.) (Adverb forming **-ly** added to **-tional** adjective.) additionally conditionally conventionally educationally emotionally exceptionally functionally intentionally nationally proportionally rationally, *etc.*

-tionary /shən-air-ē/ (adj.) cautionary deflationary discretionary evolutionary inflationary probationary precautionary reactionary revolutionary stationary; (noun) confectionary dictionary functionary revolutionary; Plural: **-tionaries,** dictionary, *dictionaries*

-tious /shəs/ (adj.) adventitious ambitious cautious conscientious contentious disputatious dissentious expeditious facetious fictitious flirtatious infectious licentious nutritious ostentatious precautious pretentious propitious rambunctious repetitious scrumptious seditious sententious superstitious surreptitious vexatious

-tiously /shəs-lē/ (adv.) (Adverb forming **-ly** added to **-tious** adjective.) ambitiously cautiously conscientiously fictitiously nutritiously repetitiously superstitiously, *etc.*

-tive /tiv/ (adj.) *[Tendency to; quality of.]* active addictive adoptive affective assertive attentive attractive conductive connective constrictive constructive contradictive deceptive deductive defective descriptive destructive detractive digestive disruptive distinctive effective elective eruptive exertive exhaustive festive furtive imperceptive inactive inattentive inductive ineffective instinctive interactive introspective inventive irrespective nonproductive objective perceptive plaintive predictive preemptive prescriptive productive prospective protective radioactive receptive redemptive reflective reproductive resistive respective restive restrictive retentive retroactive seductive selective subjective suggestive supportive susceptive unattractive unproductive vindictive vocative votive; (noun) adjective captive collective contraceptive corrective detective elective directive incentive invective objective perspective preventive subjunctive substantive

(-ative) /ə-tiv/ (adj.) ablative accumulative accusative affirmative affricative alternative appreciative augmentative calmative combative commemorative communicative comparative conservative contemplative cooperative cumulative decorative demonstrative discriminative educative elaborative exhilarative exhortative figurative formative fricative illustrative imaginative imperative inappreciative indicative informative inoperative lucrative manipulative negative nominative normative pejorative postoperative preparative provocative quantitative recuperative relative remunerative representative restorative speculative talkative tentative uncommunicative undemonstrative unimaginative vocative; /ā-tiv/ administrative authoritative creative dative hesitative imitative irritative legislative native obligative procreative qualitative vegetative; (noun) /ə-tiv/ affirmative alternative calmative comparative conservative cooperative curative derivative fricative initiative laxative narrative negative operative prerogative preservative purgative recitative relative representative sedative

(-etive) /ē-tiv/ (adj.) concretive decretive depletive; /ə-tiv/ expletive (+n) secretive

(-itive) /ə-tiv/ (adj.) acquisitive cognitive competitive definitive fugitive genitive hypersensitive inquisitive insensitive intransitive intuitive nutritive oppositive partitive photosensitive positive primitive prohibitive punitive repetitive sensitive transitive; (noun) additive fugitive infinitive positive

(-otive) /ō-tiv/ (adj.) automotive electromotive emotive locomotive motive promotive votive; (noun) locomotive motive

(-utive) /yə-tiv/ attributive consecutive contributive diminutive distributive executive retributive; (noun) diminutive executive

-tively /tiv-lē/ (adv.) (Adverb forming **-ly** added to **-tive** adjective.) collectively competitively deceptively effectively intuitively negatively objectively positively productively secretively sensitively respectively tentatively, *etc.*

-tiveness /tiv-nis/ (noun) (Noun forming **-ness** added to **-tive** adjective.) attractiveness disruptiveness effectiveness repetitiveness retentiveness talkativeness, *etc.*

-tivity /tiv-i-tē/ (noun) (Or **-tive** adjective may become **-tivity** noun.) activity conductivity creativity festivity hyperactivity inactivity insensitivity objectivity productivity radioactivity relativity retentivity selectivity sensitivity subjectivity, *etc.*

-trix /tricks/ (noun) *[One who does or makes.]* (Feminine form of a few masculine **-tor** words.] administratrix (m. administrator) aviatrix (aviator) executrix (executor) inheritrix (inheritor) testatrix (testator)

-tual /chōō-əl/ (adj.) actual conceptual contextual contractual eventual factual habitual intellectual mutual perceptual perpetual punctual ritual (+n) spiritual virtual

-tually /chōō-(ə)-lē/ (adv.) (Adverb forming **-ly** added to **-tual** adjective.) actually conceptually eventually habitually intellectually mutually spiritually virtually, *etc.*

-tuary /chōō-air-ē/ (noun) *[Pertaining to.]* actuary mortuary obituary sanctuary statuary textuary; <u>Plural</u>: **-tuaries** obituary *obituaries.*

-tude /tōōd/ (noun) altitude amplitude aptitude attitude beatitude certitude disquietude exactitude fortitude gratitude inaptitude ineptitude ingratitude inquietude latitude longitude magnitude multitude platitude pulchritude servitude solitude

-tural /cher-əl/ (adj.) agricultural architectural conjectural cultural horticultural natural scriptural sculptural structural supernatural textural

-turally /cher-(ə)-lē/ (adv.) (A few **-ture** nouns may be made into adverbs.) agriculturally architecturally conjecturally culturally naturally scripturally sculpturally structurally

-ture /cher/ (noun) acupuncture agriculture aperture architecture creature culture curvature debenture denture departure divestiture expenditure fixture forfeiture furniture future horticulture imposture investiture juncture legislature ligature literature miniature mixture moisture musculature nature nomenclature overture portraiture prefecture primogeniture scripture signature stature stricture superstructure tablature temperature texture vesture vulture; (Both noun & verb.) adventure capture caricature cloture conjecture departure feature fracture gesture indenture lecture manufacture nurture pasture picture posture puncture rapture rupture sculpture structure suture tincture torture venture; (verb) **denature disfeature enrapture;** (adj.) /tyŏŏr/ immature mature premature

-ty /tē/ (noun) *[State, condition, or quality.]* admiralty anaplasty beauty casualty certainty commonalty county cruelty difficulty frailty guaranty honesty loyalty nicety novelty penalty poverty property puberty realty royalty sacristy satiety shanty sovereignty specialty travesty trinity ubiquity uncertainty warranty; <u>Plural</u>: **-ties**, anxiety, *anxieties;* novelty, *novelties.*

(-ety) /ə-tē/ (noun) *[State, condition, or quality.]* anxiety contrariety entirety gaiety piety sobriety society subtlety /<u>sut</u>-l-tē/ variety

(-ity) /ə-tē/ (noun) *[State, condition, or quality.]* ability abnormality absurdity actuality adversity affinity agility alacrity alkalinity ambiguity amity angularity annuity antiquity artificiality asininity atonality atrocity audacity austerity authenticity authority automaticity banality barbarity bestiality bisexuality bovinity brevity brutality calamity capability capacity capillarity captivity carnality causality cavity celebrity centrality centricity charity chastity Christianity civility clarity commodity commonality community complexity complicity confidentiality conformity congeniality congruity consanguinity constitutionality contiguity continuity conventionality cordiality credulity criminality crudity crystallinity debility deformity deity density depravity dexterity dignity disparity diversity divinity domesticity duality duplicity eccentricity elasticity electricity enmity enormity entity equality equanimity equity eternity eventuality extraterritoriality extremity factuality falsity familiarity fatality fecundity felicity felinity femininity ferocity fidelity finality formality fraternity frivolity frugality generality generosity geniality gentility granularity gratuity gravity heredity heterogeneity heterosexuality hilarity historicity homogeneity homosexuality hospitality humanity humidity humility identity illegality immensity immorality immortality immunity impartiality impracticality impropriety impunity impurity inability incapacity incongruity incredulity indemnity indignity individuality inequality inferiority infidelity infinity infirmity informality ingenuity inhumanity iniquity insanity insecurity insincerity insularity integrity intentionality intensity irrationality irregularity jocularity laity laxity legality levity liberality lithotrity locality longevity majority malignity masculinity materiality maternity maturity mediocrity mentality minority modality modernity monstrosity morality morbidity multiplicity municipality disability musicality nationality nativity necessity negativity neutrality nobility nonconformity nonentity normality nudity obesity obscenity obscurity opportunity originality parity partiality paternity peculiarity periodicity perpetuity perplexity personality perversity plasticity plurality polarity polity possibility posterity practicality priority probability profanity promiscuity propensity prosperity proximity publicity punctuality purity quality quantity rarity rationality reality receptivity reciprocity regularity rigidity saccharinity sagacity salinity sanctity sanity scarcity secularity security senility seniority sensuality sentimentality serendipity serenity severity sexuality simplicity sincerity singularity solemnity solidarity solidity sonority sorority sphericity spirituality stupidity superiority susceptibility technicality tenacity territoriality tonality totality toxicity tranquillity trinity Trinity triviality ubiquity uniformity unity university utility validity vanity varsity velocity veracity vicinity vitality; <u>See</u>: **-ability** Ap. iv-17, **-arity** Ap. iv-23, **-ility** Ap. iv-35, **-osity** Ap. iv-41.

-ude /ōōd/ (verb) allude collude conclude delude denude elude exclude exude include intrude preclude seclude; (noun) etude interlude prelude prude postlude; (adj.) crude;   <u>See</u>: **-tude** Ap. iv-49.

-ule /yōōl/ (noun) *[Little, small.]* antennule barbule cellule cupule mutule spicule spinule sporule tubule valvule venule vestibule virgule (/);   <u>But</u>: /əl/ capsule ferrule

-ulence /yə-ləns/ (noun) (Noun form of **-ulent** adjective.) corpulence feculence flocculence opulence purulence succulence truculence turbulence virulence

-ulent /yə-lənt/ (adj.) corpulent opulent succulent turbulent virulent, *etc.*

-ulently /yə-lənt-lē/ (adv.) (Adverb forming **-ly** added to **-ulent** adjective.) corpulently opulently succulently turbulently virulently

-ulosity /yə-los-ə-tē/ (noun) (Noun form of some **-ulous** adjective.) meticulosity nebulosity scrupulosity; <u>But</u>; credulity > credulous

-ulous /yə-ləs/ (Remember **-du-** /joō/) (adj.) *[Tending to do; full of.]* acidulous bibulous credulous cumulous deciduous emulous garrulous globulous meticulous miraculous nebulous pendulous populous querulous ridiculous scrupulous tremulous tuberculous

-ulously /yə-ləs-lē/ (adv.) (Adverb forming **-ly** added to **-ulous** adjective.) credulously garrulously meticulously miraculously querulously ridiculously scrupulously, *etc.*

-ulousness /yə-ləs-nis/ (noun) (Another noun form of **-ulous** adjective.) garrulousness meticulousness miraculousness querulousness ridiculousness scrupulousness

-um /əm/ (**-um** is the Latin neuter singular noun ending. Its plural is **-a**: datum, *data*. Common plurals are listed; others with this plural are marked with an asterisk. Some words are transliterations of Greek words ending in neuter singular *-on*, *e.g.,* Greek *phylon* becomes Latin *phylum*.) addendum *(addenda)* agendum *(agenda)* album aluminum antebellum *arboretum *asylum candelabrum *(candelabra)* cementum centrum *(centra)* cerebellum *(cerebella)* cerebrum *(cerebra)* chrysanthemum coliseum continuum *(continua)* *corrigendum cuprum (copper) curriculum *(curricula)* datum *(data)* decorum *desideratum *dictum *diverticulum *dorsum *duodenum Erechtheum erratum *(errata)* factotum *filum *folium *forum *frustum *fulcrum hokum (slang) inoculum interregnum linoleum *lyceum magnum *mausoleum maximum *(maxima)* memorandum *(memoranda)* minimum *(minima)* *modicum momentum *(momenta)* museum nostrum *odeum optimum *(optima)* organum *(organa)* ovum *(ova)* pabulum pendulum per annum petroleum phylum *(phyla)* platinum *plectrum *plenum post-bellum postpartum quantum (quanta) *rectum referendum *(referenda)* residuum *(residua)* *reticulum *rostrum *sanctum *scrotum *scutum Scutum secundum (adv.) *septum *serum sorghum spectrum *(spectra)* *speculum *sternum stratum *(strata)* *subphylum *substratum *superstratum talcum tantrum teetotum *tympanum *ultimatum *vacuum variorum vellum;
<u>Note</u>: Although many of these words may have the Latin plural ending (-a), many use the Old English plural (-s): fulcrum *(fulcra or fulcrums)*; egesta & ejecta appear only in their plural form.

(-ium) /ē-əm/ (noun) (**-i-** is a "connective" vowel.) aquarium atrium auditorium biennium Byzantium compendium *(compendia)* condominium consortium cranium crematorium delirium delphinium diluvium dominium eluvium Elysium endocardium epicardium equilibrium euphonium geranium gymnasium harmonium herbarium honorarium medium *(media)* millennium *(millennia)* moratorium myocardium natatorium opium palladium pandemonium planetarium podium premium Presidium principium *(principia)* sanatorium solarium stadium symposium tedium terrarium trillium;

<u>Periodic Table Elements</u>: Americium Barium Berkelium Beryllium Cadmium Calcium Californium Cesium Chromium Curium Einsteinium Europium Fermium Francium Gallium Germanium Helium Indium Iridium Lawrencium Lithium Magnesium Neptunium Nobelium Palladium Plutonium Polonium Potassium Promethium Radium Rhodium Ruthenium Selenium Sodium Strontium Uranium

-ure /yŏŏr/ (noun) brochure /brō-<u>shŏŏr</u>/ coiffure /kwä-<u>fyŏŏr</u>/ cure embouchure /äm-boo-<u>shŏŏr</u>/ epicure failure /<u>fāl</u>-yer/ figure /<u>fig</u>-yer/ flexure /<u>fleck</u>-sher/ manicure manure procedure sinecure tenure /<u>ten</u>-yer/ velure verdure /<u>ver</u>-jer/ (verb) adjure conjure cure disfigure figure immure injure manicure manure obscure prefigure procure secure transfigure; (adj.) insecure obscure secure; <u>See</u>: -sure in Ap. iv-44; ture in Ap. i-40, Ap. iv-49.

-us /əs/ (noun) (**-us** is the Latin masculine singular ending. Its plural is **-i**: The Greek masculine singular **-os** suffix is often transliterated into Latin as **-us**.) abacus Aeolus *(Gk. god of the winds.)* altocumulus altostratus alumnus *(alumni)* animus annulus anus arbutus asparagus Australopithecus bacillus *(bacilli)* bonus Bosporus bronchus *(bronchi)* Brutus Bucephalus cactus *(cacti, cactuses)* caduceus calculus *(calculi)* callus campus *(campuses)* canthus cantus *(cantus)* cantus firmus Caucasus caucus *(caucuses)* census *(censuses)* chorus circumbendibus cirrus *(cirri)* cirrocumulus cirrostratus citrus circus *(circuses)* Circus Maximus coccus *(cocci)* coleus colossus comitatus consensus conspectus Copernicus corpus *(corpora)* Crassus crocus Cronus cumulus *(cumuli)* cumulocirrus cumulonimbus Cygnus Cyprus Cyrus Damascus Democritus detritus discobolus *(discoboli)* discus *(disci)* Drusus echinus elenchus embolus *(emboli)* emeritus Epicurus Erasmus Erechtheus esophagus *(esophagi)* estrus eucalyptus exodus Fabius Maximus fetus focus *(foci)* fungus *(fungi)* genus *(genera)* gladiolus gluteus gradus halitus Hesperus hiatus hibiscus homunculus Horus humerus humus Hyacinthus hypothalamus ignoramus ileus impetus incubus isthmus Jesus Josephus jus *(jura)* lapsus Leviticus litmus locus *(loci)* lotus lupus Magus *(Magi)* mandamus manus Marcellus minus (+ prep., adj.) modus *(modi)* Morpheus mucus Narcissus nautilus nexus nimbus *(nimbi)* nonplus Nostradamus nucleus *(nuclei)* octopus *(octopi)* Odysseus Oedipus Olympus omnibus onus opus *(opera)* Orpheus papyrus *(papyri)* Parnassus Patroclus Pegasus Peisistratus Peloponnesus phallus *(phalli)* phosphorus Pisistratus Pithecanthropus plexus plus (+ prep., adj.) Polyphemus posse comitatus Prometheus prospectus pus rebus rectus *(recti)* rhesus rhombus *(rhombi)* Romulus Remus rumpus Sanctus sarcophagus *(sarcophagi)* Seleucus sinus Sisyphus solus Spartacus status stimulus *(stimuli)* stratocumulus stratus streptococcus *(streptococci)* stylus *(styluses, styli)* syllabus *(syllabuses, syllabi)* Tantalus Taurus terminus tetanus thalamus thesaurus thrombus thymus tinnitus typhus umbilicus Uranus uterus valgus Venus virus *(viruses)* viscus *(viscera)* walrus Zephyrus Zeus Zinjanthropus; <u>Note</u>: Although many of these words may have the Latin plural ending (-i), many may still use the Old English plural (-s): focus *(foci* or *focuses)*. Some plurals are irregular, opus *(opera)*.

(-ius) /ē-əs/ (noun) (**-us** is the Latin masculine singular ending. **-i-** is a *connective* vowel.) Darius Delius denarius genius /<u>jēn</u>-yəs/ Lucretius /-shəs/   Marcus Antonius Marcus Aurelius Polonius radius *(radii* /rā-dē-ī/) regius Sagittarius Sibelius Vitruvius

-use /yo͞oz/ (verb) abuse accuse confuse diffuse perfuse peruse (pə-ro͞oz) use; /yo͞os/ (adj.) abstruse (ab-stro͞os) diffuse obtuse (əb-to͞os) profuse; (noun) Syracuse use /yo͞os/

-ute /yo͞ot/ minute (adj.) tribute (n) prosecute (v); /o͞ot/ absolute (adj., n) astute (adj.) brute (n) dissolute (adj.) irresolute (adj.) resolute (adj.)

-utely /o͞ot-lē/ (adv.) [Adverb forming **-ly** added to **-ute** adjective.] absolutely astutely dissolutely irresolutely resolutely

-xion /-k-shən/ (noun) (Var. of **-tion**.) complexion crucifixion defluxion flexion fluxion retroflexion

-xious /-k-shəs/ (adj.) anxious innoxious noxious obnoxious

-xiously /-k-shəs-lē/ (adv.) (Adverb forming **-ly** added to **-xious** adjective.) anxiously noxiously obnoxiously

-xiousness /-k-shəs-nis/ (noun) (Noun forming **-ness** added to **-xious** adjective.) noxiousness obnoxiousness

-y /ē/ (noun) ability acrimony actuary alimony ally armory army assembly beauty boundary bounty burglary caddy cavity ceremony charity city cogency colony company contrary controversy copy county country courtesy custody delivery deputy destiny diary embassy enemy entry envy factory faculty fairy family frequency fury gully honesty identity ignominy industry injury inquiry ivory jelly jetty jury larceny levy liberty library lily livery luxury majesty malady mastery matrimony memory mercury military miscellany misery modesty mutiny navy nicety pity plenty pony poppy prodigy progeny puppy rally remedy ruby safety salary sally scrutiny soliloquy subfamily subsidy tally testimony treaty unity vagary villainy
<u>Plural</u>: **-ies**, ceremony, *ceremonies*.

<u>See Other Noun Endings</u>: **-ability, -ancy, -arity, -ary, (-iary), -atory, -bury, -ciency, -cy, (-acy) -ency, -ey, -ibility, -ility, mony, -ory, -osity, -sivity, -tivity, -tuary, -ty (-ety), (-ity), -ulosity, -y** (Both L, Gk. & Other.);

<u>See Adverb Endings</u>: **-ably, -ally, -anely, -antly, -ardly, -arily, -arly, -ately, -cially, -ciently, -ciously, -cisely, -edly, -enly, -entally, -ently, -erly, -escently, -esquely, -etely, -fically, -ficently, -fully, -geously, -giously, -ially, -ibly, -ically, -idly, -ilely, -ily, -inely, -ingly, -iorly, -ishly, -lessly, -ly, -manly, -mentally, -orily, -osely, -ously, -quely, -sionally, -sively, -somely, -tially, -tiently, -tionally, -tiously, -tively, -tually, -turally, ulently, -ulously, -utely, wardly, worthily, -xiously;**

<u>See Verb Endings</u>: **-fy,** /fī/ **(-ify).**

<u>See Adjective Endings</u>: **-y** (OE)

-a /ə/ (noun) agora agrapha (pl.) anathema aroma asthma biota charisma cholera chroma cithara coma comma diarrhea Diaspora dogma *(dogmata)* eczema edema enema enigma erotica (pl.) magma nausea palestra plasma plethora schema *(schemata)* sciatica soma *(somata)* stigma *(stigmata)* stoa stoma *(stomata)* tiara trauma trichina

-ad /ad/ (noun) duad (2) ennead (9) Galahad gonad heptad (7) hexad (6) monad nomad octad (8) Olympiad pentad (5) tetrad (4) triad (3); /əd/ Iliad jeremiad myriad salad

-asm /az-əm/ (noun) (*Remaining after **-os** dropped from **-asmos**.) chasm *enthusiasm iconoclasm *orgasm phantasm *pleonasm *(Use of needless words.)* *sarcasm *spasm

-ast /ast/ (noun) bombast enthusiast gymnasiast gymnast iconoclast pederast

-ene /ēn/ (Chemical suffix.) bezene carotene kerosene menthene naphthalene neoprene phosphene polystyrene; <u>Others</u>: convene Hellene intervene Miocene Nazarene Neocene Nicene obscene Paleocene Pliocene scalene serene Slovene

-es /ēz/ (noun) (Often a name.) Achilles Alcibiades Andes Mts. Androcles Aristophanes atlantes Ceres Cervantes Cleisthenes Cortés /cor-<u>tez</u>/ Damocles Demosthenes diabetes Euripides feces Hades Hercules Hermes herpes Hippocrates ides /īdz/ Isocrates Miltiades mores /mor-āz/ Moses /<u>mō</u>-zis/ Orestes Pericles Praxiteles Rameses Simonides Socrates Sophocles Thales Themistocles Thucydides Xerxes

-eum /ē-əm/ (noun) (Latin transliteration of Gk. **-eion**.) atheneum coliseum Colosseum linoleum lyceum mausoleum museum petroleum

-gen /jən/ (noun) *[That which produces.]* allergen androgen antigen carcinogen estrogen hallucinogen halogen hydrogen nitrogen oxygen pathogen

-ia /ē-ə/ (noun) agraphia alexia anemia anesthesia anorexia aphrodisia arrhythmia asphyxia bacteria bronchia bulimia catatonia criteria diphtheria dyslexia encyclopedia euphoria hypochondria hysteria kleptomania megalomania melancholia myopia neuralgia nymphomania ophthalmia paraphernalia phobia pneumonia pyromania schizophrenia utopia; /yə/ ammonia; /zhə/ amnesia aphasia euthanasia magnesia

-iac /ē-ak/ (noun) amnesiac aphrodisiac cardiac (+adj.) hemophiliac hypochondriac insomniac maniac (+adj.) melancholiac Pontiac *(Indian chief.)* pyromaniac sacroiliac zodiac

-ic /ik/ (adj.) *[Pertaining to, consisting of.]* (From Greek **-ikos**.) academic allergic analgesic (+n) anarchic anemic angelic apostolic archaic atheistic atmospheric atomic barbaric basic bucolic cataleptic catastrophic catholic Catholic Cenozoic cephalic ceramic choleric chronic cleric (+n) clinic (n) colic (+n) comic conic cosmic cubic cyclic cynic (n) Cyrillic Delphic demagogic democratic demonic diabolic diatonic Doric draconic dynamic eccentric economic electrodynamic electronic embryonic encephalic encyclopedic endemic enharmonic enteric epic (+n) epidemic (+n) episodic esoteric ethic (+n) ethnic eugenic euphoric eurhythmic exoteric extrinsic forensic gastric generic geriatric Germanic Gothic graphic harmonic Hebraic hedonic Hellenic hemophilic heroic historic hydraulic hydroelectric hygienic hypodermic (+n) hysteric iambic iatric idyllic Indic Ionic irenic ironic italic Judaic laconic lethargic liturgic logarithmic logic (n) lyric magic (+n) manic mechanic (n) melodic Mesolithic mesomorphic metabolic metallic metapsychic meteoric metric mimic (n) mnemonic monolithic monosyllablic mosaic (+n) music (n) mystic (+n) Neolithic nomadic nostalgic obstetric oceanic Olympic organic pandemic Pan-Hellenic panic parabolic pedagogic pentatonic peptic periodic phallic philharmonic philippic phobic phonemic phonic physic (n) picric platonic pneumonic polemic polyphonic polysyllabic polytechnic (+n) psychedelic psychic psychopathic rhetoric (n) rhombic rhythmic scholastic seismic sophomoric spasmodic sporadic stoic (+n) strategic strobic syllabic symbolic symphonic systemic tectonic telic thermoelectric thoracic titanic tonic topic toxic tragic Triassic tropic (+n) tympanic uric; <u>Often -ics as singular noun:</u> academics aerodynamics astrophysics biodynamics bionics biophysics dynamics economics electrodynamics ethics eugenics eurythmics forensics geophysics geriatrics graphics harmonics heroics hydraulics hygienics hysterics italics liturgics mechanics metaphysics metrics mnemonics orthopedics pediatrics phonics physics polemics pyrotechnics strategics tectonics theatrics thermodynamics <u>See:</u> Latin suffix **-fic**, Ap. iv-32, **-ic** Ap. iv-33, **istic** Ap. iv-37 and Gk. suffix **-tic** Ap. iv-59.

-ical /i-kəl/ (adj.) (Gk. **-ic** + L **-al**.) alphabetical anatomical antithetical astronomical atypical Biblical biographical biological canonical categorical chemical chimerical clerical clinical comical critical cyclical cylindrical cynical dialectical diametrical ecclesiastical economical ecumenical electrical empirical encyclical ethical evangelical geographical grammatical heretical hierarchical historical hysterical hypercritical liturgical logical magical mathematical metaphysical mechanical metrical musical mystical mythical optical parenthetical periodical pharmaceutical philosophical physical political practical rhetorical rhythmical skeptical spherical surgical symmetrical tactical technical theatrical theoretical topical tropical typical typographical tyrannical; <u>See:</u> Latin suffix **-ical** Ap. iv-34.

-ically /ik-lē/ (Note dropped syllable: /ik-(ə)-lē/.) (adv.) (Gk. **-ic** + L **-al** + O.E. **-ly**.) academically acoustically aerobically aerodynamically aeronautically aesthetically allegorically alphabetically analytically anatomically antagonistically antiseptically antithetically apologetically arithmetically astronomically athletically atmospherically atomically authentically autobiographically autocratically automatically basically biblically biographically biologically bureaucratically canonically categorically chaotically characteristically chromatically chronically chronologically climatically clinically cosmetically cosmically critically cynically demonically despotically diabolically diametrically diplomatically dogmatically dramatically drastically dynamically ecologically economically ecumenically electrically electronically emphatically empirically energetically enigmatically enthusiastically epistemologically erotically esoterically esthetically ethically euphemistically fantastically frantically genetically geographically geometrically grammatically graphically harmonically

Ap. iv-55

hedonistically heroically hierarchically historically hygienically hysterically ideologically idiomatically idiotically illogically ironically lethargically liturgically lyrically logically logistically magically mathematically mechanically melodically metaphorically metaphysically methodically musically mystically mythically neurotically nostalgically optically organically paradoxically parenthetically pathetically pathologically periodically philosophically phonetically physically poetically politically practically pragmatically psychologically rhetorically rhythmically sarcastically scholastically skeptically spasmodically sporadically stoically strategically surgically symbiotically symbolically symmetrically sympathetically symptomatically synthetically systematically tactically technically theatrically thematically theoretically therapeutically tragically traumatically typically;   See: Latin -ically Ap. iv-34.

-is /is/ Adonis aegis Alcestis Atlantis clitoris epiglottis hubris mantis Paris Salamis;   See also: Latin suffix -is Ap. iv-36 and Greek suffix -sis Ap. iv-59.

-ism /iz-əm/ (noun) *[A theory, doctrine or condition.]* (From Greek *-ismos*.) agnosticism anachronism anarchism antagonism anthropomorphism anti-Semitism aphorism asceticism astigmatism atheism autism baptism barbarism catechism Catholicism chromaticism criticism cubism cynicism despotism dogmatism dynamism eclecticism ecumenism electromagnetism embolism empiricism epicureanism eroticism euphemism evangelism exorcism hedonism Hellenism hyperthyroidism hypnotism hypothyroidism lesbianism lyricism magnetism mechanism metabolism monasticism monotheism mysticism narcissism ostracism pantheism parochialism patriotism polytheism pragmatism rheumatism scholasticism skepticism sophism syllogism symbolism synergism theism;   See: Latin suffix -ism Ap. iv-36.

-ist /ist/ (noun) *[A person who does, is, or believes something.]* (From Greek *-istes*.) allergist anarchist anesthetist antagonist apologist archivist atheist Baptist bigamist botanist chemist cyclist dogmatist dramatist economist Egyptologist elegist encyclopedist etymologist eulogist evangelist hedonist Hellenist homeopathist hygienist hypnotist liturgist lyricist machinist ophthalmologist optometrist organist orthopedist pharmacist physicist plagiarist polemicist protagonist psalmist psychiatrist psychologist sophist strategist taxidermist theorist tympanist typist; See: Latin -ist.

-ite /īt/ (noun) (From Greek *-ites*.) anthracite dendrite dynamite graphite hermaphrodite hoplite meteorite parasite stalactite stalagmite;   /it/ hypocrite

-ize /īz/ (verb) (From Greek *-izein*.) acclimatize accustomize actualize agonize alphabetize anesthetize Anglicize antagonize anthropomorphize antisepticize apologize atomize authorize baptize brutalize burglarize cannibalize canonize capitalize catechize categorize cauterize centralize characterize civilize collectivize colonize commercialize concertize criticize crystallize decentralize decimalize deemphasize dehumanize dematerialize demilitarize demobilize democratize demoralize deodorize departmentalize depolarize deputize desensitize desterilize devitalize dichotomize disorganize dramatize economize editorialize empathize emphasize energize epitomize equalize eulogize evangelize extemporize externalize fantasize federalize feminize fertilize fictionalize finalize formalize fragmentize fraternize galvanize generalize glamorize harmonize Hellenize homogenize hospitalize humanize hypnotize hypothesize idealize idolize immobilize immortalize immunize impersonalize industrialize institutionalize internationalize italicize itemize jeopardize legalize legitimize liberalize lionize localize magnetize materialize maximize mechanize memorialize memorize mesmerize metastasize militarize minimize mobilize modernize monopolize moralize motorize nationalize naturalize neutralize notarize optimize organize ostracize oxidize particularize pasteurize patronize penalize personalize philosophize plagiarize pluralize polarize politicize popularize pressurize publicize pulverize rationalize realize recognize reorganize revitalize revolutionize rhapsodize romanticize sanitize satirize scandalize scrutinize secularize sensitize socialize specialize stabilize standardize sterilize stigmatize stylize subsidize summarize symbolize sympathize synchronize synthesize systematize tantalize temporize tenderize terrorize theorize tranquilize tyrannize unionize utilize vaporize verbalize victimize visualize vitalize vocalize winterize womanize; See: Latin -ise Ap. iv-36.

-ization /i-zā-shən/ (noun) *[Condition, act, or process.]* authorization brutalization characterization civilization colonization commercialization demilitarization dramatization equalization fertilization generalization harmonization hospitalization idealization industrialization liberalization legalization legitimization materialization mechanization memorization militarization mobilization nationalization naturalization neutralization organization pasteurization personalization polarization rationalization realization stabilization standardization stylization urbanization utilization visualization vitalization; Note: improvisation; See: **-ize** above for verbs that can be changed into nouns with the suffix **-ization**.

-lyze /līz/ (verb) *[To do or cause.]* analyze catalyze electrolyze hydrolyze paralyze psychoanalyze

-ode /ōd/ (noun) (Combining form from Greek *hodos,* way.) anode antipode cathode diode electrode episode geode triode [Also from Greek *hodos*: method, synod.]; (verb) (Chance endings, mainly Latin.) abode (+n) code (+n) commode (n) corrode decode encode erode explode implode mode (n) outrode overrode rode strode

-oid /oid/ *[Like or resembling.]* adenoid alkaloid android arachnoid asteroid bacteroid cancroid Caucasoid celluloid colloid conoid coralloid crystalloid cuboid cycloid cystoid deltoid dentoid dermatoid diploid discoid fibroid fungoid globoid hematoid hemorrhoid hominoid hysteroid ichthyoid keratoid lipoid lithoid lymphoid mastoid meteoroid Mongoloid Negroid neuroid ornithoid osteoid paranoid petaloid phylloid prismoid resinoid rheumatoid rhizoid rhomboid saccharoid salmonoid schizoid scorpioid sinusoid solenoid spheroid spiroid steroid tabloid thanatoid thyroid toxoid trapezoid typhoid viscoid xyloid

-om /əm/ axiom accustom (L) atom bosom (O.E.) buxom (M.E.) carom (F) custom (O.F.) hansom (Name) idiom phantom pogrom (Rus.) random (O.F.) ransom (L) seldom (O.E.) slalom (Nor.) Sodom symptom transom (L) venom (L) wisdom (O.E.); shalom /shä-lōm/ (Heb.)

-on /on/ (noun) (Greek neuter singular.) Agamemnon antiphon archon argon Armageddon automaton axon Babylon chameleon decagon decahedron decathlon electron enchiridion epsilon ganglion icon interferon ion Jason lexicon macron marathon melodeon meson micron moron neon neuron neutron noumenon omicron organon oxymoron pantheon paragon Parthenon pentagon pentathlon Phaethon phenomenon *(phenomena)* philodendron photon pi-meson plankton positron proton propylon pylon radon telamon triskelion; /ən/ colon canon demon diapason dragon eudemon Gorgon horizon melon octahedron Orion polyhedron Poseidon rhododendron siphon skeleton tendon; From other sources: /ən/ abandon Akron apron arson baron beacon beckon bison Boston bourbon Burton canton carbon cannon carrion carton cauldron chevron cinnamon citron Clinton cordon crayon crimson falcon flagon gibbon glutton heron jargon Johnson lemon lesson London mammon mason Milton Mormon mutton Newton Nixon pardon patron pennon persimmon person piston prison reckon ribbon saffron salmon Sampson Saxon season semicolon sexton silicon Solomon son squadron talon treason unison wagon wanton weapon Wisconson Zion; /on/ Aragon Avon baton bouillon /bŏŏl-yon/ capon carillon Ceylon chiffon coupon echelon Huron liaison /lē-ā-zon/ on nucleon Oregon rayon Rubicon tampon upon Yukon; /'n/ Breton Brighton Briton button cotton Eton; And: chanson /shän-sôn/ chaperon /shap-ə-rōn/ iron /ī-ern/

-os /os/ (Greek masculine, singular ending, **-oi** plural.) Athos Atropos bathos benthos chaos Delos demos epos Eros ethos hoi polloi *("The many." The common people.)* logos Logos Minos mythos *(mythoi)* omphalos Parthenos pathos Pharos Samos Talos Thanatos; /əs/: asbestos cosmos peplos rhinoceros *(rhinoceroses)*

-ose /ōs/ cellulose dextrose fructose glucose lactose; See: Latin suffix **-ose** Ap. iv-40.

-osis /ō-sis/ (noun) *[Condition, process, state of.]* acidosis *(Acid intoxication.)* alkalosis *(Excessive blood alkali.)* alphosis *(Lack of pigmentation.)* anhidrosis *(Lack of perspiration.)* ankylosis *(The fusing of bones.)* arteriosclerosis *(The hardening of artery walls.)* arthrosis *(Degeneration of the joints.)* asbestosis *(Lung disorder from inhalation of asbestos.)* avitaminosis *(A vitamin deficiency.)* cirrhosis *(A liver disease.)* coronary thrombosis *(A blood clot in a coronary artery.)* dermatophytosis *(Athlete's foot.)* diagnosis *("To know between." To recognize a disease from its symptoms.)* fibrosis *(Increase of fibrous connective tissue.)* halitosis *(Offensive breath.)* hallucinosis *(Persistent hallucinations.)* hematosis *(The formation of blood.)* hidrosis *(Excessive sweating.)* hypervitaminosis *(Sickness due to excess of vitamins.)* hypnosis *(Artificially induced trancelike state. Gk. hypno- = sleep.)* ichthyosis *(Scaly skin condition. Gk. ichthyo- = fish.)* kyphosis *(Humpback.)* melanosis *(Dark skin pigment.)* mitosis *(Chromosome division.)* metamorphosis *(A change in form or shape.)* mononucleosis *(Abnormal increase of white blood cells.)* mycosis *(A fungus growth.)* narcosis *(Drug induced stupor.)* necrosis *(Death of tissue; gangrene.)* nephrosis *(Kidney disease.)* neurosis *(Mild mental disorder.)* osmosis *(The passing of a fluid through a membrane.)* ostosis *(Bone formation.)* pediculosis *(Lice infestation.)* pneumoconiosis *(Lung disease.)* pollinosis *(Hay fever.)* prognosis *("To know before." The prediction of the outcome of a disease.)* proptosis *(Bulging of the eyeball.)* psychosis

(Severe mental disorder.) pyosis *(Formation of pus.)* pyrosis *(Heartburn.)* sclerosis *(Hardening of a tissue.)* scoliosis *(Curvature of the spine.)* siderosis *(A lung disease resulting from inhaling iron particles.)* silicosis *(A lung disease resulting from inhaling silica dust.)* stenosis *(A duct narrowing.)* symbiosis *(Sym = together; bio- = life. The beneficial association of two organisms.)* toxicosis *(A poisoning of body tissue.)* trichinosis *(An infection of the intestine by small worms.)* tuberculosis *(An infection of the lung by the tubercle bacillus.)* varicosis *(Vein dilation.)* xerosis *(Eye or skin dryness.)*

-ous /əs/ (adj.) (Greek words originally ending in **-os** transliterated to **-ous** in Latin.) amorphous analogous androgynous anomalous analogous anonymous asynchronous autonomous barbarous blasphemous cacophonous dichotomous homogeneous hydrous idolatrous leprous melanous monogamous monotonous nauseous petalous petrous phosphorous polygamous polyphonous polypous pseudonymous religious synchronous synonymous tendinous tyrannous zealous

-ously /əs-lē/ (adj.) (Adverb forming **-ly** added to **-ous** adjective.) analogously anonymously monotonously nauseously synonymously zealously, *etc.* <u>See</u>: **-ous** above.

-sis /sis/ (noun) (Plural: **-ses** /sēz/; plural of **-xis** is **-xes**. The plural of some of the most common words is given.) amniocentesis anaclisis analysis antisepsis antithesis autohypnosis axis *(axes)* basis *(bases)* catachresis *(Wrong word use.)* catharsis crisis *(crises)* diagnosis *(diagnoses)* dialysis diastalsis dieresis electrolysis elephantiasis ellipsis *(ellipses)* emesis *(Vomiting.)* emphasis *(emphases)* exegesis *(exegeses)* genesis *(geneses)* Genesis hypnosis *(hypnoses)* hypothesis *(hypotheses)* Isis mimesis nemesis *(nemeses)* neurosis *(neuroses)* oasis *(oases)* osmosis paralysis *(paralyses)* parapraxis parenthesis *(parentheses)* pathogenesis peristalsis pertussis *(Whooping cough.)* photosynthesis prognosis *(prognoses)* prosthesis psoriasis psychoanalysis psychosis *(psychoses)* ptosis *(Drooping eyelids.)* symbiosis synopsis *(synopses)* synthesis *(syntheses)* telekinesis thesis *(theses)*

-tery /ter-ē/ (noun) *[Often a place for.]* (From Greek **-terion**.) artery baptistery mystery; /tair-ē/ cemetery dysentery monastery; <u>And</u>: adultery battery effrontery upholstery

-tic /tik/ (adj.) *[Pertaining to.]* (From Greek **-tikos**.) acoustic acrobatic acrostic aeronautic aesthetic agnostic allegoristic alphabetic anachronistic anaclitic analytic anarchistic anesthetic antagonistic Antarctic antibiotic anticlimactic antipyretic antiseptic aortic apathetic aphoristic apocalyptic apologetic Arctic aristocratic arithmetic aromatic arthritic ascetic aseptic Asiatic asthmatic astigmatic atheistic athletic Atlantic attic authentic autistic autocratic automatic axiomatic ballistic biotic bombastic catalytic cathartic caustic chaotic characteristic charismatic chiropractic (n) chromatic cinematic climactic climatic cosmetic critic cybernetic cystic democratic demonic despotic diabetic (+n) diagnostic diagrammatic dialectic didactic dietetic diplomatic diuretic dogmatic dramatic drastic dynamistic dynastic dyspeptic ecclesiastic eclectic ecstatic eidetic elastic Eleatic electrolytic electromagnetic electrostatic elliptic emblematic emetic emphatic energetic enigmatic enthusiastic epileptic (+n) eristic erotic esthetic euphemistic evangelistic exotic fantastic frantic frenetic galactic genetic geodetic geostatic gigantic gnostic gymnastic hectic hedonistic Hellenistic hematic hemostatic heretic (n) hermaphroditic hermetic heuristic holistic homeostatic hydrolytic hydrostatic hypnotic iconoclastic idiosyncratic idiomatic idiotic kinetic logistic magnetic mechanistic melodramatic mimetic monastic monistic monochromatic monopolistic monotheistic mystic (+n) narcissistic narcotic (+n) neurotic noetic optic orgiastic orthodontic pancreatic pantheistic paradigmatic paralytic (+n) parasitic parenthetic pathetic patriotic pedantic peptic peripatetic periphrastic phlegmatic phonetic photosynthetic plastic (+n) pleonastic plutocratic pneumatic poetic politic polytheistic pragmatic problematic prognostic programmatic prophetic prophylactic psychoanalytic psychosomatic psychotic (+n) rheumatic (+n) sarcastic schematic schismatic scholastic sciatic semantic Semitic septic skeptic (n) Socratic somatic sophistic spastic (+n) static stigmatic stylistic styptic sycophantic syllogistic symbiotic sympathetic symptomatic synergistic synoptic syntactic synthetic systematic tactic theistic thematic theocratic theoretic therapeutic thermostatic traumatic;   <u>See:</u> **-fic** Ap. iv-32, **-ic** Ap. iv-33, **-istic** Ap. iv-37.

<u>Often **-ics** as singular noun:</u> acoustics acrobatics aesthetics athletics ballistics bionics chromatics cybernetics dialectics diagnostics didactics dramatics esthetics genetics geopolitics gymnastics homiletics kinematics kinetics logistics mathematics melodramatics optics orthopedics pharmaceutics phonetics pneumatics poetics politics prosthetics semantics tactics therapeutics

-tron /tron/ (noun) (Scientific ending from ***electron***.) cyclotron electron magnetron neutron positron

-um /əm/ (noun) (The Greek ending ***-on*** is the neuter singular of many Greek nouns; it is transliterated into Latin ***-um***; Greek *stadion* becomes Latin *stadium*.   The plural in both languages is ***-a:** stadia.*)   <u>See:</u> Latin suffix **-um** Ap. iv-51.

-y /ē/ academy agony allegory allergy amnesty anatomy androgyny anomaly apathy apology apoplexy appendectomy artery atrophy autonomy autoplasty autopsy bigamy biography biology biopsy blasphemy botany canopy category cautery celery chiropody clergy comedy crony demagogy democracy dichotomy dynasty dysentery ebony economy ecstasy elegy empathy energy entropy epilepsy Epiphany epoxy eulogy fantasy frenzy galaxy gastronomy geodesy geology geometry harmony harpy hegemony idiocy irony jealousy leprosy lethargy litany liturgy melancholy melody metallurgy monody monogamy monopoly monotony mystery narcolepsy orthodoxy palsy parody peony periphery philogyny philosophy polygamy prosody psalmody psaltery psychiatry pygmy rhapsody strategy sympathy symphony synergy synonymy tautology taxidermy taxonomy therapy tragedy treasury trophy tyranny; <u>See:</u> Greek Combining Forms in Ap. ix: **-archy, -doxy, -ectomy, -graphy, -logy, -metry, -pathy, -phony, -scopy, -tomy, -typy, -urgy.**   <u>Of interest:</u> **-y-** in Ap. i-45.

Other Suffixes

-ac /ac/ (noun) *[Having, pertaining to.]* almanac (Ar.) bivouac (F) bric-a-brac (F) cognac (F) shellac (O.E./Hind.) lilac (Per.); <u>See</u>: Greek suffix **-iac** Ap. iv-54.

-ah /ə/ (Mostly names from Hebrew.) Beulah Deborah Delilah Elijah Hannah Hephzibah Hialeah Isaiah Jehovah Jonah Josiah Judah Leah Messiah Methuselah Micah Nehemiah Obadiah Sarah Savannah Shenandoah Susannah Uriah Zachariah Zebadiah Zechariah; <u>Others</u>: Allah (Ar.) amah (Pg.) ayah (Hin.) bar mitzvah (Heb.) fellah (Ar.) hallelujah (Heb.) Hanukkah /khä-nōō-kə/ (Heb.) jubbah (Ar.) mezuzah (Heb.) Mishnah (Heb.) moolah (Slang: *Money.*) mullah (Ar.) opah (Ibo) pariah (Tamil) selah (Heb.) Shiah (Ar.) torah (Heb.) Torah zillah (Hin.); /ä/ ah (interj.) blah (interj.) Casbah (Ar.) hah (interj.) hurrah (interj.) kiblah (Ar.) mitzvah (Heb.) pah (interj.) parashah (Heb.) rah (interj.) shah (Per.) subah (Urdu) wallah (Hindi)

-ain /ān/ (verb) (Old French) brain (Slang: *To hit on the head.*) chain complain constrain detrain drain entrain explain foreordain gain ingrain lain ordain overlain (O.E.) pain preordain rain (O.E.) refrain regain remain restrain retrain slain sprain stain strain train unchain underlain (O.E.); (noun) /ən/ bargain (+v) boatswain /bō-sən/ coxswain /kok-sən/ villain; /in/ chamberlain chaplain porcelain; <u>Except nouns of one syllable, compound words, or those with the accent on the -ain syllable</u>: /ān/ blain (O.E.) bloodstain (O.E./O.F.) brain (O.E.) Cain chain chilblain (O.E.) domain drain eyestrain featherbrain gain grain lamebrain legerdemain overlain (O.E.) pain plain rain (O.E.) refrain scatterbrain slain Spain sprain stain strain swain (O.N.) terrain train twain wain (O.E.); (adj.) certain /ser-tən/ fain main (O.E) vain; (adv.) again /ə-gen/; <u>See</u>: **-tain** Ap. iv-44.

-aire /air/ (noun) (French) billionaire concessionaire doctrinaire legionnaire millionaire multimillionaire questionnaire solitaire

-ard /erd/ (adj.) (Old French, German) haggard haphazard sluggard standard; (noun) bastard billiard /bil-yerd/ blizzard buzzard collard coward custard drunkard dullard gizzard goliard /gōl-yerd/ halyard hazard laggard lanyard leopard /lep-erd/ lizard mallard mustard orchard scabbard sluggard Spaniard /span-yerd/ standard steward tankard wizard; (name) Bernard Edward Harvard Howard Richard Shepard; (noun) /ard/ backyard barnyard bard bombard (+v) boulevard canard diehard discard (+v) dockyard farmyard hard (adj.) lard leotard placard regard (+v) retard (v) yard; /or/ award (+v) reward (+v); <u>See</u>: O. E. suffix **-ward** Ap. iv-14.

-ardly /erd-lē/ (adv.) (Adverb forming **-ly** added to **-ard** word.) bastardly cowardly dastardly haphazardly hardly sluggardly, *etc.*

-art /ert/ (noun) (Variation of **-ard**) braggart stalwart; /art/ apart chart depart flowchart heart impart outsmart pushcart rampart restart smart start sweetheart underpart upstart; /ort/ athwart quart thwart worrywart

-eer /ear/ (noun) (From Fr. *-ier* < L *-arius*.) auctioneer balladeer beer buccaneer cannoneer career charioteer cheer deer electioneer engineer jeer leer mountaineer muleteer musketeer mutineer peer pamphleteer pioneer profiteer puppeteer racketeer rocketeer sneer steerage veneer volunteer weaponeer; (adj.) domineering leery queer sheer; (verb) cheer commandeer domineer jeer leer peer sneer steer veer volunteer; (interj.) cheerio; <u>Exception</u>: seer /sē-er/ (n)

-el /əl/ (noun) (Old French. Often a diminutive.) apparel barrel bezel bowel brothel (M.E.) bushel camel (Gk.) caramel carrel chancel channel chapel charnel /<u>car</u>-nəl/ chisel citadel cockerel (O.E.) colonel /<u>ker</u>-nəl/ counsel crewel cudgel (O.E.) damsel dowel (M.E.) drivel (O.E.) duel duffel (Place.) easel (Du.) enamel flannel (Welsh) funnel (L) gavel gospel (O.E.) gravel gruel handsel (O.E.) hazel (O.E.) hostel hovel (O.E.) infidel (L) jewel kennel kernel (O.E.) label level libel mackerel mantel marvel minstrel morsel mussel (L) navel (O.E.) nickel (Ger.) novel (L) panel parcel pari-mutuel (F) pickerel pimpernel pommel pretzel (Ger.) pumpernickel (Ger.) quarrel <u>reb</u>el satchel scalpel (L) scoundrel sentinel sequel shekel (Heb.) shovel (O.E.) shrapnel (Name) sorrel (F) spaniel squirrel swivel (M.E.) tassel tercel tinsel towel travel trowel tunnel vessel wastrel weasel (O.E.) yodel (Ger.) vessel vowel weasel (O.E.) yokel (Eng. dial.); /el/ caravel (Sp.) carousel cartel hotel lapel materiel morel motel *(motor + hotel)* muscatel parallel personnel; /l/ chattel model yodel (Ger.); <u>Names</u>: /əl/ Handel Hansel Hazel Hegel Immanuel Jezebel Mendel Rachel Rommel Samuel; /el/ Nobel Ravel; (verb) /əl/ apparel barrel (slang) cancel chisel (slang) disembowel dishevel duel grovel (O.N.) impanel label ravel (M.Du.) revel shrivel snivel (O.E.) trammel travel trowel tunnel /el/ compel dispel (L) impel (L) marcel propel (L) rappel (F) re<u>bel</u> repel (L); (adj.) /əl/ charnel cruel

-esque /esk/ (adj.) *[In the style of.]* (French) arabesque burlesque grotesque humoresque picturesque sculpturesque statuesque Wagneresque, *etc.*

-esquely /esk-lē/ (adv.) (Adverb forming -ly added to **-esque** adjective.) grotesquely picturesquely sculpturesquely statuesquely, *etc.*

-ess /is/ (noun) (French feminine ending.) actress adulteress adventuress authoress baroness countess deaconess duchess empress enchantress goddess governess hostess laundress lioness mistress priestess princess seamstress seductress songstress tigress waitress; <u>Other **-ess** words</u>: buttress fortress harness mattress prowess; <u>/es/ when accented</u>: ad<u>dress</u> ca<u>ress</u> com<u>press</u> con<u>fess</u> di<u>gress</u> du<u>ress</u> repos<u>sess</u>

-et[1] /it/ (noun) (French diminutive.) aglet *(Tip of shoestring.)* anklet armlet banquet baronet basset billet blanket booklet bracket budget bullet circlet closet corset couplet cruet cutlet cygnet doublet dulcet eaglet facet ferret flasket floret freshet gullet gusset hamlet hatchet helmet islet jacket locket mallet midget millet moppet nugget omelet owlet packet pallet pamphlet pellet picket plummet pocket pullet puppet retrorocket rivulet rocket russet samlet signet skillet snippet socket sonnet suet tablet tappet target toilet trinket trivet triplet trumpet turret violet whippet;

Other -et /it/ **words:** amulet basket bayonet Becket bonnet Bridget brisket bucket cabinet (Ar.) carpet casket comet (Gk.) covet cricket crumpet faucet gadget garnet garret gasket hornet ticket interpret linnet magnet market Massachuset musket Nantucket Narraganset parapet Pawtucket pellet placket planet (Gk.) prophet (Gk.) quadruplet rabbet racket (Ar.) ratchet rivet (M.Du.) scarlet (Per.) secret sennet sextuplet sherbet (Ar.) spinet sprocket strumpet tenet thicket trivet velvet wallet wicket;   See: **-let.** below.

-et[2] /et/ (noun) (Old French diminutive) bassinet brunet cadet calumet canzonet castanet(s) cellaret clarinet collaret cornet coronet duet epaulet /ep-ə-let/ minuet motet spinneret; Others: /et/ abet alphabet (Gk.) Capulet epithet (Gk.) Joliet Juliet kismet (Ar.) Knesset (Heb.) marmoset (Gk.) martinet minaret (Ar.) nyet (Rus.) octet Plantagenet quartet quintet regret reset septet sextet Soviet (Rus.) tacet Tibet tourniquet; /ət/: claret disquiet Harriet quiet; / it/ Margaret quintuplet

-et[3] /ā/ (noun) (French) ballet Benét beret Binet bouquet buffet cabaret cachet Chevrolet Courbet crochet croquet fillet gourmet Manet Massenet parquet ricochet sachet sobriquet valet

-ette[1] /et/ (noun) (French diminutive) banquette barrette briquette brochette burette cassette cigarette Colette corvette croquette curette dinette etiquette gazette Gillette Jeannette kitchenette Lafayette LaFollette layette leatherette (O.E.) lorgnette luncheonette lunette marionette Marquette musette novelette palette pipette pirouette roomette (O.E.) roulette silhouette soubrette statuette toilette vignette

-ette[2] /et/ (noun) (French feminine marker.) Antoinette bachelorette brunette coquette farmerette majorette suffragette usherette

-eur /er/ (French) carillonneur chauffeur coiffeur (Fem. *coiffeuse*) connoisseur entrepreneur liqueur masseur Monsieur poseur raconteur restaurateur saboteur voyageur voyeur;   But: amateur /am-ə-choor/,   grandeur /gran-jer/

-grad /grad/ (noun) *[City of.]* (Russian) Kaliningrad   Leningrad   Petrograd Stalingrad   Volgograd

-kin /kin/ (noun) *[Little.]* (Middle Dutch) bodkin bumpkin catkin devilkin gherkin jerkin lambkin munchkin manikin (cf. mannequin) napkin pannikin pumpkin thumbkin

let /lit/ (noun) (Old French diminutive. Added to a complete word.)   booklet bracelet brooklet driblet droplet eyelet gauntlet leaflet platelet playlet ringlet rootlet starlet streamlet wristlet;   See: **-et**[1] on previous page.

-nik /nik/ (noun) (Yiddish)   beatnik   nudnik   refusenik

-o /ō/ (noun) (Common Italian and Spanish ending.) albino alto amoroso basso basso continuo basso profundo calypso cameo campo casino Colorado cheerio combo credo crescendo desperado ditto divertimento domino duo echo ego folio gigolo hero incognito incommunicado inferno innuendo libido lingo lumbago manifesto memento Morocco mosquito mulatto Navajo Negro Nero nuncio obbligato Orlando pepo perfecto pimento placebo proviso Pueblo righto Salerno salvo solo sostenuto stiletto soprano stretto tempo tenuto tornado torpedo torso tremolo trio tyro verso veto (L. *I forbid.*) virtuoso volcano

-ot[1] /ət/ (noun) (Chance ending.) abbot (Aramaic) ascot (Place name.) ballot (It.) bigot (F) chariot (O.F.) compatriot (L) copilot (L/It.) harlot helot (Gk.) maggot (M.E.) marmot (F) mascot (F) ocelot (F) parrot (M.E.) patriot (L) pilot (It.) pivot (F) robot (Czech.) spigot (M.E.) zealot (Gk.); /ot/ apricot (Ar.) diglot phot

-ot[2] /ō/ (French) bibelot depot haricot picot Pierrot tarot

-op /əp/ (Chance ending.) Aesop bishop (Gk.) develop (F) envelop gallop (O.F.) galop (F) hyssop (Gk.) scallop (O.F.) trollop (M.E.) wallop (A.F.) Winthrop

-que /k/ (French) baroque Basque bisque brusque catafalque cheque cirque claque discotheque Dubuque macaque masque mosque odalisque opaque plaque torque

(-ique) /ēk/ antique boutique Dominique clique critique Martinique Mozambique mystique oblique opera comique physique pique technique unique; <u>See</u>: **-esque** Ap. iv-62.

-quely /k-lē/ (adverb) antiquely brusquely obliquely opaquely uniquely

-ski /skē/ (Common surname ending.) (Polish) Demowski Komorowski Paderewski Pilsudski Sikorski Sobieski, *etc.*

-sky /skē/ (Common surname ending.) (Russian) Moussorgsky Nijinsky Rimsky-Korsakov Stanislavsky Stravinsky Trotsky Tschaikowsky Vishinsky, *etc.*

-ute /o͞ot/, (Common ending.) absolute brute convolute dilute dissolute irresolute pollute parachute resolute salute; /yo͞ot/ acute attribute confute commute contribute depute dispute distribute electrocute permute prosecute tribute;   <u>Note</u>: minute /<u>min</u>-it/ & /mī-<u>nyo͞ot</u>/.

-ville /vil/ (noun) *[Village.]* (O.F. < L *villa*.) Andersonville Asheville Bougainville Danville Evansville Hicksville Huntsville Jacksonville Knoxville Louisville Nashville Somerville Steubenville, *etc.*

-y /ē/ (noun, name) *[Little.]* (Scottish) Andy Becky Betty Billy Bobby Davy doggy Jimmy Johnny Katy kitty Nicky Ronny Sammy Timmy Tommy Willy, *etc.*

Old English . . . . *A Tale of Words* . . . . Ap. v- 2

A, B, C, D, E, ... Ap. v- 3

F, G, H, I, K, L, M, ... Ap. v- 4

N, O, P, Q, R, S, ... Ap. v- 5

T, U, V, W, X, Y; . . . . **Old Norse** . A, B, ... Ap. v- 6

C → W; . . . **Middle English** . . A, B, C, ... Ap. v- 7

D → T, ... Ap. v- 8

U, W, Y; . . **Modern English** . . . . Ap. v- 9

Australian English . . . **British English** . . . . Ap. v- 9

Canadian English . . **New Zealand English** . . **Scottish** . . Ap. v-10

GERMANIC LANGUAGES: . . . **Low German** . . . . Ap. v-10

Yiddish . . . **German** . . . . Ap. v-11

Flemish . . . **Middle Dutch** . . . **Dutch** . . . . Ap. v-12

Afrikaans . . . **Danish** . . . **Norwegian** . . . . Ap. v-12

Swedish . . . **Icelandic** . . . *Grimm's Law* . . . . . . Ap. v-12

English is a Germanic language starting from the time the Angles, Saxons, and Jutes invaded the British Isles in about A. D 449. They brought with them their Germanic languages which almost completely replaced the existing Celtic. Our most basic and common vocabulary dates from this time and is illustrated by a short quasi-story, A Tale of Words. An alphabetical listing of English words deriving from Old English follows. Note many **ai, augh, -ay, dw-, ea, ee, eigh, gh, igh, kn-, -mb, oa, oo, ou, ough, shr-, spr- , str-, sw-, th, thr-, tw-, wr-** examples. <u>See also:</u> **Old English Prefixes** in Ap. iii-2 & **Old English Suffixes** in Ap. iv-4. A fondness for combining words: *bathhouse, boathouse, houseboat, birdhouse, birdbath, blackbird, blackboard, bedside, bedpost, bittersweet, bridegroom, bridesmaid, buttercup, butterfingers, butternut, etc.* can be seen by reviewing **Compound words** in Ap. ii-2. These are not repeated here. Also note the language's utility with *dent, dream, drink, drive, etc.* serving as both noun and verb; with *dark, dead, dear, deep, etc.* serving as both adjective and noun; with *foul, ground, home, & stone* serving as adjective, noun, and verb; and *down* serving as noun, adjective, verb, adverb and preposition, *etc.*

A Tale of Words

husband work sweat swear heavy shave hunt deer fox beaver bird mouse spear iron hard earth land wheat thresh oats barley herd cow calf sheep goat horse boat lake fish wife house sweep clean sew thread needle thimble knit weave wool cook fire wood stove oven pot pan food dish fork knife spoon eat bit chew meat fat ham chicken beets salt pepper apples bake bread no hunger drink water milk ale beer wine thirst not weather hot cold warm cool air rain storm cloud above dark thunder later speak walk mile see trees birch oak maple pine brown tan green berries yellow purple watch thrush sparrow summer sun light bright now night black but moon wax and wane then winter wind blow white snow ice build shelter house abode with board beam hammer nail mother father born child red head hair eyes ears nose mouth chin cheek throat neck shoulder arm hand finger thumb chest heart lung rib side boy thigh knee shin angle foot toes whole body one son another twin girl two daughter body health sleep feather bed wake weep feed wash clothes fit hat later three four five six seven eight nine ten eleven twelve enough brothers sisters grow run twist leap race fast fight knock down break bone lame play dog flea cat wild threat throw stone tie knot pull thorn out come go left right learn bell book think know teach mind write what where when why how which become men women war oath fight blood win lose life sweet bitter some dread death die leave heaven or hell others husband wife and so on

Although the Romans had invaded and conquered in A. D. 45, after the Germanic invasions most residents who had learned Latin fled across the channel. However beginning in 597 the Christian missionary, St. Augustine, introduced many Latin & Greek church terms *(altar, angel, anthem, apostle, archbishop, church, devil, hymn, martyr, monk, organ.)* The best existing example of literature in Old English is the epic poem, **_Beowulf_**, but with its inflected endings, non-evolved forms and partially discarded vocabulary, it is generally not comprehensible to the modern reader. A sentence from this literary work appears in Appendix xv-1. Although more Old English words have been lost to modern English than have been retained and at least half of our language is borrowed from other sources, English remains a Germanic language via Old English with our most commonly used words coming from these old Germanic sources.

The extent of the evolution from Old English to Modern English can be seen by comparing the modern words in the first two lines of **A Tale of Words** with their Old English sponsors:

husband *[hūsbonda]* work *[weroc]* sweat *[swāt]* swear *[swerian]* heavy *[hefig]* shave *[scafan]* hunt *[huntian]* deer *[dēor]* fox *[fox]* beaver *[beofor]* bird *[bridd]* mouse *[mūs]* spear *[spere]* iron *[īren]* hard *[heard]* earth *[eorðe]* land *[land]* wheat *[hwæte]* thresh *[ðerscan]* oat *[āte]* barley *[bærlīc]* herd *[heord]* cow *[cū]* calf *[cealf]* sheep *[scēap]* goat *[gāt]*; Note: The-*an* ending on Old English verbs indicates an infinitive; *ð* = /th/. In the following, unusual plurals of nouns, irregular verb parts, and *meanings* are in parentheses

A Listing of English Words Deriving from Old English

A a (an) abide abode about ache acorn after aftermath *("After mowing"; results.)* again against ago ahead ail alderman ale alive all almighty almost along also am (to be, are, is, was, were, been) amaze among an and answer ant anvil any ape apple are arise (arose, arisen) ark arm arrow ash ashamed aside ask aspen at ate atone *(To set at one.)* aught awake (awoke, awaked) aware away awhile ax **B** back bake balk ban bane bare bark *(A dog sound.)* barley barn bass *(A fish; a tree.)* bat *(A stick for hitting.)* bath bathe be beacon bead beam bean bear (bore, borne) bear *(An animal.)* beard beat beaver beckon become (became) bed bee beech *(A tree.)* been (am, are, is, was, were) beer beetle before beget (begot, begotten) begin (began, begun) behalf behead behest behind behold (beheld) behoove being bell belly bellows bench bend (bent) beneath bequeath bereave berry beside best better between beware beyond bid (bade, bidden) bide bill *(A beak.)* bind birch bird bit bitch bite (bit, bitten) bitter black bladder blade blast blaze bleach bleat bleed (bled) bless blind bliss blood blossom blow (blew, blown) blush boar board boat boatswain bode body boil *(A swelling.)* bold bolster bolt bone bonfire book bore born borrow bosom bottom bough bow /bō/ *(A weapon.)* bow /bow/ *(To bend.)* bowl *(A dish.)* braid brain brand brass brazen breach bread breadth break (broke, broken) breast breath breech breeches breed (bred) brew bride bridegroom bridge bridle bright brim brimstone brine bring (brought) British broad brood brook broom broth brother brow brown buck build (built) burden burg burst burn bury (buried) business busy but buy (bought) by **C** calf (calves) can (could) can *(A container.)* care carve cat cheap cheek chew chicken child (children) chill chin choke choose (chose, chosen) churn cinder clad clam clap clatter claw clay clean cleanse clench cliff climb cling (clung) clip *(A holding device.)* clot cloth clothe (clad) clothes cloud clout clove clover cluck clue cluster coal cold colt comb come (came) cool corn cottage cove cow *(An animal.)* crab *(A sea animal.)* crack cradle craft cram crane crank crave creep crib cripple crock *(A jar.)* crop crow *(A bird; to boast.)* crowd crumb crutch cud cunning **D** daft daily daisy dale dare dark darling daughter day dead deaf deal (dealt) dear death deed deem deep deer delve den dent dew did dike dill dim din dint dip ditch dive dizzy (dove, dived) do (does, did, done, doing) doe does dog dole done doom doomsday door dot dough down drain draw (drew, drawn, drawing) dreary drench drink (drank, drunk) drip drive (drove, driven) drivel drop drought drowse drudge dry (drier, driest) duck *(A bird.)* dumb dung dusk dust dwarf dwell dwindle dye (dyed, dyeing) **E** each ear early earn earnest earth ease east Easter eat (ate eaten) eaves ebb edge eel eight (eighth) eighteen (eighteenth) eighty (eightieth) either eke elbow eleven (eleventh) elf (elves) elm else ember empty end English enough errand eve even evening ever every evil eye **F** faint fair fall (fell, fallen) fall *(Autumn.)* fan fang far fare fast *(Quick; firm,)* fat father fear feather feed (fed, feed) feel (felt) felt *(A fabric.)* fern ferry fetch few fickle field fiend fifteen (fifteenth) fifth fifty (fiftieth) fight (fought) file *(A tool.)* fill film filth finch find (found) fin finger fir fire first fish fist fit *(A spasm.)* five (fifth) flax flea flee (fled) fleece fleet *(Group of ships; swift.)* flesh flicker flight flint float flock flood floor flow flutter fly (flies, flew, flown) fly *(Flies, insects.)* foal folk follow food foot (feet) for forbid (forbade, forbidden) ford fore forget (forgot, forgotten) forgive (forgave, forgiven) fork forlorn forsake forth forty (fortieth) forward foster foul four (fourth) fourteen (fourteenth) fowl fox frame free freeze (froze, frozen) French fresh fret Friday friend fright frog from frost fulfill full further **G** gallows game gang garlic gate gather gem ghost giddy gild give (gave, given) glad glass gleam glee glide glisten glove glow gnat gnaw go (goes, went, gone) goad goat god God gold gone good (better, best) goose (geese) gore *(Blood.)* gospel gossip grass gray grave *(A burial place; to carve.)* graze great greed green greet greyhound grin grind (ground) grim grip gripe grisly grist gristle grit grits groan groin ground grout grove grow (grew, grown) grunt guest guild guilt gums gut **H** hag hail *(Ice.)* hair hale *(Healthy.)* half (halves) hall hallow halter halve ham hammer hand handle hang (hung) hard hare harken harm harp harvest hassock hat hatch hate have (has, had) haven hawk hay hazel he (his, him) head heal health heap hear (heard) heart hearth heat heath heathen heave heaven heavy hedge heed heel heifer height hell helm help hem hemlock hemp hen hence her (herself, hers) herd here herring hew hide (hid, hidden) hide *(Animal skin; land measure.)* high hill him (himself, his) hind hinder hip hint hire hither hive hoard hoarse hog hold (held) hole holiday hollow holly holy hoof (hooves) hook home hone honey hood hoop hop hope horn hornet horse hose hot (hotter, hottest) hound house how hundred (hundredth) hunger hungry hunt hurdle husband **I** I (my, mine, me, we, our, ours, us) ice icicle icy idle if imp in inn inner inning iron is (was, were) island it ivy **K** keep (kept) kernel key kin kind king kingdom kiss kite knave knead knee kneel (knelt) knell *(The tolling of a bell.)* knife (knives) knight knit knock knoll knot know (knew, known) **L** ladle lady lake lamb lame land landlord landmark lane lank lap *(Of a sitting person.)* lark last latch late lath lather latter laugh laughter lay (laid) leach lead (led) lead *(A metal.)* leaf (leaves) lean leap (leaped *or* leapt) learn (learned *or* learnt) least leather leave (left) lee *(Shelter.)* leek leer left *(A direction.)* lend (lent) length Lent less let lewd liar lick lid lie (lay, lain, lying) lie *(A falsehood.)* life (lives) light (lit) light like lily limb lime limp linden line linen lip lisp listen little (littler, littlest) little (less, least) live /liv/ live /līv/ liver *(An organ.)* load loaf (loaves) loam loan loathe lock long look loom *(Weaving device.)* loot lord lore lose (lost) lot loud louse (lice) lousy love lung lust lye **M** mad (madder, maddest) maiden mail main make (made) malt man (men) mane manifold many (more, most) maple mar marrow marsh mash mast mat match *(Something similar.)* may (might) maze me (my, mine) meadow meal mean (meant) mean *(Nasty.)* meat meet (met) melt mere *(A pond.)* mermaid merry mid middle midge *(A gnat.)* midwife might *(Power.)* mild mildew milk mind mirth miss mist mistletoe mite *(A small parasite.)* moan mole Monday month mood moon moor moot more morn most moth mother mourn mouse (mice) mouth mow much murk murder must my myself **N** nail naked name nap narrow naught naughty navel near neck need needle neighbor nest nestle net never new (newer, newest) next night nimble nine (ninth) nineteen (nineteenth) ninety (ninetieth) nit no none north nose nostril not nought now nun nut **O** oak oar oath oats of oft old (older, oldest) on one (first) oneself only onto ooze open opener or orchard ordeal ore other otter ought our (ours, ourself, ourselves) out outward oven over owe owl own ox **P** pail pan path pea pear pebble pen (pent) pen *(Enclosure.)* penny pin pit play plight *(To pledge.)* plot pluck pool *(A puddle.)* pot pound *(An enclosure.)* pretty prick pride pull put **Q** quake qualm queen quell quench quick **R** rafter raid rain rainbow rake ram rare *(Partly cooked.)* rat rather raven raw reach read reap rear *(To raise.)* reckless reckon red reed reek reel *(To stagger; a dance; a spool.)* rest rib ride (rode, ridden) ridge riddle right righteous rim rind ring (rang, rung) ring *(Jewelry.)* ripe rise (rose, risen) road roar rock *(Sway.)* rod roof room roost rope rot rough row /rō/ *(A rank; to use oars.)* rudder ruddy rue *(Regret.)* run (ran) rung *(A crosspiece.)* rust rye **S** sack sad (sadder, saddest) saddle sail sake salt salve sand sap *(A juice.)* Saturday saw *(A tool.)* sawdust say (said) sea seal *(A sea animal.)* seam sear see (saw, seen) seed seek (sought) seep seldom self (selves) sell (sold) send set *(To put.)* seven (seventh) seventeen (seventeenth) seventy (seventieth) sew (sewed, sewn) shabby shackle shade shadow shaft *(A rod.)* shaggy shake (shook, shaken) shall (should) sham shame shape share sharp shave she (her, hers) sheaf (sheaves) shear (sheared, shorn) shed *(A building; to throw off.)* sheen sheep sheet shell shelter shepherd sheriff shield shift shimmer shin shine (shone) ship shire shirt shoe (shod) shoe *(Foot covering.)* shoot (shot) shop short shot should shoulder shove shovel show (showed, shown) shower shred shrine shrink shrub shun shut shutter shuttle shy sibling sick sickle side sieve sift sight sill silly silk silver sin sinew sing (sang sung) singe sink (sank, sunk) sip sister sit (sat) six (sixth) sixteen (sixteenth) sixty (sixtieth) slack slay (slew, slain) sleep (slept) sleeve sledge *(A hammer.)* slide (slid) slime sling (slung) slink (slunk) sliver slither slope slow (slower, slowest) slumber smack small smart smear smelt *(A fish.)* smirk smith smock smoke smooth smother snail snake snare snarl sneak sniff sniffle snivel snow so soak soap sock *(A stocking.)* soft some son song soon soot soothe sore sorrow sorry soul sound *(Healthy; a narrow bay.)* sour south sow (sowed, sown) /sō/ *(To scatter.)* sow /sow/ *(Female hog.)* spade span spare spark sparrow speak spear speck speak (spoke, spoken) speech speed (sped) spell *(Time period; a charm.)* spend (spent) spider spill spin spindle spire spit (spat) spoke *(A wheel part.)* sponge spoon sprawl spread spring (sprang, sprung) sprout spur spurn spurt staff stag stair stake stalk *(To approach game.)* stall stalwart stammer stand (stood) star staple *(U-shaped metal.)* stare stark startle starve stead steadfast steam steal (stole, stolen) steed steel steeple steer stem stench step stern *(Harsh.)* steward stick (stuck) stiff still sting (stung) stink (stank, stunk) stint stir stirrup stitch stock stone stool stoop stop stork storm stove straddle straight strap straw streak stream street strength stretch stick (stuck) stick *(A piece of wood.)* sting (stung) stink (stunk) straw stricken stride (strode, stridden) strike (struck) string (strung) string *(Twine.)* strip *(To denude.)* strive (strove) stroke strong stud *(Short post; male animal.)* stunt *(To impede.)* sty *(Eyelid swelling.)* such suck sulk summer sun Sunday surf swallow *(To take in food; a bird.)* swan swarm swarthy swear (swore, sworn) sweat sweep sweet swell (swelled, swollen) swelter swerve swift swim (swam, swum) swine swing (swung) sword swoop **T** tail tale tall tame tap *(A faucet.)* tape tar tart *(Sour taste.)* teach (taught) team tear (tore, torn) /tair/ tear /tear/ tease teem *(To be full.)* -teen tell (told) ten (tenth) than thank that (those) thaw the thee theft then there thick thicket thief (thieves) thigh thimble thin thing think (thought) thirst thirteen (thirteenth) thirty (thirtieth) this (these) thistle thorn thorough thought thousand (thousandth) thrash thread threat three (third) threshold thrill throat throng through throw (threw, thrown) thread thrush thud thumb thunder thus tick *(An insect.)* tide tidings tie till *(To work soil.)* timber time tin tinder tire *(To become weary.)* tired to toad today toe together token toll *(A levy.)* ton tongs tongue tonight too tool tooth (teeth) top tough tow toward town trap tray tread (trod, trodden) tree trend trim trough true truth Tuesday turf tusk twelve (twelfth) twenty (twentieth) twice twin twine twig twinge twinkle two **U** udder uncouth under underlie underneath understand (understood) up upright upward us utmost utter *(Absolute.)* **V** [The partner /f/ & /v/ sounds in O. E. were both written with *f*. Modern transliteration changes *f* to *v* when it was thought to have been voiced, *e.g.*, leaf *leaves*, wife *wives*. The following come from words originally spelled with an initial *f*.] vane vat **W** wade wake (woke, waked) wale *(A welt.)* walk walnut wan wander wane war ward ware warm warp /worp/ wart wary was wash wasp watch water wave wax way we weapon wear (wore, worn) weary weasel weather weave (wove, woven) web wed wedding wedge Wednesday weed week weep weigh weight weird welcome well Welsh went were west wet whale wharf (wharves) what wheat wheel when where whether which while whine whisper whistle white whither who whole whom why wick wide widow wife (wives) wild will (would) will *(To choose.)* willow willy-nilly *(Will I, nill I?)* win (won) wind /wind/ wind /wīnd/ (wound) wink winnow winter wipe wire wisdom wise wish wit witch with witness woe wolf (wolves) woman (women) womb wonder woo wood wool word work world worm worry worse worship worst wort worth would wound wrath wreak wreath wren wrench wrest wrestle wring (wrung) wrinkle wrist writ write (wrote, written) writhe wrong **X** [Most words beginning with *x* in modern English are from Greek with *x* being a transliteration of the Greek letter chi χ X) and is pronounced /z/ as in *Xerox, xylophone*.] **Y** [In O.E. spelling of these *y*-words began with *g*.] yammer yard yawn yea year yearn yeast yell yellow yelp yes yesterday yet yield yoke yolk you young your youth Yule

---

Old Norse

Viking invasions began about 787 and continued. Here Norse, also of Germanic origin, made its contribution to English. Because Old English and Old Norse had similar roots but different inflections (change in form to indicate case, number, person, gender, or tense), the speaker's solution was to drop them (usually endings). This led to English becoming a generally uninflected language. Sometimes Old Norse is referred to as Scandinavian.

A alike anger angry anklet awe awful awesome awhirl awkward awe **B** bag bait ball   ball peen *(A hammer type.)* band *(A bond.)* bang bark *(Tree covering.)* bask beaker berserk bewail billow birl *(To rotate.)* birling blaze *(To mark a tree.)* bleak blend blather blithering bloom bollix *(To bungle.)* boon booth bore *(A tidal wave.)* both bound *(Destined.)* bow *(The forward part of ship.)* brad brunt bulk bur bush bustle *(To hurry.)*

button bylaw **C** cake calf *(Leg part.)* call carp *(To complain.)* cart cast clip *(To cut.)* club clump clumsy clutch *(A brood of children.)* cow *(To intimidate.)* cozy crawl crook cross **D** dangle die (died, dying) dirt down *(Bird plumage.)* doze drag droop **E** ear eddy egg *(To urge; ovum.)* eider eiderdown **F** fast *(To abstain; a mooring rope.)* fellow filly flag *(Flagstone.)* flat fleck flit floe fog *(A mist.)* freckle Frigg *(Wife of Odin and goddess of marriage; Frigg's day = Friday.)* fro froth fry *(Small fish.)* fulmar *(A sea bird.)* fumble **G** gab gabble gabby gable gad *(A mining tool.)* gainly gait gap gape gasp gaunt gawk gear geld *(To castrate.)* get (got, gotten) gift girth glitter gloat gloss gosling grovel gun gust gusty **H** haggle hail *(To greet.)* happen happy hinge hit hug **I** ill **K** keel kid kindle **L** lag law leak leg lift link litmus loan loft loon loose lope low **M** mawkish meek mire mistake **N** nag *(To scold.)* nay *(No.)* niggard Norwegian nudge **O** oaf odd Odin *(God of art, culture, and the dead; Odin's [Woden's] day = Wednesday.)* **P** peen plow **R** race *(A contest.)* raft rag raise ramshackle ransack reef reindeer rid rive roe *(Fish eggs.)* root *(Plant part.)* rotten rug **S** sale same scale *(To weigh.)* scant scare scathe scold scoot scorch score scrap scrape scrub *(Rub while washing.)* scuffle seat seem simper skeet skewer ski skid skill skimp skin skirt sky slam slant slaughter sleight sludge sly slump slush snag snipe snub span-new sprint squall stack stagger spry squab squall steak stern *(Back of ship.)* swain **T** take (took, taken) tang teem *(To pour.)* tern their them they Thor *(God of thunder, and strength; Thor's day = Thursday.)* though thrift thrive thrust Thursday thwart till *(Until.)* toss trash troll trust tug tyke Tyr *(God of war; Tyr's [Tiu's] Day = Tuesday.)* **U** ugly **V** Valhalla *(Hall of the Slain.)* Valkyrie *(A maiden who chose heroes for Valhalla.}* vanadium *(A rare metallic element.)* Viking **W** wail wake *(A track.)* wand want wassail *(Be in good health.)* weak whirl whore windlass window wing

Middle English   1050-1475 A.D.

With the Norman conquest of England in 1066, French became the language of government and business. Most of this French derived from Latin, but a sizable amount retained a Norse influence. Today the fusion of Old French and the existing English is called Middle English. French importations that were accepted with little or no change at the time are listed in Appendix vi as Old French. A selection by Geoffrey Chaucer, the most famous writer in Middle English, is included in Appendix xv. With its Old English, Old Norse, Old French, Latin components, and Scandinavian influences, Middle English is a very rich language. Words from all these sources should be added to the following for a more generous listing of words descending from Middle English.

A above abroad ado ah aha ajar akimbo alack albeit alone always amid amidst ankle apron as ashore astound awl axle **B** babble babe baby backgammon bad (worse, worst) badge badger bank *(Mound of earth.)* barnacle basket batch because bat *(A flying creature.)* bawdy bawl beagle belief believe bellow *(To shout.)* belong below beseech (besought) besmirch bestow betrothal bicker big birth blab blabber bleary bloat blot blow *(A hit.)* blubber blunder blunt blur bluster boast bob *(To move up & down; haircut type.)* boisterous booth boulder bounce bounteous bout box *(To fight.)* boy brawl breathe brink bristle brittle brothel bubble bubbler bud bug bull bun bunch bunting burrow buxom **C** chap *(To become rough.)* charcoal chastise cheat cherry chestnut chink *(A crevice.)* chip chop chub clasp cleat cleft clever clog clutch cob

(A corncob.) cobweb cockney cog *(Gear tooth.)* coke *(Fuel.)* coop core cough could cower crag craw cramp craze crazy crease creek crimson cringe crinkle crud crumble crumpet cuckold cuff curd curdle curl cuff *(Sleeve end.)* cut **D** dab dabble dagger dairy dam dank dash dawn daze dazzle dearth dell depth dicker dimple dirt dismay docket dolt dormouse dote dove dowdy dowel draft drake *(A male duck.)* dread dream dredge drift drone *(To hum.)* drown drug duck *(To submerge.)* duds dull dump **E** eerie elk entangle ewer eye *(Brood of pheasants.)* **F** farther farthest feckless feud fidget fit *(Adapted to a purpose.)* flake flash flaunt flaw *(An imperfection.)* fledgling fling (flung) flout flush *(To drive from cover.)* fond former fraught freckle freak fun **G** gag ghastly gaunt gaze gill girl glare glint gloom glum gnarled gnash goal goggle gore *(To wound.)* gossamer grasp gravy grid gridiron groom grub guess gulch gull gush **H** haddock haggis hail *(To greet.)* halibut hamper *(To hinder.)* hank harbor hark harlot harrow harsh hatch hatred heckle hey hinge hiss hitch hollyhock hoot howl hue *(Outcry.)* hurry **I** inkling insure Irish irk itch **J** [J was originally written as Latin *i* /y/ as a word's first letter; in M.E. it was influenced in pronunciation by a soft French *g* /ǰ/ (/zh/ in Modern French). Since the actual shaped "J" was not invented until the 1600's, the *j's* in the following words must have been substituted for earlier spellings by later English word compilers.] jag *(A notch.)* jaw jolly jolt jowl junk **K** keg kelp kerchief ketch kick kill kilt kindle kit kitten knack knob knowledge knuckle **L** lack lad lap *(To overlie.)* lark lass leader ledge ledger lift lightning lilt linger link lint loan lob lodestar lodestone log loiter lone loop loss low lug *(To carry.)* lull lullaby lumber *(To move awkwardly.)* lump lurk **M** maggot mark market measles mellow midnight midst minnow mold *(Fungus.)* molt mop morning morrow motley muck mud muddy muddle mulberry mulch mumble munch mushroom mutter moor *(To secure a ship.)* **N** nab nag *(Old horse.)* neither newfangled nick nickname nob nod noisome nook nor notch nothing numb nunnery nutmeg **O** off often once onslaught onward outrage **P** pack packer paddle padlock palmistry parch parsnip partner pat patch pate peal peat peck *(A measure.)* peddle peddler peek peep peeve peevish peg pelt *(To strike.)* penthouse perk pert pew *(A bench.)* pick pickax pie pig pillow pimple pincers pint pitch *(To throw.)* polliwog pond pour pout prance prong prowl proxy pry *(To snoop.)* pudding puddle puff punch *(To strike.)* **Q** quaver queasy quill quite quiver **R** rabbit rabble rake *(A lewd man.)* ramble rap ready rift rig *(To equip.)* rigmarole roam rove rub rubber rubbish rugged rumble rump rustle ruthless **S** sag saunter scab scalp scatter scavenge scoff scour scout *(To search.)* scowl scream screech shatter sheer *(Absolute.)* shelter shingle shiver shock *(Sheaves of grain.)* shore shrewd shriek shrug shudder shunt sigh silt since skillet skip skit *(A small comic drama.)* skittish skulk skull slab slant slash sleek sleet slender slick slight slit slop slope sloth slug *(A gastropod.)* slut smatter smell smile smirch smolder smudge snarl *(Growl.)* snatch sneer sneeze snoot snore snort snout sob spar spigot spike spinster spot spout spray *(A flower arrangement.)* sprig sprinkle squeak squeeze squirt stab stalk *(A stem.)* stamp starch start stifle stilt stint stomp straggle straight strain *(Line of descent.)* strip *(To denude.)* stroke stubborn struggle strawberry stumble stump stutter sty *(A pig pen.)* suckle swap sway sweep (swept) swipe swirl swivel swoon **T** tadpole tag talk tallow tangle target tarry tatter taut teal thence throe *(Violent pain.)* throttle tickle tidy tight tilt tip *(To tilt.)* tithe toll *(Bell sound.)* tomorrow totter tout toy tramp trample trickle

trollop troth truce tug tumble turd tussle twilight twirl twist twitch **U** until unto upholster upon upper urchin utter *(To say.)* **W** wag waggle waist waive wallet wanton waver wealth wee welfare welt wench whence whiff whine whip whisk whisker whittle wholesale wholesome whoop whose wicked wicker widower wile wisp wizard wondrous worthy wrangle wrap wreathe wrought wry **Y** yawp *(To yelp.)* ye yeoman yonder yours

---

Modern English 1475 A.D. to present

Beginning from about 1500, English was basically a Germanic language with contributions from all the entries in this appendix: Old English, Old Norse, Middle English, German, Dutch, Danish, Norwegian, Swedish, *etc.* This language core was overlaid with a generous Latin contribution (Appendices iii, iv, & vii) and offerings of Latin's subsequent descendants: French, Italian, Spanish, and Portuguese (Appendix viii). Greek (Appendices iii, iv, & ix) and a sprinkling of loan words from other sources (Appendix x) have all made their own unique contributions to English. The most famous writer in early Modern English was **William Shakespeare**, (1564-1616). A quotation from his <u>Hamlet</u> can be found in Appendix xv-2. Although the major English speaking countries have essentially the same vocabulary, a few special-term items are evident. Some of the Australian, British, Canadian, and New Zealand contributions are given here. A similar listing of terms peculiar to the United States is given in Ap. xiii.

Australian English backblocks *(Inland farm.)* barrack *(Cheer.)* billabong *(Backwater.)* billy *(Heating pot.)* boomerang bonzer *(Sl. very good.)* bunya-bunya *(An evergreen tree.)* bushed *(Lost; confused.)* dingo *(A wild dog.)* fossick *(To look for something.)* joey *(A young kangaroo.)* kangaroo koala *(A eucalyptus eating marsupial.)* kookaburra *(A large "laughing" bird.)* outback station *(A cattle or sheep ranch.)* sundowner *(A vagrant.)* swag *(A bundle.)* swagman *(A work seeker.)* tuckerbag wallaby *(A kangaroo type.)* wallaroo *(A kangaroo type.)* within cooee *(Within calling distance.)* wombat *(A nocturnal marsupial.)* yabber *(Inf. talk, speech.)*

British English aeroplane *(Airplane.)* aerodrome *(Airport.)* Baker Street *(Home of Sherlock Holmes.)* barrow *(A pushcart.)* biffin *(Cooking apple.)* biscuit *(Cookie, cracker.)* bloody *(An intensifying word. e.g., a bloody good time.)* bobby *(A policeman.)* bounder *(An ill-mannered person.)* bowler *(A derby.)* brash *(A rain shower.)* brolly *(Umbrella.)* buttery *(Pantry.)* buttons *(Inf. a bellboy.)* cad *(An Oxford townsman.)* cheerio *(Hello, Good-by.)* chemist *(Drug store.)* chevy *(A hunt.)* chit *(A short note.)* dabster *(Inf. dabbler; bungler.)* daft *(Insane; foolish; silly.)* darbies *(Handcuffs.)* dene *(Low sandy hill.)* destructor *(An incinerator.)* double first *(University high honors in two subjects.)* Downing Street *(Home of the Prime Minister; the British government.)* down under *(Australia or New Zealand.)* draper *(A dealer in dry goods.)* duffer *(A clumsy person.)* gaol, gaoler *(Jail, jailer.)* gippy tummy *(Upset stomach.)* gramophone *(A record player.)* greengrocer *(Vegetable and fruit seller.)* grizzle *(To grumble.)* heartsome *(Cheerful.)* high tea *(An early evening meal at which meat is served.)* hoarding *(A temporary fence.)* hot pot *(Stewed meat and potatoes.)* howler *(An absurd blunder in speaking or writing.)* hustings *(A London court.)* invigilate *(To proctor an examination.)* jemmy *(A crowbar.)* kerb *(Curb.)* let *(To rent.)* lift *(An elevator.)* lorry *(A truck.)* navvy *(A laborer.)* nipper *(Inf. a small boy.)* peeler *(A policeman, after Robert Peel.)* pence *(Pl. of penny.)* petrol *(Gasoline.)* point *(Outlet, socket.)* poppet *(A beautiful child.)* post *(To mail.)* pottle *(Small fruit basket.)* pram *(< perambulator, baby carriage.)*

prepositor *(A senior school monitor.)* pub *(A tavern.)* public school *(A private school.)* rag *(Play a joke on.)* rather *(Yes indeed!)* ratten *(To harass.)* reach-me-down *(Inf. a hand-me-down.)* rise *(An increase in salary.)* righto roundabout *(A traffic circle; a merry-go-round.)* serviette *(A napkin.)* shaw *(A thicket.)* sleeping partner *(Silent partner.)* solicitor *(A lawyer.)* spot *(A portion of, e.g. a spot of tea.)* stick *(Cane.)* sticky wicket *(Difficult.)* tele *(Television.)* surgery *(A doctor's office.)* tin *(A can.)* Tommy Atkins *(Inf. a soldier.)* tosh *(Inf. nonsense.)* trade card *(Business card.)* tripper *(Inf. a tourist.)* truck *(Freight car.)* verger *(Church usher.)* vest *(Undershirt.)* wagon *(Freight car.)* weald *(A forest area.)* wherry *(A fishing vessel.)* whilst *(While.)* windle *(A basket.)* wireless *(Radio.)* wonky *(Sl. unsteady, feeble.)* z ed *(The letter Z.)*; <u>See Chapter 3, page 44 for comments on British spelling.</u> Some special British pronunciations: again /ə-gān/ docile /dō-sīl/ epoch /ē-pok/ fertile /fer-tīl/ figure /fig-er/ hostile /hos-tīl/ issue /is-yoo/ laboratory /lə-bor-ə-trē/ lieutenant /lef-ten-ənt/ nephew /nev-yoo/ patent /pāt-nt/ plateau /plat-ō/ premature /prem-ə-tyoor/ renaissance /ri-nā-səns/ route /root/ schedule /shed-yool/ sterile /stair-īl/ whilst /hwīlst/

Canadian English blinds *(Window shades.)* bronco *(An Englishman.)* carrying place *(A portage.)* fire-reel *(A fire engine.)* fringe land *(Land without railroad access.)* Grit *(Liberal Party member.)* growler *(Small iceberg.)* McGill Fence *(Radar warning system.)* outport *(Isolated village.)* pond hockey *(Unorganized hockey.)* rampike *(Fire damaged tree.)* returned man *(A veteran.)* rubaboo *(A soup.)* sault /soo/ *(A waterfall; rapids.)* scrutineer *(Poll observer.)* shinny *(Pond hockey;* from the shout *"shin ye.")* syne *(River channel.)* tap *(Faucet.)* wastelot *(A vacant lot.)*;

New Zealand English bikkis *(Cookies.)* bloke *(A man.)* cockie *(Farmer.)* fizz *(Carbonated beverage.)* hard case *(A funny person.)* hospital pass *(Disastrous rugby pass.)* lollies *(Candy.)* mate *(Friend.)* munted *(Broken.)* panel beater *(Auto body mechanic.)* piker *(One who gives up.)* rung out *(To be teased.)* sheila *(A woman.)* She'll be right *(Everything will be O.K.)* snooker *(Billiards.)* Yeah, gidday *(Hello.)*

Scottish [Scottish is the sort of English spoken in the Lowlands--southern Scotland. The Highlanders speak Scottish Gaelic, also called Erse or Goidelic.] agley *(Awry.)* ain *(Own.)* ajee *(Askew.)* argle *(Argue.)* Auld Klootie *(The Devil.)* auld lang syne *(Old long since; long ago.)* awee *(Awhile.)* baggie *(Stomach.)* bailie *(Alderman.)* bannet *(Bonnet.)* barefit *(Barefoot.)* ben *(Inner room.)* billy *(Comrade.)* blume *(To blossom.)* bonny brae *(Hillside.)* bree *(Broth.)* breeks *(Breeches)* brig *(Bridge.)* burn *(A brook.)* burnie *(A little brook.)* cairn *(Stone marker.)* canna *(Cannot.)* cauld *(Cold.)* chucky *(A little chick.)* clan collie collieshangle *(A quarrel.)* cozy curch *(A kerchief.)* daff daffy filibeg *(A kilt.)* dunderhead firth *(Arm of sea.)* glamour gruesome gumption jilt kiltie kirk *(Church.)* kirkman loch *(Lake.)* Mac- *(Son of.)* mirk *(Dark.)* pet plaid pollack pony pudgy rink runt skullduggery slogan tab stymie swirl tam tam-o'-shanter *(A cap.)* to-name *(A nickname.)* trousers vauntie *(Boastful.)* wallydraigle *(Youngest in family.)* weel *(Well.)* yank *(A sharp blow or slap.)*

Germanic Languages

Low German [The "low" here is not one of stature, but of geography; *Low German* refers to the Dutch, Flemish, and Frisian spoken in the Low Countries and the German in the lowlands of northern Germany (Plattdeutsch).] *Italics* indicates *Middle* Low German (1100-1450).

bluster clown cranberry doodle drabble *hawk* (To shout.) hump *lash mate* ogle paltry pamper *poke prank rash* rill self (selves) shaft *(Mine entrance.)* shelf (shelves) shelve shuffle *slag* slap *sled slip* smug smuggle smut snug *spool strip* (A band of cloth.) *stump* swamp sway *tackle toot trade* tram *wiggle wriggle* wobble

Yiddish
[Yiddish is derived from the German spoken in the Rhineland in the 1200's. It finally became the language of many Jews in central Europe.] bagel blintze fin *($5.00)* gefüllte fish *(Stuffed fish.)* keister kibitz kibosh *(To put the kibosh on: squelch.)* kosher *(Ritually clean.)* lox Mazl tov! *("Good luck." Congratulations!)* mazuma *(Money.)* meshuge *(Crazy.)* -nik *(Suf.: A person connected with something, e.g., beatnik, refusenik.)* nudnik *(A pest; a bore.)* pastrami Reb *(A title of respect.)* schlemiel *(An inept person.)* schmaltz *(Florid, showy.)* schmo *(A fool, jerk.)* schnozzle *(Nose.)* shtick *("Piece"; trick, gimmick.)* shul *(Synagogue; school.)* tref *(Not kosher.)* yarmulke *(Skullcap.)*

German
[PRONUNCIATION TIPS: w /v/, a /ä/, Wagner /väg-ner/; e /ā/ Weber /vā-ber/; s /sh/, ie /ē/, spiel /shpēl/ *(Play.)*; ei /ī/ heil /hīl/ *(Hail.)*; eu /oi/, Deutschland /doich-länt/ *(Germany.)* au /ow/ Hausfrau /hows-frow/ *(Housewife.)*] **A** Achtung! *(Attention!)* alpenhorn angst anschluss Aufklarung auf Wiedersehen *(Till we meet again.)* Ausgleich autobahn **B** J.S. Bach L. Beethoven Berchtesgaden Bierhaus Bismarck bismuth *(An element.)* bitte *(Please.)* blitz blitzkrieg *(Lightning war.)* bower *(Euchre term.)* boxer *(Dog.)* J. Brahms bratwurst braunschweiger Buch *(Book.)* bum bund *(A league.)* Bundersrat *(State council.)* Burgess *(Citizen.)* **C** carouse chorale cobalt **D** dachshund delicatessen deutschemark Deutschland Doppelgänger dunk **E** edelweiss erlking ersatz **F** fest *(Festival.)* fife flak fleck flügelhorn Frau *(Mrs.)* Fräulein *(Miss.)* fresh *(Impudent.)* Führer **G** Gauleiter gemütlich gestalt Gestapo Gesundheit glockenspiel Goethe /gö-tə/ Graf *(Count.)* **H** Hakenkreuz *("Hooked cross"; Swastika.)* hamster hasenpfeffer Hausfrau haversack heil heroin Herr *(Mr.)* hex hinterland humoresque **J** ja *(Yes.)* Jungfrau Junker **K** kaffeeklatsch Kaiser *(Caesar.)* Kapellmeister Das Kapital *(Book by Karl Marx.)* kaput kegler kindergarten Krieg *(War.)* Kriss Kringle kuchen **L** lager ländler langläufer Lebensraum Leibnitz leitmotif lied /lēd/ *(Song.)* Liederkranz liverwurst Luftwaffe lumpen *(A phony.)* **M** marzipan Mein Kampf *(Hitler's book: My Battle.)* Meistersinger minnesinger Mozart **N** Nazi *(National Socialist.)* nein *(No.)* nix (Ger. nichts, *nothing.)* noodle **P** panzer pfennig pinscher pitchblende Plattdeutsch plunder poltergeist poodle pretzel Privatdozent pumpernickel Putsch **Q** quartz **R** Rathaus rathskeller Realpolitik Reich Reichsbank reichsmark Reichstag rucksack **S** sauerbraten sauerkraut Schrecklichkeit Schutzstaffel *(S.S.)* schilling schottische schuss Sieg Heil Singspiel sitzbath sitzmark schnauzer snorkel spiel spitz stalag statistics stein strafe strudel stuka stunt *(A feat.)* Sturm und Drang swindle **T** taler *(Origin of dollar.)* turner *(Gymnast.)* turnverein **U** übermensch U-boat (Ger. Unterseeboot, *Under sea boat.)* umlaut Ursprache Urtext **V** vandal Vandal vandalism verboten vermouth Volkslied *(Folk song.)* von (Used in family names, *from, of;* often a title of status; *e.g., Von Braun, Von Bulow)* vorlage **W** Wagner /väg-ner/ die Walküre waltz wanderlust Weber /vā-ber/ Wehrmacht Weimar Republic Weltanschauung Wien /vēn/ *(Vienna.)* Wiener schnitzel Wiesbaden Wilhelmstrasse J. Winckelmann (An archeologist.) Wittenberg L. Wittgenstein (A philosopher.) **Y** Yiddish yodel **Z** zeitgeist Zeppelin zigzag zinc zollverein zwieback *(Twice baked.)*

Flemish [One of the official languages of Belgium; it is closely related to Dutch.] dock *(Witness box.)* grime hunk *(A large piece or lump.)*

Middle Dutch [A form of Low German spoken before the 16th Century.] booze brake brake drum bruin *(Brown bear.)* bundle bung *(A stopper.)* bushing caboose clamp clock crimp crimple croon damp damper dapper deck dock droll drum Dutch freight frump frumpish hold *(Ship area.)* golf grab huckster lathe Lollard luck mackerel margrave mart -kin *(Small.)* mesh pickle plug plump poll prate prattle prop *(A support.)* pump quack *(A pretender.)* rack rant ravel rumple rover scoop scour scow scratch scum skim sledge *(A vehicle.)* slip *(A plant cutting.)* smelt *(To reduce ores in a furnace.)* snack snap snare drum snuff *(To sniff.)* sod splice splint split stripe suds swab swamp switch tattle tip *(A point.)* trawl trip tub tubby twaddle wiseacre

Dutch ahoy aloof avast *(Hold!)* beleaguer *(To surround.)* blink bluff *(To deceive; a steep bank.)* boer *(A farmer.)* boom *(A pole.)* boor boss bowery *(A farm.)* The Bowery *(A New York City street.)* brackish brandy buck *(A sawbuck.)* bumpkin burgher bushwhack cam clinker cockatiel coleslaw commodore cookie cruise cruller domineer dope drill dud dune easel etch floss foist freight frolic furlough gherkin grab groove gruff gulp guy *(A rope, a wire.)* The Hague hanker heist hock *(To pawn.)* holster howitzer hustle iceberg kink knapsack laager *(A camp.)* landscape maelstrom manikin mite *(A small ant.)* muff nasty nip Norse pit *(A fruit stone.)* poppycock potash roster Santa Claus schipperke schnapps scrabble scram scramble skate sketch skipper *(Captain of a ship.)* slaw *(Cole slaw.)* sleigh slim sloop slurp snip snoop snuff *(Tobacco.)* Spinoza spook sputter stoop *(A small porch.)* tankard tattoo trek trigger uproar van (Used in family names, *from, of;* *e.g.,* Van Buren, Van Dyck, Van Gogh) waffle waft wagon walrus yacht yawl zee *(Sea.)*

Afrikaans [South African Dutch.] aardwolf apartheid blaubok Boer Boer War commando dingus gemsbok hartebeest kloof *(A gorge.)* kop *(A hill.)* kraal *(A village.)* laager *(A defensive enclosure.)* rand *(Monetary unit from Witwatersrand.)* springbok Taal *(Afrikaans.)* uitlander veldt waterbuck wildebeest Witwatersrand *(Region of Transvaal.)*

Danish ballast flense fog Kierkegaard krone narwhal -sen *(Son, e.g., Jensen)* skoal

Norwegian Birkebeiner *("Birch leg"; faction in 12th century civil war. Now the name of an annual ski race run in Wisconsin.)* fjord lemming ski skiing slalom slump vole *(Fieldmouse.)*

Swedish bungle gantlet mink ose *(A ridge.)* rutabaga smörgåsbord squabble tungsten Vasaloppet *(Sweden's famous annual skiing event.)* **Icelandic** geyser

---

Grimm's Law **Jakob Grimm**, 1785-1836, one of the brothers Grimm of fairy tale fame, formulated a law of consonant shift from Latin to the Germanic languages. This accounts for why certain words with similar meanings in Latin and English *appear* to be unrelated in spelling. Some of the consonant "shifts" with attendant examples are listed.

p (pater) → **f** (father)	**d** (duo) → **t** (two)	**c** (cord-) → **h** (heart)
f (frater) → **b** (brother)	**t** (tres) → **th** (three)	**g** (gen-) → **k** (kin)

Old French (From Latin) A, B, C . . . . Ap. vi-1

D, E, F, G, H, I, J, L, M, N, O, P . . . . Ap. vi-2

Q, R, S, T, U, V . . . . Ap. vi-3

Old French (Greek via Latin) . . **Old French** (Norse, Germanic) . . . Ap. vi-4

Anglo-French A → P . . . . Ap. v-4

Q → W . . . . **Middle French** . . . . Ap. vi-5

Modern French 1600 A.D. to present . . . . (See Ap. viii)

Appendix vi   The French Connection
(Old French, Middle French, & Anglo-French)

Old French   (From Latin) 850-1400

A ability able abominable abstain accomplish accord account accuse accustom ace achieve acquaint acquit address adjourn adjust administer admit admonish adore adorn adventure adversity advise advocate affirm affront age agree aid aim alliance allow amend amends amiable amorous amount anguish announce annual annul anoint antelope apiece appall apparel appeal appear appetite apply appoint approve apron arbor arch argue armor arrest arrive arrogance art ascent assault assemble assent assess assign assort assure attain attempt attend attorney audience aunt authority avail avenge avert **B** bar battle beast bounty bugle bulge **C** cabbage cable cage capital captain carpet cave celestial cell cement ceremony certain chain chair challenge champion chance channel chant chapel chaplain charge charity charter chase chaste cheer cherish chief chivalry choir citation civilian claim clarify clause clear cloak cloister close closet coast coil collar collect college color comfort commendation comment commence commission common communion companion company compass compel complain compound compress conceal conceit conceive condition confession confirm conquest conscience consent consideration consolation constrain contain continue contrast contrive converse convert cope cornet corrosion corrupt corsage cost couch count *(To list.)* counterfeit country couple courage court courtesy cover covert covet coward creature crest crevice crew cruel crime crucify crust cry cucumber current curtail curtain custom **D** dainty delay damage damn danger daub daunt debate decay decease deceive decide decline decrease decree deface default defeat defense defer defiant defile define defraud defy degrade degree delicious delight deliver deny depart depend deport depose depress deprive deputy descend deserve desire despise destiny destroy destruction detain determine device devise devote devour diamond differ dignity diligent dime diminish disarm disappoint disburse discern discharge discipline disclose discolor discomfort discontinue discord discourage discover discretion disease dishonest dishonor disloyal disobey dispense displace display displease dispose dispute disturb diverse divine division doctrine document double dozen dress due dungeon durable **E** eagle easy emperor enclose encounter encourage endanger endorse endure enemy enforce enjoy enlarge enrage enroll ensure entrance entrench envy error essay estate esteem eternal event example excel excess excite exercise exile experience expert exploit exposition expound express **F** faculty fade fail fairy false familiar fault favor feasible feast feat feature feeble felony female fester festival fierce fig finance fine finish flair flavor flourish flower flute forest forfeit form fortress fortune foundation fountain fraction frank fraud fringe front fruit fuel function funeral future **G** garment gash gavel gender general gentle gland glory glue gorge gorgeous government gown grace grain grand grease grief grocer gross gum gutter **H** habit haughty heir honest honor host hostage human **I** ignorant image immune impair impart impeach imperial impertinent imply impotent impoverish impression imprison improper impudent impulsive impurity incense incision incite incline inconvenient increase indent indifferent indignation induction indulgence inequality infant infection infinite influence inform infusion inhumanity inhabit inherit injury injustice innocent inquest inquire insatiable insist inspire instant institution instruction intelligence intend intense intent intention intercourse interest interior interpreter interval introduction invention invisible irregular isle issue ivory **J** jail jaundice jelly jeopardy jest jewel join joint journal journey joy juggle juice jurisdiction just justice **L** labor language languish lard large league leprosy lesson letter lettuce level lever levy libel liberal library lineage litter lizard loyal luxury **M** madam majesty malady male malevolent malice manger mansion mantle manual manure map marble marine marry marvel masculine mass master matter meager meddle medicine medley member memory menace mention merchant mercy meridian merit mess message metal minstrel mirror mischief miserable mister moist mold molest money monster moral morsel mortal mortify motet motion mount mountain move mule murmur muzzle mute mutiny **N** nasal nature navy neat necessity negligence nephew nice nobility noise nominative note notice noun nourish number nurse nurture **O** obedient obey obligation oblivion obscure observe obstacle obtain occupy octave odor offend offense office officer ointment omnipotent onerous onion operation opinion opportunity oppose oppress oracle ordain order ordinary origin ornament ostrich ounce overt oyster **P** pact pain paint palace pale palm palsy panel pant pardon parent parole parsley partial particular party passage passion pasture patient patron paunch pay peace peach pearl pellet pen pencil penitence pension pensive perceive perfect perform peril period perish perjury permanent perpendicular perpetual persecution perseverance personal pertain perverse petition pierce pier pigeon pint pioneer pity place plague plaintiff plank plate plea pleasant please pleasure plenty plight plunge plural point poison polish ponder poor poise porch porcupine pork porpoise porter portion pose position positive possibility posterity poverty powder power pray prayer preach preamble predecessor preface prefix prejudice presence present preserve president press pressure presume prevail prime prince prisoner probable probation proceed process procession proclamation procure profound profession progressive prohibition projection prolong promotion prompt profit pronoun pronounce proof proper property proportion propose proposition propriety prose prosper protest prove proverb providence province provision provoke prudent publish pulse punish puny pupil puppet pure purge purify purpose **Q** quail quantity quarry quart quarter quest question quilt quit **R** rage rail raisin rascal rate ratify ray razor real realm reason rebate receipt receive reception recite reclaim recluse recoil reconcile record recourse recover redemption refer reflect reform refrain refuge refund refuse regiment register regular relative release relic relief relieve religion relinquish relish rely remain remember remnant remorse remount remove rent repair repay repeal repeat repent replenish replication reply report represent reprisal repugnant request rescue resemble reservation reserve residence resign residue resist resort resound resource response restitution restoration restraint retain retention retribution return reveal revenge reverence reverse revert revile revoke revolution revulsion rigor rinse riot river roll Roman romance round route royalty ruby rude rumor **S** sacred sacrilege saint salad salmon salvation sanctuary satin satisfy sauce saucer savage save savor savory scar science scissors scout screw script scrutiny search season second secret secretion sect secular sedition see *(A religious office.)* senate senator sensible sensitive sentiment sentinel sequel sermon servant serve service sex sign simple singular sirloin skirmish slate society soil soldier sole solemn solicit solitude solution sort source space specify spine spirit spoil stability stage stain stance state stature staunch stew store strain strait strange stranger stray stress student study stuff stun sturdy subdue substance subtle suburb subversion succeed succumb suction sudden suffer summit superior supersede superstition supplant supple supply support suppose surge surmise surmount surname surplus suspend suspense sustain style **T** tablet tailor tapestry tassel tax temper tempest tempt tend tenement tenor term terrace test text tissue title toast tolerable torment torrent torture total trace tradition tragedy traitor transcript transfer transgress translate transpose travel treble tremble tremor trench trespass triangle tribe tribulation Trinity triumph trouble trowel trunk try turmoil **U** unicorn unity universe use usher usual utensil **V** valiant valley valor value vanish vanity vary vegetable vehement veil vein venom verify vermin verse very vessel vice vicious victory vigil vigor vile village villain vinegar violent violet virgin virile virtue visible vision visit vital voice volatile volume voluntary volunteer voluptuous vow vowel

Old French (From Greek via Latin)

A adamant age air arsenic austere **B** balm baptism barbaric base blaspheme
C cane carol cedar chair chart chimney choir chord clergy coffin coral cord
crocodile crystal cube cubic cycle cypress **D** date *(A fruit.)* despot dialectic diet
(Regulated eating.) dragon **E** ecstasy emerald **F** fantasy frenzy **G** galley giant goblin
govern graft *(A tree insert.)* gulf gum **H** heretic hermit hyacinth **I** idiot ink **J** jealous
L lamp lyre **M** macrocosm marble mass melody metal mosaic music **N** nymph
O ocean oil oyster **P** pain paper paragraph parish parliament parsley partridge
pedagogue periphery place planet pole pore *(An opening.)* presbytery prophecy /prof-ə-sē/
(A prediction.) prophesy /prof-ə-sī/ *(To predict.)* prophet protocol pulley **S** scorpion siren
sphere stomach surgeon surgery sycamore syllogism synagogue **T** tapestry theater
theme throne tomb tone topaz tour treasure treasury triumph turn turpentine
V vial **Z** zeal

Old French (Norse and Germanic Sources)

A array attach attack **B** bacon band bank *(A set.)* banner baste *(To sew.)* blank block
(To impede.) blue border brawn brush *(Small trees.)* **C** choice coat cramp cricket *(An
insect.)* crouch crush **D** dally dart dilly-dally **E** encroach ermine **F** filter flatter
flinch foray frank fray *(A conflict.)* frock frown furnish **G** gable gallop garland
garnish garrison gasket gauntlet gay *(Happy, merry.)* giblet glance grape grate *(To
shred.)* growl guarantee guard guide guise **H** hamlet harass hardy hash haste haunch
havoc heinous helmet herald heron hodgepodge hoe hurt hut **I** installment **J** jig
jiggle jolly **L** label lanyard lattice lecher list locket lodge lure **M** mail *(Letters.)*
maim marshal marten mason mayhem misspell morass **N** Norman **P** park paw
pledge pottery pucker putty **Q** quail **R** raffle rampant random rank rebuttal regard
regret reward rich rivet roast rob robe **S** scallop scorn screen scrimmage seize
slice spell *(To name letters of a word.)* spy stallion standard staples *(Basic items.)* stout
strand *(A line of rope.)* strife strive supper **T** tack tarnish tier towel track trip troll
trolley troop trot trumpet tuft

Anglo-French 1066-1400

[The hybrid of Old French and Old English along with more pure Old French and Old English
used in England from the Norman Conquest through about 1400.] **A** allege amenable
arraign array avoid **B** barber benefit broker bullion **C** canker canvas canvass car
carcass carriage carry case *(A box.)* catch (caught) cater caterer caterpillar cattle chisel
chive chorister chuck *(Cut of beef.)* chunk committee confound conspirator contrary
convey corner counsel count *(Nobleman.)* counter *(Table.)* county creditor croquet
/crō-kā/ crotch crown culprit curfew currant **D** descant disclaim distress dowry
E enamel engross enhance escrow exception exchange expense **F** fashion fee
G gallon *(Cel.)* garbage garden *(Gmc.)* garter *(Cel.)* griddle **H** hideous **I** incarnation
indict /in-dīt/ inhabitant **J** juror jury **L** larceny lavender **M** mangle manner
menial mischievous **O** oust orator **P** packet pensioner pretense purchase

Q quiver *(Arrow holder.)* **R** rape rebuke region rein remedy renown rush **S** salary sausage scarf scoundrel scourge scroll several slander socket spawn squeamish stay sturgeon subsidy sudden sue suffer suit sullen sum summon surgeon surrender surround survey survive suspicion sustenance syllable *(Gk.)* **T** tally toil tortuous treason trial trick tutor **V** vapor vengeance verdict victor vintage visor voidance vulture **W** wafer wage wager waif wait waive wallop warble warden *(Gmc.)* wardrobe warrant *(Gmc.)* warrior waste wreck

---

Middle French 1400-1600

A acquest acquiesce adopt advertise alter alteration amity armature assist assistant attest **B** bargain barrel bound *(To spring back.)* brisk **C** capacity capture card caress carnage casual cause cavern cavity cease cede certitude chamois /sham-ē/ charivari (chivaree) /shiv-ə-rē/ chieftain civil clairvoyant class clique colonel *(Formerly coronel.)* /ker-nəl/ combination commodity compare compliment *(Cf. complement.)* compose composition compressor compromise comrade concave concord concourse condescend conduit confection conference confess confine congeal coherent consider conserve consign consonant consort conspire constant contagion contentious control convene conversion copy coronation corporal corps /cor/ counterpoint couplet course coy credence credit crucial **D** decide defer density design detest dig disaster disband discount disembark disgrace disheveled dismantle disorder disparity disperse distinguish district divorce docile domain dome domestic dominant **E** embroider embroil expose **F** forgery **G** gallant gallivant garb gargle garment gauze gratify grumble **H** harpsichord **I** immensity impetuous incorrigible industry infest infidel influx ingenious inhuman instability install insult interview **J** jibe **K** kennel **L** lampoon **M** macaroon manufacture march maritime moralize mortuary musket **N** naturalize noble nudity **O** obscene observant offensive opportune oval **P** pacific pansy parity passport patrol peak peculiar pedigree pend penitent pernicious perspire persuade pest petrify pewter pick *(A tool.)* pike *(A spear.)* pilfer pilot platform plush poach *(A cooking term.)* popularity portable portage portal portrait post *(To mail.)* poultry premise problematic profusion progression promenade prom prosperous Protestant proximity pubescent public pulp pumpkin **Q** qualify queue **R** race *(Subdivision of mankind.)* ravage rave rebuff recent rectify redeem relay reminiscence responsible resume retard retrench review revise revive revolt ruffian rural ruse **S** salvage satire section sediment sedition sensual sentence serious severe servitude shivaree *(Var. charivari.)* situation slash sully suppliant surpass suture sylvan **T** tinsel tour transport travesty treacherous trillion **V** variety version vertical viceroy vicissitude vie vigilant visual volley **W** wig

| Appendix vii | For Latin Lovers (Latin Roots) | CONTENTS |

A	Ap. vii- 2	H	Ap. vii-17	P	Ap. vii-28
B	Ap. vii- 4	I	Ap. vii-18	Q	Ap. vii-34
C	Ap. vii- 4	J	Ap. vii-19	R	Ap. vii-34
D	Ap. vii-10	L	Ap. vii-19	S	Ap. vii-36
E	Ap. vii-12	M	Ap. vii-21	T	Ap. vii-44
F	Ap. vii-13	N	Ap. vii-25	U	Ap. vii-47
G	Ap. vii-16	O	Ap. vii-27	V	Ap. vii-48

More Latin Root Elements Ap. vii-52   **Latin: The Short Course** Ap. vii-53

Latin is a highly *inflected* language. This means that the endings of an **adjective** or **noun** change according to their *case* (nominative, genitive, dative, accusative, and ablative), *number* (singular or plural), and *gender* (masculine, feminine, and neuter). Thus the adjective, **bonus** *(good)*, has the following *declension:*

	SINGULAR			PLURAL		
	masculine	*feminine*	*neuter*	*masculine*	*feminine*	*neuter*
nominative	bonus	bona	bonum	boni	bonae	bona
genitive	boni	bonae	boni	bonorum	bonarum	bonorum
dative	bono	bonae	bono	bonis	bonis	bonis
accusative	bonum	bonam	bonum	bonos	bonas	bona
ablative	bono	bona	bono	bonis	bonis	bonis

Each **noun** has an assigned *gender* (masculine, feminine, or neuter) and is inflected with *case* endings (nominative, genitive, dative, accusative, or ablative) and **number** (singular or plural) with endings similar to the adjective declension. In the sentence, "The young boy's happy mother gave the tall teacher a good book in the dark hall." If the sentence were in Latin, the following cases would be used: *boy* (possessive) genitive; *mother* (subject) nominative; *teacher* (indirect object) dative; *book* (direct object) accusative; *hall* (object of preposition *in*) ablative. It is also necessary to note that each noun is <u>singular</u> and boy, teacher, and book are <u>masculine</u> gender, mother is <u>feminine</u> and hall is <u>neuter</u>. The adjectives *(young, happy, tall, good, and dark)* would each have the case endings of the nouns they modify. There are also other classes of adjectives and nouns with different sets of inflections. In this appendix an adjective is listed with its three gender singular nominatives: **bonus bona bonum**. A noun is listed with its nominative and genitive singulars: **amicus amici**

A **verb** may have *person*, *number*, and *tense.* : A *conjugation* of two tenses follows:

	PRESENT TENSE		PAST TENSE	
	SINGULAR	PLURAL	SINGULAR	PLURAL
first person	amo, *I love*	amamus, *we love*	amavi, *I loved*	amavimus, *we loved*
second person	amas, *you love*	amatis, *you love*	amavisti, *you loved*	amavistis, *you loved*
third person	amat, *he loves, she loves*	amant, *they love*	amavit, *he loved, she loved*	amaverunt, *they loved*

The verb *to love* is listed **amo amare amavi amatus**. These four basic verb parts translated into English are: **amo,** I love (first person, singular, present tense), **amare,** to love (the infinitive), **amavi,** I loved (perfect or simple past tense), **amatus**, loved (past participle)

Appendix vii For Latin Lovers (Latin Roots)

A

ab *(Shows motion away from.)* [prep.]   abduct absent abuse;   <u>See</u>: **ab-** as prefix in Ap. iii-6.

aboleo abolere abolevi abolitus *(To abolish.)* [v.]   abolish   abolition   abolitionism

acerbus acerba acerum *(Bitter, sour; harsh.)* [adj.]   acerbity acerbate acerb acerbic

acidus acida acidum *(Sour, tart; disagreeable.)* [adj.] acid acidity acidify acid test acidosis
acuo acuere acui acutus *(Sharpen; exercise; rouse.)* acute acuity acumen acupuncture

ad *(To, towards; against.)* [prep.]   <u>See</u>: prefix **ad-** (ac-, af-, ag-, al-, ap-, ar-, as-, at-) in Ap. iii-6.

adolesco adolescere adolevi *(Grow up; increase.)* [v.] adolescence adolescent adult adulthood

aequo aequare aequavi aequatus *(Make equal, even.)* [v.] equal equalitarian equality equanimity equate equator equilateral equilibrium equinox equivalent equivocate

aestimo aestimare aestimavi aestimatus *(To value.)* [v.] estimate estimation esteem (F)

aeterno aeternare aeternavi aeternatus *(To immortalize.)* [v.] eternal eternity eternally

aevum aevi *(Age, life-time; eternity.)* [neut. n.]   longevity   primeval   medieval

ager agri *(Field, farm; countryside; territory.)* [masc. n.] agriculture agriculturist agrarian

ago agere egi actus *(To do, to drive.)* [v.] act active action activate activist activity actor actress actual actuality actualize actually agent agency agenda agitate agitation agitator ambiguous ambiguity coagulate cogent counteract counteraction enact exact exam examine interact interaction react reaction reactor reactionary transaction

albus alba album *(White; bright.)* [adj.] albino album albumen alburnum alb alba

alius alia aliud *(Other, another; different.)* [adj.]   alien alienate alienation alias alibi

alo alere alui altus *(To nourish; promote.)* [v.] alimony aliment alimentary canal coalition

alter altera alterum *(The one, the other, next.)* [adj.] alter alteration alternative altercation alternate alternator altruism altruist altruistic alter ego alternating current alter idem

altus alta altum *(High; deep; noble; profound.)* [adj.] altitude altimeter alto alto clef contralto altocumulus altostratus altar altar boy altarpiece exalt exalted exaltation

ambo ambae ambo *(Both, two.)* [pl. n.] ambidextrous;   <u>See</u>: prefix **ambi-** in Ap. iii-7.

ambulo ambulare ambulavi ambulatus *(To walk, go, travel.)* [v.] amble ambulance ambulant somnambulist somnambulate perambulate perambulator preamble

amicus amici *(Friend.)* [masc. n.] **amica amicae** *(Friend.)* [fem. n.]
amo amare amavi amatus *(To love, like.)* [v.] amateur amateurish amorous amity amiable amicable amorist amoroso amoretto inamorata inamorato enamor amatory   amative   amour   enemy (In + amicus; *not a friend.*)   enemy alien

amplus ampla amplum *(Large, spacious; great.)* [adj.] ample amplify amplification amplifier amplitude amply amplitude modulation *(A. M. radio.)*

angusto angustare angustavi angustatus *(To make narrow.)* [v.] anguish anxiety anxious anxiously anxiousness angina angina pectoris

angulus anguli *(Angle, corner; out-of-the-way place.)* [masc. n.] angle angular angularity angled triangle triangular triangulate triangulation quadrangle quadrangular

anima animae *(Wind, air; breath; life; soul; ghost.)* [fem. n.] animate animation animal

animus animi *(Mind, soul; reason, thought; opinion.)* [masc. n] animus animosity unanimous unanimity magnanimous equanimity equanimous pusillanimous pusillanimity

annus anni *(Year.)* [masc. n.] annual annals anniversary annuity annuitant Anno Domini *(A. D.)* perennial biennial triennial triennium centennial per annum

ante *(Before.)* [prep.] antecedent antedate anteroom; <u>See</u>: **ante-** as prefix in Ap. iii-7.

antiquus antiqua antiquum *(Ancient, former, old.)* [adj.] antique antiquity antiquated

aptus apta aptum *(Suitable; joined together.)* [adj.] apt aptitude adapt adaptable adaptation adapter adaptive inept ineptitude

aqua aquae *(Water.)* [fem. n.] aqueous aquatic aquarium aquamarine aqueduct aqua

arbitror arbitrari arbitratus *(To testify; suppose.)* [v.] arbitrate arbitration arbitrator arbitrary

arcus arcus *(Bow; rainbow; arch, curve; arc.)* [masc. n.] arc arch arcade archer archery

ardeo ardere arsi arsus *(To burn, shine, be on fire.)* [v.] ardent ardor arson arsonist

argentum argenti *(Silver, silver plate; money.)* [neut. n.] argentum *(Ag = silver in Periodic Table.)* argentine Argentine Argentine Republic Argentina argent

arguo arguere argui argutus *(To prove, declare; accuse.)* [v.] argue argument argumentation argumentative argufy argumentum ad hominem *("Argument to the man"; based on emotion.)*

armo armare armavi armatum *(To arm, equip; rouse to arms.)* [v.] arms armed armament armor armory armada armadillo armature armet arms *(Weapons.)*

ars artis *(Skill, art; science, theory; virtue.)* [fem. n.] art artifact artificial artisan artist artistic

articulus articuli *(Joint, knuckle; clause; point.)* [masc. n.] articulate articulation article

audax audacis *(Bold, daring,; rash; audacious; proud.)* [adj.] audacious audacity

audio audire audivi auditus *(To hear; learn; listen.)* [v.] audio audience auditorium audible inaudible audit audition auditor auditory audio-visual

augeo augere auxi auctus *(To increase; enrich; praise.)* [v.] augment augmentation august August Augustus Caesar auction auctioneer author authority auxiliary

aurum auri *(Gold; gold plate, jewelry; money.)* [neut. n.] aurum *(Au = gold in the Periodic Table.)* auric aurous auriferous aureole Marcus Aurelius aureate oriole (OF)

avis avis *(Bird; omen.)* [fem. n.] aviate aviation aviator aviary avian aviculture auspices (F) auspicious

B

barba barbae *(Beard.)* [fem. n.] barb barber barbel *(Threadlike attachments to certain fish jaws.)*

bassus bassa bassum (Late Latin) *(Low.)* [adj.] base *(Vile.)* abase abasement debase debasement bass basso (It.) basso profundo bas-relief /bä-ri-lēf/ bassoon (F)

batuo batuere batui *(To beat.)* [v.] batter *(To beat.)* battle battery The Battery battalion abate abatement combat combatant combative debate debatable rebate

beatus beata beatum *(Happy; rich; blessed.)* [adj.] beatitude beatify beatification Beatrice

bello bellare bellavi bellatus *(To fight, wage war.)* [v.] bellicose belligerence belligerency belligerent ante-bellum rebel rebellion rebellious revel (OF) revelry

bellus bella bellum *(Pretty, handsome; pleasant.)* [adj.] embellish embellishment belle (F) Belle Isle belladonna (It.) Belvedere Belmont beau (OF) beauty beautiful beautician

bene *(Well; correctly; profitably; very.)* [adv.] benefit beneficial beneficiary benefactor benevolent benevolence benediction Benedict Benedictine

bini binae bina *(Two by two; a pair.)* [pl. adj.] binary binaural binoculars combine combination

bis *(Twice.)* [adv.] biceps bifocals bilingual bipolar bisect; See: **bi-** as prefix in Ap. iii-7.

bonitas bonitatis *(Goodness; honesty, integrity.)* [fem. n.] bounty bountiful bounteous

bonus bona bonum *(Good.)* [adj. positive.] bonus bona fide bon voyage (F) bonny bonanza (Sp.); **melior** *(Better.)* [adj. comparative.] meliorate ameliorate; **optimus** *(Best.)* [adj. superlative.] optimist optimism optimal optimum

bracchium bracchii *(An arm, a branch.)* [neut. n.] brace bracelet bracer brachial embrace

brevis brevis breve *(Short, small, shallow; brief; concise.)* [adj.] brevity breve breviary abbreviate abbreviation brief briefcase briefing abridge abridgment alla breve (It.)

bursa (Med. L.) *(A purse, a sack.)* [fem. n.] bursar bursarial bursary bursa bursitis disburse disbursement purse purser reimburse reimbursement

C

cado cadere cecidi casus *(To fall; die.)* [v.] case *(An instance.)* casual casualty casuist casuistry casus belli *(A cause justifying war.)* cadence (It.) cadenza chance (OF) cascade (F); **accido:** accident accidental; **decido:** decadent decadence deciduous decay (OF); **incido:** incident incidental incidentally incidence; **occido:** occasion occasional occasionally occasionalism occident occidental; **recido:** recidivism recidivist

caedo caedere cecidi caesus *(To cut; strike; kill.)* [v.] **-cide:** fratricide fungicide genocide germicide herbicide homicide infanticide insecticide matricide patricide pesticide spermicide suicide; **circumcido:** circumcise circumcision; **concido:** concise concision; **decido:** decide decision decisive; **excido:** excise excision; **incido:** incise incised incisive incisor incision; **praecido:** precise precisely precision; **recido:** recision

calor caloris *(Warmth, heat, glow.)* [masc. n.] calorie caloric calorimeter cauldron (AF)

calx calcis *(Pebble; lime, chalk; finishing line.)* [fem. n.] calcium calcify calcite calcimine calculate calculus calculation calculator chalk (OE)

camera camerae *(Vaulted room; arched roof.)* fem. n.] camera cameral chamber (F)

campus campi *(Plain; sports field; arena; theater.)* [masc. n.] camp campus campo (It.) campo (Sp.) campaign (F) champagne champion championship encamp encampment

cancelli cancellorum *(Grating, enclosure; barrier.)* [masc. pl. n.] cancel cancellation chancel (OF) chancellery chancellor chancery

cancer cancri *(Crab; tropical heat, south; cancer.)* [masc. n.] cancer cancerate cancroid Cancer *(A constellation, The Crab.)* Tropic of Cancer canker (AF) *(A sore.)* chancre /shang-ker/ (F)

candeo candere candui canditus *(To shine; be white hot.)* [v.] candle candor candelabra chandelier (F) candid candidate candidacy incandescence incandescent

cano canere cecini cantus *(Sing, play; recite.)* [v.] cantata cantor cantus firmus chant (OF) chanson (F) chantey accent accentuate descant enchant incantation incentive recant

capio capere cepi captus *(Take, capture.)* [v.] captive captor capture capable incapable capacity capacitance incapacitate cable case *(Box.)* casement encase encasement municipal participate emancipate; **accipio:** accept acceptance; **antecapio:** anticipate anticipation; **concipio:** concept conception conceptual conceive conceit; **decipio:** deceit deceive deception; **excipio:** except exception; **incipio:** inception incipient intercept interception; **occipio:** occupy occupant occupancy occupation occupational; **percipio:** perception perceptible perceptive perceptual perceive perceiver; **praecipio:** precept preceptor; **recipio:** reception receptionist receptive receptor receive receiver receipt recipe recipient recuperate; **suscipio:** susceptible susceptibility

caput capitis *(Head, top, extremity.)* [neut. n.] cap capital capitol capitalism capitalist capitalize decapitate captain caption capitulate recapitulate cape *(Land.)* da capo caput biceps triceps quadriceps chief (OF) chieftain mischief mischievous kerchief (ME) chapter (OF) achieve (OF) achievement precipice (F) precipitate precipitation precipitous

capra caprae *(She-goat.)* [fem. n.] caper caprice (It.) capriccio capriccioso capricious Capricorn *(A constellation, The Goat.)* Tropic of Capricorn capriole cabriole cabriolet cab

carbo carbonis *(Coal, embers.)* [masc. n.] carbon bicarbonate carbohydrate carbuncle

caro carnis *(Flesh.)* [fem. n.] carnal carnality carnage carnivore carnivorous carnival carnation carrion incarnate incarnation reincarnate reincarnation charnel (OF)

carpo carpere carpsi carptum *(Pick, pluck.)* [v.] carpet excerpt carpe diem *("Seize the day!")*

carrus carri *(Wagon.)* [masc. n.] carry career cargo charge (OF) chariot charioteer

carus cara carum *(Dear, beloved; costly.)* [adj.] caress charity (OF) charitable cherish cheer

castus casta castum *(Clean; innocent.)* [adj.] caste castigate incest chaste (OF) chastise chastity

causa causae *(Cause, reason.)* [fem. n.] cause causal causality causation causative accuse accused accusation accusative excuse excusable excusatory inexcusable

caveo cavere cavi cautus *(To beware of, guard against.)* [v.] caution cautious precautious incautious cautionary precautionary caveat caveat emptor *("Let the buyer beware!")*

cavus cavi *(Cavity, hole.)* [neut. n.] cave cavern cavity concave excavate excavation

cedo cedere cessi cessus *(Go; yield.)* [v.] cede cession; **abscedo:** abscess; **accedo:** accede access accessible; **antecedo:** antecede antecedent ancestor (OF) ancestry; **concedo:** concede concession concessionary; **decedo:** decedent decease deceased; **excedo:** exceed excess excessive; **intercedo:** intercede intercession; **praecedo:** precede preceding precedence; **procedo:** proceed proceeds procedure process procession; **recedo:** recede recess recession recessional; **secedo:** secede secession secessionism; **succedo:** succeed success successful succession successive successor

celebro celebare celebravi celebratus *(To crowd, frequent; repeat, practice; celebrate.)* [v.] celebrate celebration celebrated celebrity celebrant

celero celerare celeravi celeratus *(To quicken, hasten.)* [v.] celerity accelerate acceleration accelerator accelerando decelerate deceleration

censeo censere censui census *(Assess, take a census.)* [v.] censor census censure censorship

centum *(A hundred.)* [indeclinable number] century centennial centurion cent per cent centenarian centavo bicentennial tricentennial centimeter; See: **centi-** as prefix in Ap. iii-7.

cerebrum cerebri *(Brain; understanding.)* [neut. n.] cerebrum cerebellum cerebral cerebral palsy cerebrate cerebration cerebroside cerebrospinal

cerno cernere crevi cretus *(See, discern; separate.)* [v.] **concerno:** concern concerned concerning; **decerno:** decern decree (OF) **discerno:** discern discernible indiscernible discerning discreet indiscreet discretion indiscretion; **excerno:** excrete excretion excrement; **incerno:** increation; **secerno:** secret secrecy secrete secretion secretary

certus certa certum *(Certain, determined, definite.)* [adj.] certain certainly certainty certify certification certificate certified certitude incertitude ascertain

cesso cessare cessavi cessatus *(To stop; delay; rest.)* [v.] cease ceaseless ceaselessly cessation incessant incessantly

ceteri ceterae cetera *(The rest, the others.)* [pl. adj.] et cetera *(And the rest; and so forth.)* etc. (Abbr.) etceteras ceteris paribus *(Other things being equal.)* cet. par. (Abbr.)

charta chartae *(Sheet of paper; writing.)* [fem. n.] chart charter card cartel carton cartoon cartouche carte blanche /kart blänsh/ (F) *("White card," i.e. unrestricted authority.)* cartridge

cingo cingere cinxi cinctum *(To surround, enclose; gird.)* [v.] cincture cingulum precinct succinct succinctly surcingle

cinis cineris *(Ashes; ruins.)* [masc. n.] cinder cinerator incinerate incinerator

circa *(Approximately, about.)* [Prep. used before approximate date or figure.] *e.g.,* circa 1880

circum *(Around; surrounding.)* [prep.] <u>See:</u> **circum-** as prefix in Ap. iii-7: circumference, *etc.*

circus circi *(Circle; racecourse.)* [masc. n.] circle encircle circlet circular circulate circulation circulatory circus Circus Maximus *(Chariot arena in ancient Rome.)* search (OF) research

cis *(On this side of.)* [prep.] <u>See:</u> **cis-** as prefix in Ap. iii-7: cisalpine, cisatlantic, *etc.*

cito citare citavi citatus *(To rouse; call; appeal to.)* [v.] cite citation; **excito:** excite excitement excitable excitation excitant exciter excitor; **incito:** incite incitement; **recito:** recite recital recitation recitative; **resuscito:** resuscitate resuscitation

civis civis *(Citizen, fellow-citizen.)* [masc. & fem. n.] civic civics civil civilian civility civilization civilize civvies city (OF) city-state citified citizen (AF) citizenship citadel (It.)

clamo clamare clamavi clamatus *(To shout; call; proclaim.)* [v.] clamor clamorous claim (OF); **acclamo:** acclaim acclamation; **declamo:** declaim declamation disclaim (AF) disclaimer; **exclamo:** exclaim exclamation; **proclamo:** proclaim proclamation; **reclamo:** reclaim reclamation

clarus clara clarum *(Clear, bright, evident; famous.)* [adj.] clarity clarify clarification claret clarion declare declarative declaration clear (OF) clearly clearance clearing clerestory

classis classis *(Class, group.)* [fem. n.] class classic classical classicism classicist classify classified classification classy

claudo claudere clausi clausus *(Shut; conclude.)* [v.] clause claustrophobia; **concludo:** conclude conclusion; **excludo:** exclude exclusion exclusive; **includo:** include inclusion inclusive; **occludo:** occlude occlusion; **praecludo:** preclude preclusion; **recludo:** recluse reclusion; **secludo:** seclude secluded seclusion seclusive; close (OF)

clavis clavis *(Key.)* [fem. n.] clavichord clavier clavicle enclave exclave conclave clef (MF)

clemens clementis *(Mild, gentle, calm; merciful.)* [adj.] clement inclement clemency

clino clinare clinavi clinatus *(To lean, bend, tilt.)* [adj.] **declino:** decline declension declination declinometer; **inclino:** incline inclination disinclination; **reclino:** recline recliner

codex codicis *(Book, ledger; trunk; block of wood.)* [masc. n.] code codex codicil codify codification

cogito cogitare cogitavi cogitatus *(To think; ponder.)* [v.] cogitate cogitation excogitate cogito ergo sum *("I think, therefore I am."* Existence proof from <u>Meditations</u> by René Descartes.)

cognosco cognoscere cognovi cognitus *(To learn, understand; recognize.)* [v.] cognition cognitive cognizance cognize cognizant incognito precognition recognize recognition recognizance quaint (OF) acquaint acquainted acquaintance

collum colli *(Neck.)* [neut. n.] collar collaret collet colporteur (F) accolade decollate

colo colere colui cultus *(To cultivate, work; live in.)* [v.] cult culture cultural cultivate agriculture agriculturist subculture viniculture floriculture horticulture horticulturist

colonus coloni *(Farmer; colonist.)* [masc. n.] colony colonize colonist colonialism colonial

coloro colorare coloravi coloratus *(To give color to.)* [v.] color colored coloring colorist colorless colorable coloration colorful Colorado (Sp.) coloratura (It.)

columna columnae *(Column, pillar; pillory.)* [fem. n.] column columnar columnist colonnade (F) colonel /ker-nəl/ (It.)

com- *(With, together.)* [prefix] *(From preposition* **cum**.*)* <u>See</u>: **com-** (co-, col-, con-, cor-) in Ap. iii-8.

communis commune *(Common, general.)* [adj.] common commonalty commonplace commons commoner commonwealth commune communion community communicate communication communist excommunication communiqué (Fr) incommunicado (Sp.)

concilio conciliare conciliavi conciliatus *(Unite; win over, reconcile; bring about.)* [v.] conciliate conciliatory reconcile reconcilable reconciliation

congruo congruere congrui *(To coincide; correspond, suit; agree, sympathize.)* [v.] congruent congruity congruous incongruent incongruity incongruous

consulo consulere consului consultus *(To seek advice.)* [v.] consult consultant consultation consulting consul consulate

contra *(Against, opposite.)* [prep.] <u>See</u>: **contra-** as prefix in Ap. iii-9: contradiction, *etc.*

copia copiae *(Abundance, wealth.)* [fem. n.] copy copier copious cornucopia *(Horn of plenty.)*

copulo copulare copulavi copulatus *(To join; associate.)* [v.] copula copulate copulation copulative copulatory couple coupler couplet coupling

coquo coquere coxi coctus *(To cook, bake; parch; ripen.)* [v.] precocious concoct concoction decoct decoction biscuit (OF) *(Twice cooked.)* kitchen (OE)

cor cordis *(Heart.)* [neut. n.] cordial cordiality accord accordance accordant according accordingly concord concordance concordant core discord discordance discordant record recorder recording courage (OF) courageous encourage encouraging encouragement discourage discouraging discouragement accordion (It.)

cornu cornus *(Horn, horn-shaped.)* [neut. n.] cornet cornettist corner cornered cornea corneous unicorn Capricorn cornucopia corn *(Skin thickening.)*

corona coronae *(Garland, crown.)* [fem. n.] coronation coronet corona Corona Borealis coronal corolla corollary coroner *(Officer of the crown.)* coronary *(Encircling, e.g. heart arteries.)*

Ap. vii-8

corpus corporis *(Body; substance, flesh; corpse.)* [neut. n.] corpse corporeal incorporeal corporal corporal punishment corporation incorporation corporate incorporate incorporated corps /kor/ *(E.g., Marine Corps.)* corpuscle corpulent corpulence corpus corpus juris *(The body of law.)* corpus delicti *(The body of the offense, e.g., the victim's body.)* corpus callosum *("Hard body"; connects brain hemispheres.)* Corpus Christi corsage(OF) corset

costa costae *(Rib; side, wall.)* [fem. n.] costa costal intercostal accost coast (OF) coastal coastline coaster Costa Rica cutlet (F)

counter- *(Opposing, contrary.)* [Prefix: < **contra**] <u>See</u>: **counter-** in Ap. iii-26: counteract, *etc.*

credo credere credidi creditus *(To believe, trust, think.)* [v.] credo credible credence creed credit credential creditor accredit accreditation discredit incredible incredulous

cremo cremare cremavi crematus *(To burn, cremate.)* [v.] cremate crematory cremation

creo creare creavi creatus *(To create, produce, beget.)* [v.] create creation creative creator creature; **procreo:** procreate; **recreo:** recreate re-create recreation

crepo crepare crepui crepitus *(To rattle, creak; snap.)* [v.] crepitate crevice (OF) crevasse (F); **de + crepo:** decrepit decrepitate decrepitude; **discrepo:** discrepant discrepancy

cresco crescere crevi cretus *(To grow, thrive, increase.)* [v.] crescent crescendo (cresc.); **accresco:** accrescence accretion accrue (F) accrual **concresco:** concrete concretion concrescence concretize **decresco:** decrescent decrease (OF) decrescendo (decresc.); **excresco:** excrescent excrescence; **incresco:** increase (OF); **recresco:** recruit (F)

crimino criminare criminavi criminatus *(To accuse.)* [v.] crime criminal criminality criminology; **discrimino:** discriminate indiscriminate discriminating discrimination; **in + crimino:** incriminate incrimination; **re + crimino:** recriminate recrimination

crudus cruda crudum *(Rough; immature; bleeding.)* [adj.] crude crudely crudeness crudity recrudesce recrudescence crud (ME)

crux crucis *(Cross; gallows; torment.)* [fem. n.] crux Crux *(A constellation, Southern Cross.)* crucifix crucifixion crucify crucial crucible crusade excruciate excruciating cruise (Du.) cruiser

cubo cubare cubui cubitus *(To recline.)* [v.] incubate incubation incubator incubus; **incumbo** *(To lean on.)*: incumbent; **procumbo** *(To lean forward.)*: procumbent

culmen culminis *(Top, roof, summit; height; acme.)* (neut. n.) culminate culmination culminant

culpa culpae *(Blame, fault; mischief.)* [fem. n.] culpa culpable culprit inculpate inculpable exculpate exculpation exculpatory mea culpa *(My fault.)*

cum *(With, together.)* [prep.] cum grano salis *(With a grain of salt; with reservation.)* cum laude *(With praise.)* <u>See</u>: **com- (co-, col-, con-, cor-)** as prefixes in Ap. iii-8 complex, *etc.*

cumulo cumulare cumulavi cumulatus *(To heap up, amass.)* [v.] cumulate cumulation cumulative cumulus cumulous cumuliform cumulonimbus cumulocirrus cumulostratus accumulate accumulation

curo curare curavi curatus *(To take care of.)* [v.] cure curable incurable curator curious curiosity curio; **accuro:** accurate accuracy; **procuro:** procure procurement procurance; sinecure *("Without care"; an office with few duties.)* secure *("Without care.")* security manicure *(Manus = hand.)* pedicure *(Pes, pedis = foot.)* sure (OF) assure assurance

curro currere cucurri cursum *(To run, hasten; fly.)* [v.] current currency curriculum cursive cursory; **concurro:** concur concurrence concurrent; **decurro:** decurrent; **discurro:** discursive; **excurro:** excursive excursion: **incurro:** incur incursion; **intercurro:** intercurrent; **occurro:** occur occurrence; **praecurro:** precursor precursory; **recurro:** recur recurrence recurrent; **succurro:** succor; course (MF) concourse discourse intercourse recourse courier (MF) courante (F) corridor (It.) corsair (MF)

curtus curta curtum *(Short, broken off; incomplete.)* [adj.] curt curtail curtal curtate

custodio custodire cutodivi custoditus *(To guard, defend.)* [v.] custody custodial custodian

D

damno damnare damnavi damnatus *(To condemn, sentence.)* [v.] damn damnable damnation damndest damned damage condemn condemnation indemnity indemnify

de *(Down from; away from.)* [prep.] <u>See</u>: **de-** as prefix in Ap. iii-9: decline delude demerit, *etc.*

debeo debere debui debitus *(To owe; ought, should, must.)* [v.] debt debtor debit debenture indebted indebtedness devoirs (OF)

decem *(Ten.)* [Indeclinable adj.] December (Dec.) Decembrist decemvirate decade (Gk.) dean (OF) *(Head of ten men.)* deanery; <u>See</u>: prefixes L **dec-** Ap. iii-10 & Gk. **deca-** in Ap. iii-23.

decens decentis *(Seemly, proper; comely, handsome.)* [adj.] decent decency indecent indecency

decimus decima decimum *(The tenth.)* [adj.] decibel, *etc.* dime (OF); <u>See</u>: **deci-** Ap. iii-10.

decoro decorare decoravi decoratus *(To adorn, embellish.)* [v.] decorate decoration decorative decorator decorous decorum décor (F)

delecto delectare delectavi delectatus *(To charm.)* [v.] delectable delight (OF) delightful

delicatus delicata delicatum *(Pleasing; dainty.)* [adj.] delicate indelicate delicacy delicious

deleo delere delevi deletus *(To destroy, annihilate; erase.)* [v.] delete deletion delible indelible dele *(In editing: "Take out.")*

deliro delirare deliravi deliratus *(To be crazy; rave.)* [v.] delirious delirium deliration *(Mental derangement.)* delirium tremens *("Trembling delirium.")*

dens dentis *(Tooth; ivory; prong.)* (masc. n.) dentist dentistry denture dentine dental dentoid dentil denticle indent indentation indenture indentured trident dent *(Toothlike part.)*

densus -a -um *(Thick, dense, close.)* [adj.] dense density condense condensation condenser

desidero desiderare desideravi desideratus *(To desire.)* [v.] desire desirable desirous desiderate *(To feel the lack of.)* desideratum /di-sid-ə-rā-təm/ *(Something needed or desired.)*

destino destinare destinavi destinatus *(To appoint, determine, resolve; aim at.)* [v.] destine destiny destined destination Destinies predestine predestination predestinate

deterior deterioris *(Lower; inferior, worse.)* [adj.] deteriorate deterioration

deus dei *(A god.)* [masc. n.] deity deist deism deify Dei gratia *(By the grace of God.)* Deus vobiscum *(God be with you.)*   Te Deum laudamus *(We praise thee, O God.)* deus ex machina   /dē-əs eks mak-ə-nə/   adieu (F) /ə-dōō/ *("To God" I commend you.)*

dexter dextri *(Right, right-hand; handy, skillful.)* [adj.] dexter dexterity dexterous dextral dextrose dextrorse ambidextrous *(Ambi- = both.)* ambidexter

dico dicare dicavi dicatus *(To dedicate; make known; accuse.)* [v.] **abdico:** abdicate abdication; **dedico:** dedicate dedication; **indico:** indicate indication indicative indict /in-dīt/ indictment; **praedico:** predicament predicate predicable predication preach (OF) preacher

dico dicere dixi dictus *(To say, speak, tell; plead.)* [v.] dictate diction dictation dictionary dictum dictator; **addico:** addict addiction addictive; **condico:** condition conditional conditioner; **contradico:** contradict contradiction contradictory; **edico:** edict; **interdico:** interdict interdiction; **praedico:** predict prediction predictor; benediction (Bene = *good.*)   Benedict;   jurisdiction (Jus, juris = *law.*);   malediction (Malus = *bad.*); verdict (Veritas = *truth.*);   valedictory (Vale = *farewell.*) valedictorian; ditto (It.)

dies diei *(Day.)* [masc. & fem. n.] **diurnus diurna diurnum** *(Daily.)* [adj.] dial diary diurnal meridian per diem *(By the day.)* dismal (Dies mali, *evil days.*) carpe diem *("Seize the day!")* Dies Irae *(Day of Wrath.)*

digitus digiti *(Finger; toe; inch.)* [masc. n.] digit digital digitalis digitate prestidigitation (F)

dis- *(Apart, away from; reverse; loss of; not.)* [pref.] disable distrust, *etc.* See: **dis-** in Ap. iii-10.

disco discere didici *(To learn, be taught, be told.)* [v.]   disciple   discipline   disciplinarian

divido dividere divisi divisus *(To divide; distribute.)* [v.] divide dividend division divisor divisible divisive indivisible individual individuality devise (OF) device divvy (sl.)

divinus divina divinum *(Divine.)* [adj.] divine divination Divine Comedy *(Poem by Dante.)*

do dare dedi datus *(To give, permit, grant; put; make.)* [v.] date dated dateless datum data; **addo:** add addendum addition additional additive; **edo** (ex-): edit edition editor editorial; **perdo:** perdition; **reddo** (re-): reddition render (F) rendition surrender (AF) rendezvous (F) /rän-dā-vōō/; **trado** (trans-): tradition extradite treason (OF) traitor betray (ME)

doceo docere docui doctus *(To teach; inform, tell.)* [v.] docent docile doctor doctorate doctrine doctrinal doctrinaire document documentary documentation indoctrinate

dono donare donavi donatus *(To present, bestow; remit.)* [v.] donate donation donor donee   condone   pardon (OF) (par- = *per-.*)

doleo dolere dolui dolitus *(To suffer, grieve, pain.)* [v.] doleful dolor dolorimetry dolorous doloroso (It.) Via Dolorosa *("Sorrowful Way.")* condolence indolence indolent

domo domare domui domitus *(To tame, break in; conquer.)* [v.] domain dominate domination domineer dominance dominion dominium domino *(A hood.)* predominate indomitable   Anno Domini (A.D.) *("In the year of our Lord.")*

domus domi *(House, home; native place; family.)* [fem. n.] domestic domesticate domesticity   domicile   dome   major-domo (Sp.) *("Chief of the house," the head butler.)*

dormio dormire dormivi dormitus *(To sleep, be asleep.)* [v.] dormant dormancy dormitory   dorm   dormer   dormouse

dorsum dorsi *(The back.)* [neut. n.] dorsal *(E.g., dorsal fin.)* dorsum dorsiferous dorsiventral   dorsoventral   endorse (OF) *("On back.")*   endorsement   endorsee

dubito dubitare dubitavi dubitatus *(To doubt, hesitate.)* [v.] dubious dubitable indubitable   doubt (OF)   doubtful   doubtless   Doubting Thomas

duco ducere duxi ductus *(To lead, guide; draw; consider.)* [v.] duct ductile; **abduco:** abduct abduction; **adduco:** adduct adductor; **conduco:** conduce conducive conduct conduction conductance conductive conductivity conductor conduit; **deduco:** deduce deduct deduction deductive; **educo:** educe educt education educate educated educator educational; **induco:** induct inductance inductee inductile induction inductive inductivity inductor; **introduco:** introduce introduction introductory; **produco:** produce producer product production productive productivity reproduce reproduction reproductive; **reduco:** reduce reducer reduction reductio ad absurdum (In Logic: *"Reduction to absurdity."*) **seduco:** seduce seduction seductive; **subduco:** subduce subduction; **traduco:** traduce traduction; aqueduct viaduct douche (F)

duo duae duo *(Two.)* [adj.]   **secundus** *(Second.)* duo dual dualism duality duel (It.)   duet (It.);   See: **secundus** in Ap. vii-38 and **duo-** as prefix in Ap. iii-11.

duplex duplicis *(Double.)* [adj.]   duple duplicate duplication duplicator duplicity

durus dura durum *(Hard, harsh, rough; hardy, tough.)* [adj.] durable durance endurance dure endure during enduring duress indurate obdurate obduracy duro (Sp.) *(Silver dollar.)*

dux ducis *(Guide, leader, ruler.)* (masc. & fem. n.)   duke duchess duchy ducal ducat duce (It.) /dōō-chä/   il Duce *("The leader," Benito Mussolini.)*   See: **duco** on this page.

E
ego *(I, the self.)* [pron.] ego egotism egotist egoistic egocentric egomania egomaniac

elementum elementi *(Element; pl. first principles.)* [neut. n.] element   Table of Elements elemental   elementary   elementary school

emo emere emi emptus *(To buy, procure; win over.)* [v.] caveat emptor *("Let the buyer beware.")* adeem exempt exemption preempt preemption redemption premium prompt prompter emporium (Gk.) example (OF) *exemplar exemplary exempli gratia (e.g.)* *(By way of example.)* sample (OF) sampling sampler redeem (OF) redeemable redeeming ransom (OF)

en- *(In, into.)* [Old French form of Latin *in*; used to form verbs.] enclose;   See: **en-** in Ap. iii-26.

eo ire ivi itus *(To go, move; march; pass; proceed.)* [v.] **adeo:** adit; **ambio:** ambience ambition ambitious; **circueo:** circuit circuitry; **exeo:** exit **ineo:** initial initiate initiation; **obeo:** obituary; **pereo:** perish; **praeeo:** preterition; **transeo:** transit transient transition transitory; introit (F) trance (OF) entrance sudden (OF) sedition (F)

erro errare erravi erratus *(To wander, stray; waver.)* [v.] err erring error erroneous erratic errant errancy erratum   errare humanum est *("To err is human.")* aberrant aberration

ex *(Out of, from; lacking; former.)* [prep.]   See: **ex-** as prefix in Ap. iii-11: exclude export, *etc.*

exerceo exercere exercui exercitus *(To train, exercise.)* [v.] exercise exercised exerciser

experior experiri expertus *(To test, try; experience.)* [v.] experience experienced experiment experimental experimentalism experimentation expert expertise (F)

exter exterus *(From outside; foreign.)* [adj.] exterior external externalize exteroceptor

extra *(Outside, beyond.)* [prep.]   See: **extra-** as prefix in Ap. iii-12:   extraterrestrial, *etc.*

extremus extrema extremum *(Outermost, extreme, last.)* [adj.] extreme extremely extremism extremity extremist   extreme unction *(An anointing before death.)*

F

faber fabri *(Workman, craftsman, tradesman, artisan.)* [masc. n.] fabric fabricant fabricate fabrication prefab prefabrication prefabricate

fabula fabulae *(Story, drama, fable.)* [fem. n.] fable fabled fabulous confab confabulate

facies faciei *(Form, shape; face, looks; aspect.)* [fem. n.] face facial façade (F) deface defacement efface effacement enface enfacement surface surfacing superficial

facio facere feci factus *(To make, do; create; cause.)* [v.] fact factual factor faction factional facile facility facilitate factory faculty; **adficio:** affect affection affectionate; **conficio:** confect confection; **deficio:** defect defection defective defector deficient deficiency deficit; **efficio:** effect effective effectual efficacious efficacy efficient efficiency; **inficio:** infect infection infectious; **perficio:** perfect imperfect perfection imperfection perfectionist perfectly; **praeficio:** prefect prefecture; **proficio:** proficient proficiency; **reficio:** refectory; **sufficio:** suffice sufficient sufficiency; benefit beneficial beneficiary benefactor; malefactor *(Malus = bad.)* malfeasance (AF); artifact artifice artificial edifice *(Aedes = building.)* edification difficult *("Away from easy.")* difficulty satisfy *(Satis = enough.)* satisfaction satisfactory manufacture *(Manus = hand.)* facsimile *("Make like.")* fiat *(Let it be done.)* ipso facto *(By the fact itself.)*   See: suffixes **-fy** and **-fication** in Ap. iv-32.

fallo fallere fefelli falsus *(To deceive, cheat, betray.)* [v.] fallacy fallacious fallible infallible false falsehood falsify falsification fail (OF) failing failure fault (OF) default faultless   faulty   falsetto (It.)   faux pas (F) /fō-pä/ *("False step," mistake.)*

fama famae *(Talk, rumor; reputation, fame.)* [fem. n.] fame famous infamous infamy defame defamation defamatory

familia familiae *(Family; school.)* [fem. n.] family familial familiar familiarity familiarize

fanum fani *(Sanctuary.)* [neut. n.] fane *(Temple.)* profane profanity fanatic fanatical fanaticism

farior fari fatus *(To speak.)* [v.] affable effable ineffable preface infant infancy infantile infantilism infantry infantryman   infantile paralysis (Gk.) *(Poliomyelitis, polio.)*

fateor fateri fassus *(To confess, acknowledge; witness.)* [v.] confess confession confessional confessor profess profession professional professor professorial

fatum fati *(Divine word, divine will; fate, doom.)* [neut. n.] fate fated fateful fairy (OF)

femina feminae *(Female, woman.)* [fem. n.] female feminine femininity feminism feminist feminize effeminate effeminacy   femme fatale (F)

fendo fendere fendi fensus *(To strike, hit.)* [v.] fend fender fence fencing defend defendant defense defensible defensive indefensible offend offense offensive

fero ferre tuli latus *(To bear, carry, bring; produce.)* [v.] fertile fertility fertilization fertilize fertilizer; **adfero:** afferent; **circumfero:** circumference; **confero:** confer conference; **defero:** defer deference deferment; **differo:** differ difference different differential differentiate; **effero:** efferent; **infero:** infer inference; **offero:** offer offering offertory; **praefero:** prefer preferable preference preferential; **profero:** proffer; **refero:** refer reference referendum referent; **suffero:** suffer sufferable sufferance; **transfero:** transfer transference; **latus:** ablation ablative; collate collation; delate delation; elate elation; illation illative; oblate oblation; prelate; prolate; relate related relation relational relationship relative relativism relativity; correlate correlation; translate translation translator; legislator *(Lex, legis = law.)*

ferveo fervere ferbui fervus *(To boil, rage.)* [v.] fervent fervid fervor effervescence

fido fidere fisus *(To trust; rely on.)* [v.] fidelity fiduciary affiant affiance affidavit confide confidant confidence confident confidential diffident diffidence infidel infidelity perfidy perfidious   bona fide *(In good faith.)*   federal (F) federalism federalize federalist confederate Confederacy confederation faith (OF) faithful

figo figere fixi fixus *(To fasten, attach; pierce.)* [v.] fix fixate fixation fixings fixture affix affixture infix prefix suffix   traffic (It.)   idée fixe /ē-dā fēks/ (F) *(A fixed idea.)*

filium fili *(Thread, string.)* [neut. n.] file *(Line.)* filament profile filigree (F) filet /fī-lā/

filius filii *(Son.)* [masc. n.] filial filiate filiation affiliate affiliation

figura figurae *(Shape, form; nature, kind.)* [fem. n.] figure figured figurine effigy figment figurant figurative transfigure Transfiguration

fingo fingere finxi fictus *(To form, shape; mold, model.)* [v.] fiction fictional fictionalize fictitious feign (OF) /fān/ feigned faint feint (F) /fānt/

finis finis *(Border; end, limit; summit; death; aim.)* [masc. n.] final finale finalist finally fine fine (It.) /fē-nā/ *(In music: the end.)* finish finite infinite infinitive infinitesimal fineness finery finable finance (OF) financial financier finesse (F); affined affinity; confine confined confinement; define definition definite definitive; refine refinement refinery

Ap. vii-14

firmo firmare firmavi firmatus *(To strengthen; support.)* [v.] firm *(Strong; a business.)* firmament farm (F) farmer; **adfirmo:** affirm reaffirm affirmation reaffirmation affirmative; **confirmo:** confirm confirmation; **infirmo:** infirm infirmity infirmary

fiscus fisci *(Purse; treasury.)* [masc. n.] fisc *(The treasury of a state.)* fiscal confiscate confiscatory

flagro flagrare flagravi flagatus *(To blaze, burn.)* [v.] flagrant conflagration conflagrant

flecto flectere flexi flexus *(To bend, turn; persuade.)* [v.] flex flexible flexion flexor flexuous flexure; **deflecto:** deflect deflection; **inflecto:** inflect inflection inflexible; **reflecto:** reflect reflection reflector reflex reflexive

fligo fligere flictus *(To strike, dash down.)* [v.] **adfligo:** afflict affliction; **confligo:** conflict conflictive; **infligo:** inflict infliction; **profligo:** profligate profligacy

flo flare flavi flatus *(To blow.)* [v.] flatus flatulence afflatus conflate conflation deflate deflation deflationary inflate inflation inflationary sufflate sufflation

floreo florere florui *(To blossom, flower; flourish.)* [v.] flower flowered floweret floral florist florid floriated floriculture florescence floruit *(He flourished.)* Florida Florence florin flour (Var. flower.) floury flourish flourishing efflorescence efflorescent

fluo fluere fluxi fluxus *(To flow; overflow; drip.)* [v.] fluid flume fluent fluency fluctuate fluctuation flush flux; **adfluo:** affluent affluence afflux; **confluo:** confluent confluence conflux; **defluo:** defluxion; **effluo:** effluent effluence efflux; **influo:** influence influential influx; **profluo:** profluent profluence; **refluo:** refluent refluence reflux; **superfluo:** superfluent superfluid superfluity superfluous

focus foci *(Hearth, fire-place.)* [masc. n.] focus (Pl. foci) focal focalize fuel (OF) fusil fusillade

folium folii *(Leaf.)* [neut. n.] foliage foliate foliation folio portfolio foil trefoil tinfoil

foras *(Out, outside.)* [adv.] foreign (F) foreigner forest (OF) forestry forester forestation afforest deforest reforest foreclose foreclosure forfeit forfeiture; See: **fore-** Ap. iii-2.

formo formare formavi formatus *(To shape, fashion, form.)* [v.] form formal formality format formation formative formula; **conformo:** conform conformable conformation; **deformo:** deform deformation deformed deformity; **informo:** inform informed informer information informative informant informal informality; **performo:** perform performance performer; **reformo:** reform reformation Reformation reformed reformatory; **transformo:** transform transformation transformer unformed uniform uniformed uniformity malformed pro forma *(As a matter of form.)*

foro forare foravi foratus *(To pierce; bore.)* [v.] foramen *(An opening.)* foramen magnum *(Skull opening for spinal cord.)* perforate perforated perforation

fors fortis *(Luck, chance.)* [fem. n.] fortune fortunate fortuitous misfortune unfortunate

fortis forte *(Strong, sturdy, brave, manly.)* [adj.] fort fortification fortify fortitude fortress comfort comfortable comforter effort effortless force (F) forceful forcible enforce forte (It.) /fŏr-tā/ *(In music: loud.)* fortissimo pianoforte *("The soft-loud" instrument; the piano.)*

frango frangere fregi fractus *(To break, shatter; crush.)* [v.] fraction fractional fractious fracture diffract diffraction infract infraction refract refraction fragile fragment

frater fratris *(Brother; ally.)* [masc. n.] frater fraternity fraternal fraternize friar

frico fricare fricui fricatus *(To rub, chafe.)* [v.] friction frictional fricative dentifrice

frons frontis *(Forehead, brow; front, façade.)* [fem. n.] front frontal frontage frontier affront confront confrontation effrontery

fugio fugere fugi fugitus *(To flee, run away, escape.)* [v.] fugitive fugacious refuge refugee subterfuge fugue (It.) fugal centrifugal centrifuge (F) tempus fugit *(Time flies.)*

fundo fundare fundavi fundatus *(To establish; secure.)* [v.] fund fundamental fundament fundamentalism fundus found founder foundation profound profundity

fundo fundere fudi fusus *(To pour, shed, spill; cast.)* [v.] fuse fusible fusion; **adfundo:** affusion; **confundo:** confound confuse confusion; **diffundo:** diffuse diffusion; **effundo:** effuse effusion effusive; **infundo:** infuse infusion; **profundo:** profuse profusion; **refundo:** refund refuse refusal; **suffundo:** suffuse suffusion; **superfundo:** superfuse superfusion; **transfundo:** transfuse transfusion

fungor fungi functus *(To perform, do; discharge.)* [v.] function functional functionary functionalism defunct dysfunction dysfunctional malfunction perfunctory

futilis futile *(Worthless.)* [adj.] futile futility futilitarian

G
gelo gelare gelavi gelatus *(To freeze.)* [v.] gelatine gelation gelatinous gelid congeal congelation jell jelly jellied Jello

genero generare generavi generatus *(To procreate, breed.)* [v.] generate degenerate ingenerate regenerate generation degeneration regeneration generative generator

gens gentis *(Clan, family, race, tribe.)* [fem. n.] gentle genteel (MF) gentility gentile Gentile

genus generis *(Birth, descent, race, kind, class.)* [neut. n.] genus (Pl. genera.) general generality generalization generalize generally generic gender engender generous generosity gens ingenuous disingenuous genre (F) /zhän-r/

gero gerere gessi gestus *(To carry on, do.)* [v.] gesture gestate gestation gesticulation congest congestion congestive digest digestion digestible ingest ingestion suggest suggestion suggestible register registrar registration registry belligerent

gigno gignere genui genitus *(To beget, produce.)* [v.] genius genial congenial genitive genitals ingenious ingenuity progeny primogeniture engine (OF) engineer engineering

gradior gradi gressus *(To step, walk, go, move.)* [v.] grade gradation gradient gradual graduate graduation aggressor aggression aggressive congress congressional congressman degrade degradation degree degression digress digression digressive egress ingress ingredient progress progression progressive transgress transgression

granum grani *(Seed, grain.)* [neut. n.] granule granular granulate granary granulose grange Grange granite granivorous garner garnet pomegranate (OF) (Pome = *fruit.*)

grandis grandis grande *(Large, great, grand, strong; tall; old.)* [adj.] grand grandiose grandeur (F) grandiloquent aggrandize aggrandizement grandparent grandmother (OE) grandfather (OE) Rio Grande (Sp.) Grand Canyon Grand Prix (F) *(Grand prize.)* grand mal (F)

gratus grata gratum *(Pleasing, welcome.)* [adj.] grateful gratification gratify gratis gratitude gratuity congratulate congratulations ingrate ingratiate ingratitude grace (OF) graceful agree (OF) agreeable agreement con grazia (It.) (Music: *with grace.*)

gravitas gravitatis *(Weight; seriousness.)* [fem. n.] grave *(Important.)* gravity gravitate gravitation gravamen aggravate aggravation grief (OF) grieve grievance grievous

grex gregis *(Flock, herd.)* [masc. n.] gregarious congregate congregation congregational aggregate segregate segregation segregationist desegregate desegregation egregious

gusto gustare gustavi gustatus *(To taste, enjoy.)* [v.] gustatory gusto (It.) disgust

H

habeo habere habui habitus *(To have, hold; keep.)* [v.] habit habitual; **adhibeo:** adhibit; **exhibeo:** exhibit; **inhibeo:** inhibit; **prohibeo:** prohibit

habilis habilis habile *(Manageable, handy; suitable.)* [adj.] able (OF) unable debility debilitate disable disabled ability disability habilitate rehabilitate rehabilitation

habito habitare habitavi habituatus *(To dwell; remain.)* [v.] habitable habitant habitat habitation inhabit inhabitant inhabitancy inhabited cohabit cohabitation

halo halare halavi halatus *(To breathe; give off scent.)* [v.] exhale exhalation exhalant inhale inhalation inhalant inhalator halitosis *(Bad breath; Gk. -osis = condition.)*

haereo haerere haesivi haesitus *(To cling, stick.)* [v.] **adhaereo:** adhere adherence adherent adhesion adhesive; **cohaereo:** cohere coherence coherent cohesion cohesive; **haesito:** hesitate hesitation hesitant hesitancy; **inhaereo:** inhere inherent inherence

heres heredis *(Heir, heiress; successor.)* [masc. n.] heir heirloom heiress heredity hereditary inherit inheritable inheritor

homo hominus *(Human being, man; pl. people.)* [masc. & fem. n.] Homo sapiens *("Wise man.")* homicide (Caedere = *to kill.*) homicidal homage hombre (Sp.); See: Ap. ix-9, Gk. **homo-** *(Same.)*

honor honoris *(Honor, esteem; award; position.)* [masc. n.] honor honorable honorary honorarium honest (OF) honesty honestly

horreo horrere horui *(To shiver, shudder, tremble.)* [v.] horror horrible horrid horrify horrendous abhor abhorrence abhorrent

hospes hospities *(Host, hostess; guest, friend.)* [masc. n.] hospice hospitable hospitality hospital hospitalize hospitalization Hospitaler host hostess hostel hotel (F)

humanus humana humanum *(Human; humane, kind.)* [adj.] human inhuman humane inhumane human being humanity humanism humanist humanize humankind humanly humanitarian humanitarianism humanum est errare *("To err is human.")*

humilis humilis humile *(Low; humble; poor.)* [adj.] humility humiliate humiliation humble

humus humi *(Earth, ground, land.)* [fem. n.] humus exhume exhumation inhume inhumation

I

ibidem *(In the same place in the work or chapter just mentioned.)* [adv.] ibidem (Abbr. ibid.)

idem eadem idem *(The same.)* [pron.] identical identity identify identic identification (ID)

imago imaginis *(Likeness, picture, statue; ghost.)* [fem. n.] image imagery imagine imaginable unimaginable imaginary imagination imago

imitor imitari imitatus *(To copy, portray; imitate.)* [v.] imitate imitation imitative imitator inimitable *(Cannot be imitated.)*

impero imperare imperavi imperatus *(To rule, command.)* [v.] imperative imperious imperial imperialism imperialist empire (F) emperor

in *(Not.)* [prep.] Underline: See: **in-** as prefix in Ap. iii-12: incorrect; Also: OE **in-** *(in)*, Ap. iii-2: inside.

index indicis *(Forefinger; witness, informer; title.)* [masc. n.] index Index index finger (OE) indices indicia Related to: **indico:** indicate, indication *(To point.)*; See: **dico**, Ap. vii-11.

infernus inferna infernum *(That which comes from below.)* [adj.] infernal inferno (It.) Inferno

inferus infera inferum *(Low, below.)* [adj.] inferior inferiority inferiority complex

infra *(Below, beneath.)* [prep.] See: **infra-** as prefix in Ap. iii-15: infrared

initio initiare initiavi initiatus *(To initiate, begin.)* [v.] initial initiate initiation initiative commence (OF) commencement

insula insulae *(Island; block of houses.)* [fem. n.] insular insulate insulation insulator peninsula (Paene = *almost.*) peninsular isolate (It.) isolation isolationism isolationist

intellego intellegere intellexi intellectus *(To understand, learn.)* [v.] intelligence intelligent intellectual intellect intelligentsia intelligible intelligibility intelligence quotient (I.Q.)

integer integra integrum *(Whole, complete, intact.)* [adj.] integer integral integrity integrate integration entire (OF) entirely

inter *(Between, among, amid.)* [prep.] See: **inter-** as prefix in Ap. iii-15: interact interrupt

internus interna interum *(Inward, internal; domestic, civil.)* [adj.] internal internality intern

intra *(Within, inside.)* [prep.] See: **intra-** as prefix in Ap. iii-15: intramural intravenous

intro *(Inwards; within.)* [adv.] See: **intro-** as prefix in Ap. iii-15: introduction introvert

J <u>Note</u>: There was no *j* in classical Latin. In the 17th century copyists added a lower stroke to the initial *i* that sounded /y/. This accounts for the two "dotted" letters, *i* & *j*, being adjacent in our modern English alphabet. The following words beginning with *j* here are spelled with *i* in Latin dictionaries.

jacio jacere jeci jactus *(To throw, hurl, cast.)* [v.] **abicio** (abjacio): abject; **adicio** (adjacio): adjective *("Added to.")*: **conjecto:** conjecture conjectural; **deicio** (dejacio): deject dejected dejection; **eicio** (exjacio): eject ejection ejector; **inicio** (injacio): inject injection; **intericio** (interjacio): interject interjection; **obicio** (objacio): object objection objective objectivity objectify objectionable objectless; **proicio** (projacio): project projection projector projectionist projectile; **reicio:** (rejacio) reject rejection rejectamenta; **subicio** (subjacio): subject *(Topic; to control.)* subjection subjective subjectivism; **traicio** (transjacio): traject trajection trajectory; introjection jet (F) jetty jettison jut

judico judicare judicavi judicatus *(To judge, condemn.)* [v.] judge judicatory judicial judicate judiciary judicator judicious judgment (Or: judgement.) adjudicate adjudication prejudge prejudice prejudicial injudicious

jugum jugi *(Yoke, collar.)* [neut. n.] conjugate conjugation conjugal subjugate subjugation jugular (< **jugulum**, *collar bone.*)

jungo jungere junxi junctus *(To join, unite, harness.)* [v.] juncture junction adjunct conjuncture conjunctivitis disjunct disjunction disjunctive injunction subjunctive join (OF) joint conjoin conjoint disjoin disjoint disjointed

juro jurare juravi juratus *(To swear, take an oath.)* [v.] abjure abjuration adjure adjuration conjure conjuration perjure perjured perjury ipso jure *(By the law itself.)*

jus juris *(Law, right, justice.)* [neut. n.] just justice jury justifiable justification justify jurisdiction injure injurious injury injustice adjust adjustment

juvenalis juvenalis juvenale *(Youthful.)* [adj.] **juvenis juvenis** *(Young.)* **junior** [adj. comp.] juvenile juvenilia juvenility rejuvenate rejuvenation junior junior varsity (J.V.)

juxta *(Close by; near.)* [prep. & adv.] <u>See</u>: **juxta-** as prefix in Ap. iii-15: juxtaposition

L

labor labi lapsus *(To slide, glide; sink, fall; slip.)* [v.] lapse collapse elapse prolapse relapse lapsus linguae *(A slip of the tongue.)* lapsus memoriae *(A slip of the memory.)*

laboro laborare laboravi laboratus *(To work, toil; suffer.)* [v.] labor labored laborer laborious laboratory collaborate collaboration collaborationist elaborate elaboration

laedo laedere laesi laesus *(To hurt, strike, wound.)* [v.] collide collision elide elision

langueo languere *(To be weary, be weak, be sick, droop.)* [v.] languid languish languishing languor languorous

lapis lapidis *(Stone; milestone; tombstone; marble.)* [masc. n.] lapidary lapidate lapidify lapillus dilapidate dilapidated dilapidation lapis lazuli *("Azure stone.")*

latus lata latum *(Broad, wide; extensive.)* [adj.] latitude latitudinal dilate dilation

latus lateris *(Side.)* (neut. n.) lateral bilateral collateral equilateral quadrilateral unilateral

laudo laudare laudavi laudatus *(To praise, commend, approve.)* [v.] laud laudable laudatory allow (OF) allowable allowance allowedly

lavo lavare lavi lautus *(To wash, bathe; soak.)* [v.] lava lavatory lavender Lavabo *(Ritual hand washing.)* lavage lave laver lavish launder (OF) laundress laundromat laundry lotion

laxo laxare laxavi laxatus *(Open up; undo.)* [v.] lax laxity laxative Exlax relax relaxation

lego legare legavi legatus *(To send, charge, commission.)* [v.] legate legation legacy allege allegedly allegation delegate delegation elegant elegance relegate

lego legere legi lectus *(To gather; choose, select; read.)* [v.] legible illegible legend legendary lecture lecturer lector lectionary lectern legion legionnaire (F) college collegiate collect collection collective colleague elect election electioneer elective elector electoral electorate eligible eligibility intelligent intelligence intelligible neglect neglectful negligence negligent negligible prelect prelection prelector select selectee selection selective selectivity selectman selector legume (F) elite (F);   See: **intellego** Ap. vii-18.

levo levare levavi levatus *(To raise up; make light.)* [v.] lever leverage levee levy levitate levity leaven (OF) alleviate elevate elevation elevator relevant relevance relief (OF) relieve

lex legis *(Law, statute; rule, principle.)* [fem. n.] legal legalism legality legalize legist legit legislate legislation legislative legislator legislature legitimate legitimacy legitimize lex illegal illegality illegitimate illegitimacy loyal (OF) loyalty loyalist privilege (OF)

liber libri *(Book, register; bark of tree.)* [masc. n.] library librarian libretto (It.) librettist libel (< **libellus** diminutive of **liber**.) libeler libelee libelant libelous ex libris *(From the books of.)*

libero liberare liberavi liberatus *(To free, release.)* [v.] liberty liberate liberal liberalism liberality libertarian illiberal livery (OF) deliver delivery deliverance ad libitum *(At will.)*

libra librae *(Balance; scale.)* [fem. n.] librate libration libratory deliberate deliberation

licet licere licuit licitus *(It is permitted.)* [v.] licit illicit license licensee licentiate licentious leisure (OF)

ligo ligare ligavi ligatus *(To fasten, bind; unite.)* [v.] ligament ligature colligate oblige obligee obligatory obligate obligation obbligato (It.) religion religious religiosity league (OF) lien (F) liaison (F) /lē-ā-zon/ liable (F) liability ally (OF) allies alliance alloy (F) rally (F)

limen liminis *(Threshold, doorway.)* (neut. n.) limen eliminate elimination preliminary prelims sublime subliminal *("Under the threshold" of consciousness.)* sublimate sublimation

limes limitis *(Boundary; path, track, way.)* [masc. n.] limit limitation limited limiting limitless delimit lintel (OF)

linea lineae *(Thread; line.)* [fem. n.] **linum lini** *(Linen; thread.)* [neut. n.] lineage linear lineal delineate lineation delineation bilinear line (OE) linen lining linseed linnet crinoline

lingua linguae *(Language, speech; tongue.)* [fem. n.] lingual bilingual linguist linguistic linguistics lingo (Pg.) language (OF) lingua franca *("Language of the Franks"; jargon; pidgin.)*

linquo linquere liqui *(To leave, quit; give up, let alone.)* [v.] delinquent delinquency relinquish derelict dereliction relic (OF) relict

liquidus liquida liquidum *(Fluid, liquid, flowing.)* [adj.] liquid liquidate liquidation liquidator liquor liqueur (F) liquate liquefaction liquefy

littera litterae *(Letter of alphabet; pl. writing.)* [fem. n.] literate illiterate literacy illiteracy literal literally literary literature alliterate alliteration obliterate obliteration letter (OF) lettered

locus loci *(Place, site, locality, region.)* [masc. n.] locus (Pl. loci.) local locality locate location localism locale (F) localize locator locomotion locomotive allocate allocation dislocate dislocation relocate relocation lieu (F) /loo/ in lieu of *(In place of.)* milieu (F)

longus longa longum *(Long, vast; protracted time.)* [adj.] long (OE) longitude longitudinal longevity oblong elongate elongation prolong prolongation purloin (OF)

loquor loqui locutus *(To speak, talk, say; mention.)* [v.] loquacious loquacity allocution circumlocution colloquial colloquialism colloquy elocution eloquent eloquence obloquy soliloquy soliloquize interlocutor interlocutory somniloquy ventriloquism

luceo lucere luxi *(To glow, shine, be light; dawn.)* [v.] lucid lucidity lucent elucidate elucidation translucent translucence pellucid (Pel = per, *through.*) Lucifer *("Light bearer.")*

ludo ludere lusi lusus *(To play, frolic; joke; make love.)* [v.] ludicrous allude allusion collude collusion delude delusion elude elusion elusive illusion illusionism illusionist illusive illusory interlude postlude prelude prelusive

lumen luminis *(Light; lamp, torch; day; eye; life.)* [neut. n.] lumen *(Light unit.)* luminous luminosity luminance luminary luminescence illuminate illumination Illuminati

luna lunae *(Moon; month; crescent.)* [fem. n.] lunar lunatic lunacy Luna *(Moon goddess.)* lunation lunette *(Anything crescent shaped.)* lunisolar lunitidal loony

luo luere lui lutus *(To loosen; wash; atone for; pay.)* [v.] ablution abluent diluent dilute dilution pollute (< **polluo**: *to defile.*) pollutant polluted polluting polluter pollution

lustro lustrare lustravi lustratus *(To purify; light up.)* [v.] lustrous luster lackluster lustrate illustrate illustration illustrative illustrator illustrious lustrum

M

magister magistri *(Master, teacher.)* [masc.n.] magistrate magistracy master (OF) masterful mastery Master of Arts (M.A.) Master of Science (M.S.) master of ceremonies (M.C.)

magnus magna magnum *(Big.)* [adj.] **major** *(Bigger.)* **maximus** *(Biggest.)* magnitude magnify magnification magnificent magnificence magnifico (It.) magnum *(Bottle; bone.)* magnum opus *(Masterpiece.)* Magnificat Magna Carta magna cum laude *(With high praise.)* magnate magnanimous major majorette majority major-domo (Sp.) majesty (OF) mayor (F) mayorality maximum maximize maximal maxim

Maia Maiae *(Goddess of growth, mother of Mercury.)* [fem. n.] May Mayday mayflower Mayflower Maypole Maytime mayweed

major *(Bigger.)* [Comparative adj.] major majorette majority;   <u>See</u>: **magnus**, Ap. vii-21.

malleus mallei *(Hammer, mallet.)* [masc. n.] mallet malleus malleable malleability maul (OF) pall-mall (It.) *(A game with ball & alley.)* Pall Mall *(A street in London.)* mall (Short for *Pall Mall*.)

malus mala malum *(Bad.)* [adj.]; **pejor** *(Worse.)* [comp.]; **pessimus** *(Worst.)* [super.] malice malicious malign malignant malignancy maladjusted malady malaria (It.) *("Bad air.")* malaise /mal-āz/ malapropism malcontent malediction malefactor malevolent malevolence malfeasance malformed malfunction malnutrition malocclusion malodorous maltreatment pejoration pejorative pessimism pessimistic pessimist

mamma mammae *(Breast; teat.)* [fem. n.] mammal mamma mammalogy mammary mammatus mammilla mammillary mammiferous

mando mandare mandavi mandatus *(To command, entrust.)* [v.] mandate mandatory command commandant commandeer commander remand demand demandant countermand commend (L. **commendo,** *to recommend*.) commendation commando (Afrikaans)

maneo manere mansi mansus *(To remain, stay; stop; last.)* [v.] manor mansion manse immanent immanence permanent permanence remain (OF) remains remainder remnant (OF) menial (AF) ménage (F) /mā-<u>näzh</u>/ menagerie

manus manus *(Hand.)* [fem. n.] manual manufacture manuscript manage manageable management manager manacles maneuver manicure manifest manifestation manifesto maniple manipulate manipulation manner mannered mannerism manumit manus manure *(Applied by hand.)* emancipate emancipation legerdemain (MF) *(Sleight of hand.)*

mare maris *(Sea.)* [masc. n.] marine mariner marina maritime submarine transmarine mare nostrum *(Named "Our Sea" by the Romans; the Mediterranean.)* marinade (F) marinate (It.)

masculus *(Male; manly.)* [adj.] masculine masculinely masculinity emasculate male (OF)

marito maritare maritavi maritatus *(To marry.)* [v.] marital marry (OF) marriage married intermarry intermarriage

Mars martis *(God of war.)* [masc. n.] Mars Martian martial Martin

mater matris *(Mother.)* [fem. n.] mater maternal maternity matron matronage matronly matrimony matriculate matrix (pl. matrices) alma mater *("Nurturing mother"; school attended..)*

materia materiae *(Matter, substance; wood; theme.)* [fem. n.] material materialize materialism materialist materiality materially immaterial nonmaterial matter (OF) materiel (F)

maturus matura maturum *(Ripe, mature; timely; early.)* [adj.] mature maturity maturate maturation immature immaturity

maximus *(Biggest, very big.)* [Super. adj.] maximum maximize;   <u>See</u>: **magnus**, Ap. vii-21.

medicus medici *(Doctor.)* [masc. n.]   **medeor mederi** *(To heal.)* [v.] medicine medical medication medicate medicinal medic Medicare medico (Sp.) remedy (OF) remedial

meditor meditare meditatus *(To think over, reflect; study.)* [v.] meditate meditation premeditate premeditation

medius media medium *(Middle.)* [adj.] medium media medial median mediate mediation mediator medieval *("Middle age"; Middle Ages.)* mediocre (F) mediocrity Mediterranean Sea mean (OF) *(Middle point.)* meantime meanwhile immediate immediacy immediately intermediate intermediary intermediator intermezzo (It.) milieu (F)

melior *(Better.)* [Comparative adj.] ameliorate meliorate;   <u>See</u>: **bonus**, Ap. vii-4.

memini meminisse *(To remember, think of; mention.)* [v.] reminiscent reminisce reminiscence

memoro memorare memoravi memoratus *(To call to mind, recount; mention.)* memory memorize memorable memorial immemorial memorialize memento *("Remember!")* memorandum *("A thing to be remembered.")* memo memorabilia in memoriam commemorate commemoration commemorative remember (OF) remembrance memoir (F)

mens mentis *(Mind, idea.)* (fem. n.)   mental mentality mentally mention compos mentis *("Of sound mind.")* demented dementia dementia praecox *(Schizophrenia.)*

mensura mensurae *(Measurement; standard; amount.)* [fem. n.] mensuration commensurate dimension immense *("Not measurable.")* immensity measure (F) measurement

merces mercedis *(Wages, fee, salary.)* [fem. n.]   **merx mercis** *(Goods, wares.)* [fem. n.] mercantile mercantilism mercenary Mercury *(God of trade.)* mercury mercurial mercy merciful merciless commerce commercial commercialism merchant (OF) merchandise (F)

mereo merere merui meritus *(To deserve; earn; win.)* [v.] merit meritorious emeritus

mergo mergere mersi mersus *(To dip, immerse, sink.)* [v.] merge merger emerge emersion emergent emergence emergency immerge immerse immersion submerge submersion

migro migrare migravi migratus *(To remove, change; depart.)* [v.] migrate migrant migration migratory emigrate emigrant emigration immigrate immigrant immigration transmigrate transmigrant transmigration émigré (F)

miles militis *(Soldier, infantryman; army, troops.)* [masc. n.] military militia militant militate militarism militarist militarize militiaman military police (MP)

mille milia (pl.) *(One thousand.)* [adj. n.] millennium millennial millenarian mile *(A thousand paces.)* milage mill *(One thousandth of a dollar.)*; <u>See</u>: **milli-** *(One thousandth.)* as prefix in Ap. iii-15.

minimus *(Smallest.)* [Superlative adj.] minimal minimize;   <u>See</u>: **parvus** *(Small.)*, Ap. vii-29.

ministro ministrare ministravi ministratus *(To serve, manage.)* [v.] minister ministerial ministry administer administrant administration administrative administrator minstrel (OF)

minor minari minatus *(To jut forth, project; threaten.)*   [v.]   minatory   eminent eminence imminent imminence prominent prominence promontory

minor *(Smaller.)* [Comparative adj.] minor minority minus; <u>See</u>: **parvus** *(Small.)*, Ap. vii-29.

minuo minuere minui minutus *(To lessen, diminish, reduce.)* [v.] minute /mī-n̄ōōt/ *(Very small.)* minute /mĭn-it/ *(Time unit.)* minutia (Pl. minutiae.) minuend minuet (F) diminish diminished diminution diminutive diminuendo (It.) comminute comminution

miror mirari miratus *(To wonder at, be surprised; admire.)* [v.] mirror miracle miraculous mirage marvel marvelous admire admirable admiration

mis- *(Bad; not.)* (< *minus.*) [pref.] misfortune misjudge mistake; <u>See</u>: **mis-** in Ap. iii-3, 26.

misceo miscere miscui mixtus *(To mix, mingle, blend, join.)* [v.] mix mixer mixture mixup miscellaneous miscellany promiscuous promiscuity admix admixture commix

miser misera miserum *(Wretched, poor, pitiful.)* [adj.] miser miserly misery miserable commiserate immiscible

mitto mittere misi missus *(To send, dispatch.)* [v.] mission missionary missile missive mess (OF) message (OF); **admitto:** admit admission admissible admittance; **committo:** commit commitment commission commissioner commissar (Rus.) commissary; **compromitto:** compromise compromising; **demitto:** demit demission demise; **dimitto** (dismitto)**:** dismiss dismissal; **emitto:** emit emission; **intermitto:** intermittent intermission; **intromitto:** intromission intromissive; **omitto** (obmitto)**:** omit omission; **permitto:** permit permission permissive permissible; **praemitto** (premitto)**:** premise; **promitto:** promise promissory; **remitto:** remit remittance remiss remission; **summitto** (submitto)**:** submit submission submissive; **transmitto:** transmit transmission

mobilis mobilis mobile *(Movable; nimble; excitable.)* [adj.] mobile mobility mobilize demobilize mobilization demobilization mob automobile

modus modi *(Manner, way, method.)* [masc. n.] mode modal modality model remodel modeling moderate immoderate moderation moderator moderato (It.) modify modification modifier modulate modulation modulator module modular modulus modus modus operandi modicum modest immodest modesty modern modernize modernity mod modish modiste /mō-dēst/ (F) commodity commodious commode accommodate accommodation accommodating incommode incommodious

moles molis *(Mass, bulk, pile; dam; pier; trouble.)* [fem. n.] molecule molecular molest molestation mole *(Barricade.)* demolish demolition

momentum momenti *(Momentum; change.)* [neut. n.] momentum moment momentary momentarily momentous

moneo monere monui monitus *(To warn, advise; remind.)* [v.] monition monitor monument monumental monster (OF) monstrous monstrosity; **admoneo:** admonition admonish; **praemoneo:** premonish premonition; **summoneo:** summon summons

mons montis *(Mountain.)* [masc. n.] montane mount (OF) *(To ascend.)* mount (OE) *(A hill.)* mountain (OF) mountaineer mountainous mounted amount (OF) montage /mon-täzh/ (F) amount (OF) Montana Montclair Montevideo Montmartre Montpelier Mont Blanc

monstro monstrare monstravi monstratus *(To show; inform.)* [v.] demonstrate demonstration demonstrative demonstrable demonstrator remonstrate remonstrance

mors mortis *(Death; corpse.)* [fem. n.] mortal immortal mortality immortality mortally mortalize immortalize moribund mortify mortification mortician mortuary morgue (F) mortmain (See: manus.) mortgage /mor-gij/ (OF) *("Dead pledge.")* amortize amortization

mos moris *(Nature, manner; mood; custom, practice.)* [masc. n.] moral immoral amoral morality immorality moralist moralize morale mores /mor-āz/

moveo movere movi motus *(To move, stir; disturb; change.)* [v.] move movement movable immovable mover movie motion motionless motive motivate motivation motor motorist motorize motif (F) mutiny (MF) mutinous mutineer automotive; **commoveo:** commotion; **demoveo:** demote demotion; **emoveo:** emote emotion emotional emotive; **promoveo:** promote promotion; **removeo:** remove removal removable remote

multi- *(Many)* (< *multus*, much.) [pref.] multifarious multiply; See: **multi-** in Ap. iii-15.

multus multa multum *(Much.)* [adj.] **plus** *(More.)* [Comp. adj.] **plurimus** *(Most.)* [super. adj.] multiply multiplication multiplicand multiplier multifarious multitude multitudinous multiplicity multiple-choice plus plural pluralism pluralist plurality pluperfect surplus

munio munire munivi munitus *(To defend, secure.)* [v.] muniment munition ammunition

munus muneris *(Service, office; function; gift.)* [neut. n.] municipal municipality munificent immune immunity immunize immunology remunerate remuneration remunerative

murus muri *(Wall, city wall; dam; defense.)* [masc. n.] mural intramural immure extramural

mus muris *(Mouse, rat.)* [masc. fem. n.] mussel muscle muscled muscular musculature

muto mutare mutavi mutatus *(To alter, change, vary; shift.)* [v.] mutate mutation mutant mutual; **commuto:** commute commutable commuter commutation; **immuto:** immutable; **permuto:** permute permutable; **transmuto:** transmute transmutable transmutation

N

narro narrare narravi narratus *(To tell, relate, say.)* [v.] narrate narration narrative narrator

nascor nasci natus *(To be born; originate, grow.)* [v.] nascent natal native nativity naive /nä-ēv/ naiveté /nä-ēv-tā/ (F) renascence *("Rebirth.")* renascent renaissance /ren-ə-säns/ (F) innate

natio nationis *(Nation, tribe; race, breed; class.)* [fem. n.] nation national nationalism nationalist nationality nationalize international internationalism Internationale (F)

natura naturae *(Birth; nature, quality, character.)* [fem.n.] nature natural naturalist naturalistic naturally supernatural natured good-natured

navigo navigare navigavi navigatus *(To sail, cruise.)* [v.] **navis navis** *(Ship.)* [fem. n.] navy navigate navigation navigator navigable navicular nave

necesse *(Necessary, inevitable; needful.)* (Indeclinable adj.) necessary necessity necessarily necessitate unnecessary

necto nectere nexui nexus *(To bind, tie, fasten, connect.)* [v.] nexus; **adnecto:** annex annexation; **conecto:** connect disconnect connection disconnection connective

nego negare negavi negatus *(To say no, deny; refuse.)* [v.] negate negative negation negativism abnegate abnegation deny denial renegade renege

negotium negotii *(Business, work; trouble; matter.)* (**neg-otium,** *"Not leisure."*) [neut. n.] negotiate negotiable negotiation negotiator nonnegotiable

neuter neutra neutrum *(Neither.)* [adj.] neuter neutral neutrality neutralization neutron neutrino (It.)

nihil or **nil** *(Nothing.)* (Indeclinable noun.) nil nihil nihilism annihilate annihilation

nobilis nobilis nobile *(Known, noted, famous; noble.)* [adj.] noble nobility nobleman noblewoman ignoble noblesse oblige /nō-blĕs ō-blēzh/ (F) *("Nobility obligates.")*

noceo nocere nocui nocitus *(To do harm, hurt.)* [v.] **noxa noxae** *(Hurt, harm, injury.)* [fem. n.] noxious obnoxious nocuous innocuous innocent innocence nuisance (F)

nomen nominis *(Name.)* [neut. n.] **nomino nominare nominavi nominatus** *(To name.)* [v.] nominate nomination nominative nominee nominal nominally nominalism nomenclature misnomer binomial trinomial polynomial denominate denomination denominational denominator ignominy ignominious agnomen noun (OF) pronoun

non *(No, not.)* [adv.] <u>See</u>: **non-** as prefix in Ap. iii-15: nonfiction nonnegotiable nonsense

norma normae *(Rule, standard.)* [fem. n.] norm normal normalcy normalize normally abnormal abnormality enormous *("Out of the norm.")* enormity subnormal

noto notare notavi notatus *(To mark, write; observe.)* [v.] note notebook noted notation notable notary notarize annotate annotation connote connotation denote denotation

notus nota notum *(Known, familiar; notorious.)* [adj.] notice noticeable notification notify notion notional notorious notoriety

novo novare novavi novatus *(To renew; change.)* [v.] **novus nova novum** *(New, young.)* [adj.] nova novel *(New.)* novel *(Prose.)* novelty novelist novelette novella (It.) novice innovate innovation renovate renovation Nova Scotia nouveau rich /nōō-vō rēsh/ (F) *(" Newly rich.")*

nox noctis *(Night, darkness; obscurity.)* [fem. n.] nocturnal nocturne Nocturn noctilucent noctuid equinox noctambulation

nucleus nuclei *(Nut, kernel.)* [masc. n.] diminutive of **nux nucis** *(Nut.)* [fem. n.] nucleus nuclear nuclease nucleate nucleon nucleonics nuclide nucleoplasm

nudo nudare nudavi nudatus *(To bare, strip, uncover.)* [v.] nude nudism nudist nudity denude denudate denudation nudum pactum *("Nude pact"; an unenforceable agreement.)*

nullus nulla nullum *(No, none, not any; nonexistent.)* [adj.] null nullify nullification nullity annul annulment null and void

numerus numeri *(Number, quantity; pl. mathematics.)* [masc. n.] number numerator numerical numerous numerology enumerate enumeration innumerable supernumerary

nuntio nuntiare nuntiavi nuntiatus *(To announce, declare.)* [v.] nuncio annunciate Annunciation denunciate denunciation enunciate enunciation pronunciation renunciation announce (OF) announcement announcer denounce (OF) denouncement pronounce (OF) pronounced pronouncement renounce (F) renouncement

nutrio nutrire nutrivi nutritus *(To nourish, rear, nurse.)* [v.] nutrition nutrient nutritive nutritious nutritionist nurture (OF) nurturing nurturer nurse (OF) nursemaid nursery

O

ob *(Before; in return for; because of.)* [prep.]   See: **ob-** as prefix in Ap. iii-16: object observe

octo *(Eight.)* (number) **octavus** *(Eighth.)*   See: Latin **oct-** as prefix in Ap. iii-16 (octave octet October) and Greek **octo-** as prefix in Ap. iii-25 (octagon octopus).

oculus oculi *(Eye; sight; plant bud; darling, jewel.)* [masc. n.] ocular oculist oculomotor monocle binocular binoculars inoculate inoculation inoculum antler (OF) *("Before the eyes.")*

omen ominis *(Foreboding, omen, sign; solemnity.)* [neut. n.] omen ominous abominate abomination abominable

omnis omnis omne *(All, every, any; the whole of.)* [adj.] omnipotent omnipotence omnipresent omnipresence omniscient omniscience omnivorous omnibus

onus oneris *(Load, burden, cargo; difficulty.)* [neut. n.]   onus   onerous   exonerate

opera operae *(Effort, work; service.)* [fem. n.]   **opus operis** *(Work; book; building.)* [neut. n.] operate operation operational operative operator operable cooperate cooperation cooperative inoperable inoperative opus opera (It.) operetta inure (OF) inurement

optimus *(Best, very good.)* [Superlative adj.] optimist optimal optimum; See: **bonus**, Ap.vii-4

opto optare optavi optatus *(To choose; wish for.)* [v.] opt option optional optative coopt adopt adoption

orbis orbis *(Circle, ring, orbit; world; cycle.)* [masc. n.] **orbita orbitae** *(Rut, track, path.)* [fem. n.] orb orbit orbicular exorbitant exorbitance

ordo ordinis *(Row, rank, series, order; line.)* [masc. n.] order orderly ordinal ordinary extraordinary ordinarily ordinance ordination ordnance ordain coordinate coordination disorder disorderly disordered inordinate reorder subordinate subordinary suborder insubordinate insubordination ornery *(Alteration of ordinary.)*

origo originis *(Beginning, source; ancestry.)* [fem. n.] **orior oriri ortus** *(To rise; descend.)* [v.] origin original originally originate originality orient Orient oriental Oriental orientate orientation aborigine aboriginal abort abortion abortive

orno ornare ornavi ornatus *(To enhance, adorn; equip.)* [v.]   ornate ornament ornamental adorn adornment suborn *("Secretly equip"; to bribe; to incite evil.)*

oro orare oravi oratus *(To speak; beg; pray.)* [v.]   **os oris** *(Mouth; face; opening.)* [neut. n.]
oral orally orifice oracle orate oration orator oratory oratorio (It.) orison adore
adorable adoration exorable inexorable perorate peroration oscitancy *(Yawning.)*

oscillo oscillare oscillavi oscillatus *(To swing; fluctuate.)* [v.] oscillate oscillation
oscillator oscillogram oscillograph oscilloscope

otium otii *(Leisure, idleness; quiet.)* [neut. n.] otiose *(Lazy; futile.)* otiosely otiosity negotiate;
See: **negotium**, Ap. vii-26.

ovum ovi *(Egg.)* [neut. n.] oval ovary ovate ovum ova ovule ovulate
ovulation oviduct oviform ovipara oviparous ovoviviparous ovolo (It.)

P

paco pacare pacavi pacatus *(Pacify, conquer.)* [v.] **pax pacis** *(Peace; serenity.)* [fem. n.]
pacify pacification pacific pacifist pacifier Pacific Ocean appease (OF) appeasement
pay (OF) payment payable payday payee paymaster payroll payload payoff payola
repay repayment peace (OF) peaceful peacemaker peace-loving peacetime Pax Romana

palleo pallere pallui pallutus *(To be pale; fade; anxious.)* [v.] pale pallid pallor palish
pall appall appalling

pando pandere pandi passus *(To spread out, extend; open.)* [v.] expand expanse
expansive expansion passim *(Here and there.)*

pango pangere panxi pactus *(To drive in; fasten; fix.)* [v.] compact *(Pressed together.)*
impact impacted impinge propagate propaganda propagandist propagandize

panis panis *(Bread, loaf.)* [masc. n.] pantry pannier accompany accompanist
accompaniment appanage company companion companionship companionway

par paris *(Equal, like; a match; proper, right.)* [adj.] par parity apparel compare
comparison comparable comparative disparity disparage (OF) disparaging pair (F) peer (OF)

parens parentis *(Parent; father, mother; founder.)* [masc. fem. n.] parent parentage parental

pareo parere parui paritus *(To appear, be evident.)* [v.] apparent apparently apparition
appear (OF) appearance disappear disappearance transparent transparency viviparous

paro parare paravi paratus *(To prepare; provide; intend.)* [v.] pare parade (Sp.) parapet (It.)
parasol (It.) parachute (F) parachutist disparate prepare preparation preparatory reparable
reparation reparations repair (OF) repairman separate separation separatist separator
separable inseparable sever (OF) severance several severally spar (It.)   Semper Paratus

pars partis *(Part, share, fraction.)* [fem.n.] **partio partire partivi partitus** *(To share; divide.)* [v.]
part partly parted parting part-time parse parcel (F) partake partook partial partiality
particle particular particularity particularly participle participial participate
participation party partition partitive partisan apart apartment compart compartment
compartmentalize depart departed department departmental departure impart
impartial impartiality partite tripartite repartee (OF) repartition   ex parte *(One-sided.)*

parvus parva parvum *(Small.)* [adj.] **minor** *(Smaller.)* [Comp. adj.] **minimus** *(Smallest.)* [Super. adj.] minor minority minimum miniature minimal minimize miniskirt minus (Neut. minor.)

pasco pascere pavi pastus *(To feed, pasture; nourish.)* [v.] pasture pasturage pastor pastoral pastorate pastorale pastern repast pester (OF)

passus passus *(Step, pace, footstep.)* [masc. n.] pass passable impassable passage passenger passerby passing passport Passover password past compass encompass surpass surpassing trespass pace (F) passé (F) impasse (F) passepied (MF)

pater patris *(Father; pl. forefathers.)* [masc. n.] **patria patriae** *(Native land, hometown.)* [fem. n.] paternal paternity paternalism patrician patriarch patrimony patron patriot patriotic patriotism patron patronage patronize compatriot expatriate repatriate pater

patior pati passus *(To suffer, endure; experience; allow.)* [v.] patient (n., adj.) patience passion passionate passive passivity compassion compassionate dispassionate compatible impassion impassioned impassive impatient impatience impatiens

pecco peccare peccavi peccatus *(To make a mistake.)* [v.] peccable impeccable peccant impeccant peccadillo (Sp.)

pectus pectoris *(Breast, heart, feeling, mind.)* [v.] pectoral pecs (Short for *pectoral muscles.)* expectorate expectorant pectoral arch pectoral fin parapet (It.)

pecunia pecuniae *(Wealth, money, property.)* [fem.n.] **pecus pecoris** *(Cattle, herd, flock.)* [neut. n.] pecuniary peculiar peculiarity peculate peculium impecunious

pejor pejor perjus *(Worse.)* [Comp. adj.] pejoration pejorative; <u>See</u>: **malus**, Ap. vii-22.

pello pellere pepuli pulsus *(To drive, repel.)* [v.] pulse pulsate pulsimeter pulsar push (OF) pusher pushing pushy push-button pushcart pushover push-up; **appello:** appellant appellate appulse appeal (OF); **compello:** compel compelling compulsion compulsive compulsory; **dispello:** dispel; **expello:** expel expellant expulsion expulsive; **impello:** impel impellent impulse impulsion impulsive; **propello:** propel propellant propellent propeller propulsion; **repello:** repel repellent repulse repulsion repulsive

pendeo pendere pependi *(To hang; hover.)* [v.] pend pending pendant pendent pendulum penchant (F); **dependeo:** depend dependent independent dependence independence dependency; **impendeo:** impend impending; **propendeo:** propensity

pendo pendere pependi pensus *(To weigh; pay; ponder.)* [v.] pension (OF) pensioner pansy (MF) peso (Sp.) poise (OF); **appendo:** append appendage appendix appendectomy; **compendo:** compendium compend compendious; **expendo:** expend expendable expenditure expense expensive spend (OE); **perpendo:** perpendicular; **suspendo:** suspend suspense suspension stipend *(Stips* = coin, *"To pay in coin.")* stipendiary

penso pensare pensavi pensatus *(To weigh out; consider.)* [v.] pensive; **compenso:** compensate compensation; **dispenso:** dispense dispenser dispensable dispensation

per *(Through; thoroughly; by.)* [prep.] <u>See</u>: per- as prefix in Ap. iii-16: perfect permission

persona personae *(Mask; character, part; person.)* [fem. n.] persona personae person personable personal impersonal personage personality personalize personally personify personification personnel impersonate persona non grata *(Unwelcome person.)*

pes pedis *(Foot.)* [masc. n.] pedal pedestal (It.) pedestrian pedicure pediment biped expedite expedient expediency expedition expeditionary impede impediment impedance quadruped impeach (OF) (**impedicare** = *to entangle*; **pedica** = *fetter.*) impeachment

pessimus *(Worst.)* [Super. adj.] pessimism pessimist pessimistic <u>See</u>: **malus**, Ap. vii-22.

peto petere petivi petitus *(To seek, chase; demand, ask.)* [v.] petition petulant (OF) petulance; **appeto:** appetite appetence appetizer appetizing; **competo:** competent competence compete competition competitive competitor; **impeto:** impetus impetuous impetuosity; **repeto:** repetition repetitious repetitive repetend repeat (OF)

pingo pingere pinxi pictum *(To paint, color; decorate.)* [v.] picture pictorial picturesque (F) depict depiction pigment (**pigmentum** > **pingere**.) pigmentation pimento (Sp.)

pius pia pium *(Dutiful; holy.)* [adj.] pious impious piety impiety pietism (Ger.) Pieta /pyā-tä/ (It.) Pope Pius pity (OF) piteous expiate *(To atone for.)* expiation

placeo placere placui placitus *(To please, satisfy.)* [v.] placid placebo complacent complacency complaisant complaisance pleasant (OF) pleasantry please (OF) displease pleasing pleasure (OF) pleasurable plea (OF) pleading

placo placare placavi placatus *(To calm, appease.)* [v.] placate placable implacable

plango plangere planxi planctus *(To lament loudly, bewail.)* [v.] plaint (OF) plaintive plaintiff complain complaint complainant

planta plantae *(Sole, foot; sprout.)* [fem. n.] **planto plantare plantavi plantus** *(To plant.)* [v.] plant plantation planter displant implant supplant plantar fasciitis plantar wart

planus plana planum *(Level, flat; plain, clear.)* [adj.] plan plane *(A surface.)* plane *(A tool.)* plank plain (OF) explain explanation esplanade (Sp.) piano (It.)

plaudo plaudere plausi plausus *(To clap, beat, stamp)* [v.] plaudit plausible implausible; **applaudo:** applaud applause; **explodo** (explaudo)**:** explode explosion explosive; implode

plebs plebis *(Common people, plebeians, lower class.)* [fem. n.] pleb plebe plebeian plebiscite

plecto plectere plexi plexus *(To twist; punish, torture.)* [v.] plexus complex complexity complexion complexioned complexus perplex perplexed perplexing accomplice (F)

plenus plena plenum *(Full, sated; mature.)* [adj.] **pleo plere plevi pletus** *(To fill.)* [v.] plenty plentiful plentitude plenary plenum plenipotentiary; **compleo:** complete completion complement complementary comply (It.) compliance compliant compliment (MF) complimentary; **depleo:** deplete depletion; **expleo:** expletive; **impleo:** implement implementation; **repleo:** replete repletion replenish; **suppleo:** supply supplier supplement supplemental supplementary; accomplish (OF) accomplished accomplishment

Ap. vii-30

plico plicare plicavi plicatus *(To fold, coil.)* [v.] ply pliable pliancy pliant plait (OF) pleat (OF) pleater ploy (F) deploy employ employment employee employer; **applico:** apply misapply appliance applicable applicant application; **complico:** complicate complication complicity; **duplico:** duplicate duplication duplex; **explico:** explicit explicate explicable inexplicable exploit (OF) exploitation; **implico:** imply implicate implication implicit; **multiplico:** multiply multiplication; **replico:** reply replica replicate; **supplico:** supplicate supplicant supple (OF); display (OF) triplex triplicate

ploro plorare ploravi ploratus *(To wail, lament, weep.)* [v.] **deploro:** deplore deplorable; **exploro:** explore exploration exploratory explorer; **imploro:** implore

plumbum plumbi *(Lead; bullet; pipe.)* [neut. n.] Pb *(Periodic Table symbol for* lead.) plumb plumber plumbing plumbago plumbeous plumbism plumbiferous plumb line

plurimus *(Most.)* [Super. adj.] **plus pluris** *(More.)* [Comp. adj.] plural; See: **multus,** Ap.vii-25.

poena poenae *(Penalty, punishment, pain.]* [fem. n.] penal (OF) penalty punish (OF) punishment punitive impunity subpoena pain (OF) pained painful painkiller painstaking repent (OF) repentance repentant penitent (OF) penitence penitentiary penance (OF)

polio polire plivi politus *(To polish; improve; order.)* [v.] polish polished polite politely politesse (F)   interpolate   interpolation

pondero ponderare ponderavi ponderatus *(To weigh; reflect.)* [v.] ponder ponderous ponderable   imponderable   preponderate   preponderance   pound (OE) *(Weight unit.)*

pono ponere posui positus *(To put, place, lay, set.)* [v.] pose position positive positivism positron post *(Employment; mail.)* posture; **appono:** appose apposition; **compono:** compose composition composer composite composure compost component compound (OF); **contrapono:** contrapose contraposition; **depono:** depose deposition deposit depository depot (F); **dispono:** dispose disposition disposal; **expono:** expose exposition exponent exponential expository exposure exposé (F); **impono:** impose imposition imposing impostor; **interpono:** interpose; **juxta + pono:** juxtapose juxtaposition; **oppono:** oppose opposition opponent opposite; **postpono:** postpone; **praepono:** preposition prepositional; **propono:** propose proposition proponent proposal propound purpose (OF) provost (OF); **repono:** repose reposition repository; **suppono:** suppose supposition suppository; **transpono:** transpose transposition

pons pontis *(Bridge; gangway, deck.)* [masc. n.]   pons   pontine   pontoon (MF) pontifex *("Bridge maker.")* pontiff pontifical pontificate punt (OE) *(Boat.)* Pontine Marshes

populus populi *(People, populace, public; nation.)* [masc. n.] populus populate depopulate population populous popular unpopular popularity pop (Short for *popular.*) pop art pop culture   people (OF)   vox populi *("The voice of the people.")*

porcus porci *(Pig, hog.)* [masc. n.] pork porker porkpie porcupine porpoise porcelain (MF)

portio portionis *(Share, installment.)* [fem. n.]   portion apportion apportionment proportion proportional proportionate disproportion disproportional disproportionate

porta portae *(Door, gate, entrance.)* [fem. n.] **portus portus** *(Port, harbor, haven.)* [masc. n.] port portal porter *(Doorkeeper.)* portico portcullis (OF) *(Door grating.)* porthole opportune inopportune porch (OF) portal-to-portal pay

porto portare portavi portatus *(To carry, bear, bring.)* [v.] porter *(Luggage carrier.)* portage portable portfolio portmanteau (MF) port *(Rifle position.)* portly portamento (It.); **comporto:** comportment; **deporto:** deport deportation deportment deportee (F); **exporto:** export exporter; **importo:** import importer important unimportant importance; **reporto** report reporter reportedly; **supporto:** support supporter supportive; **transporto:** transport transportation transportable; purport (OF) disport (OF)

possum posse potui *(To be able, have power.)* [v.] posse possible; See: **sum**, Ap. vii-43.

post *(After, behind, since.)* [prep.] See: **post-** as prefix in Ap. iii-16: postgraduate postlude

potens potentis *(Able, capable; endowed; strong.)* [adj.] potent potency potential potentiality potentate potentiometer omnipotent plenipotentiary impotent impotence

prae *(Before, in front of.)* [prep., adv.] See: **pre-** as prefix in Ap. iii-17: prefer predict predate

precor precari precatus *(To beg, pray, entreat; wish.)* [v.] precatory precarious pray (OF) prayer; **deprecor:** deprecate deprecatory; **imprecor:** imprecate imprecation

prehendo prehendere prehendi prehensus *(To grasp, seize.)* [v.] prehensile prehension prison (OF) prisoner imprison pregnable (OF) impregnable; **apprehendo:** apprehend apprehension apprehensive apprentice (OF) apprenticeship apprise (F); **comprehendo:** comprehend comprehension comprehensive incomprehensible comprise (MF); **reprehendo:** reprehend reprehensible enterprise (OF) reprise (OF) reprisal surprise (OF)

premo premere pressi pressus *(To press, squeeze, compress.)* [v.] press pressing pressure pressurize print (OF) printer printing print-out imprint reprint; **apprimo:** appressed appressor; **comprimo:** compress compressed compression compressor; **deprimo:** depress depressed depressing depression depressive depressant; **exprimo:** express expression expressive expressly expressionism; **imprimo:** impress impression impressionable impressive impressionism imprimatur *("Let it be printed.")*; **opprimo:** oppress oppression oppressive; **reprimo:** repress repression repressive reprimand (F); **supprimo:** suppress suppression suppressive

pretium pretii *(Price, value, money; reward.)* [neut. n.] price (OF) prize (OF) precious (OF) praise (OF) appreciate appreciation appreciable appreciative depreciate depreciation

primus prima primum *(First, foremost; earliest.)* [super. adj.] prime primal primary primarily primer primitive primacy primeval primordial primogeniture primate primatology primitivism primrose primo (It.) prima donna (It.) primus inter pares *("First among equals.")* prima facie /prī-mə fā-shē/ *("At first view.")*

princeps principis *(First.)* [adj.]; *(Leader.)* [masc. n.] prince (OF) princess (F) principal principality

principium principii *(Beginning, origin.)* [neut. n] principium *(First principle; beginning.)* principia (pl.) *(Fundamentals.)* principle principles principled

prior prioris prius *(Former, previous; better.)* [Comp. adj.] prior *(Before; an office.)* priority

privo privare privavi privatus *(To set apart; free.)* [v.] private privacy privation privilege privileged privy (F) privity privateer deprive deprivation

pro *(In front of; on behalf of; in place of.)* [adv. prep.] <u>See</u>: **pro-** as prefix in Ap. iii-17: proceed

probo probare probavi probatus *(To approve, judge.)* [v.] probe probate probation probity prove (OF) proof (OF) probable (OF) improbable probably probability; **approbo:** approbation approve approval; **re + probo:** reprobate reprobation reprove reprieve (F)

proles prolis *(Offspring, child; descendants, race.)* [fem. n.] prolific proliferate proliferous proles *(The poor who served Rome only by having children.)* proletarian proletariat

prope *(Near.)* [prep., adv.] **propinquus propinqua propinquum** *(Near.)* [adj.] propinquity **propior** *(Nearer.)* [Comp. adj.] **proximus proxima proximum** *(Nearest.)* [Super. adj.] proximate proximity proximo approximate approximation

proprius propria proprium *(One's own; peculiar.)* proper improper properly property propriety appropriate inappropriate misappropriate appropriation expropriate

provincia provinciae *(Province.)* [fem. n.] province provincial provincialism

proximus *(Nearest.)* [Super. adj.] approximate approximation; <u>See</u>: **prope** above.

publicus publica publicum *(Public; of the state.)* [adj.] public publish republic publication publicist publicity publicize publicly Republican République (F) republication

pudeo pudere pudui puditus *(To feel or be ashamed.)* [v.] pudency pudendum; **in + pudeo:** impudent impudence impudicity; **repudeo:** repudiate repudiation

pugno pugnare pugnavi pugnatus *(To fight; disagree.)* [v.] pugnacious pugilist pugilism; **impugno:** impugn; **oppugno:** oppugn oppugnant; **repugno:** repugnant repugnance

pulmo pulmonis *(Lung.)* [masc. n.] pulmonary pulmonic pulmonate pulmonary Pulmotor

pungo pungere pupugi punctus *(To prick, sting, pierce.)* [v.] puncture punctual punctuality punctuate punctuation punctilious punctilio (Sp.) pungent; **compungo:** compunction compunctious; **expungo:** expunge expunction; venipuncture (**vena** = *vein.*)

pupus pupi *(Boy, child.)* [masc. n.] **pupa pupae** *(Girl, doll.)* [fem. n.] pupa pupate pupil *(Student.)* pupil *(Eye part;* so named because of little figure reflected there.*)* puppet (OF) puppeteer puppy pup

purgo purgare purgavi purgatus *(To cleanse, purge, purify.)* [v.]
purus pura purum *(Clear, pure, clean; plain, chaste.)* [adj.] pure impure purity impurity purify purist purely purification Puritan puritanical purée (F) purge purgatory purgative purgatorial depurate depuration; **expurgo:** expurgate expurgatory spurge (< **expurgo.**)

puto putare putavi putatus *(To think; count; trim.)* [v.] putative; **computo:** compute computation computer counter (AF) *(Table.)*; **deputo:** depute deputation deputy (OF);

disputo: dispute disputant disputable disputation; **imputo:** impute imputation; **reputo:** repute reputed reputable reputation amputate *(ambi-* around+ *puto* to trim.) amputee

Q

quadrum quadri *(Square.)* [neut. n.]   **quadrans quadrantis** *(Quarter.)* [masc. n.] quad quadrangle quadrant quadratic; See: **quad-** as prefix in Ap. iii-18: quadrilingual quadruplet

quaero quaerere quaesive quaesitus *(To seek, inquire.)* [v.] query question questionable questionnaire (F) quest; **acquiro:** acquire acquisition acquisitive; **conquiro:** conquer conqueror conquest conquistador (Sp.); **disquiro:** disquisition; **exquiro:** exquisite; **inquiro:** inquire inquiry inquisition inquest inquisitive enquire (OF) enquiry; **perquiro:** perquisites *("Perks.")* **requiro:** require requirement request requisition prerequisite

qualis qualis quala *(What kind of, what sort of.)* [adj.]   quality   qualify   disqualify qualified   qualification   disqualification   qualitative   qualitative analysis

quantus quanta quantum *(How much, how great.)* [adj.] quantity   quantify   quantitative quantitative analysis   quantum   quantum mechanics

quattuor *(Four.)* [number] **quartus quarta quartum** *(Fourth.)* [adj.] **quater** *(Four times.)* [adv.] quarantine (It.) *(Forty days.)* quart quarter quartet quarto quarry (OF) *("Square stone.")* quarter-hour quarterly quartile quatrain quire (OF) squad (It.) squadron square (OF)

quasi *(As if, nearly.)* [adv.] See: **quasi-** as prefix in Ap. iii-18: quasi-official quasi-scientific

quatio quatere quassus *(To shake, agitate, disturb.)* [v.] **concutio concussus:** concuss concussion concussive; **discutio discussus:** discuss discussion discussant; **excutio excussus:** rescue (OF) *(re + excussus)*; **percutio percussus:** percussion percussive

queror queri questus *(To complain, find fault; lament.)* [v.] quarrel querulous querimonious

quietus quieta quietum *(At rest; peaceful; neutral.)* [adj.] quiet   quietude   quiescent quit (OF) quite (ME) acquiesce acquiescence acquiescent acquit (OF) acquittal acquittance requite   requital   requiem   coy (MF)   requiescat in pace *("May he rest in peace.")* R.I.P.

quinque *(Five.)* [number] **quintus quinta quintum** *(Fifth.)* [adj.] See: **quint-** in Ap. iii-18.

quotus quota quotum *(How many?)* [adj.] quota quote quotation quotable quotient aliquot

R

radius radii *(Ray, beam; rod.)* [masc. n.] radius (Pl. radii.) ray radial radian radiant radiance radiate radiation radiator radio radioactive radium radon corradiate eradiate irradiate

radix radicis *(Root; lower extreme; source, origin.)* [fem. n.] radical   radicalism   radically radicand   radicel   radix   radish (OF)   eradicate   eradication   eradicator

rado radere rasi rasum *(To scrape, shave, scratch; erase.)* [v.] raze (OF)   razor (OF) rasp (OF) rasping rasped raspberry razz (sl.) razzberry (sl.) rascal (OF) rascality rascally abrade abrasion abrasive corrade erase (**e** < **ex-**, *out.*) eraser   erasure

rapio rapere rapui raptus *(To seize, carry off, hasten.)* [v.] rape rapacious rapine rapid rapt rapture rapturous raptorial enrapt enrapture surreptitious raven (OF) *(To devour.)* ravening ravenous ravish (OF) ravishing ravishment ravage ravine (F)

rarus rara rarum *(Rare, uncommon; thin; porous.)* [adj.] rare rarely rarity rareness rarefy rarefaction rara avis *("Rare bird." An unusual person.)*

ratio rationis *(Account, method, manner, reason.)* [fem. n.] ratio rational irrational rationale rationalism rationality irrationality rationalize rationalization ratify (OF) ratification rate (OF) prorate pro rata *(In proportion.)* rating ration (F) reason (OF) reasonable

re- *(Back; again; anew.)* [An inseparable prefix.] <u>See</u>: re- as prefix in Ap. iii-18: reform replace

recens recentis *(Recent; fresh; young.)* [adj.] recent recently recentness recency

reciprocus reciproca reciprocum *(Returning; going backwards and forwards.)* [adj.] reciprocal reciprocate reciprocity reciprocation reciprocatory

recuso recusare recusavi recusatus *(To refuse.)* [v.] recuse recusant ruse (OF) rush (AF)

rego regere rexi rectus *(To guide, direct.)* [v.] regent regimen regime regiment regimentation region reign regular irregular regularity regulate regulation regulator rectum (**rectum intestinum**, *straight intestine.*) rectus *(A straight muscle.)* rectify rectification rectifier rector rectory rectilinear rectangle rectangular rule (OF) ruler ruling rail (OF); **corrigo** (com/rego): corrigible incorrigible; correct incorrect correction; **dirigo** (dis/rego): direct indirect directly direction directive director directory dirigible *(Directable.)*; **erigo** (ex/rego): erect erector escort (F); adroit (F) (a + droit, *to right>* ad + dirigo.)

res rei *(Thing, event, affair, circumstance, fact.)* [fem. n.] real (OF) reality realize really realist realism realistic realization realizing realty realtor rebus *(A puzzle.)* republic surrealism (F)

restauro restaurare restauravi restauratus *(To repair, rebuild; restore.)* [v.] restaurant (F) restaurateur restore (OF) restoration restorative; **instauro:** store (OF)

retro *(Back, behind.)* [adv.] <u>See</u>: **retro-** as prefix in Ap. iii-20: retroactive retrograde retrospect

rex regis *(King; tyrant; leader; patron; rich man.)* [masc. n.] rex regicide realm (OF) regal (OF) regality regalia royal (OF) royalist royalty viceroy corduroy (F) (Corde du roi. *King's cord.*)

rideo ridere risi risus *(To laugh, smile; ridicule.)* [v.] **ridiculus ridicula ridiculum** *(Amusing; ridiculous.)* [adj.] ridicule ridiculous deride derision derisive

rigeo rigere *(To be stiff.)* [v.] rigid rigidity rigor rigorous rigor mortis *(Stiffness of death.)*

ripa ripae *(River bank, shore.)* [fem. n.] **rivus rivi** *(Stream, brook, channel, conduit.)* [masc. n.] riparian riparious river (OF) rivulet rival *("Those living on opposite banks.")* rivalry; arrive (OF) *("To the shore.")* arrival; derive *("From the stream.")* derivation derivative

robustus robusta robustum *(Strength, hardness; oak.)* [adj.] robust robustness robustly roble (Sp.) *(Oak types.)* roborant corroborate corroboration corroborative corroborant

rodo rodere rosi rosus *(To gnaw, nibble, erode.)* [v.] rodent corrode corrosion corrosive erode erosion erosive
Ap. vii-35

rogo rogare rogavi rogatus *(To ask, question; propose.)* [v.] **abrogo:** abrogate; **adrogo:** arrogate arrogant arrogance; **derogo:** derogate derogatory derogative; **interrogo:** interrogate interrogation interrogator interrogatory; **praerogo:** prerogative **prorogo:** prorogation; **super + ex + rogo:** supererogation; **sub + rogo:** surrogate

Roma Romae *(Rome.)* [fem. n.] Rome Roman roman *(Type.)* roman /raw-<u>män</u>/ *(French novel.)* Romans *(New Testament book.)* romance (OF) romantic romanticism romanticize romanesque Roman numerals (XI, IV, XCIII, *etc.*) Roman Empire Romance languages

rota rotae *(Wheel, disk.)* [fem. n.] rota rotate rotation rotator rotary rotund rotunda round (OF) rounded roundish roll (OF) roller roulette (F)

rubeo rubere *(To be red; blush.)* [v.] ruby rubious rubicund rubescent rubella rubellite rubric rubricate rubrician erubescence rouge /rōōzh/ (F)

rudis rudis rude *(Untaught, in natural state; rough.)* [adj.] rude rudely rudeness rudiment rudimentary erudite (**e** = **ex**, *out of.*) erudition

rugo rugare *(To become wrinkled, creased.)* [v.] ruga *(A wrinkle.)* (Pl. rugae) rugate; **corrugo:** corrugate corrugated

rumpo rumpere rupi ruptus *(To break, burst, tear, destroy.)* [v.] rupture ruptured; **abrumpo:** abrupt; **corrumpo:** corrupt corruption corruptible incorruptible; **disrumpo:** disrupt disruption disruptive; **erumpo:** erupt eruption eruptive; **interumpo:** interrupt interruption interrupted; **irrumpo:** irruption irruptive bankrupt bankruptcy rout (OF) route (OF) routine (F) rut (Var. of *route.*)

rus ruris *(Countryside; farm.)* [neut. n.] rural rurality ruralize rustic rusticate rusticity

S

sacro sacrare sacravi sacratus *(To dedicate, consecrate.)* [v.] sacred sacrament sacrifice sacrificial sacrilege sacrilegious sacristy sacrosanct consecrate consecration desecrate desecration execrate execration obsecrate sexton (OF)

sal salis *(Salt; brine, sea.)* [masc. n.] saline salinity salary salt (OE) salty salad (OF)

salio salire salui saltus *(To leap, spring, jump; gush.)* [v.] salient salience sally (OF) salmon (OF) saltant saltation saltarello (It.); **adsalio:** assail (OF) assailant assault (OF); **desultor** *(Leaper.)*: desultory; **dissulto:** dissilient; **exsulto:** exult exultant exultation; **insulto:** insult insulting; **resulto:** resilient resilience result resultant; **transulto:** transilient

saluto salutare salutavi salutatus *(To greet, wish well.)* [v.] **salus salutis** *(Health.)* [fem. n.] salute salutary salutation salutatorian salutatory salubrious

salvus salva salvum *(Safe, sound, alive, well.)* [adj.] salvage salvable salvation salver save saving safe (OF) safety savings savior saviour Saviour

sanctus sancta sanctum *(Sacred, holy, pious.)* [adj.] Sanctus sanctity sanctify sanctification sanctimony sanctimonious sanctuary sanction sanctum saint (OF) St. (Abbr.)

sainte (F) (fem. *saint:* abbr. Ste.) San (Sp.) (masc. *saint.*) Santo (It.,Por.) (masc. *saint.*) São /soun/ (Por. Before all consonants, but h.) (masc. *saint.*) Santa (Sp. It. Por.) (fem. *saint.*); Saint-Germaine St. Louis Ste. Agathe San Francisco Santa Barbara São Paulo; sanctum sanctorum *("Holy of holies.")*

sanus sana sanum *(Healthy; sane.)* [adj.] sane insane sanity insanity sanely saneness sanitary sanitation sanitize sanitarium sanatorium sanatory sanative

sapio sapere sapivi *(To taste; know.)* [v.] sapid sapor sapient sapience insipid insipience

satis *(Enough, sufficient.)* [adj., adv.] sate satiate satiable satisfy satisfactory satisfied dissatisfied satisfaction dissatisfaction asset (AF) assets

satur satura saturum *(Filled, well fed; replete; rich.)* [adj.] saturate saturated saturation saturant satire (MF) *(Sarcasm, irony; originally a discourse on a number of subjects, i.e., a full dish.)* satirize satiric satirical satirist

scalae scalarum *(Stairs, ladder.)* [fem. pl. n.] scale (In music.) escalate escalator escalade (F)

scando scandere scandi scansus *(To climb, ascend, mount; scan verses.)* [v.] scan; **ascendo:** ascend ascendancy ascendant ascent; **descendo:** descend descendant descendent descent; **transcendo:** transcend transcendent transcendental transcendentalism

scindo scindere scidi scissus *(To cut open; tear apart.)* [v.] scissors scission scissure; **abscindo:** abscission abscissa; **praescindo:** prescind; **rescindo:** rescind rescission

scio scire scivi scitus *(To know; have skill in.)* [v.] science scientific scientist; **conscio:** conscience conscientious conscious unconscious consciousness conscionable unconscionable; **omni + scio:** omniscient omniscience; **praescio:** prescience prescient

scintilla scintillae *(Spark.)* [fem. n.] scintilla scintillant scintillate scintillatingly scintillation

scribo scribere scripsi scriptus *(To write; draw.)* [v.] scribe script Scripture scribble scriptorium scrive (OF) serif (Du.); **ascribo:** ascribe ascription; **circumscribo:** circumscribe circumscription; **conscribo:** conscript conscription; **describo:** describe description descriptive; **inscribo:** inscribe inscription; **postscribo:** postscript; **praescribo** prescribe prescription prescriptive; **proscribo:** proscribe proscription **rescribo:** rescript; **subscribo:** subscribe subscript subscription; **superscribo:** superscribe superscript superscription; **transcribo:** transcribe transcript transcription

scrutor scrutari scrutatus *(To search, probe, examine.)* [v.] scrutiny scrutinize inscrutable

sculpo sculpere sculpsi sculptus *(To carve, engrave.)* [v.] sculpt sculptor sculpture Sculptor *(A constellation; The Sculptor's Workshop.)* sculpsit *("He sculptured it.")*

se, sed *(Apart; without; but.)* [conj., prep.] See: **se-** as prefix in Ap. iii-20: secrete secure select

seco secare secui sectus *(To cut, injure; divide.)* [v.] section sectional sectionalize sector sectile secant; bisect bisector; trisect trisection trisector; **disseco:** dissect dissection dissector; **exseco:** exsect exsection; **inseco:** insect insectarium insecticide insectival insectivore; intersect intersection intersectional; **proseco:** prosect prosection; **reseco:** resect resection; **trans + seco:** transect transection; segment segmentation sickle (OE)

secundus secunda secundum *(Following, next, second.)* [adj.] second *(After first.)* second *(Time unit.)* secondary secund secundine secundum *(According to.)* seconde (F); <u>From</u>: **sequor.**

sedeo sedere sedi sessus *(To sit; be in session.)* [v.] sedentary sedate sedation sedative sediment sedimentary sedimentation sedan (It.) session (F) see (OF) *(Church rank.)* size (F) siege (OF); **adsideo:** assiduous assess (OF) assessment assessor assize (OF); **dissideo:** dissident dissidence; **obsideo:** obsess obsession obsessive; **possideo:** possess possession possessive; **praesideo:** preside president presidency presidio (Sp.); **resideo:** reside residence residency resident residential residual residue residuum; **subsido:** subside subsidence subsidiary subsidy subsidize; **supersideo:** supersede supersession

semen seminis *(Seed; race, child; origin.)* [neut. n.] **semino seminare** *(To sow; produce.)* [v] semen seminal seminary seminarian seminar semination disseminate inseminate

semper *(Always, ever, every time.)* [adv.] sempiternal *(Eternal.)* semper fidelis *("Always faithful.")* semper paratus *("Always prepared.")* sempre (It.) *(Always, e.g., in music, sempre legato.)*

semi- *(Partly, not fully; half.)* [pref.] semicircle semicolon semifinal; <u>See</u>: **semi-** in Ap. iii-20.

senex sexis *(Old.)* [adj.] **senior** *(Older.)* [Comp. adj.] senior /sēn-yer/ seniority senile senility senate senator senatorial sire (OF) sir (< sire.) señor /sā-nyor/ (Sp.) señora señorita signore /sē-nyō-rā/ (It.) signora signorino signorina seignior /sēn-yer/ (AF)

sentio sentire sensi sensus *(To feel, perceive; think.)* [v] sentience sentient insentient sentiment sentimental sentimentality sentimentalize sententious sentence (OF) sentinel (It.) sentry *(Var. of sentinel.)* sense (F) nonsense nonsensical sensible insensible supersensible sensate insensate sensation sensational sensationalism senseless sensitive insensitive sensitivity sensitize desensitize sensor sensorium sensory sensual supersensual sensualism sensuality sensualize sensuous sententious; **adsentio:** assent assentation assentor; **consentio:** consent consensus consensual; **dissentio:** dissent dissenting dissenter dissension dissentient dissentious; **praesentio:** presentiment; **re + sentio:** resent (F) resentful resentment

septem *(Seven.)* [num.] **septimus septima septimum** *(Seventh.)* <u>See</u>: Pref. **sept-** in Ap. iii-20.

sequor sequi secutus *(To follow, accompany; ensue.)* [v.] sequel sequence sequent sequential sequacious sequela sequencer seq. *(sequens, the following.)* non sequitur *("It does not follow.")* non seq. *(abbr.)* sue (AF) ensue (OF) ensuing suit (AF) suitable suitcase suitor (AF) suite (F) sect (OF) sectarian nonsectarian set (OF) *(A group.)*; **consequor:** consequent consequently consequence consequential consecutive; **exsequor:** exequy *(Funeral ceremonies.)* exequies execute executor executrix execution executioner executive; **obsequor:** obsequies obsequious; **persequor:** persecute persecution; **prosequor:** prosecute prosecution prosecutor pursue (AF) pursuit; **subsequor:** subsequent subsequently subsequence; extrinsic (F) intrinsic (OF)

serenus serena serenum *(Clear, bright; serene.)* [adj.] serene serenity serenade (F) serenata (It.)

serius seria serium *(Earnest, serious.)* [adj.] serious seriously seriousness

series serie *(Row, sequence, succession.)* [fem. n.] **sero serere serui sertus** *(To join, link.)* [v.] series serial serialism serialize seriatim *(One after another.)* **adsero:** assert assertion; **desero:** desert /dez-ert/ *(Sand.)* desert /di-zert/ *(To leave.)* desertion deserter; **dissero:** dissertate dissertation; **exsero:** exert exertion exertive; **insero:** insert insertion

serra serrae *(A saw.)* [fem. n.] serrate serrated serration serriform serrulate serrulation serranoid sierra (Sp.) *(Mountain range.)* Sierra Madre biserrate

servio servire servivi servitus *(To serve, be of use to.)* [v.] serve servant server service serviceable servile servitude servo; **deservio:** deserve deserved deservedly deserving deserts (OF) *(Reward.)* dessert (F) *(After dinner sweets.);* **praeservio:** preserve preservation preservative; **subservio:** subserve subservient serf (OF) serfdom serfhood sergeant (OF)

servo servare seravi servatus *(To save, rescue; preserve.)* **conservo:** conserve conservation conservationist conservatism conservative conservatory conservator; **observo:** observe observation observable observance observant observatory; **reservo:** reserve re-serve reservation reserved reservist reservoir (F)

severus severa severum *(Strict, stern; severe; grim.)* [adj.] severe severely severity asseverate asseveration persevere perseverance

sex *(Six.)* [num.] **sextus sexta sextum** *(Sixths.)*   See: **sex-** as prefix in Ap. iii-20: sextet

sexus sexus *(Sex.)* [masc. n.] sex sexual sexuality sexology heterosexual (Gk. **hetero** = *different.*) heterosexuality homosexual (Gk. **homo** = *same.*) homosexuality asexual bisexual

sidus sideris *(Star; constellation; season; destiny.)* [masc. n.] sidereal consider consideration considerable considerate inconsiderate considering reconsider reconsideration

signo signare signavi signatus *(To mark, stamp; seal.)* [v.] sign signal signature signatory signify significant significance signet ensign (OF) sennet (OF); **adsigno:** assign assignment assignee assignation assignat (F); **consigno:** consign consignment consignee consignor; **designo:** design designate designation designedly designee designer; **insignio:** insignia insignificant insignificance; **resigno:** resign re-sign resignation

sileo silere silui *(To be still, be quiet; cease.)* [v.] silent silence silencer silent partner

silex silicis *(Flint, hard stone, rock.)* [masc. n.] silica silicon silicone silex silicate siliceous silicic silicide silicify silicosis

silva silvae *(A wood, forest; shrubbery.)* [fem. n.] silva silvan sylvan sylvatic Silvia Sylvia Pennsylvania silviculture savage (OF) savagery

similis similis simile *(Like, similar.)* [adj.] **simulo simulare simulavi simulatus** *(Imitate; pretend.)* (v.) simile similar similarity similitude simulate simulation; **adsimulo:** assimilate assimilation; **dissimulo:** dissimilar dissimilarity dissimilate dissimilation dissimilitude dissemble (OF) dissemblance dissimulate dissimulation; **re + simulo:** resemble (OF) resemblance; facsimile (**fac simile**, *make like.*) fax (Short for *facsimile.*) verisimilar verisimilitude

simplex simplicis *(Single, simple; natural.)* [adj.] simple   simplicity   simplistic   simplify simplification   simplex   simpleton   simple-minded   Simple Simon

simul *(At the same time; together.)* [adv.] simultaneous simulcast assemble (OF) assembly

sincerus sincera sincerum *(Genuine; pure.)* [adj.] sincere sincerity sincerely insincere

sine *(Without.)* [prep.]   sine qua non *("Without which not." That which is indispensable.)*
sine prole *("Without offspring.")*   sinecure *("Without care." A paid office with few duties.)*
sine die *("Without setting a day.")*   sincere (**sin-** + **caries**: *"Without decay." Thus, pure.)*

singulus singula singulum *(Single, one, one each.)* [adj.] Freq. pl.: **singuli singulae singula** single singular singularity singly singleton singleness singularize single-handed, *etc.*

sinister sinistra sinistrum *(Left; unfavorable.)* [adj.] sinister sinisterly sinistral sinistrorse

sinus sinus *(Curve, fold; curl; valley; gulf.)* [masc. n.] sinus sinusitis sinuous sinuosity sinuate   insinuate   insinuation   sine   sine curve   sinusoid   sinusoidal projection

sisto sistere stiti status *(To cause to stand, place)* [v.] **adsisto:** assist assistance assistant; **consisto:** consist consistent consistency consistory; **desisto:** desist desistance; **exsisto:** exist existence existent existentialism; **insisto:** insist insistent insistence; **persisto:** persist persistent persistence; **resisto:** resist resistant resistance irresistible resistive resistivity resistor; **subsisto:** subsist subsistent subsistence solstice

situs situs *(Situation, site.)* [masc. n.] in situ *(In its original site.)* situate situated situation site (F)

socius socii *(Comrade, ally, companion, friend.)* [masc. n.] social sociable sociability socially society socialite socialize sociology sociometry Socialist associate disassociate association disassociation associative soccer *(Alter. of association.)* dissocial dissociable social studies social contract Social Security Society of Friends Associated Press, *etc.*

sol solis *(Sun, sunlight.)* [masc. n.] solar solarium solstice solarize solarization solarimeter parasol (It.) *("Shelter from sun.")* solano (Sp.) *(Hot wind.)* solar system solar plexus

soleo solere solitu *(To be accustomed.)* [v.]   insolent   insolence   obsolete   obsolescent

solidus solida solidum *(Solid, dense, firm; whole.)* [adj.] solid solidity solidify solidarity consolidate consolidation solder /sŏd-er/ (OF) soldier /sōl-jer/ (OF) soda (It.) sodium

sollicito sollicitare sollicitavi sollicitatus *(To stir up, disturb; trouble, distress; rouse.)* [v.] solicit   solicitation   solicitor   solicitous   solicitude   Solicitor General

solor solari solatus *(To comfort.)* [v.] solace console consolation consolatory disconsolate

solus sola solum *(Alone; only; lonely, forsaken.)* [adj.] solus sole solely solo (It.) soloist solitude solitary soliloquy solipsism solitaire (F) desolate desolation

solvo solvere solvi solutus *(To loosen; free, release.)* [v.] solve insolvable solvent insolvent solvency solution soluble insoluble solubility; **absolvo:** absolve absolution absolute absolutely absolutism; **dissolvo:** dissolve dissolvent dissolution dissoluble dissolute; **resolvo:** resolve re-solve resolved resolvent resolute resolution

somnus somni *(Sleep.)* [masc. n.] somnolence somnolent somniferous somniloquy somnambulate somnambulism somnambulist insomnia insomniac

sono sonare sonui sonitus *(To sound, make a noise; speak.)* [v.] sonority sonorous sone *(Unit of loudness.)* sonic supersonic subsonic sonic boom soniferous sound (OF) soundless sound-proof sonnet (It.) sonneteer sonata (It.) sonata form sonatina; **ab + sono:** absonant *(Discordant.)*; **adsono:** assonant assonance; **consono:** consonance consonant; **dissono:** dissonance dissonant; **persono:** person *("Sounding through" actor's mask.)* persona personable personal impersonal personality personalize persona grata *("A welcome person.")* personify personification personnel (F) parson (OF) parsonage; **resono:** resonance resonant resonator resound re-sound; unison *("One sound.")*

sorbeo sorbere sorbui *(To suck up, sup up; swallow.)* [v.] sorbefacient; **absorbeo:** absorb absorbed absorbent absorption; **ad + sorbeo:** adsorb adsorption; **de + sorbeo:** desorption; **resorbeo:** resorb resorption

sors sortis *(Lot; prophecy; oracle; fate, fortune.)* [fem. n.] sort sorcery sorcerer assort assorted assortment consort consortium resort (F) re-sort

spargo spargere sparsi sparsus *(To disperse, scatter.)* [v.] sparse sparsely sparseness; **aspergo:** asperse aspersion; **dispergo:** disperse dispersion; **interspargo:** intersperse

spatium spatii *(Space, distance; room, extent; time.)* [neut. n.] spatial space (OF) spacing spacious expatiate *(To speak or write at length.)* spacecraft space probe space-time, *etc.*

species speciei *(Kind, species; appearance, form.)* [fem. n.] species subspecies specific specifically specify specification specifiable special specialist specialize specialization specialty speciality specie *(Coined money.)* spice (OF) spicy specific gravity, *etc.*

specto spectare spectavi spectatus *(To look at, watch.)* spectator spectacle spectacles spectacular; **aspecto:** aspect; **circumspecto:** circumspect circumspection; **exspecto:** expect expectation expectancy expectant; **inspecto:** inspect inspection inspector; **introspecto:** introspect introspection introspective; **perspecto:** perspective perspectively; **prospecto:** prospect prospective prospector prospectus; **suspecto:** suspect unsuspected unsuspecting; RELATED: **specio specere spexi spectus** *(To look at; behold, see.)* [v.] specimen speculate speculation speculative speculator; **conspicio:** conspicuous conspectus; **despicio:** despise despicable despite (OF) spite; **perspicio:** perspicacious perspicacity perspicuity perspicuous; **respicio:** respect disrespect respectable disrespectable respectability respecting respectfully respective irrespective; **retrospicio:** retrospect retrospection retrospective; **suspicio:** suspicion suspicious; auspex [avis, *bird* + specio.] *(Soothsayer who predicted by observing birds.)* auspices auspicious

spectrum spectri *(Specter, apparition; vision.)* [neut. n.] spectrum spectrogram spectrograph spectroscope specter spectral

spero sperare speravi speratus *(To hope, expect; trust.)* [v.] **despero:** desperate desperation desperado (Sp.) despair (OF) despairing; **prospero:** prosper prosperous prosperity

spina   spinae   *(Thorn; spine, back; fish-bone.)*   [fem. n.]   spine   spinal   spineless spiniferous   spiny   spinule   spinate   spinal cord   porcupine (**porcus** *[pig]* + **spina.**)

spiro spirare spiravi spiratus *(To breathe; be alive.)* spirit spirited spiritual spiritualism spirituality spirograph spirometer spiritoso (It.) spiracle (OF) sprite (OF) esprit /es-prē/ (F) esprit de corps; **aspiro:** aspire aspiring aspirate aspirant aspiration aspsirator; **conspiro:** conspire conspiracy conspirator conspiratorial con spirito (It.); **exspiro:** expire expiration expiratory; **inspiro:** inspire inspiration inspirit inspirational inspiratory; **perspiro:** perspire perspiration; **respiro:** respire respiration respirator respiratory; **suspiro:** suspire suspiration; **trans + spiro:** transpire (F) transpiration

splendor splendoris *(Brilliance.)* [masc. n.] splendor splendiferous splendorous resplendent

spolio spoliare spoliavi spoliatus *(To strip; rob.)*   [v.]   spoliation   spoliative spoil (OF)   spoilage   spoiler   spoilsport   spoils system   despoil (OF)   despoliation

spondeo spondere spopondi sponsus *(To promise, answer.)* [v.] sponsor sponsorship spouse (OF) spousal espouse espousal; **despondeo:** despondent despondency; **respondeo:** respond correspond respondence correspondence respondent correspondent responding corresponding response responsive responsible responsibility

statuo statuere statui statutus *(To set up, place; establish.)* [v.] statute statutory; **constituo:** constitute constitution constituent constituency; **destituo:** destitute destitution; **instituo:** institute institution institutional institutionalize; **prostituo:** prostitute prostitution; **restituo:** restitution; **substituo:** substitute substitution

stella stellae *(Star.)* [fem. n.] stellar stellate stelliferous stelliform stellular constellation

sterilis sterilis sterile *(Barren, sterile; bare.)* [adj.] sterile sterility sterilize sterilization

sterno sternere stravi stratus *(To spread; throw down.)* [v.] stratum substratum stratus stratify stratocumulus stratosphere street (OE) consternation prostrate prostration

stilus stili *(Pen; stake.)* [masc. n.] stylus style stylish stylist stylistic stylize stiletto (It.)

stilla stilae *(A drip.)* [fem. n.] still *(For distilling.)* distill distillation distilled distillery instill

stimulus stimuli *(Spur, stimulus; incentive.)* [masc. n.] stimulus stimuli stimulate stimulation stimulant stimulative

sto stare steti staturus *(To stand; persist.)* [v.] status status quo stamen stamina state (OF) [adj.v.n.] stately statement station (F) stationary stationery stable (OF) *(Animal lodging.)* stable (F) *(Firm.)* stability stabilize stance (OF) stanza (It.) stature (OF) statue (F) statuary statuesque statuette stay (AF) stage (OF) stance (OF) stanch (OF) stanchion establish (OF); **circumsto:** circumstance circumstantial circumstantiate; **consto:** constant constancy cost (OF) costly; **contrasto:** contrast (OF) contrasting; **disto:** distant distance; **exsto:** extant; **insto:** instant instance instantaneous; **obsto:** obstacle obstinate obstinacy; **resto:** rest *(Remaining.)* restless restive resistivity resistor transistor (*trans*fer + res*istor*.) arrest (OF) (ad + resto.); **substo:** substance substantial substantiate substantive consubstantiation transubstantiation; **supersto:** superstition superstitious;

stringo stringere strinxi strictus *(To bind, tighten.)* [v.] strict stricture stringent stringency stringendo (It.) strain (OF) strained strainer strait (OF) stress (OF); **ab + stringo:** abstriction; **adstringo:** astriction astringe astringent; **constringo:** constrict constriction constrictor constrain (OF) constraint; **distringo:** district districting distrain (OF) distress (OF) distressing; **obstringo:** obstriction; **praestringo:** prestige (F) prestigious; **restringo:** restrict restriction restrictive restrain (OF) restraint restrainer

struo struere struxi structus *(To build; arrange.)* [v.] structure structural; **construo:** construct reconstruct construction reconstruction constructive construe; **destruo:** destruct destruction destructive destroy (OF) destroyer; **instruo:** instruct instruction instructive instructor instrument instrumental instrumentalist; **obstruo:** obstruct obstruction obstructionist; **substruo:** substructure; **superstruo:** superstructure

studeo studere studui *(To study; strive for.)* [v.] study studied studious studio student

stupeo stupere stupui *(To be stunned, be astonished.)* [v.] stupid stupefy stupendous stupefaction stupidity stupor

suadeo suadere suasi suasurus *(To urge, exhort, advise.)* [v.] dissuade dissuasion dissuasive persuade persuasion persuasive moral suasion

sub *(Under, below, beneath.)* [prep.] See: **sub-** as prefix in Ap. iii-20: submarine submit

sui *(Of himself, of herself, of it.)* [pron.] suicide suicidal sui generis *(Unique; of one kind.)*

sum esse fui *(To be, exist.)* [v.] essence essential essentially; **absum:** absent absence absentee absenteeism; **ens** [Pres. par.]: entity; **futurus** [Fut. par.]: future futurism; **possum (potis,** *able* **+ sum.):** possible possibility posse potent puissant (OF); **praesum:** present represent presence presentable presentation representation; **prosum:** proud (OF)

summa summae *(Chief control; main part; summary.)* [fem. n.] sum summary summarize summation summit consummate consummation summa cum laude summum bonum

sumo sumere sumpsi sumptus *(To take; assume.)* [v.] sumptuous; **adsumo:** assume assumed assumption; **consumo:** consume consumer consumption consumptive; **praesumo:** presume presumption presumptuous; **resumo:** resume resumption

super *(Above, over; beyond.)* [prep., adv.] See: **super-** as prefix in Ap. iii-21: superhuman

superus supera superum *(Above; high.)* [adj.] (Rel. *super, supra.*) **superior** *(Higher.)* [comp. adj.] **supremus** *(Highest.)* [Super. adj.] superb superbly superbness superior superiority supreme supremely supremeness supremacy sovereign (OF) (< **super**) sovereignty soprano (It.) (< **supra**); See: **super-** as prefix in Ap. iii-21: superlative supersonic

supra *(Above, over, beyond.)* [prep., adv.] See: **supra-** as prefix in Ap. iii-21: supraorbital

sur *(Above, beyond.)* [prep.] (O.F. for **super**.) See: **sur-** as prefix in Ap. iii-26: surcharge surplus

surgo surgere surrexi surrectus *(To get up, rise.)* [v.] surge source (OF); **insurgo:** insurgent insurgence insurrection; **resurgo:** resurge resurgence resurgent resurrect resurrection

T

taberna tabernae *(Shed, cottage; shop; inn.)* [fem. n.]   tabernacle   tavern (OF)   taverner

tabula tabulae *(Plank; writing-tablet; map, picture.)* [fem. n.] table tablature tabloid tablet tabular tabulate tabulator tableau (F) entablature   tabula rasa *("Blank tablet";* Locke: *the mind.)*

taceo tacere tacui tacitus *(To be silent, keep silent.)*   tacet tacit taciturn reticent reticence

tango tangere tetigi tactus *(To touch, handle; strike.)* [v.] tact intact tactful tactile tangent tangential tangible intangible;   **attingo:** attain (OF) attainment attainable attainder attaint;   **contingo:** contingent contiguous contiguity contact contactor contagion (MF)   contagious   contaminate   contamination;   entire (OF)   integer

tardo tardare tardavi tardatus *(To delay.)* [v.] tardy retard retardant retardation retarded

taxo taxare taxavi taxatus *(To value, appraise; to touch.)*   (< *tango*)   [v.] tax taxation taxable   tax-free   taxpayer   taste (OF)   tasteful   tasteless   tasty   taste bud

tego tegere texi tectus *(To cover; conceal, hide; protect.)* [v.] tegmen *(A covering.)* toga (L) *("A covering.")* tog (F) tile (OE); **detego:** detect detection detective detector;   **obtego:** obtect; **protego:** protect protection protective protector protectorate protégé (F)

temno temnere tempsi temptus *(To scorn, despise; slight.* [v.] **contemno:** contemn contempt   contemptible   contemptuous

tempero temperare temperavi temperatus *(To blend, moderate.)* [v.] temper tempered temperament temperate intemperate temperance intemperance temperature tempered

templum templi *(Sanctuary; temple; open space.)* [neut. n.]   temple   templed templar Knight Templar   contemplate   contemplation   contemplative

tempto temptare temptavi temptatus *(To try, attempt; test; prove.)* [v.] tempt tempting temptation   attempt   taunt (OF)

tempus temporis *(Time; opportunity, right time.)* [neut. n.] tempo (It.) temporary temporize temporal temporality contemporary contemporize contemporaneous extemporize extemporaneous   tense (OF) *(A verb form.)*   tempus fugit *("Time flies!")*

tendo tendere tetendi tentus *(To stretch, reach, extend.)* [v.] tend tendance tendency tendentious tender *(To present.)* tense (OF) *(Taut.)* tension tensile tensor tent (F) tendril (F); **attendo:** attend attendance attendant attention attentive;   **contendo:** contend contention contentious; **distendo:** distend distensible distention detent (F) détente (F); **extendo:** extend extended extensible extent extensive extension; **intendo:** intend intended intense intensity intensify intensive intent;   **ostendo:** ostensible ostensive ostentation ostentatious;   **portendo:** portend portent portentious; **praetendo:** pretend pretended pretender pretense pretension pretentious; **subtendo:** subtend

teneo tenere tenui tentus *(To hold, keep; possess, occupy.)* [v.] tenant tenacious tenement tenable tenet tenon tenor tenure tenuto (It.) tennis (AF); **abstineo:** abstention abstinence abstinent abstain (OF) abstainer; **contineo:** content *(Contents; satisfied.)*

Ap. vii-44

contented contentment continuum (L) (Pl. continua.) continence incontinence continent *(Abstinent.)* incontinent continent *(Land mass.)* continental continue (OF) continual continuous continuance continuation continuity contain (OF) container containment countenance (OF); **detineo:** detention detain (OF) detainer; **obtineo:** obtain (OF); **pertineo:** pertinent pertinacious pertinacity pertain (OF) appertain (OF) appurtenance (AF); **retineo:** retention retentive retentivity retinue (F) retain (OF) retainer *(Keeper.)* retainer *(Fee.)*; **sustineo:** sustenance sustain (OF) sostenuto (It.); entertain (F) (enter < entre < **inter,** *between.*) entertainer entertaining entertainment; maintain (OF)

tenuis tenuis tenue *(Thin, slight, small; feeble.)* [adj.] tenuous attenuate attenuant attenuation extenuate extenuating extenuation

tergeo tergere tersi tersus *(To wipe, clean; scour.)* [v.] terse tersely terseness; **detergeo:** deterge detergency detergent detersion detersive

termino terminare terminavi terminatus *(To limit, bound.)* [v.] term terminal terminate terminus termination terminator terminology termer termor terminable interminable; **determino:** determine determined determining determiner determinism determinate determination; **extermino:** exterminate extermination exterminator; conterminous

tero terere trivi tritus *(To rub, grind; waste.)* [v.] trite triteness triturate trituration tribulation (OF) trial (AF) try (OF) trying; **attero:** attrition; **contero:** contrite contrition; **detero:** detrition detriment detrimental detritus detrital

terra terrae *(Earth, land; ground, soil; country.)* [fem. n.] terra terrace terrain terrestrial territory territorial terrier terrarium terrella terricolous terraquious terrine (F) tureen (F) inter Mediterranean Sea parterre (MF) subterranean subterrane terra firma *(Solid ground.)* terra cotta (It.) *("Cooked earth"; red kiln-burnt clay.)* terra incognito *(Unknown land.)*

terreo terrere terrui territus *(To frighten, alarm, scare.)* [v.] terror terrify terrorize terrorism terrorist terrible terrific deter deterrent

testa testae *(Shell, skull.)* [fem. n.] **testum testi** *(Earthen vessel for testing metals.)* [neut. n.] test testa testaceous tester testudo testudinal testy

testor testari testatus *(To testify, witness; prove.)* [v.] testament testacy testate intestate testator testify testimony testimonial; **attestor:** attest attestation; **contestor:** contest contestant; **detestor:** detest detestable; **protestor:** protest protester Protestant

texo texere texui textum *(To weave, intertwine; construct.)* [v.] text textile texture textured textual texualist tissue (OF); **contexo:** context contextual; **praetexo:** pretext

timeo timere timui *(To be afraid.)* [v.] timid timidity timorous intimidate intimidation

tingo ingere tinxi tinctus *(To dye, color: soak, dip.)* [v.] tinge tinct tincture tinctorial tint (It.) taint (F) intinction

titulus tituli *(Title, label, inscription; notice.)* (masc. n.) title titled titular tittle intitule intitle entitle

tolero tolerare toleravi toleratus *(To endure; support.)* [v.] tolerate toleration tolerant intolerant tolerance intolerance tolerable intolerable

torno tornare tornavi tornatus *(To twist; turn in a lathe.)* [v.] tornado (Sp.) turn (OF) return returnable tour (MF) tourist tourism tournament (OF) tourney tourniquet (F) tour de force *(A remarkable feat.)* contour (F) detour (F) attorn (OF) attorney

torpeo torpere torpui torpitus *(To be stiff; be numb.)* [v.] torpid torpor torporific torpedo

torreo torrere torrui tostum *(To scorch, parch; roast.)* [v.] torrid torrify torrent torrential

torqueo torquere torsi tortus *(To twist, wring; bend.)* [v.] torque torsion (OF) torsibility torture (OF) tortuous tort (OF) tortilla (Sp.) tortoise torment (OF) tormentor torch (OF) torticollis *("Twisted neck"; wryneck.)*; **contorqueo:** contort contortion contortionist; **distorqueo:** distort distortion; **extorqueo:** extort extortion; **retorqueo:** retort

totus tota totum *(All, whole, entire.)* [adj.] total totality totalize totalitarian totalitarianism tutti (It.) *(All.)* surtout (F) /ser/t͞o͞o/ *(Above all.)* surtout (F) /ser/t͞o͞ot/ *(Overcoat.)*

traho trahere traxi tractus *(To pull, drag; attract.)* [v.] tract *(Area; treatise.)* tractor tractable intractable trail (AF) train (OF) trainee trainer training treat (OF) entreat entreaty; **abstraho:** abstract abstracted abstraction; **attraho:** attract attraction attractive; **contraho:** contract *(Agreement; draw together.)* contraction contractor contractual; **detraho:** detract detraction detractor; **distraho:** distract distraction **extraho:** extract extraction; **protraho:** protract protractor protraction portray (OF) portrait; **retraho:** retract retraction retractor; **subtraho:** subtract subtraction subtrahend

tranquillus tranquilla tranquillum *(Calm.)* [adj.] tranquil tranquillity tranquilize

trans *(Across, over, beyond.)* [prep.] See: **trans-** as prefix in Ap. iii-21: transcontinental

tremo tremere tremui *(To tremble, quake, quiver.)* [v.] tremble tremor tremulous tremulant tremolo (It.) tremendous

trepidus trepida trepidum *(Alarmed, anxious, restless.)* [adj.] trepidation intrepid intrepidity

tres tres tria *(Three.)*; **tertius tertia tertium** *(Third.)*; **triplus tripla triplum** *(Triple.)* tertiary tertian tertial tertium quid *(One unknown related to two knowns.)* treble (OF) trellis (OF) triad triangle triplet;. See: **tri-** as prefix in Ap. iii-21, 25: triceps tripod trisect

tribuo tribuere tribui tributus *(To allot, assign, grant.)* [v.] tribute tributary; **attribuo:** attribute attribution; **contribuo:** contribute contribution; **distribuo:** distribute distribution distributive distributor distributary; **retribuo:** retribution retributive

tribus tribus *(Tribe.)* [masc. n.] tribe (< tri-, three groups: *Latins, Sabines, and Etruscans.*) tribal tribalism tribesman tribune tribunal tribunate

tricae tricarum *(Hindrances; nonsense.)* [fem. pl. n.] **tricor tricari** *(To make mischief.)* [v.] trick (AF) tricky trickery trickster; **extrico:** extricate extricable; **intrico:** intricate intricacy intrigue (F)

triumpho triumphare triumphavi triumphatus *(To triumph.)* [v.] triumph triumphant

trudo trudere trusi trusus *(To push, thrust; drive; force.)* [v.] **abstrudo:** abstruse abstrusely abstruseness; **detrudo:** detrude detrusion; **extrudo:** extrude extrusion extrusive; **intrudo:** intrude intruder intrusion intrusive; **obtrudo:** obtrude obtruder obtrusion obtrusive; **protrudo:** protrude protrusion protrusive protrusile

trunco truncare truncavi truncatus *(To cut top off; maim.)* [v.] trunk truncate detruncate truncated detruncated detruncation trunkfish truncheon (OF) trunnion (F)

tuba tubae *(War trumpet.)* [fem. n.] **tubus tubi** *(Pipe, tube.)* [masc. n.] tube tuba tubing tuber *(A tube maker.)* tubal tubate tubular tubiform tube-shaped intubate intubation

tuber tuberis *(A swelling, lump.)* [neut. n.] tuber *(E.g., a potato.)* tuberous tubercle tubercular tuberculin tuberculosis protuberant protuberance

tueor tueri tuitus tutus *(To watch, guard, protect.)* [v.] tutor (OF) tutelary tutelage tuition (OF) tutorship intuit intuition intuitive intuitionism

tumeo tumere *(To swell; be excited.)* [v.] **tumor tumoris** *(A swelling, a bulge.)* [masc. n.] **tumulus tumuli** *(A mound, hill; burial mound.)* [masc. n.] tumor tumid tumidity tumescent tumescence tumulus (Pl. tumuli.) tumulose intumesce intumescence tumult tumultuous

turba turbae *(A crowd; disorder, riot.)* [fem. n.] **turbo turbinis** *(A whirling, an eddy.)* [masc. n.] **turbo turbare turbavi turbatus** *(To disturb; make an uproar.)* [v.] turbid turbulent turbulence turbidimeter turbinal turbinate turbine turbogenerator turbojet turboprop; **disturbo:** disturb disturbed disturbance; **perturbo:** perturb perturbation

U

ulter ultra ultrum *(Far, remote.)* [adj.] **ulterior ulterioris** *(Farther, more remote.)* [Comp. adj.] **ultimus ultima ultimum** *(Farthest, most remote.)* [Super. adj.] ulterior ultimate ultimately ultimatum ultimo ultimogeniture ultima penultimate penult

ultra *(Beyond, on far side of.)* (< **ulter**) [prep., adv.]   See: **ultra-** as prefix in Ap. iii-22: ultraviolet

umbra umbrae *(Shadow, shade; ghost.)* [fem. n.] umbrage umbra umbrageous umbriferous umbrella (It.) umbel adumbrate adumbral adumbration adumbrative penumbra

umeo umere *(To be damp, be wet.)* [v.] humid humidity humidify humidor humor (OF) humorist humorous humoral humoresque (Ger.)

unda undae *(Wave, water; stream, surge.)* [fem. n.]   **undo undare** *(To surge, undulate.)* [v.] undulate undulating undulation undulant undulant fever; **abundo:** abundant abundance abound (OF); **inundo:** inundate inundation inundant inundator; **redundo:** redundant redundance redundancy redound (F); **superundo:** surround (AF) surrounding

ungo ungere unxi unctus *(To anoint; grease, smear.)* [v.]   unguent unction unctuous

unus una unum *(One, sole, single, only.)* [number, adj.] e pluribus unum *("One out of many.")* unanimous (**unus**, *one* + **animus**, *mind*.) unanimity triune *("Three in one.")* onion (OF) (Doublet of *union*.) unit united unison union uniform unify; See: **uni-** as prefix in Ap. iii-22.

urbs urbis *(City; Rome.)* [fem. n.] urban urbanize urbane suburb suburban suburbanite suburbia   interurban

utor uti usus *(To use; enjoy; practice.)* [v.] use (OF) used useful useless user usual usually utility (F) utilize utilitarian utilitarianism utensil (OF)   usury (OF)   usurer usurious usurp usurpation; **abutor:** abuse abusive; **per + utor:** peruse perusal

uva uvae *(Bunch of grapes.)* [fem. n.] uveous   uvea   uveitis   uvula   uvular   uvulitis

V

vacuus vacua vacuum *(Empty, vacant.)* [adj.] vacate vacant vacancy vacation vacationist vacuum vacuum-packed vacuous; **evacuo:** evacuate evacuation evacuee

vado vadere vasi *(To go.)* [v.] Quo vadis? *(Whither goest thou?)* **evado:** evade evasion evasive; **invado:** invade invasion invasive; **pervado:** pervade pervasion pervasive; vamoose (Sp.)

vagor vagare vagatus *(To stroll about, wander, roam.)* [v.]   vagabond   vagrant vagrancy   vague   vagary   extravagant   extravagance   extravaganza   extravagate

valeo valere valui valiturus *(To be strong, be in good health.)* [v.] vale /vā-lē/ *(Farewell.)* valedictory valedictorian valetudinarian *(A chronic invalid.)* valence valid (F) invalid /in-val-id/ *(Not valid.)* invalid /in-və-lid/ *(A sickly person.)* validate invalidate validation invalidation validity valiant (OF) value (OF) valuable invaluable valuator valued valuate evaluate (F) valuation evaluation valor (OF) valorous avail (OF) available availability countervail (AF); **convalesco:** convalesce convalescent; **praevaleo:** prevalent prevail (OF) prevailing

valles vallis *(A valley.)* [fem. n.]   valley   vale   intervale   avalanche (F. Swiss.)

vallum valli *(Rampart, fortification, entrenchment.)* [neut. n.] interval circumvallate wall (OE)

vanus vana vanum *(Empty, idle.)* [adj.] vanity (OF) vain (F) vainglory (OF) vanish (OF) vaunt; **evanesco:** evanesce evanescence evanescent   vanitas vanitatum *(Vanity of vanities.)*

vapor vaporis *(Vapor; steam; heat.)* [masc. n.] vapor vaporize vaporization vaporizer vaporific   vaporous   evaporate   evaporation

vario variare variavi variatus *(To vary, change.)* [v.] vary varied variable invariable various variety variation variant invariant variance variegate variegated variorum variform variola *(Smallpox.)*   varicella *(Chicken pox.)*   variole *(A pockmark.)*   variolate *(To vaccinate.)*

vas vasis *(Vessel; duct.)* [neut. n.] vas vase vascular   vascular bundle   vasculum vasectomy vasoconstrictor vasodilator vasomotor cardio-vascular extravasate vessel (OF)

vaso vastare vastavi vastatus *(To lay waste.)* [v.] vast vastly vastness devastate devastation

vegetus vegeta vegetum *(Quickly, lively, sprightly.)* [adj.] vegetable vegetal vegetarian vegetarianism   vegetate   vegetation   vegetative   vegetant   vegetable oil

veho vehere vexi vectus *(To bear, carry; drive, ride.)* [v.] vehicle vehement vehemence vector vectorial; **adveho:** advection; **conveho:** convection convective convex; **eveho:** evection evectional; **inveho:** invective inveigh; **proveho:** provection

velum veli *(A sail; curtain.)* [neut. n.] velum velamen velar velarium velate Vela *(A constellation, The Sail.)* veil (OF) unveil veiling; **revelo:** reveal revealing revelation Revelations

vello vellere velsi vulsus *(To pull, pick; tear up.)* [v.] **convello:** convulse convulsion convulsionary convulsive; **revello:** revulsion revulsive

vena venae *(Vein, artery; vein of metal; rivulet.)* [fem. n.] venous venosity venule venulose venipuncture venation intravenous vein (OF)

vendo vendere vendidi venditus *(To sell; betray.)* [n.] venal venality vend vender

veneror venerari *(To revere, worship.)* [v.] venerate veneration venerable venerability

venio venire veni venturus *(To come.)* [v.] venture venturous venturesome venire *(Jury summons.)* "Veni, vidi, vici." (Caesar: *"I came, I saw, I conquered."*) Venite Adoramus *("Come, let us adore.")*; **advenio:** advent Advent adventure adventuresome adventitious adventurer adventurous avenue (F); **convenio:** convene convenient convenience convent (OF) convention conventional; **contra + venio:** contravene (F) contravention; **evenio:** event eventful eventually; **invenio:** invent invention inventive inventor inventory; **intervenio:** intervene intervention interventionist; **pervenio:** parvenu (F); **praevenio:** prevent prevention preventive; **provenio:** provenience; **revenio:** revenue (F) revenuer; **subvenio:** subvene souvenir (F); **supervenio:** supervene

venter ventris *(Stomach, belly; womb.)* [masc. n.] venter ventral ventricle ventricular ventriculus ventricose ventriloquist ventriloquism *(To speak [loqui] from the belly.)* ventral fin

ventus venti *(Wind.)* [masc. n.] vent ventilate ventilation ventage ventilator ventiduct

venus veneris *(Charm, beauty; love.)* [fem. n.] Venus venereal venereal disease venereology Venus de Milo Venus flytrap Venus's-hair *(A maidenhair fern.)*

verbum verbi *(Word, saying.)* [neut. n.] verb verbal verbalize verbose verbosity verbatim verbatim et literatim *(Word for word and letter for letter.)* verbigerate *(To repeat meaningless words over and over.)* verve (F) adverb adverbial proverb proverbial Proverbs

vereor verreri veitus *(To fear; revere, respect.)* [v.] venerate venerable veneration; **revereor:** revere reverence reverent reverential Reverend Reverence

veritas veritus *(Truth, truthfulness; reality.)* [fem. n.] **verus vera verum** *(True, real, actual.)* [adj.] veritas verify verifiable verification very (OF) verily verity veritable veracious veracity verism verisimilar veridical verdict (**vere dictum**, *truly said.*) aver (OF) averment

vergo vergere versi *(To turn, incline; bend.)* [v.] (Rel. to **verto**.) verge *(To incline.)* converge convergence diverge divergence divergent

vermis vermis *(A worm.)* [masc. n.] (< **verto.**) vermin verminous vermivorous vermicelli vermicular vermiculate vermiculation vermiculite vermiform vermifuge vermilion

verto vertere verti versus *(To turn; invert; change.)* [v.] vertical vertebra (Pl. vertebrae.) vertebrate vertex (Pl. vertices.) vertigo vertiginous verse versed versemonger versify version versus verso *(Left page.)* reverso *(Right page.)* versatile versicle versicolor versant vortex (var. vertex) vortical vorticose vortiginous; **averto** (ab + verto): avert averse aversion; **adverto:** advert advertent inadvertent advertise advertising advertisement adverse adversity adversary; **converto:** convert /con-vert/ [n.] convert /cən-vert/ [v.] converter convertible conversion conversant conversation conversational conversationalist converse /con-vers/ [n. adj.] converse /cən-vers/ [v.]; **contra** (contro)+ **verto:** controvert controversy controversial; **diverto:** divert diverting diverticulum divertimento (It.) divers diverse diversify diversified diversion diversionary diversity divorce (MF) divorcé /di-vor-sā/ (F) [masc.] divorcée (F) [fem.] divorcee /di-vor-cē/; **everto** (ex + verto): evert eversion evertor; **extra** (extro) + **verto:** extrovert extroversion; **inverto:** invert invertebrate inverse inversion; **intro + verto:** introvert introversion; **obverto:** obvert obverse obversion; **perverto:** pervert /per-vert/ [n.] pervert /per-vert/ [v.] perverted perverse perversion perversity; **proverto:** prose (OF); **reverto:** revert reverse reversal reversible reversion; **subverto:** subvert subversion subversive; **transverto:** transverse transversal traverse; dextrorse *(Turn to right.)* sinistrorse *(To left.)*

vestis vestis *(Clothes, tapestry.)* [fem. n.] vest *(Garment; to confer authority.)* vested vestee vestiary vestment vest-pocket vestry vesture devest divest divestment divestiture invest investment investiture investive travesty transvestite transvestitism

vestigium vestigii *(Footprint, track, trace, sign.)* [neut. n.] vestige vestigial vestigium investigate investigation investigator

vetus veteris *(Old, aged; former; pl. the ancients.)* [adj.] veteran vet inveterate inveteracy

via viae *(Way, road.)* [fem. n.] via viaduct viator viaticum deviate deviation devious obviate obvious pervious impervious previous convey (OF) conveyance conveyer conveyor convoy (MF) envoy (OF) invoice (OF) voyage (OF) Via Dolorosa *("Sorrowful Way.")*

vibro vibrare vibravi vibratus *(To vibrate, shake; wave.)* [v.] vibrate vibration vibrant vibrancy vibrator vibratory vibrato (It.) vibrissa *(A nose hair.)* vibraphone (**phone**, Gk. *sound.*)

vicis vicis *(Change; alternation.)* [fem. n.] vicissitude vicissitudinary vicar vicarage vicarious vicarial vice versa *(Conversely.)* vice-president See: **vice-** as prefix in Ap. iii-22.

vicinus vicina vicinum *(Near, neighboring.)* [adj.] vicinity vicinage vicinal vicinal road

video videre vidi visus *(To see, observe; know; consider.)* [v.] video vision (OF) envison visionary visible (OF) invisible visibility invisibility visual (OF) visualize visit (OF) visitor visitation visor (AF) visa /vē-zə/ (F) vista (It.) visage (OF) vizard *(A mask,* alter. visor.) view (OF) interview vis-a-vis /vē-zə-vē/ (F) *("Face to face.")* voyeur (F); **advideo** (LL): advise (OF) advisable advised advisedly adviser (Also: advisor.) advisory advice (OF); **evideo** (LL): evident evidence evidentially; **invideo:** invidious envious (OF); **revideo:** revise (MF) revision review (MF) revisit revue (F); **provideo:** provide provider provided provident providence providential provision provisional proviso provisory improvise improvisation prudent (OF) imprudent prudential prudence jurisprudence; survey (AF) (**super + video.**) surveying surveyor television (**tele**, Gk., *distance.*) televise vide (Abbr. v., *See.*) vide supra *(See above.)* vide infra *(See below.)* vide ante *(See before.)* vide post *(See after.)* videlicet (Abbr. viz., *that is to say, namely.*)

villa villae *(House, villa.)* [fem. n.] villa village (OF) villager villain villainous villainy

vinco vincere vici victus *(To conquer, defeat; win.)* [v.] vincible invincible victor victory victorious vanquish (OF) vanquisher; **convinco:** convince convincing convict /con-vict/ *(Prisoner.)* convict /cən-vict/ *(To prove guilty.)*; **evinco:** evict eviction evince; Victor Victoria

vindico vindicare vindicavi vindicatus *(To avenge; protect.)* [v.] vindicate vindication vindictive vengeance (OF) vengeful avenge (OF) avenger revenge (OF) revengeful

vinum vini *(Wine.)* [neut. n.] vine vinedresser vinaceous vinery vineyard vinic vinometer vinous vinosity vinegar vinegary vintage vintner wine (OE) winery

viola violare violavi violatus *(To violate; do violence.)* [v.] violate inviolate violable inviolable violation violent violence

vir viri *(Man; hero; husband; soldier.)* [masc. n.] virile virility virilism virtue virtuous virtual virtually virtuoso (It.) virtuosity triumvirate *(Three man rule.)* virtu (It.)

virus viri *(Slime; poison; offensive smell.)* [neut. n.] virus virulent virulence virology

virgo virginis *(Maiden, girl, young woman; virgin.)* [fem. n.] virgin virginal *(Chaste.)* virginal *(Harpsichord.)* virginity Virgin Mary Virgin Islands (<u>Note</u>: Virginia < *Virginius,* a Roman clan.)

vita vitae *(Life, livelihood; way of life; career.)* [fem. n.] vita (pl. vitae) vital viable vitality vitalize devitalize revitalize vitalism vitals vitamin vitaminology Ars longa, vita brevis. *(Art is long, life is short.)*

vitium vitii *(Fault, flaw, defect, failing, vice.)* [neut. n.] **vitupero -are -avi -atus** *(To find fault.)* [v.] vitiate vitiated vitiation vitiator vituperate vituperation vituperative

vivo vivere vixi victus *(To live, be alive.)* [v.] vive (F) *(Long live!)* viva (It.) *(Long live!)* vivacious vivify vivacity vivid vivace (It.) vivarium viand vivisect vivisection vivisectionist; **convivo:** convivial conviviality; **revivo:** revive revival revivalist revivify; **supervivo:** survive (AF) survival survivor; in vivo *(Within the living organism.)*

voco vocare vocavi vocatus *(To call, summon; name; invite.)* [v.] vocal vocalist vocalize vocabulary vocation vocative vociferous; **avoco:** avocation avocatory; **advoco:** advocate advocation advocacy advocatus diaboli *(The devil's advocate.)*; **convoco:** convoke convocation; **evoco:** evoke evocation; **invoco:** invoke invocation; **provoco:** provoke provocation provocative; **revoco:** revoke revocation revocable irrevocable; equivocate equivocation intervocalic sotto voce (It.) *("Under voice"; softly.)*

volcanus volcani (Also: **vulcanus vulcani.**) *(Vulcan, god of fire; fire.)* [masc. n.] Vulcan Vulcanian vulcanite vulcanize volcano (It.) volcanology volcanic volcanism

volo velle volui *(To wish, want; will.)* [v.] **voluntas voluntatis** *(Will, wish, inclination.)* [fem. n.] volition volitional voluntary involuntary volunteer benevolent (**bene** = *good.*) malevolent (**mal** = *bad.*)

volo volare volavi volatus *(To fly; speed)* [v.] volley volleyball (ball, O.N.) volleying volatile volatility volitant volitation volant vole *(Card game term.)* volery

volvo volvere volvi volutus *(To roll, cause to revolve.)* [v.] volute voluted volution voluble volvulus volume (OF) volumeter volumetric voluminous vault (OF) *(Chamber.)* vault *(To leap.)* vaulting volti (It.) *(Turn the page.)* volt (F) *(Fencing term.)*; **circumvolvo:** circumvolve circumvolution; **convolvo:** convolute convolution convolve; **devolvo:** devolve devolution; **evolvo:** evolve evolution evolutionary evolutionist; **involvo:** involve involved involution; **inter + volvo:** intervolve; **revolvo:** revolve revolver revolution revolutionary revolutionist revolt (MF) revolting

voro varare voravi voratus *(To swallow; devour.)* [v.] voracious voraciously carnivore *(A meat eater.)* carnivorous devour herbivore *(A plant eater.)* herbivorous omnivore *(Eats all, i.e., both plants and meat.)* omnivorous

voveo vovere vovi votus *(To vow; promise; dedicate.)* [v.] vote votive votary vow; **devoveo:** devote devoted devotion devotional devotee

vox vocis *(Voice; sound; cry, call; word, saying.)* [fem. n.] voice (OF) revoice voiced voiceless voiceprint vowel vox humana vox populi vouch (OF) vouchee voucher vouchsafe

vulgus vulgi *(The mass of people, the public; crowd.)* [neut. n.] vulgar vulgarian vulgarism vulgarity vulgarize vulgate Vulgate Bible Vulgar Latin divulge divulgence promulgate promulgation

MORE LATIN ROOT ELEMENTS

aceti- *acetic acid*	**acu-** *point*	**amino-** *with* NH_2
Anglo- *English*	**antero-** *in front*	**arbori-** *tree*
-aster *little, inferior*	**avi-** (< avis) *bird*	**bacci-** *berry*
.bovi- *ox, cattle*	**calci-** *lime*	**carbo-** *carbon*
cerebro- *brain*	**cervico-** *neck*	**-cide** (< caedo) *killer*
cirro- *cirrus, curly*	**-colous** *dwelling in*	**costo-** *rib*
cupro- *copper*	**curvi-** *curved*	**duodeno-** *duodenum*
equi- (< aequo) *equal*	**Graeco-, Greco-** *Greek*	**febri-** *fever*
-ferous (< fero) *producing*	**ferri-, ferro-** *iron*	**fibrino-** *fibrin*
fibro- *fibrous*	**-fid, fissi-** *split*	**flabelli-** *fan shaped*
flexi- (< flecto) *bent*	**-florous** (< floreo) *flowering*	**fluoro-** *fluorine*
fluvio- *river*	**-folious** (< folium) *leafy*	**fronto-** *frontal bone*
Franco- *French*	**Gallo-** *Gaul, French*	**genito-** (< gigno) *genital*
Germano- *German*	**-gerous** (< gero) *producing*	**grani-** *grain*
grano- *like granite*	**hernio-** *hernia*	**igni-** *fire*
ileo- *ileum*	**imino-** *with imine*	**immuno-** *immune*
inguino- *groin*	**Judeo-** *Jewish*	**labio-** *lips*
lacto- *milk*	**lamelli-** *in layers*	**lati-** (< latus) *broad*

MORE LATIN ROOT ELEMENTS (Continued)

levo- *to the left*
magneto- *magnet*
-natured *disposition*
occipito- *occipital*
oro- *mouth, oral*
palmi- *palm*
-pede (< pes) *footed*
-petal (< peto) *seeking*
pinni- *web, fin*
pluvio- *rain*
radio *radioactive*
reni- *kidney*
scapi- *stem, shaft*
-section (< seco) *dividing*
seti- *bristle*
spini- *spine, thorn*
strati- *stratum*
tuberculo- *tuberculosis*
utero- *uterus*
ventro- *abdomen*

ligni- *wood*
muci-, muco- *mucus*
nigri- *black*
oculo- *eye*
ossi- *bone*
para- (< paro) *shelter*
pelvi- *pelvis*
pili- *hair*
pisci- *fish*
-proof (< probo) *protected*
recti- (< rego) *straight*
sacro- *sacrum bone*
sebi- *fat*
sero- *serum*
silico- *silicon*
stamini- *stamen*
sulfa-, sulfo- *sulfur*
turbo- *turbine*
vagino- *vagina*
vesico- *bladder*

lympho- *lymph*
naso- *nose*
nocti- *at night*
oleo- *oil*
ovi-, ovo- *egg*
-parous *producing*
-pennate *with wings*
pinnati- *feathered*
plumbo- *lead*
pulmo- *lung*
recto- *rectal*
sangui- *blood*
-sect (< seco) *cut, divide*
sesqui- *one and a half*
Sino- *Chinese*
stercori- *excrement*
ter- *three*
urino- *urine*
vaso- *a blood vessel*
vitri- *glass*

LATIN: THE SHORT COURSE (Bare Roots)

Review the Latin Prefixes.   They are used over and over again.

ab- *from;* ad- *to, toward;* circum- *around;* com- *with, together;* contra- *against;*
counter- (F- contre) *against;* de- *down; not;* dis- *apart;* ex- *out;* in- *in, on; not;*
inter- *between;* intra- *within;* juxta- *beside;* mis- (OF) *bad; not;* multi- *much, many;* non- *not;* post- *after;* pre- *before;* pro- *for, forward;* re- *again, back;*
retro- *again;* se- *apart* sub- *under* super- *above;* trans- *across* ultra- *beyond;*
Remember: as chameleon prefixes **ad-** may be: ac-, af-, ag-, al-, an-, ap-, ar-, as-, at-; **com-:** co-, col-, con-, cor-; **ex-:** e-, ec-, ef-; **in-:** il-, im-, ir-; **sub-:** suc-, suf-, sug-, sum, sup-, sur-, sus-

act *(To do.)* act actor actress actual action enact exact interact react
transact interaction reaction transaction enactment [< **ago** Ap. vii-2.]

aud- *(To hear.)* audio auditory audience auditorium audible inaudible
audit audition auditor auditory audio-visual   [< **audio** Ap. vii-3.]

cap *(Head.)* cap capital capitol capitalism captain caption [< **caput** Ap. vii-5.]

ceed, cede, cess *(To go.)* exceed proceed succeed concede intercede precede recede abscess access excess process recess success excessive concession intercession procession recession [< **cedo** Ap. vii-6.]

cent *(Hundred.)* cent century centennial bicentennial centipede centigrade centimeter centigram per cent [< **centum** Ap. vii-6.]

cept *(To take.)* accept concept except intercept conception deception exception inception perception reception susceptible [< **capio** Ap. vii-5.]

cide *(To kill.)* fungicide genocide homicide pesticide suicide [< **caedo** Ap. vii-5.]

cise *(To cut.)* concise excise precise precisely circumcise decision decisive excision incision incisive incisor precision [< **caedo** Ap. vii-5.]

cite *(To rouse.)* cite excite incite recite excitement incitement [< **cito** Ap. vii-7.]

claim, clam *(To shout.)* claim acclaim declaim exclaim proclaim reclaim acclamation declamation exclamation proclamation [< **clamo** Ap. vii-7.]

cline *(To lean.)* decline incline inclination recline recliner [< **clino** Ap. vii-7.]

clude, clus *(To close.)* conclude exclude include preclude seclude recluse conclusion exclusion inclusion seclusion [< **claudo** Ap. vii-7.]

cogni *(To understand.)* cognition cognitive incognito recognize [< **cognosco** Ap. vii-8.]

cord *(Heart.)* accord accordion concord discord record cordial [< **cor** Ap. vii-8.]

corp *(Body.)* corpse corporal corporation corpuscle corps /kor/ [< **corpus** Ap. vii-9.]

cred *(To believe.)* credible credit creditor discredit incredible [< **credo** Ap. vii-9.]

crim *(To accuse.)* crime criminal discriminate incriminate [< **crimino** Ap. vii-9.]

cur *(To run.)* current currency curriculum cursive cursory concur incur occur occurrence recur recurrence concurrent [< **curro** Ap. vii-10.]

dict *(To speak.)* dictate diction dictionary dictator contradict edict predict indict /in-dīt/ contradiction benediction prediction [< **dico²** Ap. vii-11.]

div *(To divide.)* divide division divisible indivisible individual [< **dividio** Ap. vii-11.]

duct *(To lead.)* duct ductile abduct conduct deduct induct product viaduct abduction conduction deduction induction introduction production reproduction reduction seduction conducive conductor [< **duco** Ap. vii-12.]

fect *(To make.)* affect defect defective effect effective infect perfect affection defection infection perfection imperfection [< **facio** Ap. vii-13.]

fer *(To bear.)* fertile confer defer differ infer offer prefer refer suffer transfer conference deference difference preference reference transference different circumference referendum [< **fero** Ap. vii-14.]

fid, fed *(To trust.)* fidelity infidelity affidavit confide confident diffident perfidious fiduciary federal confederate confederation [< **fido** Ap. vii-14.]

fin *(End.)* final fine finish finite infinite confine define refine [< **finis** Ap. vii-14.]

firm *(To support.)* firm affirm reaffirm confirm infirm infirmary firmament affirmation reaffirmation confirmation [< **firmo** Ap. vii-15.]

fix *(To fasten.)* fix fixation fixture affix infix prefix suffix [< **figo** Ap. vii-14.]

flate *(To blow.)* inflate conflate deflate inflation deflation [< **flo** Ap. vii-15.]

flect *(To bend.)* deflect inflect reflect inflection reflection [< **flecto** Ap. vii-15.]

flo *(To flower.)* flower floral florid Florida florescence [< **floreo** Ap. vii-15.]

flu *(To flow.)* fluid fluent flume fluctuate flux influx reflux flush affluence confluence influence superfluous [< **fluo** Ap. vii-15.]

form *(To shape.)* form conform deform inform perform reform transform uniform formation conformation information reformation transformation performance deformity malformed [< **formo** Ap. vii-15.]

fract *(To break.)* fraction fractional fractious fracture diffract infract refract diffraction infraction refraction [< **frango** Ap. vii-16.]

fuse *(To pour.)* fuse fusible confuse diffuse infuse profuse refuse refusal suffuse superfuse transfuse fusion confusion diffusion infusion profusion suffusion superfusion transfusion [< **fundo** Ap. vii-16.]

gest *(To carry on.)* gesture congest digest digestible ingest suggest congestion digestion ingestion suggestion suggestible [< **gero** Ap. vii-16.]

grad, -gress *(Step.)* grade gradation gradient gradual graduate graduation aggress congress digress egress ingress progress aggression digression progression transgression [< **gradior** Ap. vii-16.]

greg *(Group.)* gregarious aggregate congregate segregate desegregate aggregation congregation segregation desegregation [< **grex** Ap. vii-17.]

-here, hes *(To stick.)* adhere cohere inhere adherent coherent inherent adhesive cohesive cohesion hesitate hesitation [< **haereo** Ap. vii-17.]

ject *(To throw.)* abject deject eject inject object project reject subject traject dejected ejection injection objection projection rejection subjection trajectory adjective conjecture subjective [< **jacio** Ap. vii-19.]

jud *(To judge.)* judge judicial judiciary judicious injudicious judgment adjudicate adjudication prejudge prejudice prejudicial [< **judico** Ap. vii-19.]

junct *(To join.)* juncture junction adjunct disjunct disjunction disjunctive conjuncture injunction subjunctive conjunctivitis [< **jungo** Ap. vii-19.]

jure *(To swear.)* conjure conjurer perjure perjury abjure adjure [< **juro** Ap. vii-19.]

labor *(To labor.)* labor laborer laboratory collaborate elaborate [< **laboro** Ap. vii-19.]

lapse *(To slip.)* lapse collapse elapse prolapse relapse [< **labor** Ap. vii-19.]

late *(To bear.)* collate elate oblate prelate prolate relate correlate translate collation elation relation relational relationship relativism relativity correlation translation translator [< **fero** Ap. vii-14.]

lect *(To gather.)* lectern collect elect neglect prelect select collection collective election elective selection selective [< **lego** Ap. vii-20.]

loc *(To place.)* local locate locus loci locomotive allocate dislocate relocate location allocation dislocation relocation [< **locus** Ap. vii-21.]

mal *(Bad.)* malice malicious malign malignant malady malaria [< **malus** Ap. vii-22.]

man *(Hand.)* manual manufacture manuscript manage manager manicure manifest manipulate manner maneuver emancipate [< **manus** Ap. vii-22.]

mand *(To order.)* mandate command countermand demand [< **mando** Ap. vii-22.]

merge, mers *(To sink.)* merge merger emerge immerge submerge emersion immerse immersion submersion [< **mergo** Ap. vii-23.]

migra *(To change.)* migrate migrant emigrate immigrate transmigrate migration emigration immigration transmigration [< **migro** Ap. vii-23.]

mit, -mis *(To send.)* admit admittance commit commitment demit emit intermit omit permit remit transmit mission admission admissible commission commissioner dismiss dismissal emission intermission omission permission remission transmission [< **mitto** Ap. vii-24.]

mod *(Manner.)* mode model moderate moderation modify modulate modest modern mod accommodate commodity [< **modus** Ap. vii-24.]

mot, mov *(To move.)* motor motion motive motivate demote emote promote remote move remove movable movement movie [< **moveo** Ap. vii-25.]

mut *(To change.)* mutate mutation mutant mutual commute commuter commutable immutable permutation transmutation [< **muto** Ap. vii-25.]

nun, noun *(To announce.)* annunciation denunciation enunciation pronunciation renunciation announce denounce pronounce renounce [< **nuntio** Ap. vii-27.]

ord *(Order.)* order disorder reorder suborder ordinary ordain ordinance coordinate inordinate subordinate insubordinate [< **ordo** Ap. vii-27.]

par *(To prepare.)* pare prepare preparation reparation separate [< **paro** Ap. vii-28.]

part *(Part.)* part apart partial depart impart impartial participate particular party apartment compartment department reparation [< **pars** Ap. vii-28.]

pass *(To step.)* pass compass surpass trespass impasse [< **passus** Ap. vii-29.]

pel, pul *(To push.)* compel dispel expel impel propel repel appellant pulse compulsion expulsion propulsion repulsion [< **pello** Ap. vii-29.]

pend *(To weigh; to hang.)* pending pendulum append depend expend impend suspend impending depending suspension [< **pendeo, pendo** Ap. vii-29.]

ple *(Full.)* plenty complete deplete implement supplement [< **plenus** Ap. vii-30.]

plic *(To fold.)* application complicate duplicate explicate implicate implicit multiplication replica replicate supplicate [< **plico** Ap. vii-31.]

pose *(To place.)* appose compose depose expose impose interpose juxtapose oppose propose repose suppose transpose [< **pono** Ap. vii-31.]

port *(To carry.)* port porter portfolio portage deport export import report support transport purport exporter importer reporter supporter transporter deportation importation transportation [< **porto** Ap. vii-32.]

prehend *(To grasp.)* apprehend comprehend reprehend [< **prehendo** Ap. vii-32.]

press *(To press.)* press compress depress express impress oppress repress suppress compression depression expression impression oppression repression repressive suppression [< **premo** Ap. vii-32.]

prove *(To judge.)* prove disprove approve disapprove improve [< **probo** Ap. vii-33.]

pute *(To reckon.)* compute computer depute dispute impute repute computation deputation disputation reputation [< **puto** Ap. vii-33.]

quest, **quire** *(To inquire.)* quest question questionable conquest inquest request acquire inquire require prerequisite [< **quaero** Ap. vii-34.]

rog *(To question.)* arrogant derogatory interrogate prerogative [< **rogo** Ap. vii-36.]

rect *(To make straight.)* rectangle rectify rectum correct incorrect direct indirect director erect correction direction erection [< **rego** Ap. vii-35.]

rupt *(To break.)* rupture abrupt corrupt disrupt erupt interrupt irrupt bankrupt corruption disruption eruption interruption [< **rumpo** Ap. vii-36.]

scend *(To climb.)* ascend descend transcend ascendant descendant transcendent transcendental transcendentalism [< **scando** Ap. vii-37.]

sci *(To know.)* science conscience conscious omniscience [< **scio** Ap. vii-37.]

scrib, **script** *(To write.)* scribe script ascribe ascription describe description inscribe inscription prescribe prescription proscribe proscription subscribe subscription transcribe transcription postscript conscript conscription Scripture scribble [< **scribo** Ap. vii-37.]

sacr, **secr** *(To dedicate.)* sacred sacrament sacrifice sacrilege sacrosanct consecrate consecration desecrate desecration [< **sacro** Ap. vii-36.]

sect *(To cut.)* section sector bisect dissect exsect insect intersect prosect resect transect trisect bisection dissection insecticide intersection prosection resection transection trisection [< **seco** Ap. vii-37.]

sed, **sid** *(To sit.)* sedentary sedate sedation sediment sedan dissident president resident preside reside residual subside [< **sedeo** Ap. vii-38.]

sent, **sens** *(To feel.)* sentient sentiment assent consent dissent resent sense sensible sensitive sensation consensus dissension [< **sentio** Ap. vii-38.]

sequ, **secu** *(To follow.)* sequel sequence consequent subsequent execute persecute prosecute execution persecution prosecution [< **sequor** Ap. vii-38.]

sert *(To join.)* assert desert deserter exert insert assertion assertive desertion dissertation exertion exertive insertion [< **series** Ap. vii-39.]

serv *(To serve; to save.)* serve servant conserve deserve observe preserve reserve conservation preservation reservation [< **servio, servo** Ap. vii-39.]

sign *(To mark.)* sign assign assignment consign design ensign resign resignation insignia signal signify signature significant [< **signo** Ap. vii-39.]

simil *(Similar.)* similar simile simulate assimilate facsimile [< **similis** Ap. vii-39.]

sist *(To set.)* assist consist desist exist insist persist resist subsist assistance resistance existence insistence persistence subsistence assistant consistency insistent persistent irresistible [< **sisto** Ap. vii-40.]

soci *(Comrade.)* social sociable society socialite socialize sociology socialist associate disassociate association associative [< **socius** Ap. vii-40.]

solv, solu *(To loosen.)* solve solvent absolve dissolve resolve absolute solution absolution dissolute resolution resolute [< **solvo** Ap. vii-40.]

spect *(To look at.)* spectator spectacle aspect circumspect expect inspect introspect prospect suspect expectation inspection [< **specto** Ap. vii-41.]

spir *(To breathe.)* spirit spiritual aspire aspirations conspire conspiracy expire expiration inspire inspiration inspirational perspire perspiration respire respiration respirator transpire [< **spiro** Ap. vii-42.]

spond, spons *(To answer, promise.)* respond correspond despondent correspondent sponsor response responsible [< **spondeo** Ap. vii-42.]

stance, stant *(To stand.)* stance circumstance distance instance substance constant distant instant circumstantial substantial [< **sto** Ap. vii-42.]

stitu *(To place.)* constitute destitute institute prostitute substitute constitution institution prostitution restitution substitution [< **statuo** Ap. vii-42.]

strict *(To bind.)* strict constrict district restrict restriction [< **stringo** Ap. vii-43.]

struct *(To build.)* structure construct destruct instruct obstruct construction destruction instruction obstruction reconstruction constructive destructive instructor substructure superstructure [< **struo** Ap. vii-43.]

sum *(To take.)* assume consume presume resume assumption consumption presumption resumption consumer sumptuous [< **sumo** Ap. vii-43.]

tain, ten, tin *(To hold.)* abstain appertain contain detain entertain maintain obtain pertain retain sustain tenor tenant tenet tennis tenon tenure tendency abstention detention retention content continue continuum continent continence incontinence continuity pertinent [< **teneo** Ap. vii-44.]

tect *(To hide.)* detect detector protect detection protection [< **tego** Ap. vii-44.]

tend, **tent** *(To stretch.)* tend tendency attend contend distend extend intend portend pretend subtend attendance attention attentive contention distention extension intention pretension [< **tendo** Ap. vii-44.]

test *(To prove.)* testament attest contest detest protest [< **testor** Ap. vii-45.]

text *(To weave.)* text textile texture context contextual pretext [< **texo** Ap. vii-45.]

tort *(To twist.)* tort torture tortoise contort distort extort retort contortion distortion extortion contortionist torticollis torsion [< **torqueo** Ap. vii-46.]

tract *(To pull.)* tract abstract attract contract detract extract protract retract subtract traction abstraction attraction contraction detraction extraction protraction retraction subtraction [< **traho** Ap. vii-46.]

trib *(To grant.)* tribute tributary attribute contribute distribute distributor attribution contribution distribution retribution [< **tribuo** Ap. vii-46.]

tric *(Hindrance.)* trick trickery extricate intricate intricacy [< **tricae** Ap. vii-46.]

trud, **trus** *(To push.)* detrude extrude intrude intruder obtrude protrude abstruse extrusion intrusion obtrusive protrusion [< **trudo** Ap. vii-47.]

vad, **vas** *(To go.)* evade invade pervade evasion invasion [< **vado** Ap. vii-48.]

ven *(To come.)* advent convent event invent prevent convention invention intervention prevention subvention venture adventure [< **venio** Ap. vii-49.]

vert, **vers** *(To turn.)* vertical vertebra vertigo advertise avert convert divert extrovert introvert invert revert subvert inadvertent version versatile versus aversion conversion controversial diversion inversion perversion reversion subversion traverse [< **verto** Ap. vii-49.]

vid, **vis** *(To see.)* vision envision provision revision television visible visual visit visor vista advise improvise revise televise video evident evidence invidious provide providence [< **video** Ap. vii-50.]

voc, **vok** *(To call.)* convoke evoke invoke provoke revoke vocal vocation avocation vocabulary advocate convocation equivocate invocation provocation provocative revocation [< **voco** Ap. vii-51.]

volv, **volu** *(To roll.)* devolve evolve involve involvement revolve revolver Volvo volume convoluted evolution revolution [< **volvo** Ap. vii-52.]

French [With special pronunciations.] A, B, C . . . . Ap. viii- 1

D, E F, G, H, I, J, K, L, M, N, O, P . . . . Ap. viii- 2

R, S, T, V, W . . . . Ap. viii- 3

French [Words from Latin with Anglicized pronunciations.] A → M . . . . Ap. viii- 3

N, O, P, Q, R, S, T, U, V . . . . Ap. viii- 4

Italian . . . . . . Musical Terms . A → P . . . . Ap. viii- 4

Q → V . . Other Words from Italian . . **Spanish** A, B . . Ap. viii- 5

Spanish C → Y . . . . **Portuguese** . . . . Ap. viii- 6

Appendix viii The Romantic Romance Languages
(Modern French, Italian, Spanish, and Portuguese)

French [With special pronunciations.]

[Pronunciation hints: often **a** /ä/, **e** /ā/, **é** /ā/, **i** /ē/, **o** /ō/, **au** /ō/, **eau** /ō/, **-et** /ā/, **ch** /sh/, but your best aid remains a good dictionary.] **A** à deux *(For two.)* adieu agent provocateur à la carte à la mode à la king à la Newburg amateur amour apéritif apropos /ap-rə-pō/ arête *(A sharp ridge.)* artiste /ar-tēst/ attaché au courant *(Up to date.)* au pair au revoir avalanche (Swiss Fr.) avant-garde avoirdupois **B** ballet /ba-lā/ barrage baton beau Beaumont Beauregard belle /bel/ *(An attractive woman.)* beret Bizet /bē-zā/ blouse bonbon bon mot /bawn mō/ *(A witty saying.)* Bordeaux bouffant bouquet bourgeoisie boutonniere buffet bureau blasé bourrée brochure **C** cabaret cache cachet café caffeine caisson Calais /kal-ā/ camaraderie camouflage campaign Camus /kə-mōō/ canapé canard caprice capricious carafe caramel carbine carom *(A billiard shot.)* carousel carte *(Menu.)* carte blanche Cartier /kar-tyā/ cartouche cashier casserole cassimere catacomb cause célèbre celesta centrifuge Cézanne chaconne Chagall chagrin chaise longue chalet chalumeau *(Lower register of the clarinet.)* chamber chamfer *(To bevel.)* chamois champagne Champagne Champs Élysées /shäṅ zā-lē-zā/ *("Elysian fields"; fashionable Paris avenue.)* chancre chandelier chanson chanterelle chanteuse chantey chapeau chaperon charades chard chargé d'affaires charlatan Charlemagne Chartres /shar-tr/ chartreuse chassé chassis /shas-ē/ chateau chauffeur Chautauqua chauvinism chef chemise chenille Cherbourg Chevrolet chevron Cheyenne chez /shā/ *(At; at the home of.)* chichi chic Chicago chicanery /shi-kā-ner-ē/ chiffon chiffonier chivalry Chopin chute cigarette citrine clavier Clemenceau cliché clientele cognac /kōn-yak/ coiffure collage colleague communiqué connoisseur consommé cordon bleu corps de ballet corsage corvette *(A warship.)*

coulee (*A gulch, e.g.* Grand Coulee Dam.) coup d'état /ko͞o-dā-tä/ (*"Stroke of state"; a government seizure.*) (Abbr. coup) coupé crèche courante crème /krem/ Creole crêpe /krāp/ crêpes suzette /krep so͞o-zet/ crevasse cricket (*A game.*) critique crochet croissant croquette crouton cuisine cul-de-sac culottes cushion **D** danse macabre de (*Of, from.*) debacle debauchery debonair debris /də-brē/ Debussy debut di-byo͞o/ debutante décor dé jà vu Delacroix /də-lə-krwä/ deluxe demitasse deportee depot /dē-pō/ derrière /dair-ē-air/ DesCartes /dā-cärt/ détente dinette discothèque divorcé (m) divorcée (f) dossier /dos-ē-ā/ double entendre /do͞o-blän tän-dr/ douche /do͞osh/ **E** eau /ō/ (*Water.*) Eau Claire echelon éclair école (*School.*) egalitarian élan élite embouchure émigré encore en masse ennui en route ensemble /än-säm-bəl/ entente entrée entrepreneur envoy escargot (*Snail.*) espionage esprit de corps étude exposé **F** façade fait accompli fatigue Fauré faux pas /fō-pä/ (*"False step"; blunder.*) femme fatale fatigue fiancé (m) fiancée (f) figurine filet /fi-lā/ filet mignon /min-yon/ filigree finesse flamboyant fleur-de-lis (*"Flower of lily"; royal emblem.*) fondue Fond du Lac (*"Foot of the lake."*) Fontainebleau foreign foyer franc français frappé frère /frair/ (*Brother.*) fricassee fugue fuselage **G** gaiety garage garçon gauche /gōsh/ (*"Left-handed"; awkward; boorish.*) gavotte gendarme genre /zhän-rə/ Gide /zhēd/ gigue gigolo glair (*Egg white glaze.*) glacé gouge gourd gourmet /go͝or-mā/ grand mal (*Severe seizure.*) Grand Prix /grän prē/ grandeur grenadier grippe grotesque **H** habitué /hə-bich-o͞o-ā/ (*A frequent attender.*) harangue (Ger.) hearse hollandaise sauce hors d'oeuvres /or-dervz/ (*"Outside of work," i.e. nonessential,* thus: *appetizers.*) **I** idée fixe imbecile imbecility impasse enfant terrible Ingres /än-gr/ insouciant (*Carefree.*) Internationale intrigue inveigle **J** javelin (Cel.) je ne sais quoi /zhən se kwə/ (*An indefinable something; "I know not what."*) jonquil Juneau **L** Lafayette laissez-faire /les-ā-fair/ (*"Let do"; non-interference of state in economics.*) layette (Du.) legionnaire levee liaison licit (*Lawful.*) lieu /lo͞o/ (*Place. Now only in phrase: "In lieu of."*) lingerie liqueur liter /lē-ter/ locale loge /lōzh/ (*Theater box.*) logistics lorgnette (*Folding eyeglasses.*) lycée (*Secondary school.*) **M** machine macramé Madame (*Mrs. pl. mesdames.*) Mademoiselle (*Miss;* pl. mesdemoiselles.) maître d' /mā-trə dē/ (maître d'hôtel) majorette malaise malinger Manet maneuver maraud Mardi gras /mar-dē-grä/ (*"Fat Tuesday"; last day before Lent.*) margarine marinade marionette marquis /mar-kē/ (*A rank below duke.*) marquee massage masseur matinee mauve mayonnaise mélange memoir menagerie meringue (*"Cake of Mehringen, Ger."*) medallion mediocre melee /mā-lā/ merci /mair-cē/ (*Thank you.*) Michigan migraine (Gk.) milieu (*Environment.*) millionaire minuet mirage monde (*The world.*) Monet Monseigneur (*My lord, title of nobility;* pl. Messeigneurs.) Monsieur /mə-syer/ (*Mr.;* pl. messieurs.) montage Mont Blanc moraine (*Glacier debris; e.g..* The Kettle Moraine.) morgue motif mousse (*A dessert.*) musicale mustache mystique **N** naive /nä-ēv/ (*fem. adj.; masc.:* naif) naiveté /nä-ēv-tā/ née (*Born with the name of.*) niche Nîmes /nēmz/ noblesse oblige (*The noble are obligated.*) Noël nonchalant Notre Dame (*Our Lady.*) nougat nouveaux riches /no͞o-vō-resh/ (*Newly wealthy.*) **O** ogre opéra comique oui /wē/ (*Yes.*) **P** palette papier-mâché par excellence parimutuel (*Betting system.*) parquet /par-kā/ (*Gmc. Flooring.*) partisan pas /pä/ (*A dance step.*) passé pâté /pä-tā/ (*A little pie.*) père /pair/ (*Father.*) petite physique picayune /pik-i-yo͞on/ (*Petty.*) picturesque pièce de résistance Pierrot (*Pantomime character.*) pince-nez /pans-nā/ (*Eyeglasses.*) pinion (*Toothed wheel.*) piqué /pē-kā/ (*Corded cotton fabric.*) pirouette (*Ballet movement.*) plaque plateau pointillism pompon potage (*A thick soup.*) potpourri (*Unusual mixture.*) prairie precipice précis /prā-cē/ (Summary; abstract.) prehensile premier (First in rank; prime minister.) premiere (First performance.) prestige protégé (m) protégée (f) purée **R** ragout /ra-gōō/ raison d'être /re-zôṅ da-tə/ (Reason for being.) rappel rapport /rə-por/ rapprochement /rà-prôsh-mäṅ/ (Reconciliation.) Ravel reconnaissance régime Renaissance rendezvous /rän-dā-vōō/ Renoir /rə-nwär/ repertoire répondez s'il vous plait (R.S.V.P.) (Please reply.) restaurant résumé ricochet risqué rococo romaine (Lettuce.) romanesque rondeau rotisserie Rouault /rōō-ō/ Rouen /rōō-äṅ/ roulette Rousseau **S** sabotage sac sage (An herb.) Saint-Saëns /saṅ-säṅs/ salami saline salon saloon sashay sauté savoir faire séance sec (Dry, e.g. wines.) serenade siècle (Century.) silhouette soiree /swä-rā/ (Evening party.) soufflé souvenir suave svelte **T** tableau table d'hôte (Opposite of: à la carte.) tambourine (Ar.) tête-à-tête /tāt-ə-tāt/ (Private chat; S-shaped sofa.) technique (Gk.) Thoreau tic (Muscle twitch.) toilet toilette touché toupee tour de force triste trousseau tutu (Ballet skirt.) **V** veneer vignette vis-à-vis /vē-zə-vē/ vive la république **W** Watteau

---

French [Words from Latin with Anglicized pronunciations.]

A abolish absence abstinence absurd abuse academy accolade (Gk.) accompany accost accredit accrue acerbity action active adapt adhesion admirable admire adoration adroit affable affect (To imitate.) aggrandize agriculture agility alloy altruism ameliorate amplify angle annex aptitude artifice artisan artist assonance attack attic attitude augment **B** bankrupt barb beneficence beneficial bilious bowling **C** cab cabby cabin cabinet cad caddie cadet cajole caliber caliper calorie caloric canteen capable captive carbon careen career carnation carrot (Gk.) carton cartoon cash celery (Gk.) censure cerebral chapter charm chemical chiffon chowder cite cocktail cocoon coffer cohesion coin comedian commandant commandeer commerce communism complaint conform confront conjugal contest contestant convoke costume cravat crayon culture curb cutlass cutlet **D** damnation dandelion decadence decry defray demand democracy (Gk.) demolish denture deploy derail deranged desert (To abandon.) dessert detach deranged develop devotee dilate dine dinner discourse disengage disorient disposition distant dominion drab **E** effort effrontery elegant eligible embalm embankment embark embarrass embassy empire employ enchant enclave engage engagement evaluate exhale exist expire expression extravagance **F** fabric facet facile faction famish fanfare farce federal fetish fiber fiction fidelity figure filament final flank flask foliage folly foment forage foundry fracture frieze frisk fry fugitive furl futile furniture **G** gain gallery galop generous gerbil gibbon glacial goiter gopher gout gradation grade gravity **H** hatchet (Ger.) hotel hutch **I** immense imperceptible implant implicit import important impose impossible impostor impressionable imprint impromptu improvise incarnation incident incomparable incompetent incongruity inconstant indication indicative indigestion industrial infirmity inflammatory information ingredient instrumentation insurrection intensive intermediary intern interpret intimate introit invalid (Disabled person.) investigation invincible invite invoice **J** judicious jurist **L** lagoon lantern (Gk.) laurel lemonade liberty local **M** machine (Gk.) manicure manipulation marmot maroon (A color.) maturity Mayday (From: m'aidez: Help me.) measure medal melon (Gk.)

mental merchandise mercantile military ministerial model modify molecule mollusk moment muffle municipality mural muscle **N** nation native natural negative notoriety novel novice **O** omelet operative opt optimism orangeade outrageous oxygen ozone (Gk.) **P** pace page pair paradox (Gk.) paralyze (Gk.) parcel patriot (Gk.) petty persecute person picket picnic piston pivot platitude platoon ply polygamy (Gk.) ponderous positivism possess precede precedent precise prefer preliminary prepare preposition preside pretentious primitive principal priority production prominence pronunciation propulsion prosperity prudish **Q** quality quarrel quartet questionnaire **R** ration rectangle relate relation render rendition renounce repetition repose reprieve reprimand republic resent reside resignation resistance retract retreat reveille reverie risk roil role romantic rudiment **S** saber salute satellite satiety Saxon sense separable session signal signature silence similar sinister siphon (Gk.) site skeptic (Gk.) soar sobriety sociable solid sonnet soup spectacle station statue statute strangle (Gk.) surcharge surface surtax suspect **T** tardy taxi tenant tender tent tenure terror testament toilet tolerant trait transpire tube tweezers **U** uncle unction uniform unify union urgent utility **V** vacant vacation vagabond vague valid variation vehicle venison veracity verb verge versatile verve vest vestige viable visa vogue volition

---

Italian

[Pronunciation hints. c before e or i /ch/; a /ä/, often i /ē/, e /ā/]

Music Terms: Because most of our musical terms are from Italian and are so popular in our everyday language, these are listed together first:

A a cappella *("In chapel style," unaccompanied.)* accelerando (accel.) accordion adagio *(At ease.)* agitato al fine *(To the end.)* alla breve *(2/2 time.)* allegretto allegro alto amoroso andante *(Walking.)* animato appoggiatura *(An ornamental note.)* aria arietta ariose arioso arpeggio assai *(Very.)* a tempo **B** baritone bass basset horn basso continuo basso profundo bass viol bel canto bravo bravissimo **C** cadence cadenza cantata capo dastro *(Guitar pitch-raiser.)* capriccio capriccioso *(Fanciful.)* cello clarinet coda *(Tail. End section of a composition.)* coloratura con amore con brio *(With spirit.)* concert concertina concertino concerto concerto grosso con moto *(With motion.)* con spirito contrabass contrabassoon contralto contrapuntal counter-tenor crescendo (cresc. ◁) **D** da capo (D.C. *The beginning.*) dal segno (D.S. *From the sign.*) decrescendo (decresc. ▷) diminuendo (dim.) divertimento dolce *(Sweetly.)* doloroso *(Sorrowfully.)* duet duo **F** falsetto fantasia fermata *(Hold.* ⌒ *)* finale fine /fē-nā/ *(The end.)* forte (f) forte-piano (fp) fortissimo (ff) furioso fuga *(Fugue.)* **G** glissando grandioso grave grazioso **I** impresario intermezzo **L** largo larghetto legato lento libretto **M** madrigal maestoso maestro mandolin ma non troppo *(But not too much.)* meno *(Less.)* mezzo *(Middle, moderate.)* mezzo forte (mf) mezzo piano (mp) mezzo-soprano moderato molto mordent mosso **O** obbligato oboe ocarina octet opera (Pl. of *opus.*) operetta opus (L. *work.*) oratorio ostinato ottava **P** passacaglia pianissimo (pp) piano (p) pianoforte piccolo *(Small.)* piu *(More.)* pizzicato poco *(A little.)* poco a poco *(Little by little.)* portamento presto *(Very fast.)* prestissimo prima donna prima volta *(First time.)* primo **Q** quartet quintet **R** rallentando (rall.) ritardando (rit.) rondo rubato **S** scale scherzo seconda volta *(Second time.)* secondo semplice sempre *(Always.)* serenata sextet sforzando (sfz.) sinfonia solfeggio solo (Pl. soli.) sonata sonatina soprano sordine *(Or sordino, a mute.)* sostenuto sotto voce *("Under the voice"; softly.)* spiccato spiritoso staccato stretto stringendo **T** tarantella tenor tenuto toccata tremolo trill trio tutti **V** veloce vibrato vigoroso viola viola da gamba viola d'amore violin violoncello virtuoso vivace volante *(Swiftly.)* volti *(Turn the page.)*

Note: The musical syllables, **do, re, mi, fa, sol, la, ti, do** came from this medieval Latin hymn: **Ut** queant laxis **re**sonare fibris, **mi**ra gestorum **fa**muli tuorum, **sol**ve polluti **la**bii reatum, Sancte Iohnnes. Eventually **ut** was changed to the more singable **do** and a 7th tone, **ti**, was added.

Other Words from Italian:

A alarm (All' arme. *To arms!)* alert (All' erta. *On the watch.)* amore *(Love.)* antipasto a rivederci /ä rē-vā-*dair*-chē/ *(Until we meet again.)* arsenal artichoke (Ar.) **B** balcony ballerina balloon ballot bambino bandit banister barracks bas-relief bastion belladonna belvedere *("Beautiful view"; a building with a good view.)* Belvedere *(Part of Vatican exhibiting art works.)* ben venuto *(Welcome!)* benzene berretta bordello breve *(Short vowel mark, e.g. ă; a judicial writ; in music, a note equivalent to two whole notes.)* brigade brigand bronze buffalo buffoon bulletin buon giorno *(Good day.)* buono *(Good.)* bust (n) **C** cadre calm cameo cannon canto caricature carnival casino cavalcade cavalier cavalry Chianti ciao /chä-ō/ *(Hello; farewell.)* confetti confidant contraband contrapposto cornice corridor **D** Dante /dän-tā/ Decameron *(100 stories by Boccaccio.)* dilettante dispatch ditto duce /dōō-chā/ *(Leader; Il Duce, Mussolini.)* **E** espresso **F** fascism fiasco fracas fresco fuse (n) **G** gazette gelatin gel generalissimo ghetto gondola **I** impassion incognito inferno influenza **L** lasagna lingua franca lira Lombard lottery **M** macaroni madonna mafia malaria manage manifesto marina marinate marzipan mezzanine million minestrone miniature Monsignor motto mozzarella **N** neutrino novella **P** padre page (Gk.) pantaloons pants paparazzi *(Freelance photographers.)* parapet parakeet parasol pasta pastel pedestal pellagra perfume piazza pilot pistachio pizza pizzeria portfolio portico **Q** quarantine **R** ravioli regatta rialto rocket rotunda **S** salami saloon salvo scenario scenery Signora Signore Sistine soda sonnet spaghetti spumoni squad squadron stanza stiletto stucco studio **T** tarantula tarot *(Fortune telling card.)* tempera terrace terra cotta tint tirade torso torte traffic trampoline trecento *(1300's; 14th Century.)* tutti-frutti **U** umbrella **V** vendetta vermicelli virtu *(Rare quality.)* vista vive volcano **Z** zany zucchini

---

Spanish

[Pronunciation hints: e /ā/, i /ē/ (San Diego), j /h/ (junta), soft g /h/ (Geraldo)] Words with asterisks are from Indian sources (Arawakan, Carib, Nahuatl, Quechua & Taino). See: Ap. x-3, 6, 7.

A adios *("To God." Good-by.)* adobe aficionado *(An enthusiast.)* Alamo *(Cottonwood tree.)* Alcatraz *(Albatross.)* alfalfa alligator *(El lagarto: "The lizard.")* alpaca amigo *(Friend.)* anchovy Armada armadillo arroyo avocado a vuestra salud *(To your health.)* **B** balsa banana *barbecue barracuda barricade barrio bodega *(Wine cellar.)*

bolero bolo *(A knife.)* bonanza bracket bravado breeze brocade bronco buckaroo bueno *(Good; well.)* bunco *(Swindle.)* burro **C** caballero cabana *cacao *(Seeds to make cocoa.)* calaboose *(A jail.)* canasta *cannibal *canoe cañon *(Canyon.)* capsize carapace *(Turtle shell.)* cargo cask castanets cedila (ç) chaparejos (Chaps: *Cowboy leather leg protectors.)* chaparral *(A thicket.)* *chigger *chili chili con carne *("Chili with meat.")* *chinchilla *chocolate cigar cinch cocaine cockroach *cocoa Colorado *(Ruddy, red.)* compadre *("Godfather"; a close male companion.)* compañero *(Comrade.)* comrade *condor conga conquistador corral Cortes *(Spanish legislature.)* Cortés *(Sp. explorer.)* *coyote crusade Crusades Cuba libre *("Free Cuba," a rum drink.)* **D** demarcation desperado Don *(Sir.)* doña *(Noblewoman.)* Doña *(Madam.)* Dorado *(The Swordfish Constellation.)* El Dorado *(Legendary city of riches.)* **E** El Greco ("The Greek": *Spanish painter.)* embargo enchilada escapade esplanade **F** fandango fiesta filibuster flamenco flotilla **G** gabardine garbanzo beans garrote gaucho grenade grimace gringo *(Foreigner.)* grunion *guano *(Bird dung.)* *guava *(Jelly-producing fruit.)* guerrilla guitar **H** habanera hacienda hammock hombre /om-brā/ *(Man.)* *hurricane **I** *iguana Inca incommunicado indigo *istle *(A plant fiber.)* **J** jade *jerky junta /ho͞on-tä/ **L** lackey la cucarache *("The cockroach"; a dance.)* La Jolla /lə hoi-yə/ lariat lasso launch *(A motor boat.)* llama loco *(Insane.)* **M** machete macho madre *(Mother.)* *maize mañana *(Tomorrow.)* *manatee marijuana maroon *(To abandon.)* mascara *("Mask"; a cosmetic darkener.)* masquerade matador medico *(A doctor.)* mesa mescal mestizo mahogany minaret (Ar.) Montana *(Montaña: mountain.)* mosquito muchacha *(Girl.)* muchacho *(Boy.)* mulatto mustang **N** Navajo Negro Nevada *(Snowfall.)* Niña *(One of Columbus' ships.)* la Niña *("Girl"; Pacific Ocean's cooling.)* el Niño *("Boy"; Pacific Ocean's warming.)* **O** olio *(A collection.)* ombre *(Man; gambling game.)* **P** padre *(Father.)* palomino pampas *papaya parade peccadillo penuche *(A candy.)* peon perfecto peso *peyote picador pimento piña *(Pineapple.)* piñata Pinta *(One of Columbus' ships.)* pinto piñon platinum plaza politico poncho *potato presidio pronto pueblo *puma **Q** Quinceañera *("Fifteen years"; A young woman's coming of age celebration.)* quinine **R** ranch rancher renegade Rio Grande *(Big river.)* rodeo **S** Sacramento *(Sacrament.)* San *(Saint; fem. Santa.)* San Diego *(St. James.)* San Francisco *(St. Francis.)* San Juan *(St. John.)* San Salvador Santa Barbara Santa Clara Santa Fe Santa Maria *(St. Mary; one of Columbus' ships.)* sarsaparilla sassafras *savanna Señor Señora Señorita si *(Yes.)* sierra *(A saw; mountain range.)* Sierra Madre siesta silo sombrero spade stampede stevedore **T** *tamales tango tequila *(A Mexican liquor.)* Tijuana /tē-hwä-nä/ tilde (ñ) *tobacco *tomato toreador torero tornado tortilla tuna **V** vamoose vanilla vigilante **Y** *yucca

---

Portuguese

Words marked with an asterisk are from Tupi Indian. <u>See</u>: Ap. x-7.

A apricot **B** baroque **C** coco *(Coconut palm.)* **D** dodo *(An extinct bird.)* Dona *(Madam.)* **E** emu *(A large flightless bird.)* **F** flamingo **J** *jaguar **M** *macaw *(A parrot.)* mandarin *maraca **P** palaver **S** samba (Afr. *Brazilian dance.)* São *(Saint.)* São Paulo **T** *tanager tank *tapioca *tapir *toucan *(A large bird.)* Toucan *(A constellation.)* valorization

Appendix ix It's All Greek To Me! (Greek Combining Forms) **CONTENTS**	

The Greek Alphabet . . . . Ap. ix- 2

Notes on Greek Grammar . . . . Ap. ix- 4

Greek Combining Forms   A . . . . Ap. ix- 5

     B, C . . . . Ap. ix- 6

     D, E . . . . Ap. ix- 7

     G . . . . Ap. ix- 8

     H . . . . Ap. ix- 9

     I, K . . . . Ap. ix-10

     L, M . . . . Ap. ix-11

     N . . . . Ap. ix-12

     O, P . . . . Ap. ix-13

     R, S . . . . Ap. ix-16

     T, U . . . . Ap. ix-17

     X, Z . . . . Ap. ix-18

And Still More Greek Combining Forms A, B, C, D, E . . . Ap. ix-18

     G, H, I, K, L, M, N, O . . . . Ap. ix-19

     P, R, S, T, U, X, Z . . . . Ap. ix-20

Greek - - - The Short Course   A, B, C . . . . Ap. ix-21

     D, E, G . . . . Ap. ix-22

     H, I, L . . . . Ap. ix-23

     M, N, O . . . . Ap. ix-24

     P . . . . Ap. ix-25

     S, T, Z . . . . Ap. ix-26

The Greek Alphabet

First it would be appropriate to review the letters of the Greek alphabet since they contain spelling clues and are often used individually as mathematical and scientific symbols.

α A alpha /al-fə/ **alpha**bet **alpha** & omega *(The beginning & end.)* acropolis ameba

β B beta /bā-tə/ alpha**bet** **beta**tron basic Bible biology blasphemy bronchitis

γ Γ gamma /gam-ə/ graph **gamma** rays genealogy geography Greek gymnasium

δ Δ delta /del-tə/ democracy **delta** **delt**oid dermatology diabetes dragon dynamic

ε E epsilon /ep-sə-lon/ eclipse ecstasy embryo emphasis epigram epidemic

ζ Z zeta /zā-tə/ zealot zephyr Zeus zither zodiac zone zoology zymurgy

η H eta /ā-tə/ echo electron ethics ethos hedonism helium hemisphere

Note: There is no letter symbol for the /h/ sound in Greek. When it is to be pronounced, this sound is written as a rough breathing mark (ʹ) over an initial vowel or the second vowel in a diphthong. Thus the Greek ʹηλιος *(sun)* would be rendered *helios* in English; the prefix ʹημι– *(half)* as *hemi-;* ʹηδονη *(pleasure)* as *hedone, etc.*

θ Θ theta /thā-tə/ thanatopsis theater theory therapy theme thermal theology

ι I iota /ī-ō-tə/ iota *(A very small amount----because ι is so small.)* idea idiom ionic iris

κ K kappa /kap-ə/ kaleidoscope kinetic kleptomania krypton kudos kylix

λ Λ lambda /lam-də/ labyrinth laconic lamp laryngitis leprosy lexicon logic

μ M mu /myōō/ macron magnet megaphone melodrama metaphor metastasis

ν N nu /nōō/ narcissus narcotic nemesis neophyte neurology nostalgia nymph

ξ Ξ xi /zī/ axiom paradox xenon xenophobia xeric Xerox Xerxes xylophone
Note: Initial *x* is pronounced /z/.

o O omicron /om-ə-kron/ obelisk oligarchy oncology onomatopoeia onyx optics

π Π pi /pī/ **pi** = 3.14159...Paleolithic pandemonium paragraph parallel perimeter

ρ P rho /rō/ rhapsody rheostat rhesus rhetoric rheumatism rhodium
           rhododendron rhombus rhubarb rhyme rhythm
Note: *Rho* gives reason to the *rh* spelling. The *h* *(Rough breath mark.)* has ceased being pronounced.

σ Σ sigma /sig-mə/ saccharin sapphire sarcasm scandal schizophrenia semaphore

Note: σ is written ς at end of a word.

τ T tau /tow/ tactics talent tantalize taxonomy technology telephone titanic

υ Y upsilon /yo͞op-sə-lon/ cycle cymbal dynasty dyslexic gymnasium hyphen lyceum lyric martyr mystery myth oyster symphony sympathy

Note: -y- within a word acts exactly as an *i* would---long /ī/ or short /ĭ/ depending on open or closed syllables and accent.

φ Φ phi /fī/ philanthropy Philip philosophy phlegm phobia phonics photon photograph phrase phylum physical physician symphony telephone

Note: *ph* is the Greek spelling for the sound /f/. The English, of course, uses *f* for /f/.

χ X chi /kī/ chameleon character charisma chemistry cholera chord chorus Christ chromatic chromosome chlorophyll chronic monarch school

Note: Whereas *ch* in English based words is pronounced /ch/ *(chain)* and French based words /sh/ *(chute)*, *ch* in Greek is /k/.

ψ Ψ psi /sī/ eclipse psalm psalter pseudonym psoriasis psyche psychedelic psychoanalysis psychology psychosomatic psychotic

Note: Initial *ps-* sounds /s/ having lost the once pronounced *p*.

ω Ω omega (long ō) oasis ocean ocher ode omega *(The end.)* otology

Note: Fairly reliable markers of Greek words: **rh-** /r/, **-y-** /ĭ/ or /ī/, **ph** /f/, **ch** /k/, **ps-** /s/.

Notes on Greek Grammar

Greek grammar is a highly sophisticated system and is thoroughly inflected. There are five cases: Nominative (subject), Genitive (possessive), Dative (indirect object), Accusative (direct object), and Vocative (direct address). For example, here is the declension of the adjective agathos (αγαθος), *good:*

	SINGULAR			PLURAL		
	M	F	N	M	F	N
N	agathos	agathē	agathon	agathoi	agathai	agatha
G	agathou	agathēs	agathou	agathōn	agathōn	agathōn
D	agathō	agathē	agathō	agathois	agathais	agathois
A	agathon	agathēn	agathon	agathous	agathas	agatha
V	agathe	agathē	agathon	agathoi	agathai	agatha

And with the Greek alphabet:

	SINGULAR			PLURAL		
	M	F	N	M	F	N
N	αγαθος	αγαθη	αγαθον	αγαθοι	αγαθαι	αγαθα
G	αγαθου	αγαθης	αγαθου	αγαθων	αγαθων	αγαθων
D	αγαθω	αγαθη	αγαθω	αγαθοις	αγαθαις	αγαθοις
A	αγαθον	αγαθην	αγαθον	αγαθους	αγαθάς	αγαθα
V	αγαθε	αγαθη	αγαθον	αγαθοι	αγαθαι	αγαθα

Nouns are masculine, feminine, or neuter and generally follow their column above. However, there are other classes of nouns with their own set of inflections. For example **anēr** *(man)* has a genitive of **andros** which is the form English uses.

The Greek verbs have complete tense, mood, person, and number inflections, some irregular.

Notice Greek has separate letters for long and short e's and o's: ε = ĕ, η = ē. o = ŏ, and ω = ō. A little practice will get one used to the following substitutions: γ = g, θ = th, λ = l, μ = m, ν = n, ξ = x; π = p; ρ = r; σ = s, ς = s (at end of word), υ = y, φ = f, χ = ch, ψ = ps.   α (a), β (b), δ (d), ε (e), ζ (z), ι (i), κ (k), o (o), and τ (t) should give little trouble.

Greek Combining Forms

A

a- *(Without; not; apart.)* *[α–]* **an-** (Before vowels.) apathy anemic <u>See</u>: **a-** as prefix Ap. iii-22.

acouo- *(Hearing.)* *[acouein* ακουειν *to hear, listen.]* acoustic acoustician acoustics

acro- *(At the top.)* *[akros* ακρος *highest.]* acrobat acrobatics acronym acropolis acrostic

aero *(Air.)* *[aer* αηρ*]* aerobatics aerodynamics aerogram aeronautic aeronautics aerophagia

aesthet- *(Perception.)* *[aisthētikos* αισθητικος *perceptive.]* aesthesia; <u>See</u>: **esthet-** Ap. ix-8.

-agogue *(Leading, promoting, inciting.)* *[agein* αγειν *to lead.]* demagogue pedagogue synagogue
-agogy demagogy pedagogy;   **-agoge** apagoge isagoge *(Introduction to a field of study.)*

-algia *(Pain or disease of.)* cardialgia gastralgia nephralgia neuralgia nostalgia uteralgia

allo- *(Other; alien.)* allobar allogamy allomorph allonym allopath allopathy allotrope

amphi- *(Both; around.)* *[amphi* αμφι *on both sides; around.]* <u>See</u>: **amphi-** as prefix in Ap. iii-22.

ana- *(Up; back; anew; thorough.)* *[ana* ανα *on, upon; up.]*   <u>See</u>: **ana-** as prefix in Ap. iii-22.

andro- *(Man.)* *[ανδρος]* androgen androgynous androgyny android; **-andry** polyandry

antho- *(Flower.)* anthodium anthoid anthologize anthology anthophore anthophorous

anthropo- *(Man.)* *[ανθρωπος]* anthropocentric anthropogenesis anthropogeography
anthropoid anthropological anthropology anthropomorphic anthropomorphism
anthropomorphize anthropomorphosis anthropophilic; **-anthrope** misanthrope
Pithecanthropus; **-anthropic** misanthropic; **-anthropy** misanthropy philanthropy

anti- *(Against.)* *[anti* αντι*]* antifreeze antiseptic antitrust <u>See</u>: **anti-** as prefix in Ap. iii-22.

apo- *(Off; from; away.)* *[apo* απο*]* apology apostle   <u>See</u>: **apo-** as prefix in Ap. iii-23.

arch- */ark/* **archi-** *(Chief, ruler.)* *[archos* αρχως*]* archbishop* archdeacon* archdiocese*
archetype archfiend archipelago architect architecture archives archon; (*arch = /arch/)
-arch */ark/* *(Chief, ruler.)* hierarch matriarch monarch nomarch oligarch

archeo- *(Primitive, ancient.)* archeology archeopteryx Archeozoic archaic archaism

-archy *(Rule; government.)* anarchy hierarchy matriarchy monarchy oligarchy patriarchy

aristo- *(Best; finest.)* *[aristos* αριστος *best of its kind.]* aristocracy aristocrat aristotype

arterio- *(Artery.)* *[artēria* αρτηρια *windpipe.]* arterial arterialize arteriosclerosis artery

arthro- *(Joint.)* arthralgia arthritis arthroplasty arthrosis arthrospore arthrotomy

aster *(Star.)* **astero-** *(Related to a star.)*   aster *(A flower.)* asteriated asterisk asterism

astro- *(Pertaining to outer space.)* astrobiology astrodome astrology astronaut astronavigation astronomer astronomical astronomy astrophysics astrosphere

auto- *(Self-activating.)* autobiography autocracy autocrat autograph automat automatic automation automaton automobile automotive autonomous autonomy autopsy

B

baro- *(Weight.)* [*baros* βαρος *weight; burden; grief.*] barogram barometer isobar millibar

biblio- *(Book.)* Bible Biblical bibliographer bibliography bibliomania bibliophile

bio- *(Life.)* biochemistry biocycle biodynamics biographer biography biological biology biophysics biopsy biosphere biotic biotron biotype; **-biotic** *(Pertaining to life.)* antibiotic

C

caco *(Bad, vile.)* [κακος] cacoethes cacography *(Bad handwriting.)* cacophonous cacophony

calli- *(Beautiful.)* [*kalos* καλος] calisthenics calligraphy calliope Calliope callipygian

cardio- *(Heart.)* [*kardia* καρδια] cardiac cardialgia *(Heartburn.)* cardiogram cardiograph cardioid cardiology carditis; **-cardia** bradycardia *(Slow beat.)* diplocardia

cata- cath- *(Down; against; back.)* [*kata* κατα] <u>See:</u> **cata-** & **cath-** as prefixes in Ap. iii-23.

-cene *(New, recent.)* Eocene Pleistocene Pliocene; And: Cenozoic cenozoology

centro- *(Center.)* [*kentron* κεντρον *point, spike, spur; center.*] centroid centrosphere; **-center** epicenter orthocenter; **centric** anthropocentric homocentric *(Having same center.)* theocentric; <u>Note:</u> Gk. *kentron* became L. *centrum,* thus: central centrifuge concentric, *etc.*

cephalo- *(Head.)* cephalopod cephalous **-cephalic** brachycephalic *(Short.)* dolichocephalic *(Long.)* hydrocephalic *(Water.)* megacephalic *(Large.)* mesocephalic *(Intermediate.)*

chem- *(Dealing with chemicals.)* chemical chemist chemistry chemotherapy chemurgy; **-chemistry** magnetochemisty photochemistry radiochemisty thermochemistry

chiro- *(Hand.)* chiroplasty chiropody (podos = *foot.*) chiropodist chiropractic chiropractor

chloro- *(Light green.)* chlorine chloroform chlorophane chlorophyll chloroplast chlorosis

choreo- *(Dance.)* [*choreia* χορεια] chorea *(Nerve disease.)* choreographer choreography

chrom- *(Color.)* chromatic chromaticism chrome chromium chromophotography chromosome chromosphere; **-chromatic** orthochromatic panchromatic photochromatic

chrono- *(Time.)* anachronism chronic chronicle chronological chronology synchronize

cine- *(Movement.)* cinema cinematograph cinematography cinematographer

-clast *(Break, destroy.)* biblioclast cataclast iconoclast idoloclast osteoclast pyroclast

clino- *(Bend, slope, incline.)* cline clinic clinical clinician; <u>See:</u> Latin **clino** in Ap. vii-7.

cosmo- *(Universe.)* cosmetic cosmetician cosmetology cosmic cosmology cosmonaut cosmopolitan cosmopolite cosmos cosmoscope cosmotron macrocosm microcosm

-cracy *(Form of government.)* aristocracy autocracy bureaucracy democracy mobocracy plutocracy technocracy theocracy; **-crat** aristocrat autocrat bureaucrat democrat

-cycle *(Recurring period.)* bicycle epicycle kilocycle megacycle motorcycle tricycle; **cyclo-** cycle cyclic (or: cyclical) cyclist cyclone cyclopedia encyclical encyclopedia

D

deca- *(Ten.)* [deka δεκα] decade Decalogue decathlon <u>See</u>: **deca-** as prefix in Ap. iii-23.

-demic *(Of people.)* [dēmos δημος *the common people.*] endemic epidemic polydemic; **demo-** *(People.)* demagogue democracy democrat demography demos demotic demotics

dendro- *(Tree.)* dendriform dendrite dendritic dendrochronology dendrodate dendrograph dendroid dendrology dendron; **-dendron** philodendron trochodendron

derm- *(Skin.)* [δερμα] dermal dermatitis dermatology dermatophytosis *(Athlete's foot.)*; **-derm** ectoderm endoderm epidermis mesoderm pachyderm taxidermy; <u>And</u>: hypodermic

di- *(Two.)* [dis δις *twice.*] digraph dilemma dioxide dipole; <u>See</u>: **di-** as prefix in Ap. iii-23.

dia- *(Across; apart; completely.)* [dia δια] diagram diameter; <u>See</u>: **dia-** as prefix in Ap. iii-23.

diplo- *(Double.)* diplocardia diploma diplomacy diplomat diplomate diplomatic

dogma *(Doctrine.)* dogma dogmatic dogmaticism dogmatism dogmatist dogmatize

doxa *(Opinion; belief.)* [doxa δοξα] doxographer doxological doxologize doxology; **-dox** heterodox orthodox paradox unorthodox; **-doxy** orthodoxy heterodoxy neoorthodoxy

-drome *(Racecourse.)* airdrome dromedary hippodrome motordrome syndrome palindrome *(Same forwards as backwards, e.g. "Madam, I'm Adam." "Able was I ere I saw Elba.")*

dyna- dynamo- *(Force, power.)* dynameter dynamic dynamics dynamism dynamite dynamo dynamoelectric dynamometer dynamometry dynamotor dynasty dyne; **-dynamics** hydrodynamics magnetohydrodynamics pneumodynamics thermodynamics

dys- *(Defective; difficult.)* [dys- δυς–] dysfunction dyslexia; <u>See</u>: **dys-** as prefix in Ap. iii-23.

E

ecto- *(Outside, external.)* [ektos εκτος] ectoderm ectoplasm; <u>See</u>: **ecto-** as prefix in Ap. iii-23.
-ectomy *(A cutting away of a body part.)* adenectomy appendectomy gastrectomy hemorrhoidectomy hysterectomy mastectomy mastoidectomy pneumectomy prostatectomy thyroidectomy tonsillectomy vaginectomy vasectomy; <u>See</u>: **-tomy** Ap. ix-17.
electro- *(Electric.)* electric electrical electrician electricity electrify electrocardiogram electrocardiograph electrocute electrode electroencephalogram electrolysis electrolyte electrolyze electromagnetic electromagnetism electrometallurgy electron electronic electronics electroplate electroshock electrotechnics electrotherapeutics

-emia *(Condition of the blood.)* *[haima* ´αιμα *blood.]* anemia bacteremia copremia hyperemia hyphemia leukemia lithemia sapremia sicklemia toxemia uremia

en- *(In, into.)* *[en* εν*]* Also: **el-, em-, er-** energy engrave; <u>See</u>: **en-** as prefix in Ap. iii-23.

encephalo- *(The brain.)* encephalic encephalitis encephalogram encephalon encephaloma

endo- *(Within, inside.)* *[endon* ενδον*]* endocardium; <u>See</u>: **endo-** as prefix in Ap. iii-23.

epi- *(Upon; among; beside; in addition.)* *[epi* επι*]* episode; <u>See</u>: **epi-** as prefix in Ap. iii-23.

esthet- *(Perception.)* esthesia esthete esthetic esthetician estheticism esthetics; **-esthesia** anesthesia cryptesthesia kinesthesia telesthesia thermanesthesia

ethno- *(Race, nation.)* ethnic ethnicism ethnobiology ethnocentric ethnocentrism ethnogenic ethnogeny ethnography ethnohistory ethnolinguistics ethnology

ethos *(Character.)* *[ethos* εθος*]* ethic ethical ethically ethician ethicize ethics

eu- *(Good; well.)* *[eu-* ευ–*]* eulogy euphoria euthanasia; <u>See</u>: **eu-** as prefix in Ap. iii-24.

ex- *(Out of; from; forth.)* *[ex-* εξ–*]* exodus exorcise; <u>See</u>: **ex-** as prefix in Ap. iii-11, 24.

G

galacto- *(Milk, milky.)* galactic galactose galaxy *(Milky Way Galaxy appears as a milky strip.)*

-gamy *(Marriage.)* *[gamos* γαμος*]* bigamy misogamy monogamy polygamy

gene *(Race, kind.)* gene genealogist genealogy genesis genetic genetics geneticist genocide; **-genesis** *(Development.)* biogenesis pathogenesis psychogenesis; **-gen** *(That which produces.)* allergen androgen antigen carcinogen estrogen hallucinogen halogen hydrogen nitrogen oxygen; **-genic** *(Productive of.)* (adj.) allergenic hallucinogenic pathogenic photogenic toxicogenic; **-genetic** autogenetic monogenetic; **-geny** *(Generation of.)* (n) anthropogeny embryogeny ethnogeny; <u>See</u>: L. **genus** Ap. vii-16.

geo- *(Earth.)* *[gē* γη*]* geocentric geodesic geographer geographical geography geologic geologist geology geometric geometry geophagy geophysics geopolitical geothermal

glosso- glotto- *(Tongue.)* gloss *(Marginal note.)* glossary glossitis glossolalia glottal glottis **-glot** *(A number of languages.)* diglot monoglot polyglot tetraglot triglot

-glyph *(Carving.)* *[glyphein* γλυφειν *to carve.]* anaglyph hieroglyph petroglyph

gnosis *(Special knowledge.)* gnostic Gnostic Gnosticism "Gnothi seauton." *(Know thyself.)* **-gnosis** *(Medical knowledge.)* diagnosis misdiagnosis prognosis telegnosis

-gon *(Having angles.)* *[gōnia* γωνια *corner, angle.]* tetragram *(4)* pentagon *(5)* hexagon *(6)* heptagon *(7)* octagon *(8)* nonagon *(9)* isogon *(Equal.)* polygon *(Many.)*

-gram[1] *(Something written.)* *[gramma* γραμμα*]* anagram cardiogram cryptogram diagram electrocardiogram (EKG) electroencephalogram (EEG) epigram hologram monogram parallelogram radiogram seismogram telegram

-gram² *(A weight unit in the metric system.)* centigram (L) decigram (L) kilogram milligram (L)

graph- *(That which records.)* *[graphē γραφη representation by lines.]* graph graphic graphics graphite; **-graph** autograph barograph cardiograph digraph electrocardiograph electroencephalograph epigraph lithograph mimeograph monograph myocardiograph paragraph petrograph phonograph photograph pictograph polygraph radiograph seismograph spectrograph telegraph; **-grapher** *(The one who does the writing.)* bibliographer biographer choreographer photographer stenographer telegrapher; **-graphic** phonographic photographic telegraphic; **-graphy** *(A writing on a special subject; recording process.)* autobiography bibliography biography cacography calligraphy cartography cinematography cryptography demography geography photography polygraphy pornography seismography stenography telegraphy telephotography topography

gymno- *(Nude.)* *[gymnos γυμνος]* gym gymnasiast gymnasium *(Where Greek youth exercised nude.)* Gymnasium *(European secondary school.)* gymnast gymnastic gymnastics

gyn- *(Woman, female.)* gynecologist gynecology gyniatrics misogynist monogynist philogynist; **-gynous** androgynous; **-gyny** misogyny monogyny polygyny philogyny

gyro- *(Rotating.)* gyral gyrate gyration gyro gyrocompass gyroscope gyrostabilizer

H (Remember Greek had no "h" only a rough breathing mark: ʽ .)
hecto- *(One hundred.)* *[hecaton ʽεκατον]* hectometer; <u>See</u>: **hecto-** as prefix in Ap. iii-24.

heli-, helio- *(Sun.)* helianthus *(Sunflower.)* heliocentric heliolatry *(Sun worship.)* Heliopolis Helios *(The sun god.)* helioscope heliotherapy heliotrope heliotropic heliotropism helium

helico-, helix *(Spiral.)* helical helicoid helicon *(Tuba.)* helicopter heliport helix (Pl. helices.)

hema- hemo- *(Blood.)* hematoid hematology hematoma hemoglobin hemoid hemophilia hemophiliac hemorrhage hemorrhoid hemorrhoidectomy hemostat; <u>See</u>: **-emia**

hemi- *(Half.)* *[hēmi- ʽημι–]* hemicycle hemisphere; <u>See</u>: **hemi-** as prefix in Ap. iii-24.

hetero- *(Other; difference.)* heterodox heterogeneity heterogeneous heteronym *(Two words with same spelling, but different sound and meaning: bass [a fish] and bass [a voice].)* heterosexual

hiero- *(Sacred, divine.)* hierarch hierarchical hierarchy hieratic hierocracy hieroglyphics

hippo- *(Horse.)* hippo hippocampus hippodrome hippogriff hippopotamus

histor- *(Knowing.)* historian historic historical historicity historiography history

holo- *(Whole.)* holocaust Holocene Era holograph hologram holomorphic holotype

homeo- *(Like; similar.)* homeomorphism homeopathist homeopathy homeostasis
homo- *(Same.)* *[homos ʽομος]* homoerotism homogeneity homogeneous homogenize homologous homonym homophone homophonic homosexual homosexuality
hydro- *(Water.)* hydrocarbon hydrodynamics hydroelectric hydrofoil hydrogen hydrogenate hydroid hydrokinetics hydrology hydrolysis hydromechanics hydropathy hydrophobia hydroplane hydroponics hydrosphere hydrotherapy hydrous hydroxide

hypno- *(Sleep.)* hypnosis hypnotherapy hypnotic hypnotism hypnotist hypnotize

hyper- *(Above, over.)* *[hyper-* ὑπερ *]* hyperactive; <u>See</u>: **hyper-** as prefix in Ap. iii-24.

hypo- *(Under, beneath.)* *[hypo-* ὑπο*]* hypodermic; <u>See</u>: **hypo-** as prefix in Ap. iii-24.

hystero- *(Womb; uterine.)* hysterectomy hysteria hysterical hysterics hysteritis

I

-iatric *(Healing.)* geriatric gyniatric pediatric psychiatric; **-iatry** podiatry psychiatry

icono- *(Image.)* icon iconoclasm iconoclast iconography iconolatry iconology

ideo- *(Idea.)* *[idea* ιαεα *form.]* ideograph ideography ideologist ideology ideomotor

idio- *(One's own, individual.)* idiocy idiolect idiom idiomatic idiosyncrasy idiot idiotic

iso- *(Equal, the same.)* isobar isobath isochromatic isomer isometric isosceles isotope

-itis /ī-tis/ *(Inflammation of.)* *[-itis* −ιτις*]* adenitis *(Lymph node.)* appendicitis *(Appendix.)* arthritis *(Joint.)* blepharitis *(Eyelids.)* bronchitis *(Bronchial tubes.)* bursitis *(Bursa.)* carditis *(Heart.)* cellulitis *(Tissues.)* colitis *(Colon.)* conjunctivitis *(Conjunctiva; eyelid lining.)* cystitis *(Bladder.)* dermatitis *(Skin.)* duodenitis *(Duodenum; part of small intestine.)* encephalitis *(Brain.)* endocarditis *(Heart lining.)* enteritis *(Intestines.)* ganglionitis *(Ganglion; group of nerve cells.)* gastritis *(Stomach.)* gastroenteritis *(Membranes of stomach & intestines.)* gingivitis *(Gums.)* glossitis *(Tongue.)* hepatitis *(Liver.)* hysteritis *(Womb.)* ileitis *(Ileum; lowest part of small intestine.)* iritis *(Iris.)* keratitis *(Cornea.)* keratoconjunctivitis *(Cornea & conjunctiva.)* laryngitis *(Larynx.)* lymphadenitis *(Lymph nodes.)* mastitis *(Breast.)* mastoiditis *(Mastoid.)* meningitis *(Meninges; membranes covering brain spinal cord.)* mesenteritis *(Mesentery; a stomach membrane.)* metritis *(Uterus.)* myelitis *(Spinal cord or bone marrow.)* myocarditis *(Heart muscle.)* nephritis *(Kidney.)* neuritis *(Nerve.)* oophoritis *(Ovary.)* ophthalmitis *(Eye.)* orchitis *(Testicle.)* osteitis *(Bone.)* osteomyelitis *(Bone marrow.)* otitis *(Ear.)* ovaritis *(Ovary.)* parotitis *(Parotid; salivary glands, i.e. mumps.)* pericarditis *(Pericardium; protective bag around heart.)* perineuritis *(Perineurium; a nerve covering.)* periostitis *(Periosteum; membrane around bone.)* peritonitis *(Peritoneum; internal organ covering.)* pharyngitis *(Pharynx.)* phlebitis *(Vein.)* phrenitis *(Diaphragm.)* plantar fasciitis *(Foot sole membrane.)* polioencephalitis *(Brain gray matter.)* poliomyelitis *(Spinal cord gray matter.)* polyneuritis *(Peripheral nerves.)* pruritis *(Intense itching.)* pyelitis *(Pelvis.)* rachitis *(Rickets; bone softening.)* retinitis *(Retina.)* rhinitis *(Nose mucous membranes.)* scleritis *(Sclera; white of eyeball.)* sinusitis *(Sinuses.)* splenitis *(Spleen.)* spondylitis *(Vertebrae.)* stomatitis *(Mouth.)* synovitis *(Synovial membrane.)* tenonitis *(Tendon.)* thelitis *(Nipple.)* thyroiditis *(Thyroid.)* tonsillitis *(Tonsils.)* tracheitis *(Trachea.)* tympanitis *(Tympanic membrane.)* typhlitis *(Cecum; cavity between large & small intestines.)* urethritis *(Urethra.)* utriculitis *(Utricle; inner ear.)* uveitis *(Uvea or iris.)* uvulitis *(Uvula.)* vaginitis *(Vagina.)* valvulitis *(Valve.)*

K *(More Greek K-words listed under C.)*

kilo- *(One thousand.)* *[chilioi-* χιλιοι*−]* kilogram kilometer; <u>See</u>: **kilo-** as prefix in Ap. iii-24.

kine-, kinesi- *(Movement.)* kinematics kinescope kinesimeter kinesthesia kinetic kinetics; **-kinesis** chemokinesis photokinesis psychokinesis; **-kinesia** hyperkinesia; See: **cine-**.

L

-latry *(Worship of.)* bibliolatry demonolatry heliolatry iconolatry idolatry necrolatry

-lepsy *(Seizure, attack.)* *[lēpsis* ληπσις*]* epilepsy catalepsy narcolepsy nympholepsy

leuco- leuko- *(White.)* leucocyte leukemia leukocytosis leukoderma leukoma

-liter *(A liquid measure.)* *[litra* λιτρα*]* dekaliter hectoliter kiloliter microliter milliliter

litho- *(Stone, rock.)* lithograph lithoid lithology lithotomy lithotrity lithium;
-lith acrolith megalith monolith neolith paleolith; **-lithic** Mesolithic Neolithic Paleolithic

-logical *(Related to a specific study.)* analogical biological chronological ecological geological mythological neurological ontological pathological physiological psychological sociological technological theological zoological;
-logist *(One engaged in a specific science.)* anthropologist biologist genealogist gynecologist pathologist psychologist sociologist zoologist;
-logue *(Discourse, recitation.)* catalogue Decalogue dialogue epilogue monologue prologue travelogue
<u>Some often simplified</u>: catalog dialog monolog prolog travelog;
-logy *(Science or study of.)* analogy anesthesiology anthology anthropology archeology astrobiology astrology audiology bacteriology biology cardiology chronology climatology cosmetology cosmology criminology cryptology deontology dermatology doxology ecology Egyptology embryology endocrinology etiology etymology eulogy gastroenterology genealogy geology gerontology gynecology hematology hydrology hymnology ichthyology ideology immunology limnology lithology meteorology methodology microbiology mineralogy musicology mythology neurology numerology odontology oncology ontology ophthalmology ornithology osteology otology paleontology parapsychology pathology penology pharmacology phenomenology philology phonology phrenology physiology pneumatology proctology psychology radiology sociology technology teleology terminology theology toxicology urology zoology
logo- *(Word.)* logarithm logic logical logician logistic logistics logo logorrhea logos Logos

-lysis *(A loosening, dissolving.)* analysis catalysis dialysis electrolysis hydrolysis hypnoanalysis photolysis psychoanalysis pyrolysis urinalysis; **-lyst** anticatalyst catalyst; **-lyte** electrolyte hydrolyte; **-lytic** catalytic electrolytic hydrolytic paralytic

-lyze *(To perform; cause.)* *[lysis* λυσις *a loosening; setting free.]* <u>See</u>: **-lyze** in Ap. iv-57.

M

-machy *(A fight between.)* gigantomachy *(Giants vs. gods.)* logomachy *(Verbal contention.)*

macro- *(Large, great.)* macrocephalic macroclimate macrocosm macroeconomics macron

magnet *(Lodestone.)* magnet magnetic magnetism magnetize magneto magnetoelectricty

-mancy *(Foretelling by means of.)* chiromancy *(Hand.)* geomancy *(Earth particles.)* hydromancy *(Water.)* necromancy *(The dead.)* oneiromancy *(Dreams.)* pyromancy *(Fire.)*

-mania *(An exaggerated infatuation.)* acromania *(High places.)* bibliomania *(Books.)* dipsomania *(Alcohol.)* egomania *(Self.)* erotomania *(Sex.)* kleptomania *(Obsession to steal.)* megalomania *(Exalted opinion of self.)* monomania *(One idea.)* mythomania *(Telling lies.)* narcomania *(Narcotics.)* necromania *(The dead.)* nymphomania *(A woman's obsessive desires.)* pyromania *(Fire.),* etc. **-maniac** *(A person with a particular infatuation.)* egomaniac kleptomaniac pyromaniac, *etc.*

masto- *(Breast; chest.)* mastectomy mastodon mastoid mastoidectomy mastoiditis

mech- *(Machine.)* *[mēchanē* μηχανη *a war engine; contrivance.]* mechanic mechanical mechanics mechanism mechanistic mechanization mechanize

mega- *(Great, large.)* megacephalic megacycle megalith megameter megaohm megaphone megaton; **megalo-** *(Excessively large.)* megalomania megalosaur

melan- *(Black.)* melancholia melancholy melanin melanoid melanoma melanosis

meso- *(In the middle.)* *[mesos* μεσος *middle, moderate.]* <u>See:</u> **meso-** as prefix in Ap. iii-24.

meta- *(After, beyond.)* *[meta* μετα *among; after; behind.]* <u>See:</u> **meta-** as prefix in Ap. iii-24.

-meter *(Measuring device.)* altimeter ammeter barometer calorimeter centimeter diameter kilometer micrometer micomillimeter millimeter odometer ohmmeter parameter pedometer perimeter psychrometer pulsimeter seismometer taximeter thermometer voltmeter wattmeter; **-metric** asymmetric barometric diametric geometric isometric metric photometric psychometric symmetric trigonometric; **-metry** asymmetry geometry hydrometry hygrometry optometry psychometry symmetry trigonometry

micro- *(Very small.)* microbe microcircuit microcosm microfilm micron Micronesia microorganism microphone microscope microscopic microsecond microwave

miso- *(Hating.)* *[misein* μισειν *to hate.]* misogamist misogamy *(Of marriage.)* misogynist misogyny *(Of women.)* misologist misology *(Of debate.)* misoneist misoneism *(Of change.)*

mono- *(One, single.)* *[monos* μονος *alone, forsaken.]* <u>See:</u> **mono-** as prefix in Ap. iii-24.

morph- *(Having the form of.)* morpheme Morpheus *(God of dreams.)* morphine morphology **-morph** allomorph ectomorph *(Lean person.)* endomorph *(Heavy person.)* isomorph mesomorph *(Muscular person.)* polymorph pseudomorph; **-morphic** anthropomorphic metamorphic; **-morphosis** anthropomorphosis metamorphosis

myria- *(Very many.)* *[myrias* μυριας *numberless, countless.]* myriad myriadfold myriadly myriad-minded myriapod

mytho- *(Myth.)* myth mythical mythicize mythological mythologize mythology mythos

myo- *(Muscle.)* myocardiograph myocarditis myoid myology myoma myopia myosin

N

narco- *(Torpor; insensibility.)* *[narkē* ναρκη *stiffness, numbness.]* narcolepsy narcomania narcosis narcosynthesis narcotic narcotism narcotize

naut- *(Sailor.)* nautical nautical mile nautilus Nautilus *(First atomic-powered submarine.)*
-naut aeronaut aeronautic aeronautics aquanaut Argonaut astronaut

necro- *(Corpse; death.)* [*nekros* νεκρος *corpse.*] necrolatry necrology necromancy necrophagous necrophile necrophilia necropolis necropsy necrosis necrotomy

neo- *(New, recent.)* [*neos* νεος *young, new.*] neoclassic; <u>See</u>: **neo-** as prefix in Ap. iii-25.

neuro- *(Nerve.)* neural neuralgia neurectomy neurilemma neuritis neurology neuroma neuron neuropath neuropathology neuropsychiatry neuropsychosis neurosis neurotic

nomo- *(Science of.)* [*nomos* νομος *law, custom.*] nomograph nomology nomothetic
-nomy *(Science of.)* agronomy anthroponomy antinomy astronomy autonomy Deuteronomy economy gastronomy heteronomy isonomy

O

octo-, octa- *(Eight.)* [*oktō* οκτω] octagon octopus; <u>See</u>: **octo-** as prefix in Ap. iii-16, 25.

-ode *(Way, path.)* [*hodos* 'οδος] anode cathode diode electrode period tetrode triode

odonto- *(Tooth.)* odontalgia odontoid odontology; **-odontics** endodontics *(Root canals.)* orthodontics periodontics prosthodontics; **-odontist** orthodontist periodontist

oligo- *(Few.)* [*oligos* ολιγος *few; small.*] oligarch oligarchy oligopoly Oligocene

-oma *(Cancer, tumor.)* [*-ōma* –ωμα *tumor.*] carcinoma encephaloma fibroma glaucoma hematoma leukoma melanoma myoma neuroma osteoma sarcoma trachoma

onto- *(Being; existence.)* ontology ontologist ontogeny ontogenetic ontological

-onym *(Name.)* acronym antonym cryptonym homonym pseudonym synonym

ophthalmo- *(Eye.)* ophthalmia ophthalmic ophthalmitis ophthalmologist ophthalmology

-opia *(Defect of the eye.)* diplopia myopia; **-opsis** *(Having the appearance of.)* thanatopsis *(Meditation on death; Thanatos, Greek god of death.)*; **-opsy** biopsy necropsy
optic- *(Of the eye.)* optic optical optician optics optometer optometrist optometry

-orama *(A view.)* [*horama* 'οραμα *a view, scene.*] cosmorama cyclorama diorama panorama

organo- *(Implement.)* organ organic organism organist organization organize organography organology organon organum

ornitho- *(Bird.)* ornithoid ornithology ornithopter ornithosis

ortho- *(Straight; in line.)* orthodontics orthodontist orthodox orthodoxy orthopedics

-osis *(State or condition of.)* [*-ōsis* –ωσις] hypnosis neurosis; <u>See</u>: **-osis** as suffix in Ap. iv-58.

osteo- *(Bone.)* [*osteon* οστεον] osteoid osteology osteoma osteomyelitis osteopath osteopathy osteoplasty osteoporosis osteotomy

P

pachy- *(Thick; massive.)* pachyderm *(Thick skin: elephant. etc.)* pachysandra

paleo- *(Ancient, old.)* Paleocene paleolith Paleolithic paleology paleontology Paleozoic

pan- *(All, the whole.)* panacea Pan-American panchromatic pancratium pancreas pandemic pandemonium panegyric Pan-Hellenic panoply panorama pantheism pantheon; **panto-** pantomime;   Note: panic *(The god, Pan, was thought to cause sudden, unfounded fear.)*

para- *(Beside; beyond.)* [para παρα *beside; beyond; toward.*] See: **para-** as prefix in Ap. iii-25.

patho- *(Suffering; disease.)* [pathos παθος] pathological pathologist pathology pathos; **-pathy** *(The treatment of disease; feeling.)* allopathy antipathy homeopathy hydropathy idiopathy naturopathy osteopathy sympathy telepathy; **-path** allopath neuropath osteopath psychopath; **-pathetic** pathetic sympathetic; **-pathic** psychopathic

ped- *(Child; education.)* [pais, paidos παις παιδος *child, daughter, son.*] encyclopedia pedagogue pedagogy pedant pedantry pederast pederastry pediatrician pediatrics pedophilia pedophiliac; Not to be confused with: L. **pes, pedis** *(Foot.)* in Ap.vii-30.

penta- *(Five.)* [pente πεντε] pentagon pentameter; See: **penta-** as prefix in Ap. iii-25.

peri- *(Around; near.)* [peri περι] perimeter periscope; See: **peri-** as prefix in Ap. iii-25.

petro- *(Rock, stone.)* [petra πετρα] Peter petrification petrified petrify petrochemistry petroglyph petrograph petrol (Brit. *gasoline.*) petroleum (L. oleum = *oil.*) petrolic petrology

phanero- *(Visible.)* fancied fanciful fancy fantasia fantasize fantasy phantasm phantasmagoria phantasmal phantom;   **-phane** cellophane

phago- *(Eating.)* phagedena *(A spreading ulcer.)* phagocyte; **-phagous** anthopophagous bacteriophagous carpophagous *(Fruit.)* coprophagous *(Dung.)* entomophagous *(Insects.)* geophagous *(Soil.)* ichthyophagous *(Fish.)* myrmecophagous *(Ants.)* necrophagous *(Carrion.)* omophagous *(Raw flesh.)* polyphagous *(Excessive food.)* zoophagous *(Animals; L. carnivorous.)*; **-phagia** aphagia *(Loss of swallowing ability.)* dysphagia *(Difficulty swallowing.)*

pharmaco- *(A drug.)* pharmaceutical pharmaceutics pharmacist pharmacology pharmacy

phil- *(Loving; fond of.)* Philadelphia philander philanthropy philately *(Stamp collecting.)* philharmonic philodendron philogyny philology philosopher philosophical philosophize philosophy; **-phile** Anglophile bibliophile Francophile Germanophile necrophile, *etc..*

-phobia *(An exaggerated fear of.)* acrophobia *(Heights.)* agoraphobia *(Open places,* originally the market place, αγορα .) androphobia *(Men.)* arachnophobia *(Spiders.)* claustrophobia *(Enclosed places.)* cynophobia *(Dogs.)* gamophobia *(Marriage.)* gynophobia *(Women.)* hemophobia *(Blood.)* hydrophobia *(Water.)* musophobia *(Mice.)* necrophobia *(Dead bodies.)* ochlophobia *(Crowds.)* ophidiophobia *(Snakes.)* pyrophobia *(Fire.)* thanatophobia *(Death.)* triskaidekaphobia *(Number 13.)* xenophobia *(Strangers.)*;. **-phobic** acrophobic agoraphobic claustrophobic, *etc.* **-phobe** *(One who fears.)* acrophobe agoraphobe claustrophobe necrophobe pyrophobe, *etc.*

phono- *(Voice, sound.)* [phonē φωνη *a sound, tone.*] (n) phone phoneme phonetic phonetics phonic phonics phonograph phonology; **-phone** allophone Dictaphone homophone megaphone microphone saxophone (A. J. Sax.) sousaphone (John Philip Sousa.)

Ap. ix-14

telephone vibraphone xylophone; -**phonic** (adj.) homophonic monophonic polyphonic stereophonic; -**phony** *(Type of sound.)* *n.* acrophony antiphony cacophony homophony polyphony symphony;   Related: dysphonia *(Difficulty in uttering sounds.)*

photo- *(Light.)* [*phōs, phōtos* φως, φωτος *light, daylight.]* phot photo photocopy photoelectric photoelectron photogenic photograph photographic photography photometer photon photophilous photophobia photostat photosynthesis phototherapeutic; And: phosphorus

physico- *(Nature.)* [*physis* φυσις *inborn quality, mind, nature.]* physic physicist physical physical education physical therapy physician physicochemical physics physiognomy physiography physiological physiology physique; And: hyperphysical microphysics, *etc.*

-**plasm** *(Inner fluid of an organism.)* archiplasm bioplasm cataplasm cytoplasm deutoplasm ectoplasm endoplasm metaplasm neoplasm protoplasm trophoplasm; And: plasma

-**plasty** *(Operation on body part.)* angioplasty *(Blood vessel.)* genioplasty *(Chin.)* hernioplasty *(Rupture.)* heteroplasty *(Graft from another person.)* keratoplasty *(Cornea.)* neoplasty *(Plastic surgery.)* osteoplasty *(Bone.)* rhinoplasty *(Nose.)* staphyloplasty *(Soft palate.)* stomatoplasty *(Mouth.)* thoracoplasty *(Chest.)* zooplasty *(Grafting an animal part to a human.)*

-**plegia** *(Paralysis.)* cycloplegia *(Eye muscle.)* hemiplegia *(One side of body.)* monoplegia *(One body part.)* paraplegia *(Legs.)* quadriplegia *(Arms & legs.);* And: paraplegic quadriplegic

pluto- *(Wealth.)* [*plutos* πλουτος *wealth, riches.]* plutocracy   plutocrat   plutocratic

pneuma *(Breath; soul, spirit.)* pneuma pneumatic pneumatics pneumatology pneumatotherapy; **pneumo-** *(Lung.)* pneumectomy pneumobacillus pneumococcus pneumoconiosis pneumology pneumonectomy pneumonia

pod- *(Foot.)* [*pous, podos* πους ποδος *a foot;* pl. *claws; talons.]* podagra *(Gout.)* podiatry podium podophyllin; -**pod** *(Having so many or kind of feet.)* amphipod bipod hexapod megapod myriapod polypod tripod; Also: Oedipus *(Swollen-footed.)* platypus *(Flat foot.)*

polio- *(Gray matter of brain and spinal cord.)* [*polios* πολιος *gray.]* polio polioencephalitis *(Inflammation of the brain.)* poliomyelitis *(Inflammation of the spinal cord.)*

polis *(City.)* [*polis* πολις *citystate.]* acropolis Annapolis Indianapolis metropolis Minneapolis Persepolis police policy politic political politician politics. polity

poly- *(Many.)* [*polys* πολυς *much; many.]* polyandry polychromic polyester polygamous polygamy polyglot polygon polygraph polyhedron polynomial polyp polyphonic polyphony polysyllabic polytechnic polytheism polyunsaturated

pro- *(Before; forward.)* [*pro* προ *before.]* program prologue; See: **pro-** as prefix in Ap. iii-25.

proto- *(First in rank.)* protocol protohuman proton protoplasm prototype protozoan

pseudo- *(False.)* [*pseudēs* ψευδης *lying.]* pseudo pseudoclassic pseudomorph pseudonym

psycho- *(Mind; soul.)* psyche -psychedelic psychiatrist psychiatry psychic psychoanalysis psychoanalyst psychoanalyze psychodrama psychokinesis psychological psychologist psychology psychometry psychoneurosis psychopath psychopathic psychosis psychosomatic psychotherapy psychotic

pyro- *(Fire.)* pyrochemical pyroelectric pyrogenic pyrography pyrology pyrolysis pyromancy pyromaniac pyrometer pyrophoric pyrosis *(Heartburn.)* pyrotechnics

R

rheo- *(Current, flow.)* rheobase rheology rheometer rheoscope rheostat rheotaxis

rhino- *(Nose, nasal.)* rhinitis rhino rhinoceros rhinology rhinoplasty rhinoscope

-rrhea *(Abnormal discharge.)* diarrhea gonorrhea logorrhea pyorrhea Related: hemorrhage

S

-saurus *(Lizard.)* Allosaurus Ankylosaurus Brontosaurus Megalosaurus Paleosaurus Stegosaurus Titanosaurus Tyrannosaurus; <u>And</u>: dinosaur *(Terrible lizard.)*

schisto- schizo- *(Split, divided.)* schism schismatic schizoid schizophrenia schizophrenic

-scope *(Instrument for observation.)* fluoroscope gyroscope horoscope kaleidoscope kinescope microscope oscilloscope otoscope periscope proctoscope spectroscope stethoscope stroboscope telescope; **-scopic** macroscopic microscopic orthoscopic telescopic; **-scopy** *(Observation.)* bioscopy fluoroscopy gastroscopy horoscopy laryngoscopy microscopy radioscopy spectroscopy telescopy tracheoscopy

seismo- *(Earthquake.)* seismic seismograph seismography seismology seismometer

somato- *(Body.)* soma (Pl. somata) somatic somatology; **-some** centrosome chromosome

sophos *(Wise.)* sophism sophist sophisticate sophisticated sophistication sophistry sophomore sophomoric; **-sophy** *(Specific knowledge.)* philosophy physiosophy theosophy

sperm *(Seed.)* sperm spermatic spermatoid spermatophore spermophile sperm whale

sphere *(Globe, ball.)* [sphaera σφαερα] atmosphere bathysphere biosphere hemisphere ionosphere sphere spherical spherics spheroid stratosphere thermosphere troposphere

spiro- *(Spiral; coiled.)* spiral spire *(A whorl, twist.)* spiroid spirula spiry (In Latin **spiro-** is breath.)

spore *(Seed.)* sporadic spore sporiferous sporogenesis sporogony sporophore sporozoan sporozoite; **-spore** arthrospore endospore microspore tetraspore zoospore

-stat *(A device that makes constant.)* aerostat chemostat coelostat cryostat heliostat hemostat photostat pyrostat rheostat siderostat thermostat; <u>And</u>: static statics

steno- *(Tight; narrow.)* stenograph stenographer stenography stenosis stenotropic

stereo- *(Solid; three-dimensional.)* stere stereo stereophonic stereoscopic stereotype

stoma- *(Mouth.)* stomatodynia stomatoglossitis stomatology stomatomy stomatomycosis stomatoplasty; **-stomy** *(Making an opening.)* colostomy cystostomy enterostomy gastroenterostomy ileostomy pyeloureterostomy tracheostomy

syn- Also **syl-, sym, sys-** *(With, together.)* *[syn* συν *with.]*   See: **syn-** as prefix in Ap. iii-25.

T

tauto- *(Same.)* tautologism tautologize tautology tautomericism tautonym tautonymy

-taxis *(Order; arrangement.)* chemotaxis geotaxis homotaxis hydrotaxis hypotaxis

techno- *(Art; skill.)* technical technicality technician Technicolor technique technocracy technological technology;   But: tectonics *(Building construction;* τεκτων = carpenter.*)*

tele- *(Far off; at a distance.)* *[tēle* τηλε *far away.]* telecast telecom. telecommunications telegram telegraph telegraphy telekinesis telemetry telepathy telephone telephoto teleprinter Teleprompter (TN) telescope telescopic Teletype (TN) televise television

teleo- telo- *(Final; complete.)* *[telos* τελος *completion, fulfillment.]* teleology telesis *(Progress toward a goal.)*   telestich *(An acrostic at the ends of lines.)*

tetra- *(Four.)* *[tetra-* τετρα-*]* tetrachord tetrarcy;   See: **tetra-** as prefix in Ap. iii-25.

theo- the- *(God; a god.)* theocentric theocracy theocrat theologian theological theologize theology theomachy;   **-theism** atheism monotheism pantheism polytheism

-therapy *(Treatment of disease.)* chemotherapy heliotherapy hydropherapy hypnotherapy phototherapy physiotherapy psychotherapy;   And: therapeutic therapy

thermo- *(Heat.)* *[thermē* θερμη*]* therm thermae *(Hot springs.)* thermal thermocouple thermodynamics thermoelectric thermometer thermos thermostat thermotherapy; **thermal** geothermal isothermal;   **-thermia** hyperthermia hypothermia;

-thesis *(Formal proposition; treatise.)* antithesis biosynthesis chemosynthesis diathesis epenthesis hypothesis metathesis parenthesis photosynthesis prosthesis synthesis

-tomy *(Cutting; incision.)* arthrotomy colostomy craniotomy dichotomy gastrotomy herniotomy hysterotomy lobotomy phlebotomy tracheotomy; See: **-ectomy** Ap. ix-7.

tono- *(Tension.)* tonal tonality tone tone-deaf toneless tone poem tone row tonic

topo- *(A place, region.)* topographer topography topology;   And: isotope utopia

toxico- *(Poison.)* toxemia *(Blood poisoning.)* toxic toxicide toxicity toxicologist toxicology toxicophobia toxicosis toxin;   And: intoxication intoxicated

tri- *(Three.)* *[tri- < trias* τρι- τριας*]* See: **tri-** as both Latin & Greek prefix in Ap. iii-21, 25.

-type *(Class type; in printing.)* archetype ectype electrotype linotype prototype stereotype teletype; **type- typo-** type typecast typesetter typewrite typewriter typical typify typist typo typographer typographical typography typology;   And: atypical

U

-urgy *(Work with a material.)* chemurgy electrometallurgy hydrometallurgy liturgy *(Religious ritual; "work with people.")* metallurgy micrurgy pyrometalurgy thaumaturgy theurgy

X   (Initial x is pronounced /z/.)

xero- *(Dry, dryness.)* xeric xeroderma xerography xerophilous xerophyte xerosis Xerox (TN)

xylo- *(Wood.)* xylem xylograph xylography xyloid xylophagous xylophone xylotomy

Z

-zoa *(Zoological group.)* Hydrozoa Mesozoa Protozoa; **-zoan** heliozoan hydrozoan metazoan protozoan; **-zoic** Archeozoic Cenozoic Mesozoic Paleozoic Proterozoic; **zoo-** *(Animal.)* zoo (Short for *zoological garden.*)   zooid zoolatry zoological zoology

---

And Still More Combining Forms

A

acantho- *thorn*	**actino-** *radiate*	**adeno-** *gland*
-agra *seizure*	**agro-** *agriculture*	**amylo-** *starch*
anemo *wind*	**angio-** *blood vessel*	**aniso-** *unequal*
anklo- *bent; crooked*	**areo-** *Mars*	**asco-** *bag*
atmo- *vapor*	**azo-** *nitrogen*	

B

bacterio- *bacteria*	**batho-** *depth*	**bathy-** *deep*
-biosis *manner of living*	**-blast** *growth; sprout*	**blepharo-** *eyelid*
brachlo- *arm*	**brachy-** *short*	**brady-** *slow*
-branch *having gills*	**bromo-** *containing bromine*	**broncho-** *windpipe*

C

-carpo *fruit*	**-cele** *tumor; hernia*	**cene-** *new, recent*
ceno- *common*	**cerato-** *horn*	**cero-** *wax*
chaeto- *hair*	**chalco-** *copper; brass*	**chilo-** *lip*
chloro- *chlorine*	**chole-** *gall, bile*	**chondro-** *cartilage*
-chore *plant distribution*	**-chroous** *having certain color*	**chryso-** *gold, golden*
climato- *climate*	**cleisto-** *closed*	**cocci-** *berry*
-coccus *berry-shaped*	**coelo-** *cavity*	**colo-** *colon*
conio *dust*	**cono-** *cone*	**copro-** *dung*
coralli- *coral*	**cranio-** *cranium*	**cryo-** *cold*
crypto- *secret*	**crystallo-** *crystal*	**cteno-** *comb*
cyano- *bluish*	**cymo-** *wave*	**cyano-** *blue*
cyprino- *carp*	**cysto-** *bladder; cyst*	

D

dactylo- *finger; toe*	**demono-** *demon*	**deutero-** *second*
dicho- *in pairs*	**dino-** *terrible*	**dodeca-** *twelve*
-dolicho- *long*	**dromous** *running*	**duodeno-** *duodenum*

E

echino- *spiny; prickly*	**elaio-** *oil*	**embryo** *embryo*
entero- *intestine)*	**entomo-** *insect*	**eo-** *earliest*
ergo- *work*	**erythro-** *red*	**eury-** *wide, broad*

G

galacto- *milky*
-gamous *marriage*
gastro- *stomach*
geronto- *old age*
glyco- *sweet*
-gnathous *having a jaw*
gonio- *angle; corner*
-gony *production of*

gameto- *gamete*
-gamy *marriage*
-genous *generating*
giganto- *gigantic*
glypto- *carved*
-gnomy *knowledge*
-gonium *reproductive cell*
-gynous *female, of women*

gamo- *sexually joined*
ganglio- *ganglion*
-geny *generation*
glauco- *bluish gray*
gnatho- *jaw*
-gon *with so many angles*
gono- *procreative; sexual*

H

hagio- *sacred*
-hedral *with a number of sides*
histo- *tissue*
hygro- *wet*
hypso- *height*

halo- *salt, sea*
-hedron *w. a number of sides*
hyalo- *glass*
hylo- *matter*

haplo- *simple; single*
hepato- *liver*
hyeto- *of rain*
hymeno- *membrane*

I

iatro- *medicine*
iodo- *iodine*

ichthyo- *fish*
irido- *iris of the eye*

icosi- *twenty*

K

karyo- *nucleus; nut*

kerato- *horn, cornea*

L

laparo *loins; flanks*
lepto- *fine, slender*
lymphato- *lymphatic*

laryngo- *larynx*
lipo- *fat*
lympho- *lymph*

lepido- *scale, as of a fish*
lopho- *crest*
lyo-, lysi- *a loosening*

M

malaco- *soft*
mero- *part, partial*
metro- *the uterus*
myco- *fungus*
myxo- *slimy*

-mantic *foretelling*
-merous *having so many parts*
metro- *measure*
myelo- *spinal cord*

-mere *part, division*
meth- *methyl*
-mycete *class of fungi*
myrmeco- *ant*

N

nano- *exceedingly small*
nemato- *thread; filament*
nitro- *containing NO₂*
nycto- *night*

-nastic *plant responses*
nepho- *cloud*
noso- *disease*
nympho- *nymph; bride*

-nasty *automatic response*
nephro *kidney*
noto- *back*

O

-odont *toothed*
-oidea *zoological suffix*
oneiro- *dream*
ophio- *snake, serpent*
orchio- *testicle*
oxa- *containing oxygen*

-odynia *chronic pain*
ombro- *rain*
oo- *(ὄον ῳον) egg*
-opsia *condition of sight*
oro- *mountain*
oxy- *sharp; oxygen*

oeno- *wine*
-ome *group; mass; body*
oophoro- *ovary*
orchido- *orchid*
oto-*ear*

P

phanero- *visible*
-phany *appearance*
pharyngo- *throat*
-phasia *speech defect*
pheno- *related to benzine*
phlebo- *vein*
-phore *bearer of, producer of*
phospho- *phosphorus*
phreno- *mind; brain*
-phyceae *seaweed*
phyco- *seaweed*
phyllo- *leaf*
-phyllous *having leaves*
phylo- *tribe; species*
-phyre *rock type*
-phyte *plant kind*
phyto- *plant*
picro- *bitter*
piezo- *pressure*
plagio- *oblique; slanting*
plano- *roaming*
-plasia *growth*
-plasm *viscous material*
plasmo- *plasma*
-plast *living cell*
-plastic *growing*
platy- *flat*
pleuro- *pleura, side*
-ploid *number of chromosomes*
pneumato- *air; breath-*
poietic *making*
procto- *rectum*
prostato- *prostate gland*
psychro- *cold*
ptero-, -pterous *wing*
pyeloo- *pelvis*
pyo- *pus*

R

rhizo- *root*
-rrhaphy *surgical sewing*

S

saccharo- *sugar*
sapro- *decomposition*
sarco- *flesh*
scato- *dung*
scoto- *darkness*
scypho- *cup*
seleno- *moon*
sialo *saliva*
sidero- *iron*
sito- *food*
sclero- *hard*
-speleo *cave*
spheno *wedge-shaped*
sphygmo- *pulse*
splanchno- *viscera*
spleno- *spleen*
spondylo- *vertebra*
sporo- *seed; spore*
-sporous *having spores*
staphylo- *uvula*
stato- *position*
stauro- *cross*
sterno- *the sternum*
stetho- *breast; chest*
-stichous *having rows*
stomato- *mouth*
-stome, -stomous *mouth*
staphylo- *uvula*
stylo- *pillar*
syndesmo- *ligament*

T

tachy- *speed*
tarso- *ankle*
tauro- *bull*
-taxis *order, arrangement*
teno- *tendon*
terato- *a wonder; monster*
tetarto- *fourth*
thalasso- *the sea*
thanato- *death*
thaumato- *a wonder; a miracle*
thio- *sulfur*
thoraco- *thorax*
thyro- *thyroid*
toco- *child, birth*
tracheo- *trachea*
trachy- *rough, uneven*
tricho- *hair*
-trope *that which turns*
tropho- *nutrition*
typhlo- *blindness*
typho- *typhus*

U

urano- *the heavens*
uretero- *the ureter*
urethro- *the urethra*
-uria *condition of urine*
urico- *uric acid*
uro-[1] (ουρον) *urine*
uro-[2] (ουρα) *tail*

X

xantho- *yellow*
xeno- *strange; foreign*
xiphi- *sword*

Z

zygo- *yoke; pair*
zymo *fermentation*

Greek---The Short Course

Review the Greek Prefixes. Like the Latin Prefixes, they are used again and again.

a- *not;* ana- *up, back;* amphi- *both, around;* anti- *against;* apo- *off, away;* cata- *down, against;* deca- *ten;* di- *two;* dia- *across, apart;* dys- *defective, difficult;* ecto- *outside;* endo- *inside;* ex- *out of, from;* en- *in, into;* ennea- *nine;* epi- *upon, beside;* eu- *good, well;* hecto- *one hundred;* hemi- *half;* hepta- *seven;* hexa- *six;* hyper- *above;* hypo- *under;* kilo- *one thousand;* meso-*middle;* meta- *after, beyond;* mono- *one;* neo- *new, recent;* octo- *eight;* para- *beside, beyond;* penta- *five;* peri- *around, near;* pro- *before, forward;* syn- *with, together;* tetra-*four;* tri-*three.* Remember: as a chameleon prefix **syn-** may also be **syl-, sym,** or **sys-.**

The reference at the end of each entry indicates where more examples may be found.

A

acro *(At the top.)* acrobat acrobatics acronym acropolis acrostic [Ap. ix-5.]

anthro *(Man.)* anthropology anthropoid misanthrope philanthropy [Ap. ix-5.]

arch *(Chief, leader.)* archbishop archetype architect architecture archives archipelago matriarch monarch patriarch oligarch [Ap. ix-5.]

-archy *(Government.)* anarchy hierarchy matriarchy monarchy oligarchy [Ap. ix-5.]

ast- *(Star.)* aster asterisk astronaut astrology astronomer astronomical astronomy astrodome astrophysics astrosphere [< **aster, astro-** Ap. ix-5-6.]

auto *(Self.)* autobiography autocrat autograph automatic automation automobile automotive autonomous autonomy autopsy [Ap. ix-6.]

B

biblio *(Book.)* Bible Biblical bibliographer bibliography bibliophile [Ap. ix-6.]

bio *(Life.)* biographical biography biological biology biopsy antibiotic biochemistry biophysics biosphere biotron [Ap. ix-6.]

C

cardio *(Heart.)* cardiac cardiogram cardiograph cardiology [Ap. ix-6.]

chem *(Chemical.)* chemical chemist chemistry chemotherapy [Ap. ix-6.]

chrom *(Color.)* chromatic chrome chromium chromosome [Ap. ix-6.]

chron *(Time.)* anachronism chronic chronicle chronology synchronize [Ap. ix-6.]

cosmo *(Universe.)* cosmos cosmology cosmopolitan cosmonaut cosmetic cosmetology macrocosm microcosm [Ap. ix-7.]

-cracy *(Government.)* aristocracy autocracy bureaucracy democracy [Ap. ix-7.]

-crat *(Government member.)* aristocrat autocrat bureaucrat democrat [Ap. ix-7.]

cycle *(A recurring period; wheel.)* bicycle cycle cyclic cyclist cyclone encyclopedia kilocycle motorcycle tricycle megacycle [Ap. ix-7.]

D

dem *(People.)* democracy democrat demagogue demography epidemic [Ap. ix-7.]

derm *(Skin.)* dermatitis dermatology epidermis pachyderm taxidermy [Ap. ix-7.]

diplo *(Paper folded double.)* diploma diplomacy diplomat diplomatic [Ap. ix-7.]

dogma *(Doctrine.)* dogma dogmatic dogmatism dogmatist [Ap. ix-7.]

dox *(Opinion, belief.)* doxology orthodox paradox unorthodox [Ap. ix-7.]

drome *(Running.)* dromedary hippodrome palindrome syndrome [Ap. ix-7.]

dyn- *(Force, power.)* dynamic dynamite dynamo dynasty dyne [Ap. ix-7.]

E

-ectomy *(Cutting out.)* appendectomy mastectomy tonsillectomy [Ap. ix-7.]

electro *(Electric.)* electric electrical electrician electricity electrify electrocute electrode electrolysis electron electronic [Ap. ix-7.]

G

-gamy *(Marriage.)* bigamy misogamy monogamy polygamy [Ap. ix-8.]

gene *(Race, kind.)* gene genealogy genetics geneticist genocide [Ap. ix-8.]

-gen *(Produces.)* hydrogen nitrogen oxygen allergen antigen androgen carcinogen estrogen hallucinogen halogen [Ap. ix-8.]

geo- *(Earth.)* geocentric geographer geographical geography geologic geologist geology geometry geophysics geothermal [Ap. ix-8.]

-gon *(Angle.)* hexagon octagon pentagon polygon tetragon [Ap. ix-8.]

gram *(Written; weight.)* gram diagram telegram cardiogram centigram kilogram hologram milligram parallelogram anagram [Ap. ix-8.]

graph *(Recorded.)* autobiography autograph bibliography biographer calligraphy cardiograph choreographer digraph electrocardiograph graph graphic graphics graphite lithograph mimeograph phonograph photograph photography polygraph pornography seismograph stenographer telegraph telegraphy [Ap. ix-9.]

gym *(Exercise.)* gym gymnasium gymnast gymnastics [< **gymno-** Ap. ix-9.]

gyn *(Woman.)* gynecology gynecologist misogyny misogynist philogyny philogynist monogyny polygyny androgynous [Ap. ix-9.]

gyro *(Rotating.)* gyro gyrate gyration gyrocompass gyroscope [Ap. ix-9.]

H

hema, hemo *(Blood.)* hematology hematoma hemoglobin hemophilia hemophiliac hemorrhage hemorrhoid hemorrhoidectomy [Ap. ix-9.]

homo *(Same.)* homogeneity homogeneous homogenize homonym homophonic homosexual homosexuality (Note: in Latin **homo** = *man.*) [Ap. ix-9.]

hydro *(Water.)* hydrogen hydrocarbon hydroelectric hydrofoil hydrolysis hydrotherapy hydrous hydrology hydrophobia hydroxide [Ap. ix-9.]

I

-iatric *(Medical.)* geriatric gyniatric pediatric psychiatric [Ap. ix-10.]

-itis *(Inflammation.)* appendicitis arthritis bronchitis bursitis conjunctivitis dermatitis encephalitis gastritis gingivitis hepatitis laryngitis meningitis neuritis phlebitis poliomyelitis tenonitis tonsillitis [Ap. ix-10.]

L

lith *(Stone.)* monolith megalith Paleolithic Mesolithic Neolithic lithology lithium lithoid lithograph lithotomy lithotrity acrolith [Ap. ix-11.]

logo *(Word.)* logarithm logic logical logician logistics logo logos [Ap. ix-11.]

-logy *(Study of.)* analogy anesthesiology anthology anthropology astrology bacteriology biology cardiology chronology cosmetology cosmology criminology dermatology doxology ecology Egyptology embryology endocrinology entomology epistemology ethnology etymology eulogy genealogy geology gerontology gynecology ideology Kremlinology lithology meteorology methodology microbiology mineralogy musicology mythology neurology numerology oncology ornithology paleontology pathology pharmacology physiology psychology radiology sociology technology terminology theology toxicology zoology [Ap. ix-11.]

-logist *(One who studies.)* biologist geologist sociologist, *etc.* (See above list.)

-logue *(Discourse.)* catalogue dialogue epilogue monologue prologue [Ap. ix-11.]

M

-mania *(Obsession.)* bibliomania egomania kleptomania megalomania necromania nymphomania pyromania dipsomania [Ap. ix-12.]

mech *(Machine.)* mechanic mechanical mechanics mechanism mechanistic mechanization mechanize [Ap. ix-12.]

mega *(Large.)* megacyle megalomania megaphone megaton [Ap. ix-12.]

melan *(Black.)* melancholia melancholy melanin melanoma melanosis [Ap. ix-12.]

meter *(Measure.)* altimeter barometer centimeter diameter kilometer meter micrometer millimeter odometer ohmmeter pedometer perimeter seismometer thermometer voltmeter wattmeter [Ap. ix-12.]

-metry *(Measurement.)* geometry optometry symmetry trigonometry [Ap. ix-12.]

micro *(Very small.)* microbe microphone microscope microwave [Ap. ix-12.]

morph *(Form.)* amorphous anthropomorphic ectomorphic endomorphic mesomorphic metamorphic metamorphosis morphine [Ap. ix-12.]

N

naut *(Sailor.)* nautical nautilus aeronautics Argonaut astronaut [Ap. ix-13.]

neuro *(Nerve.)* neuralgia neuritis neurology neuron neurosis neurotic [Ap. ix-13.]

-nomy *(Science of.)* agronomy astronomy autonomy economy [Ap. ix-13.]

O

odont *(Tooth.)* endodontics endodontist odontology orthodontics orthodontist periodontics periodontist prosthodontics [Ap. ix-13.]

-oma *(Cancer.)* carcinoma encephaloma glaucoma hematoma leukoma melanoma myoma neuroma osteoma sarcoma trachoma [Ap. ix-13.]

-onym *(Name.)* acronym antonym homonym pseudonym synonym [Ap. ix-13.]

ophthalmo *(Eye.)* ophthalmitis ophthalmologist ophthalmology [Ap. ix-13.]

optic *(Of the eye.)* optic optical optician optics optometrist optometry [Ap. ix-13.]

organo- *(A tool; body organ.)* organ organic organism organist organize organization organography organology organon organum [Ap. ix-13.]

ortho- *(Straight.)* orthodontics orthodontist orthodox orthodoxy orthography orthopedics orthopedist [Ap. ix-13.]

P

paleo- *(Ancient.)* paleontology paleolith Paleolithic Paleozoic [Ap. ix-14.]

pan *(All.)* panacea Pan-American pancreas pandemic pandemonium panoply panorama pantheism pantheon pantomime [Ap. ix-14.]

path- *(Feeling, suffering.)* pathetic pathological pathologist pathos psychopath antipathy sympathetic sympathy telepathy [Ap. ix-14.]

ped- *(Child; education.)* pediatrician pediatrics pedagogue pedagogy pedant pedantry pederast pedophilia encyclopedia [Ap. ix-14.]

petro *(Rock.)* Peter petrified petroglyph petroleum petrology [Ap. ix-14.]

pharmaco *(Medicine.)* pharmacy pharmacist pharmacology [Ap. ix-14.]

phil- *(Loving.)* philosophy philosopher philosophical philanthropy philharmonic Philadelphia philodendron bibliophile [Ap. ix-14.]

phobia *(Exaggerated fear.)* phobia acrophobia agoraphobia claustrophobia arachnophobia gamophobia hemophobia triskaidekaphobia [Ap. ix-14.]

phone *(Sound.)* phone phonics polyphony megaphone microphone saxophone sousaphone symphony telephone xylophone [Ap. ix-14.]

photo *(Light.)* photo photocopy photogenic photograph photographer photography photon photostat photosynthesis phot [Ap. ix-15.]

physi- *(Nature.)* physical physician physicist physics physique [Ap. ix-15.]

pneum- *(Breath, lung.)* pneumatic pneumonia pneumology [< **pneuma** Ap. ix-15.]

pod *(Foot.)* podium tripod podiatry podiatrist bipod megapod [Ap. ix-15.]

polis *(City.)* acropolis metropolis Annapolis Indianapolis Minneapolis police policy political politician politics polity [Ap. ix-15.]

poly *(Many.)* polyandry polyester polygamous polygamy polyglot polygon polygraph polyhedron polynomial polyp polyphonic polyphony polysyllabic polytechnic polyunsaturated [Ap. ix-15.]

proto *(First in rank.)* protocol proton protoplasm protozoan [Ap. ix-15.]

psych *(Mind.)* psyche psychedelic psychiatrist psychiatry psychic psychoanalysis psychoanalyst psychoanalyze psychological psychologist psychologize psychology psychometry psychopath psychosis psychosomatic psychotherapy psychotic [Ap. ix-15.]

S

saur *(Lizard.)* dinosaur Brontosaurus Megalosaurus Tyrannosaurus [Ap. ix-16.]

scope *(See.)* microscope microscopic telescope telescopic periscope gyroscope horoscope fluoroscope oscilloscope stroboscope fluoroscope radioscopy fluoroscope kaleidoscope [Ap. ix-16.]

soph *(Wise.)* sophomore sophomoric sophist sophisticated sophistication sophisticate sophistry philosophy [< **sophos** Ap. ix-16.]

sphere *(Globe.)* sphere spherical spheroid atmosphere biosphere hemisphere ionosphere stratosphere bathysphere [Ap. ix-17.]

T

tech *(Skill.)* technique technical technicality technician Technicolor technology technological technocrat technocracy [< **techno-** Ap. ix-17.]

tele *(Distance.)* telephone television telescope telegram telegraph telegraphy telecast telepathy telecom telecommunications telekinesis teleprinter Teleprompter (TN) teletype televise [Ap. ix-17.]

theo *(A god.)* theology theological theologian theocracy theocentric atheism monotheism pantheism polytheism theomachy [Ap. ix-17.]

therapy *(Treatment.)* therapy chemotherapy heliotherapy hypnotherapy phototherapy physiotherapy psychotherapy therapeutic [Ap. ix-17.]

therm *(Heat.)* therm thermal thermometer thermostat thermos geothermal hyperthermia hypothermia isothermal [< **thermo-** Ap. ix-17.]

thesis *(A proposition.)* thesis (Pl. theses) antithesis hypothesis (hypotheses) parenthesis (parentheses) synthesis (syntheses) photosynthesis prosthesis (prostheses) metathesis (metatheses) [Ap. ix-17.]

toxic *(Poison.)* toxic antitoxin toxicity toxicology toxicologist toxin toxemia toxicide toxicosis toxicophobia [< **toxico-** Ap. ix-17.]

type *(Type.)* type typewriter typical typify typist typo typography archetype atypical linotype prototype stereotype teletype [Ap. ix-17.]

Z

zoa *(Animal.)* zoo zoology zoological zooid zoolatry Proterozoic Paleozoic Mesozoic Cenozoic protozoa protozoan [< **-zoa, zoo-** Ap. ix-18.]

African . . Algonquin . . American Indian . . Arabic . . . . Ap. x-2

Aramaic . . Arawakan . . Assyrian . . Athapascan . . . . . Ap. x-3

Bosnian . . . Cambodian . . . Carib . . . Celtic . . . . . . Ap. x-3

Chinese . . . Chinookan . . . Creole . . . Czech . . . . . . Ap. x-4

Dakota . . Egyptian . . Eskimo-Aleut . . Finnish . . . . . . Ap. x-4

Gullah . . . Haitian . . . Hawaiian . . . Hebrew . . . . . . Ap. x-4

Hindi . . . Hungarian . . . Icelandic . . . Irish . . . . . . Ap. x-5

Iroquoian . . . . Japanese . . . . Malay . . . . Ap. x-6

Malayalam . . . . Maori . . . . Marathi . . . . Ap. x-6

Moorish . . . . Muskogean . . . . Nepali . . . . Ap. x-6

Persian . . . Polish . . . Polynesian . . . Quechua . . . . . Ap. x-6

Russian . . . . Sanskrit . . . . Singhalese . . . . Ap. x-7

Siouan . . . . Tagalog . . . . Taino . . . . Tamil . . . . . Ap. x-7

Tibetan . . . . Tonga . . . . Tupi . . . . Ap. x-8

Turkish . . Uto-Aztecan . . Vietnamese . . Welsh . . . . . Ap. x-8

African banana banjo chimpanzee cola dengue (Swahili: *A tropical disease.*) gnu (Xhosa: *Antelope.*) goober (Bantu: *Goober peas; peanuts.*) gumbo (Bantu: *Gumbo soup with okra.*) impala *(Antelope.)* juba *(A dance.)* juju *(Fetish or talisman.)* jumbo *(Very large; the name of one of P.T. Barnum's elephants.)* Kwanzaa (Swahili: *First Fruit.*) kwashiorkor *(A nutritional disease.)* marimba (Bantu) Mau Mau (Kikuyu) Mt. Kilimanjaro mumbo jumbo okra potto samba tote (As in *tote bag.*) tsetse (Bantu: *Tsetse fly.*) voodoo (Ewe) yam (Senegal) zebra (Bantu) zombie

Algonquian [See **American Indian**.] caribou caucus *(Advisor.)* chipmunk Connecticut *(Mohican: Quinnehtukquet; Beside the long tidal river.)* Eskimo(Abnaki: Eskimantsic; *Raw-meat eaters.*) hickory hominy Illinois (From Iliniwek: *Tribe of superior men.*) Iroquois kinnikinic Kiwanis *(To make oneself known.)* mackinaw Manitou *(He is god.)* Manitoba (Cree: manito, *Great spirit +* wapow, *narrows.*) Massachusetts *(At the big hill.)* Menominee *(Wild rice.)* Michigan *(Great water.)* Mississippi (Misi sipi; *Big river.*) moccasin Mohegan *(Wolf.)* moose mugwump *(Great man.)* muskellunge (Abbr. muskie.) musquash (Alter. muskrat.) Ojibwa *(Roast until puckered; ref. to moccasin seams.)* opossum *(White animal.)* papoose *(Child.)* pecan persimmon Pocahontas pone *(Pone bread.)* possum *(An opossum.)* powwow *(He dreams.)* punk *(Decayed wood.)* Quebec (Kebek: *Strait, narrows.*) raccoon Saskatchewan (Cree: *Swiftly flowing.*) Shawnee *(Southerners.)* skunk squash *(Eaten raw.)* squaw *(Woman.)* succotash *(Ear of corn.)* tamarack toboggan tomahawk totem pole wampum *(White string of beads.)* wigwam *(Their dwelling.)* Wisconsin (Chippewa, Wees-konsan: *Gathering of the waters.*) woodchuck

American Indian [Some language **families** and some of their **members** are listed here.] Many have become familiar as street, city, river, *etc.* names.] **Algonquian:** Algonquin, Arapaho, Blackfoot, Cheyenne, Cree, Chippewa (Ojibwa), Delaware, Fox, Illinois, Kickapoo, Manhattan Massachusett, Menominee, Miami, Micmac, Mohegan, Mohican, Narragansett, Ottawa, Potawatomi, Sauk, Shawnee; **Athapascan:** Apache, Navajo **Chinookan:** Chinook; **Eskimo-Aleut:** Aleutian, Greenlandic, Innuit (Eskimo); **Hokan:** Mohave, Shasta, Yuma; **Iroquoian:** Cherokee, Erie, Huron, Mohawk, Oneida, Seneca, Susquehanna, Tuscarora; **Muskhogean:** Alabama, Chickasaw, Choctaw, Creek, Natchez, Seminole; **Siouan:** Biloxi, Catawaba, Crow, Dakota (Sioux), Iowa, Mandan, Missouri, Omaha, Winnebago; **Uto-Aztecan:** Aztec (Nahuati), Comanche, Hopi, Pima, Shoshoni, Ute; Yaqui; **Zuñian:** only Zuñi. Note: **Pueblo** is a social structure term and may apply to groups as diverse as the Anasazi, Hohokam, Keres, Tano, and Zuñi who do not necessarily speak the same language.

Arabic admiral al- *(The.)* alcazar *(The castle.)* alchemy *(The transmutation.)* alcohol *(The fine powder.)* alcove *(The vaulted chamber.)* algebra *(The reunion of broken parts; bonesetting.)* alfalfa *(The best kind of fodder.)* alfaqui *(The Muslim teacher.)* Algol *(The demon; a star in Perseus.)* algorism (Surname of early Arab mathematician; *The Arabic computation system.*) Alhambra *(The red house; Moorish palace at Granada.)* alkali *(The ashes of saltwort, an acid neutralizer.)* Alkoran *(The Koran.)* Allah *(The one supreme being.)* Almagest *("The Greatest Work" by Ptolemy.)* almanac Alpheratz *("The mare," a star in Andromeda.)* Alsirat *(The road; the correct way of religion.)* amber amir *(Ruler.)*

ariel *(Gazelle.)* arsenal artichoke assassin *("Hashish eaters," a killer.)* assassinate attar *(Flower petal extract.)* azimuth *("The ways.")* azoth *(Mercury.)* azure banyan *(Fig tree.)* Betelgeuse *("Shoulder of the giant," giant red star.)* borax Bwana *(Sir, master.)* caliber caliph caliphate camise *(Loose shirt.)* camphor candy carat caraway carob Casbah check *(Per.)* cipher coffee cork cotton dinar *(Gold coin.)* Druse elixir emir emirate fakir Fomalhaut *("The whale's mouth," one of 20 brightest stars.)* garble gazelle ghoul Gibraltar *(Rock of Tarick.)* hadj hadji hafiz harem hashish *(Hasheesh, "hash.")* hazard Hegira *(Hejira.)* henna ihram imam Imam imaret Islam jar *(A container.)* jihad *(Religious war.)* jinni *(Genie.)* Kaaba *("Cube," Muslim shrine at Mecca.)* kabob kismet Koran lemon lilac lime *(A fruit.)* lute *("The piece of wood," stringed instrument.)* macramé magazine mascara masjid *(A mosque.)* mattress Mecca Medina minaret mohair monsoon mosque muezzin mufti mullah mummy Muslim *(Moslem; one who submits.)* nacre nadir Ramadan ream *(A bundle.)* The Rubáiyát *(A poem by Omar Khayyám.)* safari saffron Sahib salaam *(A salutation.)* sash sayid sequin sheik sherbet *(A drink.)* Shiah Shiism Shiite sofa spinach Sufi Sufism sugar sultan sultana sultanate sumac Sunna Sunni Sunnite sura *(A chapter of the Koran.)* Swahili syrup tabby *(Striped cat; striped fabric.)* talisman tambour *(A drum.)* tarboosh *(A red felt cap.)* tariff tripe ulema vizier xebec yashmak *(Double veil.)* zenith Zinj *(Eastern Africa; as in Zinjanthropus.)*

Aramaic [One of the ancient **Semitic** languages. Aramaic is reputed to be the language spoken by Jesus.] Abba *(Father.)* abbot abbey abbess Gethsemane *("Oil press," Garden near Jerusalem.)* Golgotha *("Skull," Calvary.)* Kaddish *("Holy;" a prayer.)* Maccabees *("Hammer"; A family of Jewish patriots.)* mammon *(Riches.)* "Mene, mene, tekel, upharsin." *("Numbered, numbered, weighed, divided.")* Pharisee rabboni *(My great master.)*

Arawakan [A family on Indian languages spoken in Bolivia.] mahogany

Assyrian [One of the ancient **Semitic** (which see) languages.] ziggurat *("Mountain top," a terraced, pyramidal temple, e.g., The Hanging Gardens of Babylon.)*

Athapascan [See **American Indian**.] hogan *(Navajo dwelling.)* Apache Hupa Navajo *(Navaho)* Sarsi

Bosnian Sarajevo /sä-rä-ye-vô/

Cambodian
Angkor *(12th Century empire.)* Khmer Rouge Lon Nol Norodom Sihanouk Phnom Penh Pol Pot

Carib [South American and Caribbean Indians.] Carib *("Brave;" cannibal in Sp.)* Caribbean *(Caribbean Sea.)* cavy *(A rodent.)* cayman *(Crocodile.)* chigger *(Itchy mite larva.)* hurricane iguana manatee papaya papaw savanna tobacco yaws *(A skin disease.)*

Celtic abroach avon *(River.)* Avon bard beak bin brat broach brooch coomb *(Combe, narrow valley.)* crag cranny dover *(Water.)* Dover druid galliard gallon garter German glean glen gob goblet gravel lance lawn menhir *(Prehistoric monument.)* mine *(Excavation.)* miner mutt mutton tor *(A craggy hill.)* truant vassal

Chinese Beijing bohea *(A black tea.)* chop suey chow *(District.)* Chiang Kai-shek chow mein congou *(A black tea.)* fan-tan *(A game.)* Fo *(Buddha.)* Foism ginseng gung ho hong *(Warehouse.)* kowtow tea kumquat Kuomintang mahjong Mao Tse-Tung (Mao Zedong) Ming *(A dynasty.)* oolong *(A dark tea.)* pekoe *(A fine tea.)* pidgin *(A mixed language; Chinese word for business.)* sampan *(Flat-bottomed boat.)* samshu *(A rice liquor.)* Taiping *(Great peace.)* Tao /dow/ *(The Way, road.)* Taoism Tiananmen Square tycoon yamen *(An office.)* yen *("Opium;" desire.)* yuan *(Money.)* yin/yang *(Listing of opposites.)* Zhou (Chou) Enlai

Chinookan [See **American Indians**.] high-muck-a-muck skookum *(Excellent.)*

Creole (French and English) jazz *(Jass = coition. Jazz originated in the brothels of New Orleans.)*

Czech pistol polka robot *(Forced labor.)*

Dakota tepee

Egyptian ankh *(Life.)* ba *(Soul.)* ibis *(Wading bird.)* ka *(The spiritual self.)* Pharaoh *("The great house;" monarch in ancient Egypt.)* Ra *(The supreme deity.)*

Eskimo-Aleut: [See **American Indian**] anorak *(Hooded jacket.)* Alaska (Aleut: *Mainland* or Eskimo: *Great land.*) Iditarod *(Alaskan sled dog race.* After Iditarod River, meaning either *Clear River* or *Distant Place.)* igloo kayak mukluk parka tupik umiak Yukon *(Clear water.)*

Finnish Kalevala *(Collection of ancient poems and myths: the national epic of Finland.)* sauna

Gullah [Gullah or Geechee speech; still spoken along the Atlantic coast of Georgia and South Carolina. It is creolized African and English.] banjo buckra *(A white man.)* cooter *(A turtle.)* goober *(A peanut.)* gumbo juba *(A dance.)* juke joint (Jook, *disorderly;* juke house, *brothel.*) okra pinder *(A peanut.)* tote voodoo Note: Many of these terms also appear under African. See also: Ap. xiv: Black English Vernacular.

Haitian cacique /kə-sēk/ *(A chief.)* mambo *(A dance.)*

Hawaiian aalii *(A tree.)* aloha *("Love"; hello; good-by.)* hula lanai /lä-nä-ē/ *(A veranda.)* lehua /lā-hoo-ä/ *(A myrtle tree.)* lei /lā/ luau /loo-ow/- muumuu /moo-moo/ poi ukulele

Hebrew Abraham *(Exalted father of multitudes.)* Adonai *(Lord.)* Adam *(Man of red earth.)* alpha *("Ox"; first letter of Greek alphabet: α.)* Amen *(Verily; so it is.)* Armageddon *(World's end battle of good and evil.)* Baal *(Phoenician god; idol, false god.)* bar mitzvah *(Son of the commandment; a boy's coming-of-age ceremony.)* Beelzebub *(Lord of flies; prince of demons, the devil.)* behemoth *(A colossal beast.)* beta *("House;" second letter of the Greek alphabet: β.)* bethel *(House of God.)* Bethlehem *(Place of food.)* B'nai B'rith *(Sons of the Covenant; a fraternal organization.)* cabal *(An intrigue.)* cabala *(An occult religious system.)* cabalistic Chassidim *(Jewish sect.)* cherub chutzpah (Hutzpah; *effrontery.*) cider cinnamon Dagon *("Fish;" a god of the Philistines.)* David *(Beloved.)* Eden *(Delight.)* Elohim *(God.)* Essene *(Pious ones.)* Eve *(Life.)* Gehenna *(Valley of Hinnom; refuse dump.)* Haggadah *("To tell;" the nonlegal elements of the Talmud.)* Halakah *("To walk;" the legal elements in the Talmud.)* hallah (Challah, *braided bread.*) hallelujah *("Praise Jehovah!")* halutz (Chalutz, *"Vanguard," pioneer Jewish farmer.*) Hanukkah (Chanukah)

Hasidim (Chassidim, *a mystic sect.*) Hebrew *("From beyond the Jordan.")* hora *(A round dance.)* hosanna *(Praised be the Lord!)* Isaiah *(Salvation of God.)* jasper Jehovah *(JHVH; Yahweh.)* Jerusalem *(City of peace.)* Jew *(Of Judah.)* Jonah *(Dove.)* Jordan River *(Flowing downward.)* jubilee *(Ram's horn which announced the jubilee year.)* kibbutz (Pl. kibbutzim. *Collective farm.)* Knesset *("Gathering," Constituent Assembly of Israel.)* kosher *(Ritually clean.)* manna *("What is it?" Food from heaven.)* Mary Masora *(O.T. reading aids.)* matzo *(Unleavened bread.)* Menorah *(Seven branched ceremonial candelabrum.)* Messiah *("Anointed.")* Midrash *(O.T. commentaries.)* Mishnah *("Oral law," first part of Talmud.)* mitzvah *(Commandment.)* mogen David *(Shield of David.)* Moses *(Son.)* Nazarene Nazareth Noah *(Comfort.)* Pasch *(Feast of the Passover.)* rabbi *("My master," community spiritual head.)* Rosh Hashana *("Head of the year," Jewish New Year.)* Sabbath *("To rest;" seventh day of the week.)* Sanhedrin *(Ancient council.)* Satan *("To plot against;" the Devil.)* Semite *("Descendant of Shem," Jews and Arabs.)* Semitic seraph (Pl. seraphim; *Highest order of angels.)* Shalom *("Peace.," a greeting and a farewell.)* shekel *("To weigh;" money unit.)* sheol *(Hell.)* shibboleth *("Ear of grain;" test word: enemy could not pronounce /sh/.* O.T. Judges xii-4-6.) shiva *(Period of mourning.)* Shoah *(Holocaust.)* shofar *(Ritual ram's horn.)* siddur *(Prayer book)* Simchath Torah *(Jewish holiday; "The rejoicing over the law.")* Talmud *("Instruction.")* teraphim *(Small idols.)* Torah *(Instruction; law.)* Yahweh *(YHWH; God.)* yeshiva *(A seminary.)* yom *(Day.)* Yom Kippur *(Day of Atonement.)* Zion *(Hill.)*

Hindi [Sanskrit based language of northern India; used by Hindus.] Amritsar ayah *(A nurse.)* bandanna bangle Bombay bungalow cheetah chintz chit *(A voucher.)* chop *(Official stamp.)* chutney *(Fruit dish.)* cot dinghy *(Dingey, small boat.)* doolee *(A litter.)* dungaree *(Coarse cotton cloth.)* dungarees Gandhi gharry *(A carriage.)* Garibi Hatao! *(Remove poverty!)* gunny *(A coarse hemp material)* gunny sack guru hartal *(Closing business as passive resistance.)* howdah *(A seat to ride an animal.)* keddah *(Elephant enclosure.)* lacquer lungi *(A loincloth.)* maharaja *(A prince's title.)* maharani *(Wife of a maharaja.)* mahatma myna bird Nehru New Dehli pachisi *(Parcheesi.)* Punjab raj *(Sovereignty.)* rajah *(Hindu prince.)* Rama Ramachandra *(Hindu hero.)* rani *(Wife of a raja.)* rupee *(Money unit.)* sari *(A garment of Hindu women.)* shampoo Sikh *(Disciple.)* sirdar *(Chief, lord.)* sitar *(Stringed instrument.)* tam-tam thug tom-tom topi *(A sun helmet.)* Urdu *(A variety of Hindustani.)* veranda yoga yogi; See: **Sanskrit** Ap. x-7.

Hungarian (Magyar) coach czardas goulash hussar paprika shako

Icelandic geyser

Irish [A Celtic language.] banshee biddy bog bother brogan *(Heavy shoe.)* brogue *(Accent; shoe.)* ceilidh /kā-lē/ *(An enlightening dialogue.)* colleen *(A girl.)* crannog *(Lake dwelling.)* curse Drogheda /draw-ə-də/ *(Town destroyed by Cromwell in 1649.)* esker *(A ridge.)* galore gossoon *(A lad.)* leprechaun machree *(My heart; my love.)* mavourneen *(My darling.)* O' *(Son of, e.g., O'Neill, O'Ryan, O'Riley, O'Shaughnessy, O'Shea.)* puss *(A face.)* shamrock shebang shenanigan shillelagh Sinn Fein *("We ourselves.")* slob smithereens spleuchan *(A tobacco pouch.)* spunk tory trousers ulster *(A long, loose overcoat.)* whiskey Yeats

Iroquoian [See **American Indian**.] Hiawatha *(Mohawk chief who organized the Five Nations: Mohawks, Cayugas, Oneidas, Onondagas, & Senecas. He was the hero of Longfellow's poem, The Song of Hiawatha.)* Kentucky *(Great meadows.)* Mohawk haircut Ohio *(O-he-yo: Great river.)* Ontario *(Beautiful lake.)* sequoia *(Tree; National Park; from Sequoyah, Cherokee Indian who invented Cherokee alphabet.)* Tennessee *(Tenassee: ancient capital of the Cherokees.)*

Japanese banzai *(Battle cry.)* Bon *(Feast of Lanterns.)* bonze *(Buddhist monk.)* bushido *(Way of the warrior.)* daimio Mt. Fuji geisha ginkgo go *(A game.)* haiku hari-kari *("Belly cut.")* hibachi Hirohito Hiroshima Issei Isuzu judo jujitsu kabuki *(A stylized play.)* kakemono kamikaze karate kimono koto mikado Mitsubishi moxa Nagasaki Nisei no *(Noh, Classical drama.)* Nissan obi /ō-bē/ *(A broad sash.)* origami rickshaw *(Jinriksha.)* sake /sä-kē/ *(Rice liquor.)* samurai sayonara Shinto shogun shoji soy *(Bean; sauce.)* Subaru sukiyaki sumo *(Wrestling)* sushi Suzuki *(Piano & string method.)* Tojo Tokyo Toyota yen *(Money.)* Zen

Malay [Official language of Indonesia.] amuck (to run *amuck*) bamboo cockatoo compound *(An enclosure.)* gingham gong junk *(A boat.)* mango orangutan sarong

Malayalam [A local language of India.] atoll copra *(Coconut kernel.)* teak

Maori [Native language of New Zealand.] kakapo kiwi moa *(Extinct flightless bird.)*

Marathi [A local language of India.] mongoose

Moorish Gibraltar *(Rock of Tarick.)*

Muskogean [See **American Indian**.] Alabama (Choctaw: *alba amo: Thicket clearers.*) bayou /bī-ōō/ (Choctaw) Oklahoma (Choctaw: *Red people.*) tupelo *(Tree type.)*

Nepali [The language of Nepal.] panda

Persian arsenic Ahriman *(Spirit of evil.)* Ahura Mazda (Ormuzd, *Principle of good.*) Avesta *(Sacred writings of Zoroastrianism.)* Babism *(Religious system.)* bazaar caravan check checkmate chess cinnabar cummerbund dervish divan Gheber *(A fire worshiper.)* jackal julep (As in *mint julep.*) khaki *("Dust;" cotton cloth.)* lemon Magi *("Priests;" The Three Wise Men.)* Ormuzd *(The supreme deity.)* padishah *(Title of the shah of Iran.)* pajamas paradise Parsee percale peri *(Elf.)* naphtha pilaf *(A rice dish.)* Rook *(Chess piece.)* sepoy shah shawl saraband satrap seersucker *("Milk and honey;" a cotton fabric.)* tabor *(Small drum.)* tulip turban van (From caravan.) Zend *(Commentaries on the Avesta.)* Zoroaster (Zarathustra, *religious reformer.*)

Polish britzska *(A carriage.)* mazurka Sejm Zloty *(Money.)*

Polynesian mana *(Supernatural power.)* tattoo Tiki *(Creator of the first man.)*

Quechua [An Incan language of Peru. All words listed here have come into English through Spanish.] calisaya *(Bark containing quinine.)* charqui (Jerky, *dried meat strips.*) chinchilla coca condor guano Inca llama puma quinine vicuña *(A small wool-producing animal.)*

Russian babushka balalaika Bolshevik *("One in majority.")* borscht boyar Brezhnev Cheka *(One time secret police.)* Cominform Comintern commissar czar *(Tsar, tzar.)* czarevitch czarina da *(Yes.)* demokratizatsyia *(Multiple candidates.)* duma glasnost *(Openness.)* Gorbachev Gosplan gulag intelligentsia Komsomol *(Young Communist League.)* kopeck Kosygin Kremlin *("Citadel.")* Khrushchev kulak kvass *(Fermented drink.)* Lenin mammoth Menshevik *("One in minority.")* mir *(Peace; commune.)* Molotov NKVD *(People's Commissariat for Internal Affairs.)* nomenklatura *(The privileged class.)* nyet *(No.)* oblast perestroika *(Restructuring economy.)* pogrom Politburo Pravda *("Truth;" Russian news agency.)* Rasputin ruble sable Sakharov samovar Solzhenitsyn soviet Sputnik Stalin steppe sterlet *(Small sturgeon.)* Tass *(Russian news agency.)* tovarisch *(Comrade!)* troika tundra ukase *(An official decree.)* vodka volost *(A district.)* Yeltzin zemstvo *(Elective district.)*

Sanskrit [The ancient and classical language of Hindi speakers.] ahimsa *("Noninjury." The doctrine that life in any form is sacred.)* Aryan *("Noble." Prehistoric people or their descendants who spoke Indo-European; a term misused by the Nazis.)* atman *(In Hinduism: the soul.)* avatar *("Descent"; the incarnation of a god.)* Bhagavad-Gita *("Song of the Blessed One: Krishna"; Hindu text on caste duties and yoga doctrines.)* bodhisattva *("Knowledge + essence;" a future Buddha.)* Brahma *(Absolute essence, universal soul; supreme creator.)* Brahman *(First of four Hindu castes.)* Brahmin *(A highly cultured person.)* Buddha *("The Enlightened;" Gautama Siddhartha, the founder of Buddhism.)* Devi *("Shining one." In Hinduism: great mother goddess.)* dharma *(Right behavior.)* ginger Hindi Hindu India Indus juggernaut jute karma Krishna *(A Hindu god.)* loot maharaja mahatma mahout *(Elephant driver.)* mantra *(An incantation.)* nirvana opal punch *(A drink.)* pundit puttee Rajput *(A Hindu caste.)* saccharin Sanskrit Siva *(Or Shiva: Hindu god of destruction and reproduction.)* sutra *(A maxim.)* swami swastika *("Well-being;" ancient religious symbol; appropriated by the Nazis.)* til *(Sesame.)* toddy Trimurti *(The triad of Brahma, Vishnu, and Siva.)* Upanishad *(Treatise on the nature of the universe.)* Veda Vishnu *(A member of the Hindu trinity.)* wanderoo *(A monkey.)* yoga *("Union.")* yogi *(One who practices yoga.)*

Singhalese [A language of Sri Lanka; an Indic language.] anaconda beriberi *(Beri = weakness.)* bo tree *("Tree of perfect knowledge;" once shaded Buddha.)* dagoba *(Buddhist shrine.)*

Siouan [See **American Indian**.] Arkansas *("Downstream people.")* Iowa *("Beautiful land.")* Kansas *(After the Kansa people.)* · Minnesota *("Cloudy water.")* Missouri *("The people of the long canoes.")* Nebraska *(Nebrathka: "Flat water.")* Omaha *("Those going upstream.")* tepee *(From Dakota tipi; ti = to dwell, pi = used for.)*

Tagalog [The official language of the Philippines; in the Indonesian group.] boondocks

Taino [Language of an extinct Indian tribe probably first encountered by Columbus in the West Indies. The words listed here were borrowed by the Spanish and finally Anglicized.] barbecue canoe maize potato yucca *(A large plant found in SW United States; state flower of New Mexico.)*

Tamil [A language of southern India and Sri Lanka (formerly Ceylon).] catamaran coolie curry *(A sauce.)* pagoda pariah *(Member of low caste; a social outcast.)*

Tibetan lama polo *("Ball.")* yak yeti *(The abominable snowman.)* Sherpa *(A member of a Tibetan tribe famous as mountain guides.)*

Tonga [a Polynesian language] taboo

Tupi [Language spoken by a group of South American Indian tribes in what is now Brazil. Many of the following words have come into English by way of Portuguese.] ani *(Cuckoo.)* buccaneer (F) cashew Guarani *("Warrior;" southern branch of the Tupis.)* jaguar macaw maraca petunia (F) piranha tanager tapioca tapir toucan Tupi *("Comrade.")*

Turkish aga *(Leader; lord.)* Balkans *(Mountains.)* bey *(Lord.)* bosh *(Nonsense.)* dey *(Governor's title.)* effendi *(Sir.)* horde Khan kiosk kurbash *(A whip.)* odalisque *(A concubine.)* pasha *(Bashaw, honorary title.)* shish kebab scimitar softa *(A mosque student.)* turquoise yogurt yurt *(A tent.)*

Uto-Aztecan [See **American Indian**. Unless marked otherwise, entries here are from Nahuatl /nä-wät-l/, the language spoken by the Aztecs, and have come into English via Spanish.] Arizona *(Papago: "Little spring.")* cacao *(A tree whose seeds are used to make cocoa.)* chicle *(Juice from sapodilla tree used to make chewing gum.)* chili chocolate cocoa (Alter. of cacao.) coyote Idaho *(Shoshoni, Ee-dah-how: "The sun is coming down from the mountain tops."* kachina *(Hopi: Spirit ancestor.)* kiva *(Hopi: Room for religious ceremonies.)* ocelot (F) peyote tamales teocalli *(A temple.)* tomato Utah (After Ute: *"The hill dwellers."*)

Vietnamese
Annam *(French Central Vietnam.)* Bao Dai *(Last emperor.)* Cochinchina *(French Southern Vietnam.)* Danang Dienbienphu Haiphong Hanoi Ho Chi Minh *(North Vietnamese leader, "Father of his country.")* Hmong *(A people of Laos who disrupted the Ho Chi Minh Trail.)* Hué *(Ancient imperial capital.)* Mekong delta Mylai Saigon Tet *(Lunar New Year.)* Tonkin *(French Northern Vietnam.)* Tonkin Gulf Trung sisters Vietcong Vietnam

Welsh [The language of Celtic origin spoken in Wales. A few entries, as elsewhere, are only probable.] bald eisteddfod *(An assembly of poets and musicians.)* flannel pendragon *(A ruler, chief.)* penguin Taliesin /tal-ē-es-n/ *("Shining Brow;" Frank Lloyd Wright's residence.)* Wales

| Appendix xi | Odds and Ends | **CONTENTS** |

Abbreviations . . . . Ap. xi- 2

Acronyms . . . . Ap. xi- 2

Akin To . . . . Ap. xi- 3

Alterations . . . . Ap. xi- 3

Apheresis . . . . Ap. xi- 4

Aphesis . . . . Ap. xi- 4

Back Formations . . . . Ap. xi- 4

Coined Words . . . . Ap. xi- 4

Contractions . . . . Ap. xi- 5

Doublets . . . . Ap. xi- 5

Homophones . . . . Ap. xi- 6

Imitations . . . . Ap. xi- 8

Initials . . . . Ap. xi- 8

Interjections . . . . Ap. xi-10

Reduplications . . . . Ap. xi-10

Short For . . . . Ap. xi-11

Trade Names . . . . Ap. xi-12

Variants . . . . Ap. xi-12

Word Blends . . . . Ap. xi-13

Abbreviations

ab ex. (From without.) [L. *ab extra.*]

e.g. (For example.) [L. *exempli gratia.*]

et al. (And others.) [L. *et alii.*]

fl. (He flourished.) [L. *floruit.*]

id. (The same.) [L. *idem.*]

i.q. (The same as.) [L. *idem quod.*]

loc. cit. (In the place cited.) [L. *loco citato.*]

Mrs. (Mistress.) [O.F. *maistresse.*]

non seq. (It does not follow.) [L. *non sequitur.*]

op. cit. (In the place cited.) [L. *opere citato.*]

Q. E. D. (Which was to be demonstrated.) [L. *Quod erat demonstrandum.*]

Sr. (Senior.) [L. *senior.*]

cf. (Compare.) [L. *confer.*]

et al. (And elsewhere.) [L. *et alibi.*]

etc. (And other things.) [L. *et cetera.*]

ibid. (In the same place.) [L. *ibidem.*]

i.e. (That is.) [L. *id est.*]

Jr. (Junior.) [L. *junior.*]

Mr. (Mister.) [L. *magister.*]

Ms. (Miss or Mistress.) [O.E. *miss.*]

viz. (Namely.) [L. *videlicit.*]

Acronyms [An *acronym* is a pronounceable word formed from the first letter or letters of words meaningfully grouped. This "new" word is a convenient way to indicate the meaning of the whole word group.]

AID *(Agency for International Development.)* AIDS *(Acquired Immune Deficiency Syndrome.)*

Amvets *(American Veterans of W. W. ii & Korea.)* Awol *(Absent Without Leave.)*

CARE*(Cooperative for American Relief Everywhere.)*Conelrad*(Control of Electromagnetic Radiation.)*

CORE *(Congress of Racial Equality.)* DEW *(Distant Early Warning.)*

Eurail Pass *(European Railway Passenger.)* FEMA *(Federal Emergency Management Agency.)*

Gestapo *(Ger. Geheime Staats Polizei.)* HUAC *(House Un-American Activities Committee.)*

HUD *(Housing and Urban Development.)* Jaycees *(U.S. Junior Chamber of Commerce.)*

Jayvee *(Junior Varsity.)* Jeep *(General Purpose Vehicle.)*

Laser *(Light Amplification by Stimulated Emission of Radiation.)* Lem *(Lunar Excursion Module.)*

Loran *(Long Range Navigation.)* Nabisco *(National Biscuit Company.)*

NAFTA*(North American Free Trade Agreement.)*NASA*(National Aeronautics & Space Administration.)*

NATO *(North Atlantic Treaty Organization.)* Navar *(Navigation Radar.)*

Nazi *(Ger. Nationalsozialist.)* NOW *(National Organization for Women.)*

OPEC *(Organization of Petroleum Exporting Countries.)* OSHA *(Occupational Safety & Health Adm.)*

PAC *(Political Action Committee.)* Radar *(Radio Detection and Ranging.)*

ROTC /rot-sē/ *(Reserved Officers' Training Corps.)* Seabee *(Construction Battalion.)*

Scuba *(Self-Contained Underwater Breathing Apparatus.)* SALT *(Strategic Arms Limitation Talks.)*

SEATO *(Southeast Asia Treaty Organization.)* Shoran *(Short Range Navigation.)*

Snafu *(Situation Normal, All Fouled Up.)* Sonar *(Sound Navigation and Ranging.)*

SNCC /snik/ *(Student Nonviolent Coordinating Committee.)* SWAT *(Special Weapons Action Team.)*

UNESCO *(United Nations Educational, Scientific and Cultural Organizations.)*

UNICEF *(United Nations International Children's Education Fund.)* Veep *(Vice-President.)*

VISTA *(Volunteers In Service To America.)* WAC *(Women's Army Corps.)*

WAVES *(Women Accepted for Voluntary Emergency Service.)* WHO *(World Health Organization.)*

Zip Code *(Zone Improvement Plan.)*

Akin To Words [*Akin to words* derive from a common root.]

bake batch
band bind
beacon beckon
bite bait

blast blow
bloom blossom
break breach brick
breed brood

broom bramble
broth brew
bundle bind
burn brand

boulevard bulwark
brother pal
cam comb
clamber climb

cob cobble
corral kraal
crib cratch
crone carrion

cruel crude
daft deft
dale dell
dander dandruff

deal dole
dialogue dialect
dig dike ditch
dune down *(A sand hill.)*

flake flag *(Flagstone.)*
glad glade
glamour grammar
glimpse gleam

grope grip
guard ward
heath heathen
hinge hang

horn corn *(As on foot.)*
host guest
jam champ *(To chew.)*
kind kin

lace lash latch
lake leach leak
lather laved
lattice lath

law lay
lift loft
malt melt
marsh morass

mayhem maim
minx mensch
pick pike
pith pit *(A kernel.)*

powder pollen
price praise
remark mark
reward regard

road ride
robe rob
rubble rubbish
sale sell

scant skimp
scape scepter
scatter shatter
scoot shoot

scrap scrape
sit set *(To place.)*
skirmish scrimmage
skirt shirt

slaughter slay
slug slag
soak suck
sovereign soprano

spigot spike
sponge fungus
stark starch
streak strike

sugar saccharin
snout schnozzle
swamp sump
swan swain

talk tell tale
tax task
team teem
thrift thrive

together gather
trade tread
truce trust true
vast waste

verb word
wafer waffle
wain wagon
warble whirl

ware warn
watch wake
web weave weft
weal well *(Favorably.)*

whir whirl
whole hale *(Healthy.)*
wind wand
wrench wrinkle

Alterations [An *alteration* is a changing of a particular word to another form, sometimes keeping the same meaning, but often producing a new word with an entirely different meaning. The first word listed is the original, the second the alteration.]

Andy dandy
association soccer
baluster banister
Bethlehem Bedlam

bicycle bike
brother bub
candle cannel
cariole carryall

cartouche cartridge
charivari shivaree
charqui jerky
chassé sashay

chemise shimmy
chigoe chigger
christcross crisscross
crunch scrunch

damn darn
emptyings emptins
Eskimo Husky *(A dog.)*
eternal tarnal

fable fib
godfather gaffer
gallant gallivant
God golly

God gosh
godmother gammer
hocus hokum
housewife hussy

kraal crawl *(A fish pen.)*
lithesome lissome
marble mib
mistress missis

ordinary ornery
paver pavior
partner pardner
Richard hick

rosin resin
satin sateen
sauce sass
sawer sawyer

sumptuous scrumptious
triumph trump
vermin varmint
visor vizard

waggle wangle
weld well *(To flow forth.)*

Apheresis /ə-<u>fair</u>-ə-sis/ [*Apheresis* is the dropping of an unaccented <u>syllable</u> or sound from the beginning of a word. (Gk. *aphairein,* to take away.) adj. *apheretic*]

advantage vantage	adventure venture	beneath 'neath	croquet roque
defense fence	defend fend	display splay	disport sport
distain stain	encyclopedia cyclopedia	engine gin *(A machine.)*	university varsity

Aphesis /<u>af</u>-ə-sis/ [*Aphesis* is the loss of a short or unaccented <u>vowel</u> from the beginning of a word. (Gk. *aphienai,* a letting go.) adj. *aphetic.*]

abut butt	affray fray	amend mend	arrear rear
attaint taint	attend tend	attire tire	avant-garde vanguard
Egyptian Gypsy	estate state	esquire squire	establish stablish

Back Formations [A *Back Formation* is the creation of a new word from an existing word. The first word listed is the earliest form of the word. By analogy to other word pairs, it was assumed the second word must exist.]

automation automate	aviation aviate	botanical botany
burglar burgle	celebration celebrate	cognizance cognize
darkling darkle	demarcation demarcate	diagnosis diagnose
difficulty difficult	donation donate	editor edit
emotion emote	enthusiasm enthuse	escalator escalate
extradition extradite	fluorescence fluoresce	frivolous frivol
gambler gamble	gentrice gentry	gnarled gnarl
hazy haze	injury injure	isolated isolate
jelly jell	kibitzer kibitz	landscape scape
loafer loaf	logrolling logroll	luminescent luminesce
manipulation manipulate	mixed mix	nit-picking nit-pick
peddler peddle	peevish peeve	perplexed perplex
preemption preempt	recognizance recognize	reminiscence reminisce
resurrection resurrect	retroactive retroact	scavenger scavenge
sculpture sculpt	snivel sniff	statistics statistic
summation summate	swindler swindle	tampion tamp
tatting tat	tweezers tweeze	unity unit
upholsterer upholster	valuation valuate	vivisection vivisect
WAVES WAVE	wiretapping wiretap	

Coined Words [A *Coined Word* is usually the invention of one person or committee to name a new item or concept. Many trade names (which see) and new ideas in science are identified by coined and invented words even though some elements of the new word may be recognized as existing elsewhere; e.g., the Greeks did not have *telephones* or *telescopes* but they did use *tele, phone,* and *skopos* as language elements. Karl von Linné (L. Carolus Linnaeus), (1707-78), Swedish taxonomist, named many plant and animal organisms using Latin and Greek elements.]

bazooka beamish blatant chortle circumbendibus doodad doohickey Ebonics ecdysiast ester eugenics gobbledygook googol heebie-jeebies momism nambypamby palooka quark rayon schooner spoof sylph transmogrify whodunit witticism yahoo

Contractions

[A *contraction* is a conflation of at least two words with missing elements being marked by an apostrophe ('). Usually a contraction (L. "A drawing together.") is the combination of some of the most common and well used words in the language as the result of oral language "shortcut" and "hurryup" (To *coin* a word!).]

ain't (Dial. *am not, are not, is not, has not, have not*) aren't *(are not)*   can't *(cannot)*

couldn't *(could not)*   didn't *(did not)*   doesn't *(does not)*   don't *(do not)*

hadn't *(had not)*   hain't (dial. *have not; has not*)   hasn't *(has not)*

haven't *(have not)*   he'd *(he would; he had)*   he'll *(he will)*   here's *(here is)*

he's *(he is; he has)*   his'n (dial. *his*)   I'd *(I would; I had)*   I'm *(I am)*

it'd *(it would; it had)*   I'll *(I will; I shall)*   isn't *(is not)*   it'll *(it will; it shall)*

it's *(it is; it has)*   I've *(I have)*   let's *(let us)*   ma'am *(madam)*

mightn't *(might not)*   mustn't *(must not)*   needn't *(need not)*   ne'er *(never)*

o'clock *(of the clock)*   o'er *(over)*   one's *(one is)*   sha'nt *(shall not)*

she'd *(she would; she had)*   she'll *(she will)*   she's *(she is; she has)*

shouldn't *(should not)*   that'd *(that would; that had)*   that'll *(that will)*

that's *(that is)*   there'd *(there would; there had)*   there's *(there is)*

they'd *(they would; they had)*   there'd *(there would; there had)*

there'll *(there will)*   these'll *(these will)*   they'll *(they will)*   they're *(they are)*

they've *(they have)*   this'll *(this will)*   those'll *(those will)*   'tween *(between)*

'twas *(it was)*   'twere (Poetic, *it were*)   'twill *(it will)*   'twixt *(betwixt)*

wasn't *(was not)*   we'd *(we would; we had)*   we'll *(we will)*   we're *(we are)*

weren't *(were not)*   we've *(we have)*   what'd *(what would; what had)*

what'll *(what will)*   what's *(what is)*   where'er *(wherever)*

who'd *(who would; who had)*   who'll *(who will)*   who're *(who are)*

who's *(who is; who has)* won't *(will not, Middle English: woll not)*   wouldn't *(would not)*

you'd *(you would; you had)*   you'll *(you will)*   you're *(you are)*

you've *(you have)*

Doublets

[A *doublet* is a pair of words derived from the same source but entering English through different routes, e.g., *papyrus* directly from L. & Gk., but *paper* from L. & Gk. by way of O.F.]

amiable amicable   anthem antiphon   antic antique   aptitude attitude

arc arch   area are *(A land measure.)* armor armature   army armada

arista arris   avow avouch   balm balsam   blame blaspheme

bourdon burden *(Something often repeated.)*   burgess bourgeois   camera chamber

canal channel   canker chancre   captain chieftain   captive caitiff

card chart   cattle chattel   chair cathedra   cavalier chevalier

cavalry chivalry   challenge calumny   chance cadence cadenza

charge carry   chase catch   chorus choir   circus cirque

clock cloak   complaisant complacent   composite compost

constrain constringe   convey convoy   cord chord   corsair hussar

costume custom   count compute   court cohort   cream chrism

coy quiet   crate grate *(A framework.)* crimson carmine   crypt grotto

daffodil asphodel   dainty dignity   dame duenna   debt debit

diamond adamant · differ defer · dish dais desk disk · display deploy
domain demesne · dram drachma · employ imply · entire integer
envious invidious · escritoire scriptorium · essay assay · example sample
expand spawn · fabric forge · fact feat · fashion faction
feature facture · fidelity fealty · frail fragile · gender genus genre
gentle genteel gentile · guitar cithara zither · hanaper hamper (A covered basket.)
history story · hospital hotel hostel · hyacinth jacinth · inch ounce
influence influenza · jealous zealous · journal diurnal · lesson lection
liquor liqueur · lobster locust · locus lieu · lodge lobby loge loggia
loyal legal · Madonna madam · male masculine · mangle mangonel
mansion menage · mart market · mayor major · memory memoir
metal medal · minimum minim · module mold (A form.) monastery minster
money mint · muscle mussel · native naive · oration orison
pale pallid · palsy paralysis · papa pope · paper papyrus
parabola parable parole palaver · pass pace · peon pawn (Chess piece.) person parson
phantom phantasm · place plaza piazza · pigment pimento · plack plaque
plum prune · poison potion · poor pauper · porch portico
priest presbyter · private privy · property propriety · prove probe
provide purvey · purse burse · radish radix · rail rule
rank range · ransom redemption · ration ratio reason rapine raven (To ravage.)
ray radius · rebel revel · recognizance reconnaissance regal royal
regime regimen · release relax · round rotund · sacristan sexton
scandal slander · sect set (A group.) · secure sure · signet sennet
sinus sine · sleuth slot (Animal trail.) species spice · sprite spirit
status state · strange extraneous · strict strait · suffix soffit
suit suite · syrup sherbet · tache tack · ticket etiquette
title tittle · trait tract · tradition treason · treasure thesaurus
treble triple · tureen terrine · union onion · valet varlet
vocal vowel · vote vow · voyage viaticum · wage gage
wallop gallop · warden guardian · warranty guaranty · zero cipher

Homophones [Homophones are "sound alike" words with different spellings & meanings.]

add ad · ads adz · ail ale · air heir · all awl
allowed aloud · alter altar · ant aunt · ark arc · ascent assent
assistance assistants · ate eight · away aweigh · bail bale · bait bate
ball bawl · band banned · bard barred · bare bear · bark barque
base bass · bases basses basis · be bee · beach beech · bearing baring
beat beet · beau bow · been bin · beer bier · bell belle
berry bury · better bettor · birth berth · bite byte · blue blew
board bored · boarder border · bolder boulder · born borne · borough burro burrow
bough bow · bowl boll · boy buoy · bread bred · break brake
bridal bridle · brood brewed · bruise brews · build billed · bullion bouillon
but butt · by buy bye · callus callous · cane Cain · cannon canon

canvas canvass   capital capitol   carol Carol carrel   carrot carat caret   cash cache
cast caste   ceiling sealing   censor sensor   cents sense   cereal serial
chased chaste   cheap cheep   chic sheik   chilly chili   choose chews
choral coral   clause claws   climb clime   close clothes   coal cole
coarse course   colonel kernel   complement compliment   coop coupe   cord chord
core corps   corral chorale   council counsel   cousin cozen   creak creek
cruise crews   cue queue   current currant   cursor curser   die dye
dine dyne   discreet discrete   do due dew   done dun   dough doe do *(In music.)*
ducked duct   ducks ducts   duel dual   earn urn   emerge immerge
eyelet islet   facts fax   faint feint   fair fare   feet feat
feign fain   find fined   flair flare   flea flee   flew flu flue
flower flour   for four fore   forward foreword foul fowl   fourth forth
frank Frank franc   fryer friar   fur fir   Gail gale   gate gait
glare glair   gorilla guerrilla   great grate   groan grown   guest guessed
guilt gilt   guys guise   hail hale   hair hare   hall haul
hanger hangar   have halve   hay hey   heal heel he'll   heart hart
hear here   heard herd   heed he'd   high hi hie   higher hire
him hymn   hole whole   holy holey wholly   hoard horde horse hoarse
hostile hostel   hue hew   hurts Hertz   I eye aye   idle idol idyl
I'll aisle isle   in inn   instance instants   intense intents   its it's
jam jamb   knit nit   lamb lam   lane lain   lay lei
lead led   leak leek   lean lien   least leased   lesson lessen
levy levee   liken lichen   lie lye   Lou lieu   load lode
loan lone   locks lox   loot lute   made maid   mail male
main Maine mane   maze maize   mall maul   manner manor   mantel mantle
martial marshal   mast massed   me mi *(In music.)*   meat meet mete   medal meddle
might mite   minor miner   mist missed   moan mown   mode mowed
morn mourn   muscle mussel   naval navel   nay neigh   need knead
new knew gnu   night knight   no know   none nun   not knot
one won   or oar ore   oral aural   our hour   owed ode
owe oh   packs pacts   pail pale   pain pane   pair pear pare
palette palate pallet   past passed   patience patients   pause paws   peace piece
peak peek pique   peel peal   pearl purl   pedal peddle   peon paean
per purr   phase faze   picnic pyknic   pie pi (π)   pier peer
pious Pius   pigeon pidgin   pilot Pilate   pistol pistil   plain plane
planter plantar   plate plait   please pleas   plum plumb   pole poll
pour pore   pray prey   premiere premier   principal principle   profit prophet
rabbit rabbet   rack wrack   rain rein reign   raise rays raze   ray re *(In music.)*
reed read   red read   real reel   reek wreak   rest wrest
right write rite ring wring   road rode rowed   roll role   root route
rose rows   row roe   rude rued   rung wrung   rye wry
sale sail   sects sex   seen scene   seed cede   sell cell
seller cellar   senate sennet sennit   sent cent scent   session cession   shear sheer

shoe shoo   shoot chute   shown shone   side sighed   sight site cite
sign sine   simian Simeon slay sleigh   slight sleight   slew slue
so sew sow sol (In music.) some sum sore soar   soul sole   stare stair
stares stairs   stayed staid   steak stake   stationary stationery steal steel
step steppe   style stile   straight strait sun son   surf serf
sweet suite   symbol cymbal tail tale   taper tapir   tare tear
taught taut   tax tacks   tea tee ti (In music.) tease teas team teem
there their they're there's theirs through threw throne thrown tick tic
tide tied   tier tear   tighten Titan   tigress Tigris   timbal timbale
timber timbre time thyme Tyme to too two toad towed   toe tow
told tolled   toxin tocsin   tracks tracts   trooper trouper trust trussed
turn tern   vain vane vein veil vale   Venus venous   very vary
vice vise   viscous viscus wade weighed wait weight   wane wain Wayne
war wore   waste waist   wave waive   way weigh *whey ways weighs
we wee   weather *whether weave we've weed we'd   week weak
we're weir   wet *whet   *whale wail   *wheel we'll weal *where wear ware
*which witch *while wile   wine *whine   whose who's   wood would
worst wurst   wrap rap   wrote rote   yolk yoke   you'll Yule
you yew ewe   your you're   *Not strictly a *homophone* if pronounced with an unvoiced /hw/.

Imitations [*Imitations* are attempts to mimic an actual sound through the use of appropriate phonetic combinations. Naturally, there is much difference of opinion on which attempts actually accomplish their mission. The technical word for this is *onomatopoeia* (Gk. "to make a name").]

baa biff blare bobwhite bong boohoo boom bop bow-wow bump burp buzz cackle caw chatter cheep chitchat chuckle chug clack clang clank clash click clink clop cock-a-doo-dle-doo crash creak croak crunch cuckoo ding ding-dong fizz flap flick flip flip-flop giggle guffaw ha-ha haw-haw hiccup jabber jingle jumble meow moo mum ping pitapat plop plunk pop puff purr put-put quack racket rat-a-tat-tat rattle rap roar scrunch shoo shush splash squeal strum swish ta-dah te-hee throb thump tick tick-tock ting-a-ling tingle tinkle titter tom-tom twang tweet twitter ugh wham whew whippoorwill whish whiz woof yak yip zing zip

Initials [Where *acronyms* produce a pronounceable letter combination, mere *Initials* listings do not, but they are, nevertheless, just as useful. The "Alphabet Soup" of government agencies is legendary. Some of the most often used *Initial* combinations are listed here.]

AA (*Alcoholics Anonymous.*)   AAA (*American Automobile Association.*)
ABC (*American Broadcasting Company.*)   AC (*Alternating current.*)
ACLU (*American Civil Liberties Union.*)   ACT (*American College Testing Program.*)
A.D. (*Anno Domini.*)   ADD (*Attention Deficit Disorder.*)
ADHD (*Attention Deficit-Hyperactivity Disorder.*) AFL (*American Federation of Labor.*)
ALS (*Amyotrophic lateral sclerosis, Lou Gehrig's disease.*)   AM (*Amplitude modulation.*)
A.M. (*Ante Meridiem,* Before noon.)   ASAP (*As soon as possible.*)
BBC (*British Broadcasting Company.*)   B.C. (*Before Christ.*)
BLT (*Bacon, lettuce, and tomato sandwich.*)   BMOC (*Big man on campus.*)

Ap. xi-8

CAT scan *(Computerized axial tomography.)*   CB *(Citizens' band radio.)*

CBS *(Columbia Broadcasting System.)*   CCC *(Civilian Conservation Corps.)*

CD *(Compact disc.)*   CIA *(Central Intelligence Agency.)*

CIO *(Congress of Industrial Organizations.)*   COD *(Collect on delivery.)*

DA *(District Attorney.)*   DC *(Direct current.)*

DDT *(Dichlorodiphenyltrichloroethane.)*   DJ *(Disc jockey.)*

DMZ *(Demilitarized zone.)*   DNA *(Deoxyribonucleic acid.)*

DOA *(Dead on arrival.)*   E.D. *(Emotionally Disabled.)*

EEG *(Electroencephalogram.)*   EKG *(Electrocardiogram.)*

EPA *(Environmental Protection Agency.)*   E.R. *(Emergency Room.)*

ERA *(Equal Rights Amendment.)*   ESL *(English as a second language.)*

ESP *(Extrasensory perception.)*   ETA *(Estimated Time of Arrival.)*

ETO *(European Theater of Operations.)*   FBI *(Federal Bureau of Investigation.)*

FM *(Frequency Modulation.)*   GAO *(General Accounting Office.)*

GI *(Government Issue,* An American soldier.*)*   GM *(General Motors.)*

GMT *(Greenwich Mean Time.)*   GNP *(Gross national product.)*

H.S. *(High School.)*   HVAC *(Heating, Ventilation, & Air Conditioning.)*

IBM *(International Business Machines.)*   ICC *(Interstate Commerce Commission.)*

ICBM *(Intercontinental Ballistic missile.)*   I.C.U. *(Intensive Care Unit.)*

ID *(Identification card.)*   IDA *(International Dyslexia Association.)*

IEP *(Individual Education Plan.)*   IHS *(Jesus,* Greek: ΙΗΣΟΥΣ.*)*

IOC *(International Olympics Committee.)*   IOU *(I owe you.)*

IMC *(Instructional Materials Center.)*   I.N.D. *(In the name of God,* Latin: In nomine Dei.*)*

I.N.R.I. *(Jesus of Nazareth, King of the Jews,* Latin: Iesus Nazarenus, Rex Iudaeorum.*)*

I.P.A. *(International Phonetic Alphabet.)*   IQ *(Intelligence quotient.)*

IRS *(Internal Revenue Service.)*   IWW *(Industrial Workers of the World.)*

JV *(Junior varsity.)*   JC *(Junior Chamber of Commerce.)*

KGB *(Commission of State Security,* Russian: Komissia Gosudarstsvennoy Bezopasnosti.*)*

KIA *(Killed in action.)*   KKK *(Ku Klux Klan.)*

KO *(Knock out.)*   KP *(Kitchen Police.)*

L.A. *(Los Angeles.)*   L.A.F. *(License Applied For.)*

LD *(Learning Disabled.)*   LDA *(Learning Disabilities Association.)*

LP *(Long playing record.)*   LSD *(Lysergic acid diethylamide.)*

M.C. *(Master of Ceremonies.)*   M.D. *(Doctor of Medicine,* Latin: Medicinae Doctor.*)*

MIA *(Missing in action.)*   M.I.T. *(Massachusetts Institute of Technology.)*

MS *(Multiple sclerosis.)*   NAO *(North Atlantic Oscillation.)*

NAACP *(National Association for the Advancement of Colored People.)*

NBC *(National Broadcasting Company.)*   NCAA *(National Collegiate Athletic Association.)*

NCO *(Noncommissioned Officer.)*   NEA *(National Education Association.)*

NRA *(National Recovery Administration.)*   NRA *(National Rifle Association.)*

NPR *(National Public Radio.)*   OK *(All correct.)*

PA *(Public address system.)*   PET scan *(Positron emission tomography.)*

PBS *(Public Broadcasting System.)*   PDQ *(Pretty darn quick.)*

Ph.D. *(Doctor of Philosophy,* L: Philosophiae Doctor.*)*   P.M. *(Post Meridiem,* Afternoon.*)*

PO *(Post Office.)*
POW *(Prisoner of war.)*
PTA *(Parent Teachers Association.)*
PX *(Post Exchange.)*
RMC *(Resource Materials Center.)*
R.S.V.P. *(Please respond,* F. Répondez s'il vous plait.*)*
SAT *(Scholastic Aptitude Test.)*
SOS *(Distress signal:* "Save our ship."*)*
TGIF *(Thank goodness it's Friday!)*
TNT *(Trinitrotoluene.)*
UCLA *(University of California at Los Angles.)*
USA *(United States of America.)*
VFW *(Veterans of Foreign Wars.)*
WASP *(White Anglo-Saxon Protestant.)*
W.W. II *(World War Two.)*
YMCA *(Young Men's Christian Association.)*

P.O.D. *(Pay on delivery.)*
P.S. *(Postscript.)*
PTO *(Please Turn Over.)*
R.I.P. *(Rest in peace,* L. Requiescat in pace.*)*
R.N. *(Registered Nurse.)*
RV *(Recreational vehicle.)*
SATB *(Soprano, Alto, Tenor, Bass.)*
S.R.O. *(Standing room only.)*
TLC *(Tender loving care.)*
TV *(Television.)*
UFO *(Unidentified flying object.)*
VD *(Venereal disease.)*
VIP *(Very important person.)*
W.W. I *(World War One.)*
WPA *(Work Projects Administration.)*
YWCA *(Young Women's Christian Association.)*

Letters Used Descriptively: A-frame house   H-beam   H-girder   I-beam   S-curve   S-wrench   T-shirt   T-square   T-bar   T-bone   T-hinge   U-bolt   U-turn   V-formation   V-neck   Y-level   Z-bar   Z-beam   Z-iron

Other Letter Uses: A battery   ABC's   A-bomb   A-OK   A-one   D-day   3-D   G-man   G-string   H-hour   K-12   K ration   P's & Q's   Q-tip   On the q. t.   The 3 R's   Rh factor   Rx   Model-T   U-boat   V-E Day   V-J Day   V-mail   X-chromosome   X-axis   X-ray   Y-axis   Y-chromosome   Y2K (Year Two Thousand [Kilo-]; Computer problem dealing with year 2000.)   Y to Y (Yellowstone to Yukon land mass.)

Interjections [An *interjection* is an expression of emotion or exclamation.   An *interjection* (L. "To throw between.") is one of the eight parts of speech.]

aha ahem ahoy alack alas aw bah boo boy boy-o-boy bravo bravissimo bully *(Well done.)* bye bye-bye by cracky damn drat egad eh? encore /äng-kor/ eureka faugh fie gad gee gee whiz gee whillikers Gesundheit /ge-zŏont-hīt/ *(Ger. To your health!)* golly good-by gosh ha hah ha-ha hallelujah halloo haw haw-haw heck heigh heigh-ho hello hey hi hip hist hm hoicks hooray hosanna hoy how (Indian greeting.) huh? hum humph hurrah hushaby ick icky indeed jeez law lo look lordy man mercy nuts o oh oho oi OK ouch ow oyez *(Hear Ye!)* pah phew pish poh pooh prosit *(L. May it benefit.)* prost pshaw psst pugh rah rah-rah rockaby rot shucks shoo skiddoo skoal *(Scand. To your health.)* so tallyho te-hee thanks timber! tush tut ugh what whew whist whoa whoopee wow yah yipe yoicks yoo-hoo yuck yucky zounds; [Also, any form of swearing is an *interjection*.]

Reduplication [*Reduplication* is the doubling of all or part of a word, often with a vowel or consonant change. *Reduplication* appeals to one's delight in alliteration, assonance, and rhyme.]

boohoo	boogie-woogie	bric-a-brac	chitchat	diddle-daddle
dilly-dally	ding-dong	fiddle-faddle	flimflam	flip-flop

fuddy-duddy	flub-a-dub	hanky-panky	harum-scarum	heebie-jeebies
hee-haw	heigh-ho	helter-skelter	higgledy-piggledy	highty-tighty
hobnob	hocus-pocus	hodgepodge	hoity-toity	hokeypokey
holus-bolus	hootchy-kootchy	hotchpotch	hubble-bubble	hubbub
huggermugger	hullabaloo	humdrum	Humpty-Dumpty	hurdy-gurdy
hurly-burly	hurry-scurry	knickknack	kowtow	mishmash
mollycoddle	mumbo jumbo	namby-pamby	niminy-piminy	nitwit
peewee	pell-mell	picnic	ping-pong	pit-a-pat
pitter-patter	pompon	powwow	razzle-dazzle	rickrack
riffraff	riprap	roly-poly	seesaw	shilly-shally
sing-song	skimble-scamble	shipshape	slipslop	superduper
teeny-tiny	teeny-weeny	teeter-totter	ticktack	ticktock
ting-a-ling	tiptop	tit for tat	tittle-tattle	topsy-turvy
tricktrack	tutti-frutti	tweedledum & tweedledee		twittle-twattle
walkie-talkie	whim-wham	wigwag	willy-nilly	wishy-washy
yoo-hoo	zig-zag			

Short For [*Short For* is a time-saver where an identifiable part of a longer word is used as a substitute for that longer word. This is informal abbreviation without a period.]

abs abdominals   ad advertisement   ad-lib ad libitum   ag agriculture

auto automobile   automat automatic   beck beckon   bike bicycle

blitz blitzkrieg (Ger.)   bop bebop   bra brassiere   br'er brother (So. U.S.)

burger hamburger   bus omnibus (L. *For all.*) cab cabriolet (F)   canter Canterbury

caper capriole (F)   champ champion   chap chapman   chaps chaparajos (Sp.)

chat chatter   chick chicken   chow chow-chow (Chin.) chute parachute

cinema cinematograph   coed coeducational compo composition   confab confabulation

con contra *(Against.)*   con convict   con man confidence man   coon raccoon

co-op cooperative   cortisone corticosterone   cuke cucumber   curio curiosity

deb debutante   doc doctor   dorm dormitory   dropsy hydropsy

dynamo dynamoelectric machine   el elevated train   exam examination

fan fanatic   fancy fantasy   fax facsimile   fed federal

fest festival   flu influenza   frank frankfurter   frat fraternity

fridge refrigerator   Frisco San Francisco   gas gasoline   gator alligator

G-man government man   Godspeed God speed you.   grad graduate

gym gymnasium   hi-fi high fidelity   gent gentleman   hippo hippopotamus

hood hoodlum   hood neighborhood   hydro hydroelectricity

hypo hypodermic injection   hypo hypochondriac   incog incognito (L)

info information   intercom intercommunications system   intro introduction

jetsam jettison   lab laboratory   legit legitimate   limo limousine

lube lubricant   lunch luncheon   magneto magnetoelectric machine

mall pall-mall   mart market   math mathematics   memo memorandum

metro metropolitan railroad   mike microphone   miss mistress

mitt mitten   mod modern   movie moving picture mum chrysanthemum

muskie muskellunge mutt muttonhead   Nam Vietnam
noncom noncommissioned officer   nonsked nonscheduled obit obituary
oleo oleomargarine ordnance ordinance   pants pantaloons   pard partner
pater paternoster   pecs pectorals   pen penitentiary   penult penultima
pep pepper   percent per centum   perk percolate   perks perquisites (L)
photo photograph   phone telephone   piano pianoforte   pike turnpike
pix pictures   pip pippen   plane airplane   plebe plebeian
polio poliomyelitis pop popular   possum opossum
prefab prefabricated structure   prelims preliminary exams
prep preparatory   pro professional   prof professor   prom promenade
promo promotion   prop propeller   props properties   pup puppy
quad quadrangle   quint quintuplet   ratch ratchet   razz razzberry
ref referee   rep representative   rep reputation   rev revolution
rhino rhinoceros   roach cockroach   sax saxophone   scope telescope
scope microscope   scram scramble   sculpt sculpture   scurry hurry-scurry
semi semitrailer   sferics atmospherics simp simpleton   sis sister
specs spectacles   spot spotlight   staph staphylococci stereo stereophonic
sub substitute   sub submarine   super superintendent super superior
tarp tarpaulin   taxi taxicab   taxicab taximeter cab teen teenager
tie necktie   toady toadeater   tram tramroad   trig trigonometry
trump triumph   tux tuxedo   twaddle twittle-twattle
typo typographical error   upper upper berth   van caravan
van vanguard   varsity university   vet veteran   vet veterinarian
wig periwig   Yank Yankee   zoo zoological garden

Trade Names [A catchy name for a commercial product is money in the bank. A few are listed here. A really successful trade name often becomes part of the popular vocabulary, e.g., jello, kleenex, nylon, ping-pong and Scotch tape.]

Actifed   Advil   Aleve   Afrin   Alka-Seltzer   Allerest   Ameritech   Amyutal   Arrid   A & W Band-Aid   Benadryl   Bufferin   Caladryl   Celluloid   Cēpocol   Certs   Cheerios   Citgo   Clorets Coca-Cola   Comtrex   Correctol   Cracker Jack   Crisco   Cut-Rite   Dacron   Demerol   Denorex Dentyne   Desitin   Di-Gel   Dilantin   Dimetapp   Dixie-Cup   Dramamine   Dristan   Ecotrin Efferdent   Ethyl   Excedrin   ex-lax   Fiberglas   Fixodent   Flexall   Formica   Freedent   Freon Frigidaire   Gas-X   Gatorade   Ibuprofen   Imodium   Jif   Kit-Kat   Kodak   Kool-Aid   Lanacane Laundromat   Librium   Liederkranz   Listerine   Lysol   Mace   Maalox   Masonite   Metamucil Microsoft   Midol   Mimeograph   M & M's   Motrin   Murine   Mylanta   Neosporin   Nestea Novocaine   Nico-Derm   Noxzema   Orlon   Orudis   Ouija   Panasonic   PediaCare   Pedialyte Pentothal   Pennzoil   Pepsi   Pepto-Bismol   Photostat   Playtex   Plexiglas   Polaroid   Poli-Grip Popsicle   Pringles   Prozac   Pulmotor   Pyrex   Q-tips   Rayovac   Ritalin   Robitussin   Rogaine Rolaids   Saran wrap   Scrabble   Selsyn   Seven-Up   Silex   Sine-Aid   Sinutab   Sominex Styrofoam   Sucrets   Sudafed   Technicolor   Teflon   Teleprompter   Texico   TheraFlu   Timex Tums   Tylenol   Valium   Vaseline   Viagra   Visine   Wheaties   Windex   Xanax   Xerox   Yahtzee   Ziploc

Variants [A *variant* is a slight variation of a word due to a term need, population isolation, or some unknown consideration. The original word and its *variant* are often more similar in meaning than are an *alteration* pair. The second word listed is a *variant* of the first.]

band *(Flexible strip.)* bond baton batten *(Wood strip.)* bleat blat | borough burg

bound *(Made fast.)* bounden | bowl boll | broach brooch

Brahman Brahmin | bulge bilge | burn bourn | butt *(To bump.)* bunt

carat karat | carol carrel | casino cassino | chap *(A jaw.)* chop *(A jaw.)*

char *(A task.)* chore | chatter chitter | chrism chrisom | chuck *(A cut of beef.)* chunk

cipher sypher | clench clinch | clew clue | clot clod

club clump | cockscomb coxcomb | coin quoin | cole kale

courtesy curtsy | curse cuss | dab dap | dint dent

discreet discrete | disk disc | dint dunt | dough duff *(Flour pudding.)*

engrain ingrain | errant arrant | flip fillip | further farther

gabble gobble *(Turkey sound.)* | gargle gurgle | gullet gully

haggle higgle | halloo holler | hatch *(Cover or grating.)* hack *(A frame.)*

hatchel hackle | haul hale *(To compel to go.)* | ho whoa | hobble hopple

hoist heist | hub hob | jet *(A sudden spurt.)* jut | kevel gavel

knob nob *(The head.)* | knurled gnarled | metal mettle | nock nick

peak pike *(A pointed hill.)* | pendant pendent | pert peart *(Lively.)* | plait plat

plash splash | pond pound *(An enclosure.)* | price prize | puppet poppet

put putt | quit quite | quave quiver | quoin coign *(A corner.)*

rack *(Bank of clouds.)* wrack *(Bank of clouds.)* | robustious rambunctious | roil rile

scion cion | scrimmage skirmish | scrouge scrounge | scum skim

send *(Flow of waves.)* scend | shard sherd | shred screed | shrub scrub

shebeen shebang | skiver skewer | slabber slobber | slug *(A heavy blow.)* slog

sniff snifter | snicker snigger | snout snoot | squash squish

squeeze squeegee | strop strap | stub stob | swelter sultry

sweep swipe | temper tamper | thresh thrash | through thorough

tinkle tingle | tiny teeny | tone tune | tousle tussle

travail travel | trigonal triagonal | voodoo hoodoo | weather wither

Word Blends [Two associated words are sometimes blended together. This blending process is called *portmanteau*.]

bit *(binary, digit)*

blimp *(Type B-Limp)*

blotch *(blot, botch)*

brunch *(breakfast, lunch)*

chunnel *(channel, tunnel)*

dumfound *(dumb, confound)*

flurry *(flutter, hurry)*

gerrymander *(Elbridge Gerry, salamander)*

guesstimate *(guess, estimate)*

modem *(modulator, demodulator)*

moped *(motor, pedal)*

motel *(motor, hotel)*

motorcade *(motor, cavalcade)*

napalm *(naphthenic-palmitic acids)*

paratroops *(parachute troops)*

prissy *(prim, sissy)*

rustle *(rush, hustle)*

skylab *(sky, laboratory)*

smog *(smoke, fog)*

splatter *(splash, spatter)*

splutter *(splash, sputter)*

squiggle *(squirm, wriggle)*

tangelo *(tangerine, pomelo)*

tarnation *(tarnel* [eternal], *damnation)*

telethon *(television, marathon)*

travelogue *(travel, monologue)*

Appendix xii   Who? Where? (Words from Names & Places)   CONTENTS

Words from Names (Nomenyms)

A, B . . . . Ap. xii-1   C . . . . Ap. xii- 2

D, E, F . . . . Ap. xii-3   G, H . . . . Ap. xii- 4

J, K, L, M . . . . . . Ap. xii-5   N, O, P . . . . . . Ap. xii- 6

Q, R, S, T . . . . . .   Ap. xii-7   U, V, W, Y, Z . . Ap. xii- 8

Words from Places (Toponyms)

A, B . . . . Ap. xii- 8

C, D, E . . . . Ap. xii- 9

F, G, H, I, J, L, M . . . . Ap. xii-10

N, O, P, Q, R, S . . . . Ap. xii-11

T, V, W . . . . Ap. xii-12

Appendix xii   Who? Where? (Words from Names & Places)

Words from Names (Nomenyms)

A

Achilles' heel, Achilles' tendon (The character, Achilles, in Homer's Iliad, ninth cent. B.C.)
Addison's disease *[Disease of adrenal glands.]* (Thomas Addison, 1793-1860, Eng. physician.)
Adonis *[A man of rare beauty.]* (Gk. myth; Adonis was loved by Aphrodite for his beauty.)
Amazon *[S.A. river.]* (Gk.myth. Amazon, *["Without breast"* to aid in use of bow] female warrior.)
America, americium *[Radio active element.]* (Amerigo Vespucci, 1451-1512, It. explorer.)
Amish *[A Mennonite sect.]* (Jacob Ammann, a 17th century Mennonite, founded this sect.)
ampere *[Unit of electrical current.]* abampere, ammeter (André Ampére, 1775-1836, Fr. sci.)
aphrodisia *[Excessive sexual desire.]* aphrodisiac (Aphrodite, Greek goddess of love, beauty.)
Appian Way *[Road from Rome to Brundisium, begun 312 B.C.]* (Appius Caecus, Roman consul.)
Argyle plaid   *[Design of solid diamonds.]* (Similar to the Campbell's of Argyll county, Scot.)
atlas *[A volume of maps.]* Atlantic Ocean (Atlas; Gk. mythology: Atlas held up the heavens.)
August *[8th month of the year.]* (Augustus Caesar, 63 B.C.-14 A.D., first Roman emperor.)

B

bacchanal *[Drunken reveler.]* Bacchanalia *[Roman festival]* (Bacchus, Roman god of wine.)
Bakelite *[A heat resistant plastic.]* (Leo Hendrik Baekeland, 1863-1944, American chemist.)

Baldwin *[Red winter apple.]* (Loammi Baldwin, 1740-1807, Am. engineer who developed it.)
Baltimore oriole *[A bird; male with orange & black colors.]* (Like Lord Baltimore's coat of arms.)
Bartlett *[A variety of pear.]* (Dev. in Eng. about 1870;Enoch Bartlett intro. it to America.)
Beau Brummell *[A dandy; a fop.]* (George "Beau" Brummell, 1778-1840, English dandy.)
begonia *[A flower.]* (Michel Bégon, 1638-1710, French colonial gov. of Santo Domingo.)
bel *[Sound intensity measure.]* (Alexander Graham Bell, 1847-1922, American inventor.)
Bernoulli's principle *[Liquid pressure/velocity rule.]* (Daniel Bernoulli, 1700-1782, Swiss math.)
billy club *[A short club used as a weapon, usually by policemen.]* (Billy, nickname for William.)
Bloody Mary *[Vodka, tomato juice drink.]* (Epithet for Mary I, Queen of England 1553-1558.)
bloomers *[Woman's undergarment.]* (Mrs. Amelia Bloomer, 1818-1894, American feminist.)
bobby *[British policeman.]* (Sir Robert "Bobby" Peel, 1788-1850; introduced police reforms.)
bogey *[In golf: one stroke over par on a hole.]* (Colonel Bogey, an imaginary faultless golfer.)
Bolivia *[S. American country.]* (Simón Bolívar, 1783-1830, Venezuelan soldier & statesman.)
Bowie knife *[A unique hunting knife.]* (Invented by James Bowie, 1799-1836, Am. soldier.)
boycott *[Refusal to cooperate.]* (First used against Capt. Boycott, land agent, Ireland, 1880.)
Boyle's law *[Gas volume varies inversely with pressure.]* (Robert Boyle, 1627-91, Eng. chemist.)
boysenberry *[Hybrid of three other berries.]* (Rudolph Boysen, 20th Cent. Am. horticulturist.)
braggadocio *[A boaster.]* (Character in Faerie Queene, poem by Edmund Spenser, 1552-99.)
Braille *[Raised dot writing for the blind.]* (Louis Braille, 1809-1852, Fr. educator and inventor.)
Bright's disease *[A disease of the kidney.]* (Dr. Richard Bright, 1789-1858, English physician.)
Broca's region *[Area of the brain assoc. with language.]* (Pierre Broca, 1824-1880, Fr.surgeon.)
Brownian movement *[Random molecular mvt.]* (Robert Brown,1773-1858, Scottish botanist.)
Browning rifle, Browning machine gun (John Moses Browning, 1855-1926 Am. inventor.)
Buddhism *[A religious faith.]* (Gautama Siddhartha, about 563-463 B.C.; called Buddha.)
bunk *[Nonsense.]* (Buncombe County, N.C. whose congressman made empty speeches.)
Bunsen burner *[Type of gas burner.]* (Robert Wilhelm Bunsen, 1811-1899, German chemist.)

C

Cadillac *[A car.]* (Antoine de la Mothe Cadillac, 1657-1730, Fr. explorer, founded Detroit.)
calliope *[Musical instrument played by steam.]* (Calliope, Gk. Muse of eloquence and poetry.)
calypso *[An orchid; improvised song.]* (Calypso, nymph in the *Odyssey;* imprisoned Odysseus.)
camellia *[Glossy leaved shrub with variegated flowers.]* (G. J. Kamel, 1661-1706, Jesuit traveler.)
cardigan *[Sweater opening down the front.]* (The seventh Earl of Cardigan, 1797-1868, Eng.)
Celsius scale *[Water freezes 0°, boils 100°.]* (Anders Celsius, 1701-44, Swedish astronomer.)
cereal *[Grains: rice, wheat, rye, oats, etc.]* (Ceres, the Roman goddess of grain and harvests.)
cesarean section *[Childbirth by cutting.]* (Julius Caesar, 100-44 B.C., who was born this way.)
charlotte *[A dessert of fruit, whipped cream, etc.]* (Charlotte, given name; feminine of Charles.)
chauvinism *[Excessive devotion.]* (Nicholas Chauvin, an overzealous supporter of Napoleon.)
Chippendale *[Furniture style.]* (Thomas Chippendale, 1718-1779, English cabinetmaker.)
Christian, Christianity, christen, christcross, Christchurch (Jesus Christ of Nazareth.)
Cleopatra's Needle *[Obelisk in London or New York.]* (Cleopatra, 69-30 B.C., queen of Egypt.)
Colt *[Trade name; pistol with revolving-cylinder.]* (Samuel Colt, 1814-1862, American inventor.)
Columbia, Columbus *[A city in many of the United States.]* (Christopher Columbus,1446-1506.)
Comstock Lode *[Rich vein of silver & gold.]* (Henry Comstock, 1820-1870, Am. prospector.)
condom *[A contraceptive.]* (Dr. Condom or Conton, 18th Century English physician.)

Copernican system *[Solar system view.]* (Nicholas Copernicus, 1473-1543, Pol. astronomer.)
coulomb, abcoulomb *[Measure of electrical current.]* (C.A. de Coulomb, 1736-1806, Fr. sci.)
curie *[Unit of radioactivity.]* curium *[Element.]* (Marie Curie, 1867-1934, Pol. born F. physicist.)
Cyrillic alphabet *[A Slavic alphabet based on Greek.]* (St. Cyril, 827-869, Christian missionary.)

D

dahlia *[A perennial plant.]* (Anders Dahl, Swedish botanist, dev. this plant about 1789.)
dandy *[A man interested in an elegant appearance.]* (Alter. of Andy, nickname for Andrew.)
Darwinism *[Evolution by natural selection.]* (Charles Darwin, 1809-1882, English naturalist.)
Davis Cup *[International Lawn Tennis trophy.]* (Dwight Davis, 1879-1945, began tournament.)
Derby *[Horse race at Epsom Downs in Surrey, England.]* (Founded by the 12th Earl of Derby.)
derrick *[A hoisting apparatus.]* (Derrick, 17th Century, hangman in London, England.)
derringer *[A short-barreled pocket pistol.]* (Henry Deringer, 1786-1868, Am. gunsmith.)
Dewey decimal system *[Library book classification.]* (Melvil Dewey, 1851-1931, Am. librarian.)
dickey *[Blouse front worn under a jacket.]* (dickey < Dicky < Dick < Richard.)
diesel engine *[Oil injected internal-combustion engine.]* (Rudolph Diesel, 1858-1913, German.)
Doberman pinscher *[A breed of dog.]* (Ludwig Dobermann, 19th Century, Ger. dog breeder.)
doily *[Ornamental surface protector.]* (Doily or Doyley, fl. 1712, English draper.)
doll *[Plaything resembling a human figure.]* (doll < Dolly < Dorothy.)
Doppler effect *[Pitch difference with changing sound source.]* (C. J. Doppler, 1803-53, German.)
Douglas fir *[A Pacific coast timber pine tree.]* (David Douglas, 1798-1834, Scottish botanist.)
Down's syndrome *[Mongolism.]* (John Langdon-Down, 19th Century, English physician.)
Draconian *[Severe, inflexible.]* (Draco, 7th Century B.C., wrote first Athenian code of laws.)
dukes *[Slang: the fists.]* (Short for: Duke of Yorks; a rhyme for *forks* meaning fingers or fist.)
Duncan Phyfe *[A furniture style.]* (Duncan Phyfe, 1768-1854, born Scot., Am. cabinetmaker.)
dunce *[An ignorant person.]* (Dunsman, follower of John Duns Scotus, enemy of Humanism.)

E

Eiffel Tower *[Iron tower in Paris.]* (Alexandre Eiffel designed tower for 1889 Exposition.)
einsteinium *[Radioactive element.]* (Albert Einstein, 1879-1955, Ger. born, Am. physicist.)
Electra complex *[Strong attachment of daughter to father.]* (Gk. legend, Agamemnon's daughter.)
Elgin marbles *[Gk. sculpture from Acropolis.]* (Earl of Elgin, took these to England 1803-12.)
epicure *[A sensualist, a gourmet.]* epicurean [adj.] (Epicurus, 342-270 B.C., Gk. philosopher.)
Euclidean geometry *[Early developer of geometry.]* (Euclid, fl. 300 B.C., Gk. mathematician.)
Eustachian tube *[Between pharynx & middle ear.]* (Bartolomeo Eustacio, d. 1574, It. anatomist.)

F

Fahrenheit scale *[Water freezes 32°, boils 212°.]* (Gabriel Fahrenheit, 1686-1736, Ger. physicist.)
Fallopian tubes *[Ducts from the ovary to the uterus.]* (Gabriello Fallopio, 1523-62, It. anatomist.)
faraday *[A quantity of electricity.]* (Michael Faraday, 1791-1867, English chemist & physicist.)
fedora *[A soft felt hat.]* ("Fédora", a play by Victorien Sardou, 1831-1908, Fr. dramatist.)
fermi *[Measurement unit for atomic particles.]* (Enrico Fermi, 1901-54, It. physicist, active U.S.)
Ferris wheel *[Amusement park ride.]* (George Washington Gale Ferris, 1859-96, Am. engineer.)
filbert *[Edible nut.]* (St. Philibert, d. 684, Frankish abbot, feast day Aug. 20 when nuts ripen.)
forsythia *[A shrub native to China.]* (William Forsyth, 1737-1804, botanist, brought it to Eng.)
Franklin stove *[Cast-iron, fireplace-like stove.]* (Benjamin Franklin, 1706-90, Am. patriot, *etc.*)

Freudian *[Conforming to Freud's teaching.]* (Sigmund Freud, 1856-1939, Austrian neurologist.)

fuchsia *[A primrose plant with four-petaled flowers.]* (Leonhard Fuchs, 1501-66, Ger. botanist.)

Fulbright Act *[Teacher & student scholarships.]* (James William Fulbright, b. 1905, U.S. Sen.)

G

galvanize *[To stimulate muscles with electricity.]* (Luigi Galvani, 1737-98, It. physiologist.)

gardenia *[Shrub with large white flowers.]* (Alexander Garden, 1730-1791, American botanist.)

Gargantuan *[Huge.]* (Gargantua, giant prince, title character in Rabelais romance of 1534.)

Gatling gun *[Early machine gun.]* gat *[Sl.: gun.]* (R. J. Gatling, 1818-1903, American inventor.)

Geiger counter *[Radiation detector.]* (Hans Geiger, 1882-1945, German physicist.)

gerrymander *[Unfair altering of voting district.]* (Elbridge *Gerry*, Am. V.P. 1813 + sala*mander*.)

Gibson girl *[Idealized Am. girl.]* (Charles Dana Gibson, 1867-1944, Am. illustrator & painter.)

gilbert *[Unit of electromagnetic force.]* (William Gilbert, 1540-1603, English physicist.)

gloxinia *[Plant with large bell-shaped flowers.]* (Benjamin Gloxin, 18th C. physician & botanist.)

golliwog *[A grotesque doll or person.]* (In children's books by Bertha & Florence Upton, 1895.)

goon *[Sl. hoodlum, dolt.]* (Alice the Goon, in an E.C. Segar, 1894-1938, comic strip.)

Gordian knot *[A great problem.]* (Gordius, king of Phrygia, knot cut by Alexander the Great.)

Gothic *[Uncouth, barbarous.]* (Goths, Germanic people, invaded the Roman Empire.)

Gothic architecture *[Style of European arch. 1200-1500, pointed arches, ribbed vaulting.]* (As above.)

graham *[Unsifted whole-wheat flour.]* (Sylvester Graham, 1794-1851, American vegetarian.)

Gregorian calendar *[Calendar now in general use.]* (Offered by Pope Gregory XIII in 1582.)

Gregorian chant *[Church plainsong.]* (Pope Gregory I, pope 590-604, intro. church reforms.)

Grimm's Law *[Consonant shifts between Indo-European & German.]* (Jakob Grimm, 1785-1863.)

grog *[Rum.]* groggy *[Dazed.]* (Adm. Vernon, "Old Grog", wore a grogram cloak; rationed rum.)

Guarnerius *[A fine violin.]* (Guarneri, a family of It. violin makers, esp. Guiseppe, 18th C..)

Guggenheim Fellowship *[Research & arts grants.]* (John Guggenheim, 1867-1941, industrialist.)

guillotine *[Beheading machine.]* (Joseph Guillotin, 1738-1814, Fr. physician during revolution.)

gun *[A weapon.]* (Nickname for Gunnhildr, a feminine given name, ON.)

guppy *[Tropical fish.[* (R.J. Lechmere Guppy, Trinidad; gave specimens to British Museum.)

guy *[Fellow; grotesque person.]* (Guy Fawkes, 1570-1606, plotted against King James I.)

gypsy *[A wandering person originally from India; often musician or fortune teller.]* (Egyptian.)

H

hades *[Euphemism for hell.]* (Gk. myth: Hades, brother of Zeus, ruler of the underworld.)

hallmark *[A mark of excellence.]* (A *mark* stamped on articles at Goldsmiths' *Hall*, London.)

Harvard University *[Eastern Am. Univ.]* (John Harvard, 1607-38, Eng. clergyman, endowed it.)

henry, abhenry *[Units of electrical inductance.]* (Joseph Henry, 1797-1878, Am. physicist.)

herculean *[Having great strength; gigantic.]* (Hercules, myth. son of Zeus, performed 12 labors.)

hermetic *[Airtight.]* (Hermes Trismegistus, Gk. name for Egyptian Thoth, alchemy founder.)

hertz *[Unit of electromagnetic wave freq.]* (Heinrich Rudolph Hertz, 1857-94, German physicist.)

hick *[Having unsophisticated manners.]* (Alteration of name, Richard; nickname for Richard.)

hijack *[To seize a cargo or vehicle illegally while in transit.]* ("Hi Jack!" Robber's greeting to victim.)

Hodgkin's disease *[Enlargement of lymph nodes, spleen.]* (Thos. Hodgkin, 1798-1966, Eng. phy.)

hooligan *[Sl. a young hoodlum.]* (Hooligan, name of a particular upstart in London about 1898.)

Hudson River *[N.Y. river.]*, Hudson Bay *[Inland lake, Can.]* (Henry Hudson, d. 1611. Eng. exp.)

hyacinth *Plant with bell-shaped flowers.]* (Hyacinthus, killed by Apollo; his blood flowered.)

J

jack *[A laborer, e.g., jack-of-all-trades, lumberjack; a device for lifting.]* (Jack, nickname for John.)

Jacob's ladder *[Ladder from heaven to earth; an herb.]* (Jacob, son of Isaac; father of 12 tribes.)

January *[First month of the year.]* (Janus, Roman mythology, god of beginnings and endings.)

jimmy *[Burglar's crowbar; to pry open.]* (Jimmy, diminutive of James, a personal name.)

jockey *[A horse racer.]* (Diminutive of Jock, Scottish form of Jack < French Jacques.)

John Hancock *[One's signature.]* (John Hancock, 1737-93, Declaration of Independence signer.)

jovial *[Good-natured.]* (Jove or Jupiter, Roman mythology, the chief god. Like Gk. Zeus.)

jug *[A bulging narrow-necked container for holding liquids.]* jug *[Sl. jail.]* (Jug, nickname for Joan.)

July *[Seventh month of the year.]* (Julius Caesar, 100-44 B.C. Roman general & statesman.)

jumbo *[A large person, animal, or thing.]* (Jumbo, name of P.T. Barnum's large circus elephant.)

June *[Sixth month of the year.]* (Junius, a Roman clan name.)

Jupiter *[Fifth planet from sun.]* (Jupiter, Roman mythology, the chief god; the Greek Zeus.)

K

knickers *[Pants gathered beneath the knee.]* (Knickerbocker, early Dutch settler name in N.Y.)

Köchel *[Opus numbering in Mozart's music.]* (L. von Köchel, 1800-77, Austrian music editor.)

L

leotard *[Close-fitting dance or acrobat garment.]* (Jules Léotard, 19th Century, French aerialist.)

Levis *[Denim trousers with reinforcing rivets.]* (Levi Strauss, American manufacturer.)

lothario *[Deceiver; seducer.]* (Lothario, character in N. Rowe's play The Fair Penitent, 1703.)

lynch *[Killing by mob action, usually hanging.]* (Charles Lynch, 1736-96, Virginia magistrate.)

Lutheran Church *[Protestant church, founded in Ger.]* (Martin Luther, 1483-1546, theologian.)

M

Maginot /mazh-ə-nō/ line *[French fortifications.]* (André Maginot, 1877-1932, Fr. statesman.)

magnolia *[A flowering shrub.]* (Pierre Magnol, 1638-1715, French botanist.)

malapropism *[The absurd misuse of words.]* (Mrs. Malaprop in Sheridan's play, The Rivals, 1775.)

March *[Third month of the year.]* (Mars, Roman mythology, god of war; the Greek Ares.)

marionette *[Doll-like figure moved by strings.]* (Dim. of Marion, dim. of Marie; image of Mary.)

Mars *[Fourth planet from the sun.]*, martial *[Pertaining to war.]*, Martian *[Person from Mars.]* (Mars.)

martin *[A type of swallow.]* (Bird said to depart on Martinmas, honor of St. Martin, 316-397.)

martini *[Gin & vermouth cocktail.]* (Martini and Rossi, name of a company making vermouth.)

Marxism *[A humanitarian socialism.]* (Karl Marx, 1818-83, Ger. philosopher & pol. theorist.)

masochism *[Enjoyment of pain.]* (Leopold von Sacher-Masoch, 1835-95, Austrian novelist.)

Mason-Dixon line *[Boundary div. Penn. & Md.; drawn 1763.]* (Charles Mason & Jeremiah Dixon.)

maudlin *[Excessively sentimental or emotional.]* (Mary Magdalen, cried for brother, Lazerus.)

mausoleum *[A stately tomb.]* (King Mausolus of Caria, his burial vault one of Seven Wonders.)

maverick *[An unbranded animal; one with different ideas.]* (S. Maverick did not brand his cattle.)

May *[Fifth month of the year.]* (Maia, Roman mythology, goddess of spring.)

McCarthyism *[Unsubstantiated accusations.]* (Joseph McCarthy, 1909-57, US senator, WI.)

McGuffey readers *[Children's texts.]* (William Holes McGuffey, 1800-73, Am. educator.)

Macintosh *[An eating apple.]* (John Macintosh, Ontario, Canada; discovered it about 1796.)

Mender's Laws *[Laws of genetics.]* (Groggier John Mended, 1822-84, Austrian monk, botanist.)

Mennonite *[Member of this Protestant Christian church.]* (Menno Simons, 1492-1559, founder.)

mentor *(Teacher or guide.)* (Mentor, guardian of Telemachus, character in Homer's <u>Odyssey</u>.)
Mercator projection *[Grid-like map.]* (Gerardus Mercator, 1512-94, Flemish cartographer.)
mercerize *[To increase strength & gloss of cotton cloth.]* (John Mercer, 1791-1866, Eng. inventor.)
Mercury *[Planet nearest sun.]* (Mercury, Roman myth., messenger of the gods; god of skill.)
mesmerize *[To hypnotize.]* (Franz Anton Mesmer, 1733-1815, German physician.)
Messerschmitt *[W.W. II Ger. aircraft.]* (Wilhelm Messerschmitt, b. 1898, Ger. aircraft designer.)
milquetoast *[A very meek person.]* (Casper Milquetoast, cartoon character by H.T. Webster.)
Möbius strip *[A strip with only one side.]* (August F. Möbius, 1790-1868, Ger. mathematician.)
molotov cocktail *[Gasoline filled bottle with a rag wick.]* (Vyacheslav Molotov, Rus. diplomat.)
Morse code *[An alphabet of dots & dashes.]* (Samuel F. B. Morse, 1791-1872, Am. inventor.)
Murphy bed *[A bed that folds into a closet.]* (William L. Murphy, 20th Century, Am. inventor.)

N

napoleon *[A rich pastry.]* (Napoleon Bonaparte, 1769-1821, military conqueror, Fr. emperor.)
narcissism *[Excessive self-love.]* (Narcissus, Greek mythology, fell in love with his own image.)
narcissus *[Flowering plant of the amaryllis family, including the daffodil and jonquil.]* (Narcissus.)
nelson *[Full and half nelsons are wrestling moves.]* (Prob. first used by a wrestler named Nelson.)
Neptune *[Eighth planet from the sun.]* (Neptune, Roman myth., god of the sea; Gk. Poseidon.)
nicotine *[Addictive substance found in tobacco.]* (Jean Nicot, 1530-1600, intro. it into France.)
nobelium *[Radio active element.]* (Alfred B. Nobel, 1833-96, Sw. industrialist, inv. dynamite.)
Nobel Prizes *[Awarded in physics, chemistry, medicine, literature, and promotion of peace.]* (Nobel.)

O

obsidian *[Glassy volcanic rock.]* (Obsidius, named as its discoverer by the Roman author Pliny.)
odyssey *[A long, wandering journey.]* (Homer's, <u>Odyssey</u>, detailing the journeys of Odysseus.)
Oedipus complex *[Son-mother attachment.]* (Oedipus, Gk. myth, killed father, married mother.)
ohm, abohm *[Units of electrical resistance.]* (Georg Simon Ohm, 1787-1854, Ger. physicist.)
ottoman *[A cushion footrest or armless sofa.]* (Ottoman, a Turk, or Ottoman Empire 1300-1919.)

P

pamphlet *[An unbound printed work.]* (Pamphilet, dim. <u>Pamphilus</u>, 12th C. Latin love poem.)
pander *[To arrange sexual partners.]* (Pandare, character in Chaucer's <u>Troilus and Criseyde</u>.)
panic *[An overpowering fear.]* (Panikos, Gk. "of Pan"; god of forests; caused sudden fears.)
Pap test *[Uterine cancer test.]* (George Papinicolaou, 1884-1962, Am. physician born in Gr.)
Parkinson's disease *[A paralysis w. tremors.]* (James Parkinson, 1755-1824, Eng. physician.)
Pascal's Wager *[Best to opt for a God; win either way.]* (Blaise Pascal, 1623-62, Fr. math. phil.)
Pasteurize *[Fermentation prevention by heating above 140° F.]* (Louis Pasteur, 1822-95, Fr. chem.)
Petri dish *[Bacteria culture holder.]* (Julius Petri, 1852-1922, German bacteriologist.)
Pluto *[Ninth planet from the sun.]* (Pluto, god of the dead in Greek and Roman mythology.)
poinsettia *[Plant w. small green flowers, red bracts.]* (Joel Poinsett, 1779-1851, U.S. diplomat.)
pompadour *[Straight back from forehead hair style.]* (Marquise de Pompadour, 1721-64, Fr.)
praline *[A pecan candy.]* (Marshal Duplessis-Praslin, 1598-1675, Fr., whose cook invented it.)
Ptolemaic system *[Sun & planets revolve around earth.]* (Ptolemy, 2nd C. Gk. astronomer.)
Pulitzer Prize *[In writing, music, & art.]* (Joseph Pulitzer, 1847-1911, newspaper publisher.)
Pullman *[Railroad coach convertible to sleeping car.]* (George Pullman, 1831-97, Am. inventor.)
Pyrrhic victory *[A victory at ruinous cost.]* (Pyrrus, king of Epirus, defeated Romans 279 B.C.)

Q

quisling *[One who betrays his country.]* (Vidkun Quisling, 1887-1945, Nor. Nazi and traitor.)
quixotic *[Overly chivalrous & romantic.]* (<u>Don Quixote</u>, a novel by Cervantes 1547-1616.)

R

ragamuffin *[Child in ragged clothes.]* (Ragamoffyn, demon in Langland's <u>Piers Plowman</u>, 1393.)
ritzy *[Classy.]* (César Ritz, 1850-1918, founded Ritz-Carlton Hotel in New York City.)
robin *[Bird with reddish brown breast.]* (Robin, diminutive of Robert.)
Rorschach *[Personality test with inkblots.]* (Hermann Rorschach, 1884-1922, Swiss psychiatrist.)

S

sadism *[Pleasure in hurting others.]* (Marquis Comte de Sade, 1740-1814, French novelist.)
salmonella *[A bacteria causing food poisoning.]* (Daniel Salmon, 1850-1914, Am. pathologist.)
sandwich (4th Earl of Sandwich, 1718-92, who ate it without leaving his gambling table.)
Sanforize *[Treatment of cloth to prevent shrinking.]* (Sanford L. Cluett, Am. process inv. 1928.)
Saturn *[Sixth planet from sun.]* (Saturn, Roman mythology, god of agriculture; Greek Cronus.)
saxophone *[A reed metallic instrument.]* (Antoine J. Sax,1814-94, Belgian, instrument maker.)
Schick test *[Test for diphtheria susceptibility.]* (Dr. Béla Schick, 1877-1967, Hungarian.)
sherlock *[Sl. a detective.]* (Sherlock Holmes, character created by Arthur Conan Doyle.)
sequoia *[Gigantic evergreen tree.]* (Sequoyah, 1770-1843, invented Cherokee alphabet.)
Shakespearean sonnet *[Rhyme scheme of abab-cdcd-efef-gg.]* (Wm. Shakespeare, 1564-1616.)
shrapnel *[Anti-personnel projectile.]* (Henry Shrapnel, 1761-1842, British artillery officer.)
shylock *[A high-rate money lender.]* (Shylock, usurer in Shakespeare's <u>Merchant of Venice</u>.)
sideburns *[A man's side whiskers.]* (A. E. Burnside, 1824-81, Union general in Am. Civil War.)
silhouette *[Shadow cast by a figure.]* (Étienne de Silhouette, 1709-67, Fr. minister of finance.)
sousaphone *[A marchable tuba.]* (John Philip Sousa, 1854-1932, Am. bandmaster-composer.)
spinet *[A small harpsichord.]* (Giovanni Spinetti, fl. 1503, Venetian spinet maker.)
spoonerism *[Sound transfer: "tons of soil" for "sons of toil."]* (Wm. Spooner, 1844-1930, Oxford.)
Stetson *[Felt hat with high crown and wide brim.]* (John B. Stetson, 1830-1906, Am. hatmaker.)
Stradivarius *(A fine violin.)* (Antonio Stradivari, 1644-1737, Italian violinmaker.)

T

tam *[A Scottish cap.]* (<u>Tam O' Shanter</u>, poem by Robert Burns; Tam is a paranoid drunk.)
Tammany Hall *[Meeting place of N.Y.C. Dem. party.]* (Alter. Tamanend, Delaware Indian chief.)
tantalize *[To torment; tease.]* (Gk. myth: Tantalus was tied w. food and water just out of reach.)
tarzan *[Strong, athletic man.]* (Edgar Rice Burroughs, 1875-1950; hero in his series of novels.)
tawdry *[Showy, cheap.]* (Tawdry lace, alter. of St. Audrey's lace; silk sold at fair in Ely, Eng.)
Tay-Sachs disease *[A congenital disease.]* (Warren Tay, Eng. phy. & Bernard Sachs, Am. neur.)
teddy bear *[Toy doll-like animal.]* (Teddy, nickname of Theodore Roosevelt, 26th U.S.pres.)
Teddy-boy *[Br. sl., Edwardian dressing delinquent youth.]* (Teddy-boy, nickname Edward VII.)
titanic *[Of very great size.]* (Titans, Gk. race of giant gods, vanquished by the Olympian gods.)
Titanic *[Eng. ocean liner; hit an iceberg and sunk on its maiden voyage, April 14, 1912.]* (as above.)
Tom, Dick, and Harry *[Everyone, people in general.]* (Nicknames: Thomas, Richard, & Henry.)
Tom & Jerry *[A drink.]* (Corinthian Tom & Jerry Hawthorn in Egan's book, <u>Life in London</u>.)
tommy *[A British soldier.]* (Tommy Atkins, fictitious name used in British Army regulations.)
tommy gun *[A submachine gun.]* (John T. Thompson, d. 1940, invented it with John Blish.)
Tom Thumb *[A midget.]* (Eng. folklore, son of a plowman no bigger than his father's thumb.)

U

Uncle Sam *[Personification of the U.S.A.]* (Samuel Wilson, 1766-1854, businessman, Troy, N.Y.)
Uncle Tom *[Black man anxious to please whites.]* (Harriet Beecher Stowe's Uncle Tom's Cabin.)
Uranus *[7th planet from the sun.]* (Uranus, Gk. myth., husband of Gaea [earth], father of Titans.)
uranium *[A heavy, white radioactive element; found only in combination; source of radium.]* (Uranus.)

V

valentine *[Greetings sent to a loved one on Feb. 14th.]* (St. Valentine, 3rd C. Christian martyr.)
(But custom more often thought to come from Lupercalia, Roman fertility rite, Feb. 15th.)
Van Allen radiation belt *[Charged atomic particles circling earth.]* (James Van Allen, Am. sci.)
vandal *[A property destroyer.]*, vandalism (Vandals, a Germanic tribe, pillaged Rome in 455.)
Vandyke beard, collar, brown (Anthony Van Dyck, 1599-1641, Flemish painter.)
Venus *[Second planet from the sun.]* (Venus, Roman myth: goddess of love and beauty.)
vernier scale *[For fine tuning precision measurements.]* (Pierre Vernier, 1580-1637, Fr. math.)
Victorian *[Prudish, conventional.]* (Alexandria Victoria, Queen of England, 1837-1901.)
volt, abvolt, voltage *[Units of electromotive force.]* (Alessandro Volta, 1745-1827, It. physicist.)

W

Wagnerian *[Grand; in the style of an opera by Wagner.]* (Richard Wagner, 1813-83, Ger. comp.)
watt, abwatt *[Units of electrical power.]*, wattage (James Watt, 1736-1819, Scottish, inv.)
Wedgwood *[A fine pottery w. classical figures in cameo relief.]* (Josiah Wedgwood, 1730-95, Eng.)
wisteria *[A shrub, elongated pods, flower clusters.]* (Caspar Wistar, 1761-1818, Am. anatomist.)

Y

yahoo *[A bumpkin.]* (Yahoo one of the brutish beings in Jonathan Swift's Gulliver's Travels.)
Yankee *[New Englander; northerner in Civil War; an American.]* (Jan Kees, a Hollander in N.Y.)

Z

zeppelin *[A dirigible.]* (Count Ferdinand von Zeppelin, 1838-1917, Ger. general & aviator.)
zinnia *[An herb with showy flowers.]* (Johann G. Zinn, 1727-59, Ger. physician & botanist.)

Words from Places (Toponyms)

A

Airedale *[A large tan terrier with black markings.]* (Airedale, the Aire river valley, England.)
ammonia *[Colorless, pungent gas NH4.]* (Temple of Ammon in Libya where gum plants grew.)
angora *[The silky wool from goats in central Turkey.]* (Angora [Ankara], Turkey.)
angora cat, angora goat, angora rabbit, angora wool, angora cloth (As above.)
artesian well *[A well drilled to such a depth that water above it will force a flow.]* (Artois, France.)
ascot *[A fancy, wide tie.]* (Ascot, England where men dress well for the horse races there.)

B

babel *[A confusion of voices.]* (Tower of Babel, Babylon, builders spoke many languages.)
Babylonian captivity (Jews where exiled to Babylon in 597 B.C. by Nebuchadnezzar.)
badminton *[A game where a shuttlecock is hit over a net.]* (Badminton, Duke of Beaufort's estate.)
balkanize *[To break a region into small states.]* (Balkan Peninsula, S. Europe, site of conflict.)
baloney, boloney, bologna *[A highly seasoned sausage.]* (Bologna, province, north central It.)

bantam *[A small domestic fowl.]* bantamweight *[A light athlete.]* (Bantam, first Dutch town, Java.)
Bard of Avon *[William Shakespeare.]* (Avon river; Stratford-on-Avon, Shakespeare's birth pl.)
bayonet *[A sword-like weapon attached to firearm.]* (Bayonne, France, where it was first made.)
béarnaise sauce *[A variation of hollandaise sauce with chopped parsley & vinegar.]* (Béarn, France.)
bedlam *[Noisy confusion.]* (Bedlam, hospital for the insane, London, England.)
Bermuda shorts *[Knee-length walking shorts for both men & women.]* (Bermuda, island in Atlantic.)
bikini *[A scanty swimsuit.]* (Bikini, atoll in the Marshall Islands; site atomic bomb tests, 1946.)
bohemian *[Leading an unconventional lifestyle.]* (Bohemia, province in former Czechoslovakia.)
bolivia *[A twilled woolen fabric with a plush finish.]* (Bolivia, South America.)
boston *[A card game; a waltz.]* Boston brown bread, Boston cream pie, Boston rocker (Boston.)
Brussels sprouts, Brussels carpet, Brussels lace (Brussels, capital of Belgium.)

C

calico *[Cotton cloth printed in print colors.]* (Calicut [Kozhikode], a city in southwest India.)
Camembert *[A rich, creamy cheese.]* (Camembert, France.)
cantaloupe *[A muskmelon.]* (Cantalupo, Italian castle where it was first grown in Europe.)
canter *[An easy gallop.]* (Canterbury gallop, leisurely pace in pilgrimages to Canterbury.)
carioca *[A South American dance.]* (Serra de Carioca, a mountain range near Rio de Janeiro.)
cashmere *[A fine goat wool; a dress or shawl made of cashmere.]* (Kashmir, India.)
Castile soap *[A hard white odorless soap.]* (First made in Castile, a region in northern Spain.)
Caucasian *[A division of the human species.]* (Caucasus Mt. range, skull found establishing type.)
caucus *[Strategy planning meeting.]* (Caucus Club, Boston <Algonquin, *caucawasu*, adviser.)
chablis /shə-blē/ *[A dry, white Burgundy wine.]* (Chablis, a town in north central France.)
champagne *[A sparkling white wine.]* (Champagne, a region and former province of France.)
charleston *[A 4/4 time dance popular in the 1920's.]* (Charleston, South Carolina.)
Cheddar *[A white or yellow hard cheese.]* (Cheddar, Somerset, England where first made.)
chianti /kē-an-tē/ *[A dry, red wine.]* (Monti Chianti, small range of the Apennines Mts., Italy.)
chihuahua /chi-wä-wä/ *[A small dog, smooth fur, pointed ears.]* (Chihuahua, a Mexican state.)
china *[Fine porcelain or ceramic ware, sometimes called chinaware.]* (China, has ¼ world's pop.)
clink *[Slang, jail, prison.]* (Clink prison, London, England.)
cologne *[A perfumed liquid, alcohol & aromatic oils; cologne water; eau de Cologne.]* (Cologne Ger.)
Colossians *[A book of the New Testament; Paul's letter.]* (Colossae, ancient city in Asia Minor.)
Concord grape *[Dark blue cultivated grape.]* (Concord, Massachusetts.)
Cro-Magnon *[Upper Paleolithic European man.]* (Cro-Magnon, a cave near Les Eyzies, Fr.)

D

delftware *[White or blue glazed earthenware.]* (Delft, Holland; first made here about 1310.)
delphic, delphian *[Obscure; ambiguous.]* (Delphi, ancient Gk. city; home of Apollo's oracle.)
denim *[A firm durable twilled cotton fabric.]* (French: serge de Nimes; serge of Nimes, France.)
daiquiri /dak-er-ē/ *[A cocktail made of rum, lime juice, and sugar.]* (Daiquirí, Cuba.)
douai Bible *[English trans., 1610, of St. Jerome's Latin version, 405; used by Catholics.]* (Douai, Fr.)
Dresden china, Dresden ware *[Porcelain with dainty design & ornate decoration.]* (Dresden, Ger.)
duffel *[Coarse woolen fabric napped on both sides.]*, duffel bag (Duffel, town near Antwerp, Bel.)

E

Edam cheese *[A mild curd cheese usually coated with red paraffin.]* (Edam, Holland.)
Eton jacket *[A short jacket cut off square at the hips.]* (Eton College, boys' school, Eton, Eng.)

F

fez *[Red felt cap with a black tassel worn by Egyptian men, formerly by Turkish men.]* (Fez, Morocco.)
frankfurter *[A smoked reddish beef or pork sausage, bigger than a wiener.]* (Frankfurt, Germany.)

G

gauze *[A transparent open weave material used in bandages.]* (Gaza [Ghazzah], Gaza Strip, Israel.)
Gila /hē-lə/ monster *[Large, venomous lizard w. a stout orange & black body.]* (Gila River, Arizona.)
gin *[Aromatic alcoholic liquor distilled from various grains, esp. rye.]* (Short for Geneva, Switzerland.)
Gouda cheese *[Edam-like mild yellow cheese.]* (Gouda, town in Netherlands where first made.)
Greenwich mean time *[Time as determined from the meridian at Greenwich.]* (Greenwich, Eng.)
Guernsey *[Tan & white cattle producing rich yellowish milk.]* (Guernsey, Br. Island in Eng. Chan.)

H

Hague Tribunal *[A court of arbitration.]* (The Hague, Netherlands, first int. peace conf. 1899.)
hamburger, burger *[A cooked ground beef patty in a bun.]* (Hamburg, chief port of Germany.)

I

Indian *[Citizen of India; aborigine of North America.]* (Columbus thought he had reached India.)

J

java *[Coffee.]*, Java Man *[Pithecanthropus small-brained hominid.]* (Discovered near Trinil, Java.)
jean *[Trousers of overalls made of a sturdy twilled cotton cloth.]* (French Gênes for Genoa, Italy.)
Jersey *[Breed of small cattle; milk rich in butterfat.]* (Jersey, British island in the Eng. Channel.)
jimsonweed *[Tall, course, poisonous weed.]* (Alter. Jamestown weed, first found Jamestown, Va.)
jodhpurs *[Riding breeches, close at calf, with strap under foot.]* (Jodhpur, India.)
Jurassic *[A geological period of the Mesozoic era.]* (Jura mountain range between Fr. & Switz.)

L

laconic *[Brief, concise.]* (Lakonia, ancient Gk. state, capital Sparta; citizens were taciturn.)
lesbian *[A homosexual woman, gay.]* (Lesbos, Gk. island, here poet Sappho & followers gay.)
Leyden jar *[A static electricity gatherer.]* (Leiden [Leyden], Holland where it was invented.)
lima bean *[Large flat edible seed; a vegetable.]* (Lima, Peru.)
Limburgher cheese *[Strong odored soft, white cheese.]* (Limburg, Belgium.)
limerick *[A five-lined humorous verse.]* (Limerick county, Munster province, Ireland.)
limousine *[A large car w. open driver's seat under a projecting roof.]* (Limousin, region in France.)
lyonnaise *[To prepare a food such as potatoes with onions.]* (Lyonnaise, fem. Fr., *of Lyons,* Fr. city.)

M

magenta *[A purplish red dye.]* (Magenta, Italy; discovered here after Fr. victory in 1859.)
Maltese cat, Maltese dog, Maltese falcon, Maltese cross (Malta, an island south of Sicily.)
manila cigar, manila hemp, manila rope, manila paper (Manila, Luzon, Philippine Islands.)
marathon *[26.2 mile race.]* (Marathon, Gk. victory over Persia here; news was run to Athens.)
meander *[To take a wandering route.]* (Meander River, Turkey, takes uneven, winding course.)
mecca *[Center of importance.]* (Mecca, Saudi Arabia, birthplace Mohammed; Islam's holy city.)
meringue /mə-rang/ *[Beaten egg whites.]* (Mehringen, Ger.; cake of Mehringen; Fr. meringue.)
milliner *[A maker of women's hats.]*, millinery *[Women's hats.]* (Milaner, one from Milan, Italy.)
mocha *[A choice, pungent coffee; flavoring of coffee & chocolate.]* (Mocha, a port city in Yemen.)

monadnock *[A single mass of rock rising above a plain.]* (Mount Monadnock, New Hampshire.)

Moselle *[A light, dry wine.]*(Moselle River, chiefly Luxembourg, but also Germany & France.)

Mousterian *[A culture of Middle Paleolithic Era whose artifacts found.]* (Le Moustier, Fr. village.)

muslin *[A sturdy, plain-weave cotton fabric used for sheets.]* (Made in Mosul, Iraq; mousseline [F].

N

Neanderthal man *[Extinct species of man; Paleolithic Era.]* (Neanderthal [Neander Valley], Ger.)

Neapolitan ice cream *[Chocolate, strawberry, & vanilla flavored.]* (Neapolitan, of Naples, Italy.)

O

oxford shoe *[A low laced shoe.]*, Oxford don *[Head fellow.]*, oxford gray (Oxford Univ., Eng.)

P

Parmesan cheese *[A hard, dry cheese usually grated to flavor spaghetti.]* (Parma, Italy.)

Pekingese dog *[A dog with snub nose, short legs, silky hair.]* (Peking [Bejing], China.)

pilsner *[A light, Bohemian beer with a strong hop flavor.]* (Pilsen [Plzeň], Bohemia, Czech Rep.)

Piltdown man *[Elaborate fraud; based on skull pieces & animal bones.]* (Piltdown, E. Sussex, Eng.)

Podunk *[A small, uninteresting, isolated town.]* (Podunk, Massachusetts or Podunk, Conn.)

Q

quonset hut *[A rounded, prefabricated metal building; for U.S. armed forces use.]* (Quonset, R. I.)

R

Rhineland, Rhinestone, Rhinegold, Rhinewine (Rhine River, Germany.)

romaine *[Lettuce.]*, roman *[Type, style; type of old French literature.]* Roman calendar *[Lunar cal.]*
Roman candle *[Fireworks device.]*, Roman Catholic Church, romance *[A love affair; literature.]*
Romance Languages *[Those deriving from Latin: French, Italian, Portuguese, Spanish, Rumanian.]*
Roman collar *[A clerical collar.]*, Roman Empire *[Est. by Augustus in 27 B.C.; ended A.D. 395.]*
Romanesque architecture *[A heavy, thick wall, rounded arches church arch. 11th to 13th Centuries.]*
Roman law, Roman mile, Roman nose, Roman numerals, Romano cheese (Rome.)

Roquefort cheese *[Blue-mold type cheese.]* (Roquefort, France.)

Rosetta stone *[Tablet with demotic hieroglyphics, hieratic hieroglyphics, & Greek.]* (Rosetta, Egypt.)

Rugby *[Type of football game, fifteen men teams try to get ball over others goal.]* (Rugby, England.)

S

sauterne *[A sweet, white wine.]* (Sauternes, a district in SW France.)

Seltzer water *[A mineral water containing much free carbon dioxide.]* (Nieder Selters, Germany.)

shanghai *[To drug and kidnap a person for ship duty; to do by force or deception.]* (Shanghai, China.)

shangrila *[Utopia or paradise.]* (Shangrila, setting for Lost Horizon, by James Hilton, Eng.)

Shetland pony *[Small shaggy pony.]*, Shetland wool *[Thin, loose yarn.]* (Shetland Islands, Scot.)

shillelagh /shi-lā-lə/ *[A stout stick made of oak.]* (Shillelagh, Ireland; famed for its oak trees.)

sodomy *[Unnatural sexual relations.]* (Sodom, Biblical city, destroyed for wickedness.)

spa *[A resort, usually with mineral waters present.]* (Spa, Belgium.)

spaniel *[A breed of dog with long drooping ears and long silky hair.]* (Spain.)

Springfield rifle *[W.W. I .30 caliber bolt-operated rifle.]* (U.S. arsenal, Springfield, Mass.)

spruce *[An evergreen tree with dense foliage.]* (Pruce: a form of Prussia.)

stogy *[A slender cigar; a heavy boot.]* (Constoga Wagon, smoking drivers wore heavy boots.)

suede *[A leather with a soft finish.]* (French: *gants de Suède*, Swedish gloves.)

T

Tabasco sauce *[A red pepper sauce.]* (Tabasco, a Mexican state.)

tangerine *[A small orange-like fruit.]* (Tangier, Morocco.)

telemark *[A type of turn in skiing to stop or change direction.]* (Telemark, Norway.)

tequila *[A liquor distilled from the agave /ə-gā-vē/ plant.]* (Tequila, Jalisco, Mexico.)

Tokay *[A special white or reddish blue grape.]* (Tokay, Hungary.)

troy *[System of weights where one pound equals twelve ounces.]* (Weight used at fair in Troyes, Fr.)

turkey *[Short for turkey cock, guinea fowl; erroneously applied to Am. bird.]* (The country, Turkey.)

tuxedo *[A man's semiformal dress suit.]* (first worn at the country club in Tuxedo Park, N. Y.)

tweed *[A soft woolen fabric with a plaid pattern.]* (Tweed River, Scotland.)

V

valance *[A short board or drapery across the top of window.]* (Valance, a textile district SE Fr.)

Venetian blind, Venetian carpet, Venetian glass, Venetian School (Venice, Italy.)

Vichy water *[A mineral water.]* vichyssoise *[Cold potato cream soup.]* (Vichy, France.)

W

Waterloo *[A final defeat.]* (Waterloo, Belgium where Napoleon lost his last battle in 1815.)

Weimar Republic *[Post-W.W. I German Republic.]* Weimaraner *[Breed of dog.]* (Weimar, Ger.)

wiener, wienerwurst *[A beef or pork sausage.]*

Wiener schnitzel *[Veal cutlet.]* (Vienna, Austria; Wien [Ger.].)

worsted *[A smooth compact yarn with a hard twist.]* (Worsted, former parish in Norfolk, Eng.)

Americanisms English Peculiar To The United States . . . . . . Ap. xiii-1

Informal American Everyday usage . . . . Ap. xiii-3

Notes on the Term MIND . . . . Ap. xiii-8

American Slang Extreme Informality . . . . Ap. xiii-9

Appendix xiii   Only In America!
(Americanisms, Informal American, American Slang)

Americanisms English Peculiar To The United States

A acclimate   air coach   all-round   alter *(To castrate.)* alumna alumnus   American League apartment house   armory   assistant professor   associate professor   automat
B baby carriage   baby sitter   backhouse *(A privy.)* backstop backtrack bailiwick *(Area of competence.)* ballcarrier ballplayer barbecue or barbeque bayou /bī-ōō/   beach buggy bleachers *(Outdoor seating.)* Bloody Mary   blue laws   bogus bonanza boom *(Economic spurt.)* boost booster bootleg bossism brain-injured brash break *(Attempt to escape.)* bronco buckaroo bullpen bunny hop burlesque bushwhack bushwhacker buster *(Little boy.)*
C caboose cafe campus can *(Container.)* careen carport casket cavort   chain store check in   check on   check out   chief of staff chifforobe chore chuck wagon claim jumper clambake   class day   class *(Grade in school.)* closet cobbler *(A fruit pie.)*   coffee break Congressional district   dumbwaiter   cookie   Corn Belt   corn husking   corn shuck cotillion   cotton belt   coulee *(Deep gulch.)* covered wagon   cowboy   cracker crapshooter   crawler *(Insect.)* crew cut   crosstie *(Railroad track support.)*
D davenport   deck *(Of playing cards.)* deer lick   degree mill Democrat dessert dicker *(To haggle.)* dime novel dishtowel district court dollar-a-year man double-decker double-header   drawn butter   dropout   dude   dude ranch   duplex apartment
E elevator   end table   escalator clause   Executive Mansion   executive officer executive session   eye opener
F Fair Deal fall *(Autumn.)* fender filibuster filling station firebreak firebug firehouse fire sale firewarden first-class *(Mail.)* first floor *(Ground floor.)* first lady fix *(To prepare food.)* flapjack   flatcar   forty-niner   the four hundred   frappé   freight train full professor
G gas station general delivery glare *(Smooth.)* glary *(Slippery.)* God's country go-devil *(Hauling sled.)* go-kart gondola car   goober *(A peanut.)* grab bag grader *(E.g., 3ʳᵈ grader.)* graft graham cracker grain elevator Grange *(Agricultural association.)* grip *(Suitcase; stage hand.)* grits *(Hominy grits.)* grocery gulch gumdrop

H haberdasher hackman hallway hard-core *(Inflexible.)* haze *(To initiate in a humiliating manner.)* headcheese henchman highball *(A drink.)* hobo homestead hoodlum Hoosier hootenanny House of Representatives hung jury husking bee

I indicia /in-<u>dish</u>-ə/ *(Envelope marking replacing stamp.)* interlocutor intermission

J jellybean jog *(Turn in road; surface projection.)* johnnycake joint resolution jump bail junket

K kangaroo court key club

L ladies' auxiliary laker land bank laundromat laid off *(Fired from job.)* legal holiday levee lieutenant governor lightning bug lobby *(To exert influence on representatives.)* loyalty oath lyceum

M major *(Area of study.)* major league manual training marina meat packing Memorial Day midyear *(An exam.)* midterm minor *(Secondary area of study.)* minor league Model T mortician motel mush *(Porridge.)*

N National League nickelodeon nightstick nip and tuck *(Very close.)*

O one-night-stand on hand outhouse overly oxford *(Shoe.)*

P packing plant pandowdy pants *(Trousers.)* parish patio Peace Corps phase out picayune piggybacking *(Truck bodies on railroad cars.)* pitcher *(Liquid holder.)* plain people platter *(A dish.)* pocket veto pole cat *(Skunk.)* porter post *(Local veterans' organization.)* potato chip prairie schooner predicate *(Base an argument on.)* primary *(Election.)* private school prowl car pry *(With a lever.)* public school

Q quack grass quadrillion quintillion

R rain check raise *(To rear children.)* raising bee ranch house range *(Grazing land.)* raring *(Eager.)* Realtor Reconstruction period released time reminisce report card Republican rewrite man riffle *(A shoal.)* right-to-work-law robe *(Blanket.)* roller coaster rooming house roommate rope *(A lasso.)* rotgut *(Inferior whisky.)* roughrider Rough Riders roundup rowboat rush *(Fraternity consideration.)*

S salesclerk salesgirl saloon salt lick seafood sectional *(Sofa; athletic contest step.)* section gang security risk senior high school septillion sextillionth shade *(Window covering.)* shivaree shoofly sideman sidewalk side wall *(Car tire.)* sit in on skulduggery slicker *(Coat.)* slumlord slush fund small change sneak preview soapbox derby social *(Informal gathering.)* social security social studies solitaire *(Card game.)* space heater special delivery spectator sport speed trap spoils system sportscaster square-dance state part State policeman State trooper steam table stickball stickpin stoop *(Platform at door.)* store *(A shop.)* stretchpants subway summer theater sundown suspenders swatter *(Good ball hitter.)* swimming hole swimming pool

T take-home pay taxi dancer teachers college team teaching ten-gallon hat Thanksgiving Day thruway thumbtack tie *(Timber for railroad track.)* toilet traffic circle treasury note trolley car truant officer truck farm tuxedo twister *(A tornado.)*

U underpants underpass unemployment insurance

V vacant lot variety store vest Veterans Day veterinarian vigilance committee vigilante vocalise

W warden wiener wildcat bank wine whey wrangle *(To herd cattle.)*

A across the board   acres *(A large amount.)*   act *(A pose.)*   act up   ad   add up *(Make sense.)*   ad-lib *(Improvise.)*   alibi *(An excuse.)*   all thumbs   almighty *(Extreme.)*   almighty dollar   along about   also-ran   angel *(A financial backer.)*   argufy   auto

B babe *(Inexperienced person.)*   bach it *(Live as a bachelor.)*   bag and baggage   ballyhoo   bamboozle   bang *(Spurt of activity.)*   bank on   bark *(To cough.)*   bark up the wrong tree   barnstorm   bash *(To hit; a party.)*   baste *(To thrash.)*   beat *(Fatigued.)*   Beat Generation   beatnik   beat up   be in for it   bellhop   bellybutton   belt *(To strike.)*   be on easy street   be onto   bends *(Caisson disease.)*   better half   be up against   be up on   bib and tucker   bighead   big top   bigwig   bike   billy goat   bite *(A light meal.)*   blat *(To blurt out.)*   bleed *(Take excess money.)*   blimp *(A dirigible; a large person.)*   blind date   blockbuster   blow *(To melt a fuse.)*   blow a fuse *(Lose self control.)*   blow hot and cold *(Vacillate.)*   blow up *(Lose one's temper.)*   bluegrass   blue streak   bobble *(To fumble.)*   bobbysoxer   boondoggle   booster shot   booze   boozer   bosh *(Nonsense.)*   boss   botheration   bounce *(Vivacity.)*   bound *(Resolved.)*   boy friend   bra   brain child   brainstorm   brass tacks *(Basic facts.)*   bread and butter *(Livelihood.)*   break *(An opportunity.)*   break even   break up   breather   brick *(A fine person.)*   bromide *(A platitude.)*   bromidic *(Trite.)*   broncobuster   bruiser   brunch   bub   buck *(Carefree young man.)*   buck *(To object.)*   buck fever   buck up   bud *(Young man or boy.)*   buddy   bug *(A germ.)*   bullpen   bull session   bunch *(A group.)*   bunco *(A swindle.)*   bunk *(Bed.)*   burg *(A small town.)*   burgle *(To commit burglary.)*   burnout   burp   bus *(To do the work of a bus boy.)*   bushed   butt   butter up   buzz *(To fly an airplane low; to call on the telephone.)*   by the skin of one's teeth

C cabby   caboodle *(Collection.)*   calaboose *(A jail.)*   call down *(To reprimand.)*   call girl   card *(Witty person.)*   carhop   carry the ball   cash in on   catch on   cave man *(A brutal man.)*   channel surfing   charley horse   cheap *(Stingy.)*   cheeky *(Impudent.)*   chesty *(Proud.)*   chintzy *(Cheap, trashy.)*   chip in   chipper   choosy   chuck *(To throw away.)*   chucklehead   chummy   chump   chunk *(Stocky person.)*   chute *(A parachute.)*   circus *(Uncontrolled situation.)*   civvies   clamp down *(Become stricter.)*   clean up *(To finish.)*   clear out   cleavage   cliffhanger   close call   close shave   cock-and-bull story   cockiness   cocky   coed   cold shoulder   cold storage   colossal *(Beyond understanding.)*   combo   come through   come up with   come-at-able *(Accessible.)*   comeback   comer *(One who shows promise.)*   comeuppance *(Deserved punishment.)*   coming-out *(Presenting a debutante to society; a homosexual from the closet.)*   complected *(Complexioned.)*   commie *(A Communist.)*   confab   conk out   connect *(Hit a ball.)*   connected *(To have influential friends.)*   conniption fit   contraption   cookout   cook up *(Invent, concoct.)*   coon's age *(A very long time.)*   co-op   cop *(A policeman.)*   corky *(Lively.)*   corral *(To capture.)*   cotton to   cotton up to   cowpuncher   cox *(Coxswain.)*   coz *(Cousin.)*   crab *(To find fault.)*   crack *(To break down; break into; find a solution; a resounding blow; an attempt; witty or sarcastic remark; a moment; a skilled person; an illegal drug.)*   crackdown   cracked *(Crazy.)*   crack shot   crackup *(Mental breakdown.)*   crank *(Grouchy person.)*   crash a party   crash course   crazy *(Unpredictable.)*   crib notes   crick *(Creek.)*   critter   crosspatch   cup of tea *(Favorite activity.)*   cuss   cussed *(Mean.)*   cut *(A criticism.)*   cut a class   cut down *(Berate.)*   cute   cutie   cutoffs *(Shorts.)*   cutup *(A joker.)*

D dad   daddy   daffy   daft   damned *(Very.)*   damndest   dander   dandy   dang *(Damn.)*   darn *(Damn.)*   darndest   date *(Social appointment; person met with.)*   dawdle   deadhead   deadwood   debunk deliver the goods deuce *(The devil; bad luck.)* dickens *(The devil.)* diddle didy *(Diaper.)* dig *(A slur.)* dig in dingbat dingus *(A gadget.)* dinky dirty work *(Deceit.)* dish *(An enjoyment.)* disk jockey disremember dive *(A cheap place.)* do-gooder dog's life do-it-yourself dollop *(A serving.)* done for done in doodad doodle doodlebug doohickey do over dope addict dope ring dope sheet dopey dorm *(Dormitory.)* dose *(Amount of something.)* do time double up double date double-decker *(Sandwich.)* double-date doughboy *(W.W. I soldier.)* douse down *(Depressed; to swallow quickly.)* down on drag one's feet dratted dressing-down *(A scolding.)* dressy drive *(Energy.)* duds Dutch treat *(Each pays own way.)* **E** eat crow *(To back down.)* ego *(Self-centeredness.)* el *(Elevated train.)* elbow grease emcee *(M.C., master of ceremonies.)* emote empty *(Hungry.)* enthuse euchre *(To outwit.)* every so often every which way exam *(Examination.)*

F fake fall down on *(To fail in.)* fall for *(Be deceived by; to fall in love with.)* fall guy falsies faze *(Disturb.)* feel like feisty fetching fifty-fifty figure *(To think; believe.)* fill someone in on fill the bill finagle a fine how-do-you-do fire *(To dismiss.)* firebug first-rate first sergeant fistful fit *(Suitable.)* fiver *($5.00.)* fix *(To repair; to prearrange outcome.)* fixings flabbergast flapper flapjack flat *(Airless car tire.)* flats *(A woman's shoes.)* flimflam *(To trick.)* flip-flop flop *(Failure.)* floppy flu *(Influenza.)* flunk flustrate folks folksy fool around fool away fool with forty winks frank frat *(Fraternity.)* frazzle Frenchy fresh *(Impudent.)* fridge *(Refrigerator.)* frill Frisco *(San Francisco.)* fuddy-duddy funnies funny papers fuss-budget **G** gab gabby gadabout galley west *(Out of position.)* game *(Lame.)* gas *(Gasoline.)* gatecrasher gawk gay *(Homosexual.)* get *(To understand; obtain advantage.)* get a load of get a move on get a rise out of *(To get a reaction from.)* get around get around to get by get even get it *(Understand; be punished.)* get one's dander up get on one's nerves get on the bandwagon get the goods on get the hang of get there get through get-together get under one's skin get-up GI GI Joe ginger *(Pep.)* girl friend giveaway give it a tumble give the cold shoulder to gob go bad gobbledygook go Dutch go for *(To attack; to be attracted to.)* go-getter go haywire goings on gold mine *(Great profit.)* goodies go off on a tangent go off the deep end go on *(To chatter.)* go one better than go steady go straight *(To reform oneself.)* go to bat for go to pieces gouge *(To cheat)* go with *(To date.)* grad *(A graduate)* grand *(Excellent.)* granddad grandma grandpa grand slam *(Home run with bases loaded; take all the tricks in bridge.)* grandstand play granny graveyard shift great *(Excellent.)* greenhorn green light *(Approval.)* grill *(Cross-examine.)* grind *(Hard work.)* gripe *(Complain.)* groggy grouch grouse grubstake gumption guy gym *(Gymnasium.)* gyp *(To swindle,* prejudicial term.*)* **H** hack *(Taxicab.)* hades *(Hell.)* hair-raiser halfcocked ham *(Radioman.)* hangover hangup hanky-panky hard *(Verified;* e.g., "The hard facts."*)* hard-hat hard sell hard-shell hard up has-been have a skeleton in the closet have it in for someone have it made have-nots have someone's number have something on someone 3 *(A detective.)* hellion he-man hick hickey hide-out high *(Intoxicated.)* high and mighty highbrow highfalutin high sign hike up hillbilly hippety-hop hippo *(Hippopotamus.)* hit the high spots hit the road hock *(To pawn.)* hockshop hoe-down hog *(Glutton.)* hog-tie hold down a job hold out for holdover holdup *(A robbery.)* hold water *(Be valid.)* holler holier-than-thou homer hook, line, and sinker *(Entirely.)* hooky hoot *(Insignificant amount;* e.g., "I don't give a hoot."*)* horse sense host *(To entertain.)* hot *(Controversial; very new.)* hot cakes *(Disposed of quickly;*

E.g., "They went like hot cakes.") hot dog hound *(To pester.)* howdy huddle *(Small conference.)* humming *(Very active.)* hunch hunk *(Lump; a good-looking man.)* hush money husky hypo *(Hypodermic injection, a syringe; sodium thiosulfate used in developing photographs.)*

I iffy *(Uncertain.)* immy *(A marble.)* in *(Position of favor.)* in a bind *(In a difficult situation.)* in cog *(Incognito.)* in Dutch *(In trouble.)* in-law *(A relative by marriage.)* in step *(In agreement.)* intercom in the buff *(Naked.)* in the clear in the hole *(In debt.)* in the raw in the red *(Operating at a loss.)* in trouble *(Pregnant & unmarried.)* it beats me *(It baffles me.)* It's me. *(It is I.)*

J jalopy jam *(Trouble.)* jamboree jam-packed jam session jaw *(To talk.)* jawbreaker jayvee *(Junior varsity.)* jaywalk jazz up jeans jell jerkwater jibe with *(Agree.)* jiffy Johnny-come-lately Johnny-on-the-spot joiner jollify joy ride judgmatic junk *(To discard.)* junk food

K keep in with keep it under your hat kick *(To complain.)* kick around kick in kick upstairs kid *(Youngster; to joke with.)* knock about knock off know-how know-it-all know the ropes *(To be familiar with.)* know the score K ration

L lab *(Laboratory; labrador retriever.)* lame duck land-office-business land-poor last word *(Most fashionable.)* lay for *(Be ready to attack.)* lay it on thick lay off lay over layout lazybones legwork let on letdown let off steam let someone have it letterman letup level best lick *(To defeat.)* a lick and a promise lickety-split lie low light into the limit *(To an outrageous extent.)* loads *(Much.)* loan shark loblolly *(Mudhole.)* loco *(Crazy.)* logy /lō-gē/ *(Lethargic.)* lone wolf long johns long shot looby *(A lout.)* looks *(Appearance.)* look up *(Locate someone; visit.)* loony lose out on lot on the ball lounge lizard lummox lunkhead

M ma mad *(Angry.)* mad about *(Infatuated.)* maitre d' make a pass make the fur fly make the grade make-up *(Second exam.)* make up to man-sized massacre *(Crushing sports defeat.)* maverick maw medic mean *(Nasty.)* medico meet up with memo menace *(Troublesome person.)* menfolk me-tooism metro middy *(A midshipman; a blouse.)* middling miffed mike *(Microphone.)* missis missy mister mixer *(A dance.)* mix-up *(A fight.)* mob *(Gang of hoodlums.)* mom moniker *(One's name.)* monkey around monkey wrench *(A disruption in normal procedure.)* monumental moony *(Dreamy.)* moppet motorbike moviegoer mule *(Stubborn person.)* mule skinner mum *(Ma'am)* mumbo jumbo Murphy's Law *(Whatever possibly can go wrong, will.)* mushy muss mussy muzzy *(Muddled.)*

N nab *(Catch; arrest.)* Nam *(Vietnam.)* nanny *(Female goat; Brit. child's nurse.)* natural *(Having a special gift.)* neck of the woods needle *(To tease.)* nervy new wrinkle *(An ingenious idea.)* nightcap night crawler nights *(At night.)* nightspot nighty nit-pick nobody's fool noggin no go no great shakes noncom nonsked noodle *(The head.)* nosher *(Junk food eater.)* no spring chicken nosy not bat an eye notch *(Level, degree.)* nothing doing not worth a whoop nub *(Core point.)* number one nylons

O obit *(Obituary.)* off of *(No longer using.)* off the beam old codger old maid old-timer on account of one-horse town one-track mind on the go open-and-shut on target on the beam on the button on the double on the level on the make on the rebound on the spot on the wagon *(Off of alcohol.)* on top of the world oodles operative *(Secret agent.)* outfit out from under out of this world out of sorts outsmart over a barrel

P pa paddywhack painkiller pal pan *(Criticize.)* panhandle pass out pass the buck pass up payoff peanut *(Small person.)* pee *(Urine.)* peewee peg *(To throw.)* pep peppy pep talk perk *(Percolate.)* perks *(Perquisites.)* persnickety pesky peter out phone photo

Ap. xiii-5

pickle *(Difficulty.)*   pick a fight   pick at   pick-me-up *(A drink.)*   pick on   pickup *(Renewed activity; something that stimulates.)*   piffle   pigskin *(A football.)*   pinch-hit *(Substitute.)*   in the pink   pinkie *(Little finger.)*   pins *(Legs.)*   pip-squeak   pitch in   platter *(Phonograph record.)*   play ball   playboy   play hooky   play the field   play up *(Emphasize)*   play up to   plug *(Worn-out horse.)*   plug along   plunk   Podunk *(Dull small town.)*   polio *(Poliomyelitis.)*   politick   pot *(Sum of money.)*   possum *(Opossum.)*   potboiler   powwow *(A meeting.)*   preachify   prep *(Preparatory.)*   pressure *(To compel.)*   pretty *(To a degree, e.g. pretty big.)*   priceless   prima donna *(Vain person.)*   prissy   private eye   pro *(Professional.)*   prof *(Professor.)*   prom *(Promenade.)*   pronto (Sp.)   prop *(Propeller.)*   props *(Properties in a stage show.)*   punch line   pushy   pussy *(Cat.)*   put a crimp in   put over *(Accomplish.)*   put-up *(Prearranged.)*

Q   quad *(Quadrangle.)*   quit *(To resign.)*

R   rack up   railroad *(Rush without deliberation.)*   raise the devil   raise the dickens   raise hell   raise the roof   raise a rumpus   rambunctious   rat's nest   rattle *(Confuse.)*   raving   real *(Very, e.g., real tired.)*   real buy *(A bargain.)*   real-life   reckon   redeye express   red-handed   register *(Make an impression.)*   renege /ri-nig/   revenuer   ride *(To tease.)*   rile *(To vex.)*   roast *(Criticize; ridicule.)*   rob the cradle   roll in *(Congregate.)*   roll up *(Amass.)*   romance *(To woo; make love to.)*   romp *(An easy win.)*   rooter *(Supporter.)*   rope in *(Deceive.)*   rot *(Nonsense.)*   rotten *(Worthless.)*   rough out *(Make preliminary sketch.)*   rough up   roundup   roust   roustabout   rumpus   runaway *(An easy victory.)*   run rings around   rustle *(Steal cattle.)*

S   sacred cow *(Something above criticism.)*   sad *(Pitiful.)*   sail into *(Proceed to action.)*   saleslady   salt *(A sailor.)*   salt away   sandwich man *(A man wearing advertising boards.)*   sashay   sass   say uncle   sax   say-so   scab *(A striker's replacement.)*   scads   scalawag   scalp *(Resell tickets at a profit.)*   scary   scat   schoolmarm   scoot   scorcher   script (v)   sculpt   sea legs   second-string   see stars   sell someone on   sellout   semi *(A semitrailer.)*   send to the showers   send up *(To sentence to prison.)*   sense *(To comprehend.)*   setup   sexy   shack   shake a leg   shake down   shake up   shape up   sharpie   shellout   shenanigans   shimmy *(A chemise.)*   shinny *(To climb.)*   shoo-in   shot *(Injection; portion of liquor; rocket firing; ruined; worn out.)*   show *(Theatrical performance.)*   showoff   show up *(To outdo.)*   shuck *(To take off.)*   shucks   shut up   shy *(Lacking.)*   shy of *(A little less.)*   sidewalk superintendent   simmer down   sis   sissified   sissy   sit on *(To suppress information.)*   sit tight   sitting duck   sitting pretty   six-shooter   sizzler   sixty-four dollar question   size up   skedaddle   skunk *(Hateful person.)*   skyman *(An aviator.)*   slack-off   slather *(Daub thickly.)*   sleeper *(Unexpected success.)*   sleuth   slew *(Large number of.)*   slick *(Clever.)*   slip-up   slob   sloppy   slow *(Dull witted.)*   slowpoke   slug *(To hit.)*   slumgullion *(A stew.)*   small potatoes   smart aleck   smashing *(Impressive.)*   smidgen   smithereens   smoke *(Use a cigarette.)*   smoothie   snap *(Easy.)*   snap out of it   sneaker *(Sports shoe.)*   sniffy   snip   snippy   snit   snoop   snoopy   snoot   snooty   snooze   snort *(Laugh.)*   snuff out   sniffles   snuffles   so *(Very; apparently.)*   so-and-so   socialite   socialize   soft *(Easy.)*   soft-pedal   soft sell   soft-soap   softy   solid *(Certain support.)*   someplace *(Somewhere.)*   sonny   sore *(Offended.)*   sore spot   sort of   soupy *(Sentimental.)*   sow one's wild oats   spark plug *(Group leader.)*   specifics   specs   spell *(Distance; of weather; of illness.)*   spike *(Add alcohol.)*   spill the beans   spitting image   spit and polish   splash *(Striking impression.)*   splashy   splurge *(Spend money lavishly.)*   sponge *(One who lives off of others.)*   spoof   spook   sport *(To show off clothes.)*   sporting chance   spot *(To recognize.)*   spotter *(Official observer.)*   spread *(A feast.)*

spud *(A potato.)* spunk spunky squally *(Threatening trouble.)* square *(Honest.)* square deal square meal square shooter squeak by squelch squirt *(Young person.)* squish staffer stag line stall *(Delay.)* standee standoff *(A tie, as in a game.)* standout stay put step on *(Subdue.)* step on it step out stick *(Dull person; conductor's baton; mast of ship.)* sticker *(A puzzle.)* stick-in-the-mud the sticks *(Obscure rural district.)* stick up for stinks *(Bad quality.)* stone-broke stooge stop off stop over story *(A lie.)* storyteller *(A liar.)* straddle *(To favor both sides.)* straight *(A heterosexual.)* straight from the shoulder straightman straight-out *(Unreserved; very busy.)* strapper strapping straw boss strike it rich string along strings *(Conditions to a gift.)* string up striper *(One whose uniform has a certain number of ranking stripes.)* strobe light strong-arm stuck on stuck-up study up on stuff stuffed shirt stuffy stump *(To baffle.)* stunner stunt *(A feat.)* sub *(Substitute; submarine; sandwich.)* sure-enough sure-fire swap swear off sweat it out sweet potato *(An ocarina.)* swell *(First rate.)* swig swing *(Manage a deal; execute by hanging; n., big band jazz.)* swing shift

T tacky tad tail *(To follow.)* tailgate party tails *(Reverse side of coin; dress suit.)* take a shine to take it easy take it out on take-in *(To cheat; to visit on a tour.)* takeoff *(Caricature; depart.)* takedown *(Humiliate.)* take up with talking-to *(A scolding.)* talking through your hat tan *(To flog.)* tangle with tarp *(Tarpaulin.)* tear down tear into teeny tell off tell on tenderfoot termer thingamabob thingamajig throw in the sponge throw in the towel thumbs down thumb a ride thump *(To beat.)* tickle *(To amuse.)* tidy sum tie into tie-up *(Connection.)* tip-off tipster tiptop to-do *(Confusion.)* togs *(Clothes.)* top dog top-drawer topnotch top sergeant tossup tote *(To carry.)* tote bag tother *(The other.)* tough *(Unfortunate.)* touristy tout traffic cop traipse trimming *(A defeat.)* trip *(A drug experience.)* tripe *(Nonsense.)* triple threat trounce trustbuster tryout tunesmith tune-up turn down turn in turn loose turnoff *(Road exit; something highly uninteresting.)* twit two bits *(25¢)* two-fisted tycoon tyke typo

U ugly *(Quarrelsome.)* under the weather undies up and around up a tree up in the air upped *(Made better or larger.)* upper *(Top berth.)* uppish upper crust up the creek up to snuff

V vacate vacuum *(To use a vacuum cleaner.)* vamp *(To seduce.)* vet *(Veteran; veterinarian.)* visiting fireman *(An important visitor to a city shown special treatment.)* vittles

W wad *(Large amount.)* wagon *(Patrol wagon.)* walking papers walkout *(A strike.)* walkout on walk-up *(Apartment with no elevator access.)* wallop wallflower wangle want ad war horse washed-out *(Exhausted.)* way back weasel out welcome mat well-fixed weenie *(A wiener.)* wetback wet blanket whack whang what's what whiffet whip *(To defeat.)* whip up whirl *(Brief trip; an attempt.)* whistle stop whodunit whole kit and caboodle whop *(To strike.)* whopper wild and woolly windbag windfall wishy-washy witch hunt workout wow wrap-up *(A summary.)* write-in write-up wryneck

Y yammer *(Whimper.)* Yank yarn *(A doubtful story.)* yawp *(Yawn audibly.)* yeah *(Yes.)* yen *(Desire.)* yep *(Yes.)* yes man

Z zing zip *(Energy.)* zippy

Notes on the term MIND

Ever since the French philosopher, René Descartes (1596-1650), made his famous BODY (extended--*takes up space*) and MIND (unextended--*takes up no space*) distinction (*dualism*), philosophers and psychologists have struggled with the concept. The mind is not the brain said Descartes, since the brain takes up space and is therefore part of the body. Language philosophers have long looked to how a word is used in a language for clues to its real meaning. I think the following term listing will illustrate that no real insight into the concept of "mind" can be gleaned from such a listing. It seems "mind" usage only seeks to cover up our ignorance and in this single case seems to confound the language philosophers. These expressions are all idioms. Their meanings are apparent, but taken literally these expressions are, to say the least, puzzling.

You've **changed your mind**? I'm sorry; it **slipped my mind**. I've had it **on my mind** all day, in the **back of my mind** all night. I **have a mind to** leave! I'll **keep it in mind**. **Keep your mind on** the road. I think I'm **losing my mind**! Surely he is **out of his mind**. I'd say definitely not in his **right mind**. Finally, **peace of mind**. He gave her a **piece of his mind**; I hope he could spare it! You know, she has a **mind of her own.** Whose else might it be? We are of **one mind.** I'm **of two minds** on the subject. You might say a **divided mind** or **split mind**. I have **a good mind to** tell all! But then I have **half a mind** to say nothing. Come on--**make up your mind!** **Bear in mind** that nothing happens without a cause.. Wow! That **blows my mind.** His **mind-set** really will not allow it. She went to a **mind reader.** Why bother? I can **read her mind** like a book. I wish I had had the **presence of mind** to say the right thing. Please keep an **open mind** on this. How **open-minded** can I be? **Close-minded** is more like it. I have concluded that he is very **narrow-minded.** She is more **broad-minded** than most. That proves it; your **mind's in the gutter.** Yep, I got a **dirty mind**, sometimes even a **filthy mind.** He was the **master mind** of the crime, but the **tough-minded** police will get him. Even though they are both very **strong-minded**, they had a true **meeting of minds.** That's a **mind-altering** drug. Really, I'd say **mind-expanding.** Whatever, his **mind is wasted.** **A mind is a terrible thing to waste** (in more ways than one). That's a **mind-bender.** I can see it in my **mind's eye.** Who knows the **mind of man** (or of woman)? **Cultivated minds** are rare. **Liberal minds** have their place. Einstein had one of the **great minds** of our century. She has a very, very **good mind.** Yes, a **fine mind** and I'd add a **discerning mind** to that too. It takes a **logical mind** to do mathematics. Yes, the boy has a **keen mind.** More than that---a **razor-sharp mind.** They didn't get along; she had a **renaissance mind**, he a **medieval mind.** Further than that, he boasted a **crude mind.** Oh well, let's say it: a **Neanderthal mind.** Sad. Another case: she had a **scientific mind**, he a **musical mind.** He has a really **sick mind**; possibly a **perverted mind.** If not those, certainly a **twisted mind** or if you prefer, a **warped mind.** He's in a bad **frame of mind. Mind** the children. **Mind** your manners. **Mind you** now, not a word. Do you **mind** the noise? **I don't mind** at all. How many times do I have to **remind** you? That was a **mindless** act! Be more **mindful** next time. **Divine Mind** is omnipresent. Note: That the **brain** and **mind** are different concepts, can be shown by trying to substitute "brain" for "mind" in the above expressions. It just doesn't work!

A ace in the hole *(A hidden advantage.)* all-fired *(Excessive.)* all wet *(Quite wrong.)* ambulance chaser *(A lawyer who persuades an injured person to sue.)* ammo *(Ammunition.)* angle *(Selfish motive.)* ante *(Pay one's share.)* apple polisher *(One who seeks favor by flattery.)* applesauce *(Nonsense.)* ash can *(A depth bomb.)*

B babe *(A girl.)* bagman *(Money collector for racketeers.)* baloney *(Nonsense.)* bang *(Enjoyment.)* bangtail *(A race horse.)* bang-up job *(Did excellent work.)* barfly *(One who hangs around taverns.)* barker *(A sideshow announcer.)* barrel along *(Move fast.)* bash *(A party.)* bats *(Batty.)* bats in the belfry *(Crazy.)* battle-ax *(A nagging woman.)* battlewagon *(A battleship.)* batty *(Crazy; odd.)* bawl out *(To scold.)* bean *(To hit on the head.)* beat it *(Get out!)* beaut *(Something outstanding.)* beef *(A complaint; muscle.)* behind the eight ball *(To be in an awkward situation.)* be in the money *(To have lots of money.)* bellyache *(Complain.)* bellyful *(All one can endure.)* bender *(A drinking spree.)* be on the ball *(To be very competent.)* be on the up and up *(To be honest.)* better half *(Spouse.)* biddy *(A gossipy woman.)* biff *(A blow.)* big blow *(A boaster.)* big gun *(An important person.)* big house *(A penitentiary.)* big shot *(An important person.)* bilge *(Stupid talk.)* binge *(A drunken spree.)* bitch *(To complain.)* blah *(Nonsense.)* blooper *(A mistake.)* blowhard *(A braggart.)* blow one's top *(To get very angry.)* blowout *(Big party.)* blow this place *(Leave.)* blow off steam *(To express pent-up emotions.)* boner *(A blunder.)* bone up *(Study hard.)* boob *(A simpleton.)* booboo *(An error.)* booby hatch *(Mental hospital.)* boot *(Dismissal.)* boondocks *(Unsophisticated area away from the city.)* bootlick *(A flatterer.)* bop *(To hit.)* borscht circuit *(Summer resorts in the Catskill Mountains.)* bottom dollar *(One's last bit of money.)* bounce *(Check rejected; eject someone.)* bouncer *(One who ejects unruly persons.)* brain *(An intelligent person; v. to hit on the head.)* brass hat *(A high official.)* brawl *(An extended fight.)* breadbasket *(The stomach.)* breeze *(An easy task; v. go quickly.)* the briny *(The sea.)* broad *(A woman.)* Bronx cheer *(Expelling air with the tongue out.)* brush off *(v. to dismiss abruptly.)* brush-off *(n.)* buck *($1.00)* buck for *(To try for.)* buck private *(A private in the U.S. Army.)* buffalo *(To hoodwink; deceive.)* bug *(An enthusiast; a minor defect; a wiretap; v. to annoy.)* bug-eyed *(Very surprised.)* buggy *(Crazy.)* bughouse *(An insane asylum.)* bull *(Nonsense.)* bulldoze *(To bully.)* bum *(A tramp.)* bummer *(An offensive, unwanted event.)* bump *(To displace.)* bump off *(To murder.)* a bundle *(Much money.)* bunk *(Nonsense.)* burn *(Electrocute; to cheat.)* burn up *(Become enraged.)* bush leaguer *(Mediocre person.)* bust *(Burst.)* button your lip *(Shut up.)* by the numbers *(To do in precise order.)*

C can *(A jail; a toilet; v. to fire from a job.)* canned music *(Recorded music.)* caper *(A crime.)* carry the torch for *(To love someone who does not love you.)* case *(Look over.)* cash in *(Die.)* champ *(Champion.)* con *(Convict.)* cheesy *(Inferior.)* chew out *(Admonish.)* chew the fat *(To converse at length.)* chew the rag *(To converse at length.)* chick *(A young woman.)* chicken *(Coward.)* chicken out *(Back out of an intended action.)* chicken feed *(Very little money.)* chill out *(To calm down.)* chisel *(To cheat.)* chopper *(A helicopter.)* chow *(Food.)* chowhound *(One who loves to eat.)* divvy up chutzpah /hŏŏts-pə/ *(Brazen effrontery.)* cinch *(Easy; sure.)* clam up *(To be quiet.)* class *(Elegance.)* classy *(With style.)* clean house *(To reform.)* clean up *(Make a big profit.)* clink *(Prison.)* clinker *(A mistake, esp. in music.)* clip *(To cheat.)* clip joint *(A business establishment where prices are too high.)* clobber *(To beat.)* cockeyed *(Ridiculous.)* coke *(Cocaine.)*

cold turkey *(To stop drugs abruptly.)* come across *(Do what is requested.)* comeback *(Smart retort.)* come-hither look *(Flirting.)* conchy *(Conscientious objector.)* con game *(A swindle.)* conk *(To hit on the head.)* cool *(Excellent.)* con man *(Confidence man.)* cootie *(A louse.)* cop-out *(Back down.)* copper *(Policeman.)* corker *(Astonishing.)* corking *(Excellent.)* corny *(Trite.)* corn-fed *(Healthy, but rustic.)* crack a book *(To study.)* crack a smile *(To smile.)* crackerjack *(Excellent.)* crackpot *(An eccentric person.)* crack up *(Be convulsed with laughter.)* cramp one's style *(To hamper one's ordinary way of doing things.)* crap *(A lie; junk; excrement.)* cream *(To defeat.)* cream puff *(A weakling.)* creep *(A repugnant person.)* croak *(Die.)* a crock *(Nonsense.)* crocked *(Drunk.)* crony *(Friend.)* crud *(Rubbish.)* crummy *(Inferior.)* crust *(Insolence.)* cuckoo *(Crazy.)* cushy *(Comfortable.)* cut out *(Leave.)* cut up *(Be unruly.)* a cut *(A share.)*

D daylights *(Consciousness, e.g., "To shake the daylights out of him.")* deadbeat *(One who doesn't pay his bills.)* dick *(Detective.)* dig *(To like; understand.)* dimwit *(A stupid person.)* dink *(A dope.)* dip *(Pick pockets.)* dippy *(Crazy.)* discombobulate *(To get all mixed up.)* dish *(An attractive woman.)* dish it out *(To punish or reprove.)* ditch *(Avoid; get rid of.)* divvy up *(To divide equally.)* dogface *(Infantryman.)* do in *(Kill.)* dope *(A drug; dull-witted person; inside information.)* dope out *(Figure out.)* dose *(Venereal infection.)* double in brass *(Adept beyond one's specialty.)* double whammy *(An extra hardship.)* drag *(A puff on a cigarette; something boring; special influence.)* drip *(Uninteresting person.)* drippy *(Stupid; silly.)* duffer *(A clumsy old man.)* dukes *(Fists.)* dumbbell *(A stupid person.)* dumb cluck *(A stupid person.)* dump *(A shabby place.)*

E eager beaver *(One enthusiastic in a certain endeavor.)* easy touch *(One who will loan money with little thought.)* eats *(Food.)* egghead *(An intellectual.)* erase *(To kill.)*

F face the music *(To accept the consequences of one's actions.)* fanny *(The buttocks.)* far-out *(Involving daring thinking.)* fat cat *(A wealthy person.)* fed up *(Disgusted with the situation.)* -fest *(Gabfest, slugfest, Oktoberfest, etc.)* filthy lucre *(Money.)* fin *($5.00)* finger *(To turn into police.)* fink *(Jerk; strikebreaker.)* fireball *(Energetic person.)* fix *(A corrupt prearranged outcome; a heroin injection; v. to neuter an animal.)* fix someone's wagon *(To ruin.)* flack *(Criticism.)* flap *(A crisis.)* flasher *(A public exhibitionist.)* flatfoot *(A policeman.)* flivver *(An old, battered car.)* flummox *(To confuse.)* floozy *(A dizzy woman.)* fly-by-night *(A debtor who departs secretly.)* fly the coop *(To escape.)* fork over *(To pay or give up something.)* foul up *(To make a mess of things.)* fourflusher *(A fake; cheat.)* frame *(To set someone up.)* freeloader *(One who lives at the expense of others.)* fresh out of *(The product is sold out.)* fried *(On drugs.)* frisk *(To search someone.)* frosh *(Freshman.)* on the fritz *(Inoperative.)* fruity *(Effeminate.)*

G gaff *(n. ridicule.)* gag *(Joke.)* gaga /gä-gä/ *(Foolish.)* gal *(A girl.)* galoot *(An awkward fellow.)* gam *(Leg.)* gang up on *(A group attacking one person.)* a gas *(Something out of the ordinary.)* gasbag *(Talkative person.)* gat *(Gun.)* geek *(A weird person.)* geezer *(A crusty old man.)* gelt *(Money.)* gent *(Gentleman.)* get a fair shake *(Get just treatment.)* get away with murder *(To do the worst kind of deeds without getting caught.)* get back at *(To get revenge.)* get in someone's hair *(To continually bother someone.)* get one's goat *(To antagonize someone.)* get the gate *(To be rejected.)* get the jump on *(To have a head start.)* get the sack *(Be fired.)* get the shaft *(To be tricked or cheated.)* gig *(A demerit; musician's employment.)* gimmick *(A special consideration to make an endeavor more effective.)* gimmicky *(Overly complicated.)* gimpy *(Having a limp.)* gink *(An odd person.)* gin mill *(A saloon.)* gismo *(Special gadget, gimmick.)*

give someone the eye *(To look admiringly.)* glad eye *(Flirtatious glance.)* glad hand *(Insincere greeting.)* glad rags *(One's best clothes.)* goat *(Scapegoat.)* gob *(Sailor.)* go easy on *(Use with moderation.)* go great guns *(Work efficiently, quickly.)* goldbrick *(One who avoids work.)* gold digger goo good egg good Joe gooey goof goof off goofy gook goon goop goose *(A playful prod.)* goose egg *(A zero; a bump on the head.)* go peddle your papers *(Mind your own business.)* gopher *("A go-for", helper.)* go places *(Succeed.)* go to town *(Act with speed.)* grand *($1,000)* gravy train *(Profitable, easy work.)* grease monkey *(Car mechanic.)* grease the palm greaser greasy spoon Greek *(A member of a fraternity or sorority.)* grifter *(A swindler.)* grind *(Hip gyration.)* grub *(Food; v. to scrounge.)* guck guesstimate guff gumshoe *(A detective.)* gum up *(Spoil.)* gun an engine gung ho *(Chin. zealous.)* gun moll gutsy

H hackie hail Columbia hairy half a buck *(50¢)* half pint *(Little guy.)* ham *(Actor.)* hand it to *(Give praise.)* hang around hang one on *(Get drunk.)* hangout hanky-panky hardhat hash house hash mark hash slinger have a ball have a piece of *(Have a financial interest in.)* have a screw loose *(Crazy.)* have kittens *(Be very upset.)* have rocks in the head haywire *(Broken.)* haymaker hayseed heck heebie-jeebies heist hellbender *(Drunken spree.)* hell-bent heller hen party hep *(Hip; not square.)* highball *(To speed.)* hijack hijacker hinder /hīnd-er/ *(Ger. the buttocks.)* hip *(Aware.)* hipped on hippie hipster hitch a ride hit someone for a loan hit the bottle hit the deck hit the hay hit the sack hit the silk *(To parachute.)* hit the spot hog wild hokum hold your horses hombre *(Sp.)* honky-tonk hooch *(Whiskey.)* hood *(Hoodlum; neighborhood.)* hooey hoofer hooked *(Addicted.)* hooker *(A prostitute.)* hooligan hoopla hoosegow *(Jail.)* hootchy-kootchy hornswoggle horny horse *(Heroin.)* horse around horse opera *(Cowboy movie.)* hot *(In demand; exciting; lustful; skillful; lucky; stolen goods; dangerous.)* hot air hot rod hot seat huckster humdinger humungous *(Very large.)* hung up hunky-dory hypo *(Hypochondriac.)*

I in a spot in cahoots with *(Affiliated with.)* in drag *(A man dressed as a woman.)* in nothing flat in the chips in the groove in the soup *(In difficulty.)* an invite

J jazz *(Exaggerated talk; liveliness.)* jazz it up jerk the jig is up jinx the jitters jitterbug jive job *(Robbery.)* jock *(An athlete.)* jockstrap *(Athletic supporter.)* john *(Toilet.)* josh jug *(Jail)* juice *(Electricity; gasoline; strength.)* jump the gun jungle *(The inner-city.)* junk *(Narcotics.)* junkie

K kayo *(K.O., knockout.)* keep your shirt on keen *(Excellent.)* keister kickback kick the bucket *(Die.)* kick the habit kick *(A thrill.)* kiddy kill-joy kinky Knock it off! *(Stop it!)* knock off *(Kill.)* knock oneself out *(Make great effort.)* a knockout *(An impressive person.)* knock up *(Make pregnant.)* know from nothing know it cold

L lady-killer *(A man attractive to the ladies.)* lambaste lay an egg *(Fail.)* lay low lay off *(Stop teasing.)* leave *(Let.)* lefty legit *(Legitimate.)* lemon *(A bad product.)* let one's hair down *(To lose one's inhibitions.)* lick *(A jazz improvisation.)* lie down on the job lifer line *(Glib manner of speech.)* lip *(Impudent talk; sass.)* lippy litterbug live up to loaded *(Wealthy; intoxicated.)* lollapalooza *(Something very unusual.)* longhair *(One into classical music.)* looker *(A good looking person.)* look-see *(To take a close look.)* lose ones shirt louse *(Contemptible person.)* louse up *(To bungle.)* lousy *(Mean; worthless.)* lousy with *(Having plenty of, e.g. money.)* lulu lush *(A drunkard.)*

M mad money main drag make a stink make like make out malarkey masher

Ap. xiii-11

mazuma *(Money.)* mean *(Excellent.)* mib *(A marble.)* Mickey Finn *(Drugged drink.)* mig *(A marble.)* mitt *(Boxing glove.)* mix it up *(To fight.)* mobster moll *(Gangster's girl friend.)* monkey business monkeyshine monkey suit mooch moolah moon *(Expose the buttocks.)* moonlighting mop the floor with mosey mossback mouthpiece *(Lawyer.)* muckrake mug *(Face.)* mugger murder *(To defeat.)* murphy *(A potato.)* muscle in mutt muttonhead

N nail *(To catch; arrest.)* nark neat *(Wonderful.)* neck *(Kiss and caress; pet.)* necking necktie party nick someone for *(To cheat.)* nifty nighthawk nincompoop ninny nippers *(Handcuffs.)* nix *(No.)* nob *(Head.)* nobby *(Flashy.)* nope no picnic no soap no sweat not hay nudnik *(Yid.)* number *(A cute person.)* nut *(Crazy person; a head.)* nuts *(Crazy.)* nutty

O offbeat off the cuff off the hook Okie old hat old lady *(Mother; wife.)* old man *(Father; husband.)* once-over on deck on the fly on the lam on the nose on the q. t. *(Quietly; secretly.)* on the skids on the town oomph out of whack *(Out of order.)*

P pack rat paddy wagon paint the town red palooka pansy panty waist pap *(Privileges of public office.)* pard *(Partner.)* park *(To set or place.)* paste *(To hit.)* patsy pay off *(To bribe.)* payola pay through the nose peach *(Beautiful person or thing.)* peachy peanut gallery peanuts *(Small amount.)* pen *(Penitentiary.)* pet *(Kiss and caress.)* phony *(Fake.)* pickled pickup pie *(Political graft.)* pig *(A woman of loose morals.)* piker pile *(Much money.)* pill *(A bore.)* pin *(To give a fraternity pin to.)* pinch *(Arrest.)* pin on *(Accuse.)* pinhead pinko *(Communist.)* pinup pip *(Admirable person.)* pipe down pitch *(A talk to influence.)* pitchman pix *(Pictures.)* pixilated *(Drunk.)* plant *(Leave false evidence.)* plug *(Shoot a bullet into; push for a cause.)* plug-ugly plush *(Luxurious.)* poky *(Jail.)* pony *(A language translation.)* pooch *(A dog.)* pooped pork barrel pot *(Potbelly; marijuana.)* potted *(Drunk.)* powerhouse prexy *(President.)* prick *(Contemptible person.)* protection money prune *(Stupid person.)* pull *(n., influence.)* pull a gag on pull off *(Carry out; do.)* pull rank pumping iron *(Weight lifting.)* pump up *(Build muscle.)* punk *(Inferior; hoodlum.)* push *(To sell drugs.)* pusher *(Drug dealer.)* pushover puss *(Face.)* put down put on *(To deceive.)* put-on *(A hoax.)* put-put /pu̇t put/ *(Small engine.)* put the screws on *(To put pressure on someone.)* put to bed *(Go to press.)*

Q queer *(Homosexual; to spoil.)*

R rag *(Tease; scold.)* railroad *(Imprison on false charges.)* raise Cain *(Cause a disturbance.)* rake off *(Illegitimate commission.)* raspberry *(Razzberry, Bronx cheer.)* rat *(Cowardly betrayer.)* rat on rat race rattletrap razzle-dazzle real McCoy *(Authentic.)* redeye *(Inferior whiskey.)* reefer *(A marijuana cigarette.)* rep *(Representative; reputation.)* retard *(Dummy.)* riot *(Amusing person or situation.)* rip-roaring rip-roarious ripsnorter ritzy rod *(A pistol.)* roll *(Wad of money; to rob a drunk.)* roll in *(Arrive.)* rookie roughhouse roughneck rounder *(Drunkard.)* rubber check rubber *(A condom.)* rubberneck rubber-stamp rube rub it in rub out rub the wrong way ruckus rumble *(Gang fight.)* rummy *(A drunkard.)* runaround *(Deception.)*

S sack out sad sack saphead savvy sawbones sawbuck *($10.00)* sawed-off *(Less than average height.)* scat *(Meaningless syllables in jazz singing.)* schlemiel *(A bungler.)* schmaltz *(Something extremely sentimental.)* schmo *(A naive person.)* schnook *(An unimportant person.)* schnozzle *(Nose.)* shtick scoop *(Early news story.)* scram scrap *(A fight.)* scrapper scratch sheet screamer *(Headline.)* screw *(Prison guard; v. to cheat.)* scrounge scrub *(Cancel.)* scrumptious scuttlebutt *(Rumors.)* secondstory man *(A burglar.)* sell out *(Betray.)* send *(To fill with joy.)* setup *(An arranged victory.)* shackup shake *(To get away from.)* shakedown *(n., v., swindle.)* shark *(One with special skill.)* sharp *(Smart.)* shavetail *(Young 2nd lieutenant.)* shekel shellac *(To beat.)* shellacking sherlock *(A detective.)* shill *(Gambler's assistant.)* shindig shindy *(A quarrel.)* shine up to shiner *(A black eye.)* shiv *(Knife, razor.)* shooting iron shoot off one's mouth shoot the works shoot up *(Inject drugs.)* shucking bee shutterbug shuteye shylock *(A relentless creditor.)* shyster *(Unscrupulous business man or lawyer.)* sidekick simoleon *($1.00)* simp sing *(Confess to a crime.)* sinker *(A doughnut.)* skiddoo skid row skirt *(A young woman.)* skivvy shirt skunk *(To defeat soundly.)* slam *(Criticize.)* slap happy slugfest slurp smack-dab smalltime smeller smashed smooch snafu *("Situation normal, all fouled up.")* snatch *(To kidnap.)* snifter snitch snort *(A drink.)* snot snotty snow job soak *(Overcharge; a drinker.)* sob sister sob story sock *(To hit.)* soda jerk sorehead soup *(Fog; nitroglycerin.)* soup up soupy sourpuss souse speakeasy spiel *(Speech; sales talk.)* spiffy spot *(Spotlight; currency denomination, e.g., ten spot.)* spring *(To get someone out of jail.)* square *(Uninformed; unsophisticated.)* squeal *(To betray.)* squirrely stage-door Johnny stand up for stash *(Hide money.)* The States steady *(A regular date.)* steal *(A bargain.)* stewed *(Drunk.)* stick around stickup stiff *(A corpse.)* stinker stir *(A jail.)* stir crazy stoned stonewall stool pigeon string along stripper stud stumblebum sucker *(One easily deceived.)* suck in suck up to suds *(Beer.)* sugar *(Sweet one.)* sugar daddy super superduper swank swanky swing *(Have a full life.)* swinger wipe *(To steal.)*

T tab *(Total bill.)* tailgate *(Drive too closely.)* tailgate party *(Picnic at car before football game.)* take *(n., receipts; v., cheat)* take a dive take a powder *(To run away.)* take the rap talk big talk turkey tear-jerker teenybopper that's the ticket three sheets to the wind throw a fight throw a party throw in the towel throw the book at ticker *(Heart.)* tie the knot tight *(Drunk.)* tightwad tinker's damn *(Smallest bit.)* tinkle *(Urinate.)* tin lizzie tizzy toots tootsy top banana top kick topper *(A top hat.)* touch *(Ask for a loan.)* trap *(Mouth.)* trigger-happy trigger man turkey *(A failure.)* turn on *(v., to take drugs.)* turnon *(n., an excitement.)* turnoff *(A disappointment.)* twerp, twirp twit two-bit two cents' worth twofer *(Two for the price of one.)* two-time two-spot *(Unimportant person; two-dollar bill.)*

U Uncle Tom *(Having the personality of the lead character in Harriet Beecher Stowe's "Uncle Tom's Cabin.")* unmentionables *(Undergarments.)* uptight *(Anxious, tense.)*

V vamoose *(Command to leave quickly.)*

W wacky *(Irrational, screwy.)* wagon *(Battleship.)* ward heeler *(Helper to a political boss.)* wash *(Dry river bed.)* washout *(Failure.)* washed-up *(No longer successful.)* WASP *(White Anglo-Saxon Protestant.)* water rat *(A waterfront thief.)* way-out weirdo *(A freakish person.)* well heeled *(Wealthy.)* whammy *(Hex.)* wharf rat wheeler-dealer whizbang whole hog whole shebang whoop it up whoop-de-do willies wino wise up wiseacre wisecrack wisecracker woozy work over *(To beat up.)* to wow wrangle

Y yak *(To chatter.)* yap *(To jabber.)* yegg *(A safe-cracker.)* yellow-bellied you bet *(Certainly.)* yuk *(A loud laugh; expression of disgust.)* yummy yuppie *(Young Upward Professional.)*

Z zip gun *(A homemade pistol.)*

Whether one believes Black English Vernacular (recently dubbed *Ebonics*) to be a dialect of Standard English or a separate language entity, it remains true that B.E.V. has a very special and individual grammar most often associated with many African languages. Since the majority of American blacks grow up speaking B.E.V. and come to American schools speaking B.E.V., it would seem prudent for teachers to readily accept this and communicate to their students a warm and genuine appreciation for this special language presentation. After all, the language of home and parents for any world citizen gives him or her the earliest and deepest appreciation of self and self-worth. Teacher: "Let's not give up our Black English Vernacular, but let's also learn the useful language of business, education, and government, most often called Standard English." A profitable class exercise would be the occasional comparing and contrasting of these two expressional modes.

What are some of the differences? Consider the Shona (spoken in Zimbabwe) sentence, "Vakomana *(boys)* vatatu *(three)* avo *(these)* vakanka *(they good)*." "These three boys, they are good." Observations: 1. No double consonants in one syllable. 2. Plural marker is a prefix. 3. There is subject repetition. 4. No verb for being. 5. No "th" sound. 6. No internal "r". Notice in the following comparison, how these considerations along with others reappear in B.E.V.

A COMPARISON

B.E.V. RULE	STANDARD ENGLISH	BLACK ENGLISH VERNACULAR
Simplify consonant blends:	fact, left, kept, desk, wasp, test, told, land	fac, lef, kep, des, wahs, tes, tol, lan

Note: Only in unvoiced (-ct, -ft, -pt, -sk, -sp, -st) and voiced (-ld, -nd) blends is one consonant dropped. Words ending in a voiced-unvoiced pair are not affected: *milk, help, belt, dump, lunch, link, cent.*

Plurality expressed once:	two boys four cents	two boy four cent

Note: However, if -s remains after a consonant pair is simplified, add -ses for a plural

	desk, desks; test, tests	des, desses; tes, tesses

3rd person singular simplified:	She sees it. He walks fast.	She see it. He walk fas.
Subject repetition; "To be" verb missing:	Joe is late. Mary's gone now.	Joe, he late. Mary, she gone now.
Initial voiced "th" is pronounced /d/:	this, that, those	dis, dat, dose

B.E.V. RULE	STANDARD ENGLISH	BLACK ENGLISH VERNACULAR
Initial unvoiced "th" is pronounced /t/:	thin, think, theme	tin, tink, teem
Medial voiced "th" is pronounced /v/:	brother, breathe	bruvver, breve
Final or medial unvoiced "th" is pronounced /f/:	with, south, bath math, mouth birthday, breath, nothing	wif, souf, baf maf, mouf birfday, bref, nuffin'
-ing becomes -in':	doing, going, sleeping	doin', goin', sleepin'
"r" omitted finally or medially:	door, four, more court, during, terrific	doe, foe, moe coat, du'in', te'ific
i /ī/; /ah-ē/ = /ah/:	I, I'm, right, fight	Ah, Ah'm, raht, faht
/en/ and /in/ both become /in/:	pen, pin men, ten, tin	pin, pin min, tin, tin
Special words:	ask, street	aks, skreet
Some verb forms:	The house is cold The house is usually cold The house is always cold. The house has been cold.	Da house cole. Da house be cole. Da house bees cole. Da house bin cole.

Note: The B.E.V. words given above are spelled phonetically and might not necessarily be spelled that way by a student. In any case, these pronunciation differences can lead to spelling errors in Standard English. Happily, when a student's spelling and pronunciation are accepted as one way of doing things, but is told that we also want to learn the Standard English way too, a student can and will do both. It's called "code switching." A speaker of Black English Vernacular might exhibit only some of the above listed characteristics or incorporate still others. This is only a brief introduction to the subject. The verb forms especially are quite complicated.

The Greeks Had a Word For It!

apheresis	X_____.	(initial drop)	except > 'cept
syncope	____X___.	(medial drop)	terrific > te'ific
apocope	_____X	(final drop)	test > tes'
metathesis	___→←___.	(letter transposition)	ask > aks

It is also common in both Latin and Greek to drop the "to be" verb.

Ap. xiv-2

Most of the languages of Europe seem to stem from a common source, Indo-European, which flourished about 6,000 B.C. No trace remains of this mental construct language, but the similarities of Germanic, Celtic, Latin, Greek, Balto-Slavic, and Indo-Iranian languages attest to its existence. Note these similarities:

Modern Eng.	Old Eng..	German	Dutch	Latin	Greek	Sanskrit
mother	mōdor	mutter	moeder	mater	mētēr	mātr
father	fæder	vater	vader	pater	patēr	pitr

So English, too, must claim Indo-European as its ancestor since English is basically a Germanic language with huge borrowings from Greek and Latin, all of which are family languages from Indo-European. Latin has its own particular family members (Romance Languages): French, Spanish, Italian, Portuguese, and Romanian. Dutch, Norwegian, Swedish, Danish, along with English are Germanic descendants. English has borrowed freely from its cousin languages. The original inhabitants of the British Isles were Celts. Celtic descended directly from Indo-European finally with its own family members of the Irish, Welsh, Highland Scots, Manx, Cornish, and Bretons. Some high points in the development of English with word acquisition examples follow.

The British Celts *bard broach crag gallon tor vassal Avon* (River.) *Dover* (Water.)

55 B.C. Roman invasion led by Julius Caesar. Latin: *Chester Manchester Rochester Winchester Gloucester Leicester;* (chester, cester from *castra* = camp.)

43 B.C. Roman invasion; Tiberius Claudius is emperor in Rome. Thus far Latin had had little influence on the Celtic vernacular.

A. D. 449 Invasion of Jutes, Angles, & Saxons OLD ENGLISH *child work bird father hat earth one eat brown with knee eye weave goat what where hard* (Celtic, except for place and given names, disappears from conquered lands.)

597 St. Augustine, Christian missionary, introduces Greek & Latin church terms: *angel disciple litany martyr mass shrine psalm.*

The Eighth Century poem, **Beowulf**, author unknown, is the most famous remaining literature in Old English. It is unintelligible to the modern, casual English reader because the poem is highly inflected, some vocabulary has dropped from today's language, and today's familar words may not be recognized because of their spellings.

"Hwæt, we Gar-Dena in geardagum, þeodcyninga þrym gefrunon,
hu ða æþelingas ellen fremedon!" [Opening sentence of Beowulf. þ & ð = th.]

"Lo, we have heard of the glory of the Spear-Danes in days past, of the chieftain-kings, how these princes performed valor!"

787   and on. **Viking invasions.** Norse: *bag both bush club ear get happen happy ill take.* Norse and English have common Germanic source, but <u>inflected endings differ</u>. Solution? Drop the endings! This is where English became a much less "inflected" language and came to rely more on word order to indicate the function of a word.

1066 **Norman Conquest** MIDDLE ENGLISH These conquerors, although originally Norse and retaining some Germanic elements in their language, spoke mostly old French (Latin based). They imposed their language on government and business. Latin was used in the church and school. The common people still spoke English. Old French: *companion nation onion pressure property second sturdy.* After 1200 and hostilities with France, English is more widely used. Most famous writer in Middle English: **Geoffrey Chaucer** (1340-1400).

"A Clerk ther was of Oxenford also, That un-to logik hadde longe y-go. As lene was his hors as is a rake, And he nas nat right fat, I undertake; But loked holwe, and ther-to soberly." [The Clerk in Chaucer's <u>The Canterbury Tales</u>.]

"There also was a clerk from Oxford who long ago studied logic, His horse was as lean as a rake and the clerk wasn't very fat either, as I see it; but he looked hollow, and furthermore, sober."

1475 **Printing Introduced in England** by William Caxton (1422-1491). MODERN ENGLISH   Here begins the **English Renaissance.** Spellings become more standardized. The most famous writer in early Modern English was **William Shakespeare** (1564-1616).

"To be, or not to be: that is the question: Whether 'tis nobler in the mind to suffer the slings and arrows of outrageous fortune, or to take arms against a sea of troubles, and by opposing end them?"   [Shakespeare's <u>Hamlet</u>.]

Borrowings from Greek: *anatomy climax dialogue drama comedy paragraph scene theater*

Borrowings from Latin: *education exist industry item major position protest series solid*

Borrowings from French: *casserole corsage garage grotesque machine menu omelet parade*

Scientific words coined from Latin & Greek: *antibiotic protein radio stereophonic television*

That's all folks!

/thăts awl fŏks/

THE LONG VOWEL SONG

Words by Jean Osman & Paula Rome*

Music by Thomas B. Jon

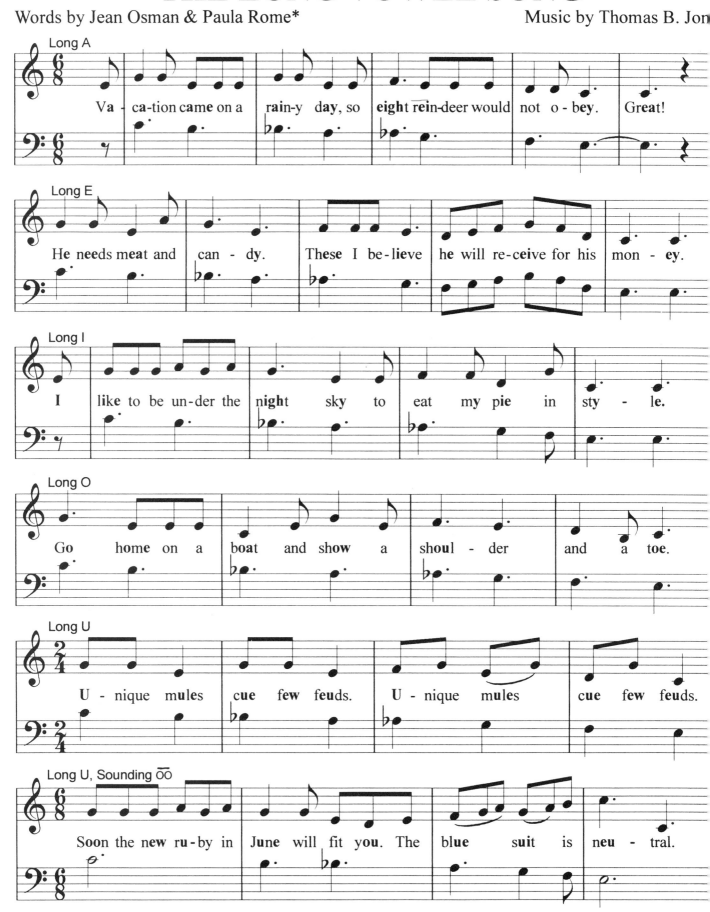

*From **Language Tool Kit,** Educators Publishing Service, Inc.

a	t d ☺	m n	c (hard)
p b ☺	r l	f v ☺ ph	s z ☺
h w	j	k g ☺	i
-ck	qu x	y-	o
e	-ff -ss -zz -ll	-ing -ang -ung -ink -ank -unk	ch sh th wh
a-e e-e i-e o-e u-e y-e	bl- cl- fl- gl- pl- sl- dw- sw- tw-	br- cr- dr- fr- gr- pr- shr- thr- tr- wr-	u

1. a /ă/ (voiced) Test word: **at**
ă (short a) at cat fat bat
ā (long a) ate late mate
ä (ah) father ma calm want

2. t /t/ **d** /d/ ☺
t (unvoiced) at tan tap tax
d (voiced) dad fad had mad

3. m /m/ **n** /n/
m (voiced) am ham mad
n (voiced) an can pan ran
ñ /ny/ cañon mañana

4. c /k/
c (hard; unvoiced)
cab can cap cat

5. p /p/ **b** /b/ ☺
p (unvoiced) pan pal pat
b (voiced) bat bad bag ban

6. r /r/ **l** /l/
r (voiced) ran rap rat ram
l (voiced) lap lab lag lax

7. f /f/ **v** /v/ ☺
f (unvoiced) fad fan fat Fax
v (voiced) van vat

8. s /s/ **z** /z/ ☺
s (unvoiced) sat sad sap
z (voiced) zap zip
s /z/ (voiced) as has his does

9. h /h/ **w** /w/
h (unvoiced) had him hit
w (voiced) wag wax win
(But **h** and **w** are not partners.)

10. j /j/
j (voiced) jam Jan jab
jazz Jack Jill

11. k /k/ **g** /g/ ☺
k (unvoiced) kit kin Kip
g (voiced) gas bag gag lag
nag rag big dig pig

12. i /ĭ/ (voiced) Test word: **it**
ĭ (short i) if in is it did hit
ī (long i) lion side night
i /ē/ (before vowel) radium

13. -ck /k/ (after short vowel)
back deck dock sick sock
hack rock tick wick Jack
Dick Rick kick quick sack

14. qu /kw/ **x** /ks/
qu quit quack quick
quiz quill quell quake
x ax fix six ox box

15. y /y/ (voiced)
y yak yam yap yes yet
you your Yale yank
yell yard yon

16. o /ah/ (voiced) Test word: **ox**
ŏ (short o) box fox mom pop
ō (long o) go no hope note
ô /aw/ dog fog off smog toss

17. e /ĕ/ (voiced) Test word: **Ed**
ĕ (short e) bed get led let
ē (long e) these theme eve
é /ā/ (French) café passé

18. -ff /f/ **-ss** /s/ **-zz** /z/ **-ll** /l/
-ff gaff miff tiff
-ss hiss pass miss less
-zz jazz buzz -ll ill hill

19. sing sang sung
ring rang rung
/ingk/ sink; /angk/ sank;
/ungk/ sunk bunk hunk

20. ch sh th wh
ch chat chill chip chop
sh shall shell ship shop
th that them; wh whip whiz

21. Silent e: a-e /ā/, etc.
at ate hat hate them theme
hid hide twin twine cop cope
not note cut cute; type style

22. -l, -w Blends:
black clap flag
glad plan sling
dwell swim twin

23. -r Blends:
brass crash drill frame
grass press shrink
thrill track write

24. u /ŭ/ (voiced) Test word: **up**
ŭ (short u) but cup cut sun
ū /yōō/ (long u) cube cute
ū /ōō/ (alternate long u) tune

ch j ☺ -tch dge ☺	g (hard) g (soft)	sc– sk– sm– sn– sp– squ– st–	-ct -ft -ld -lk -lp -lt -mp -nch -nd -nt -pt -sk -sp -st
spl- scr- spr- str-	c (hard) c (soft) sc (hard) sc (soft)	-all -oll	ar or -ar -or
ai- -ay	ee	er ir ur	oi- -oy
au- -aw	ou- -ow	oo	oa-
ea	-igh	eigh	ie
ear	-ild -ind -old -ost	eu- -ue -ui- -ew	ei ey

25. **ch j -tch** /ch/ **-dge** /j/
ch /ch/ chin chill chest
j /j/ jam jet job jug Jim
judge badge pitch ditch

26. **g** /g/ **g** /j/
g /g/ gain go gum great
g /j/ (Often before *e, i,* or *y.*)
age gem ginger gym

27. Beginning s- Blends
scale skin smell
snake spell
squish step

28. Ending Blends
fact gift **held** milk **help**
belt lamp **bunch** land
lint kept desk gasp fast

29. **splash split splotch**
scrap scratch script scrub
sprain spring sprout sprawl
strap straw street struck

30. **c** /k/ can cot cup
c /s/ cell cinch cyst
sc /sk/ scale scold scum
sc /s/ scent science scythe

31. **-all** /awl/ **-oll** /ōl/
-all ball call fall hall
small stall tall wall
-oll poll roll stroll toll

32. **ar** /are/ bar barn car card
or /or/ or for form short
-ar /er/ collar dollar
-or /er/ doctor actor

33. **ai-** /ā/ **-ay** /ā/
aid ail aim bait brain chain
gain jail mail paid paint
bay clay day hay may way

34. **ee** /ē/
beef beet bleed creep
deep fee feed feel feet
flee keep knee teen

35. **er** /er/ **ir** /er/ **ur** /er/
er fern germ clerk serve
ir bird birth shirt third
ur blur burn fur turn

36. **oi-** /oi/ **-oy** /oi/
oil boil coil coin join
joint moist soil spoil
boy joy toy destroy

37. **au-** /aw/ **-aw** /aw/
fault haul launch Paul taunt
draw jaw law raw saw
crawl scrawl dawn lawn

38. **ou-** /ow/ **-ow** /ow/
out loud; now cow down
<u>But</u>: /ōō/ youth; /ə/ young;
/ō/ soul; show snow low

39. **oo** /ōō/ **oo** /oo/
oo /ōō/ boot cool food hoop
mood moon pool root spoon
oo /oo/ book cook good took

40. **oa** /ō/
boat coach coal coat
foam goal loaf loan
road soap float boast

41. **ea** /ē/ eat heat each teach
beach beam dream meat neat
/ĕ/ dead bread breath health
<u>Exceptions</u>: /ā/ great steak break

42. **-igh** /ī/
high sigh light might
night right sight tight
fight flight fright bright

43. **eigh** /ā/
"Eight neighbors weigh the
freight on the sleigh."
<u>Exception</u>: height /hīt/

44. **ie** /ē/ /ī/
/ē/ chief field grief piece
shield thief yield believe
/ī/ die lie pie tie

45. **ear**
/er/ earn earth heard learn
/air/ bear pear wear *tear*
/ear/ ear dear fear clear *tear*

46. **-ild** /īld/ child mild wild
-ind /īnd/ bind find kind mind
-old /ōld/ old fold hold told
-ost /ōst/ most /awst/ cost lost

47. **eu- -ue -ui- -ew**
/yōō/ **feud eulogy; cue argue;**
few hew; /ōō/ **neutral Zeus;**
blue true; fruit juice suit

48. **ei** /ā/ vein veil rein their
/ē/ either ceiling receive seize
ey /ā/ they prey hey obey
/ē/ key hockey money valley

gn kn mb mn rh wr	-ly	-ture	-du -tu
-alt -alk	gh- -gh	y- -y- -y	-ed
wa war qua quar	-ough	-sion	-ion
oe wor	augh	-tion	-age

-ial -ian -ient -ious -iate	French: -age é ç ch eau -et
-cial -cian -cient -cious -ciate	-ate -ace
-que -ique -gue -igue	-less -let -ness
-ble -dle -fle -gle -kle -ple -stle -zle	ar-r er-r ar-v er-v

52. gn, kn, mb, mn rh, wr
gnash **gn**aw **kn**ee **kn**ife
li**mb** co**mb** autu**mn** colu**mn**
rhyme **rh**ythm **wr**ite **wr**ist

51. -alt /awlt/, **-alk** /awk/
-alt halt malt salt exalt
-alk talk walk chalk stalk

50. wa /wä/ wash want
war /wor/ ward warn
qua /kwä/ quality quantity
quar /kwor/ quart quarter

49. oe /ō/ foe hoe toe
Joe oboe Monroe Poe
wor /wer/ word work
world worm worse worth

56. -ly /lē/ [Forms adverb.]
closely costly daily deadly
fairly freely friendly fully
gladly kindly lately softly

55. gh- /g/, **-gh** /f/
gh- /g/ ghost ghastly ghetto
-gh /f/ enough rough tough
cough laugh

54. ough /aw/ bought thought
ough /ō/ dough though furlough
ough /ow/ bough drought plough
ough /əf/ enough rough tough

53. augh /aw/
caught taught daughter
haughty naughty
slaughter distraught

60. -ture /cher/
capture culture fixture
future lecture mixture
moisture nature picture

59. y- /y/ [consonant] yes yet
-y- [vowel] /i/ gym myth bicycle
-y- [vowel] /ī/ hyphen type style
-y [vowel] /ī/ dry my; /ē/ history

58. -sion /shən/ tension mission
admission depression pension
-sion /zhən/ confusion division
occasion version vision

57. -tion /shən/ action caution
fiction mention option infection
-ation nation notation citation
-ition addition ambition tuition

64. -du /jo͞o/ educate gradual
graduate individual residual
-tu /cho͞o/ actual fortune
fluctuate habitual statue

63. -ed /id/ /t/ /d/
/id/ [after t & d] acted pointed added
/t/ [after other unvoiced] asked fixed
/d/ [after other voiced] armed banged

62. -ion /yən/
million billion trillion
onion companion opinion
rebellion union reunion

61. -age /ij/
damage dosage drainage
garbage hostage luggage
message package sausage

68. -ial /ē-əl/ material trivial
-ian /ē-ən/ guardian; **-ient** /ē-ənt/
lenient; **-ious** /ē-əs/ tedious;
-iate /ē-āt/ radiate deviate

67. -cial /shəl/ partial; **-cian** /shən/
musician, **-cient** /shənt/ ancient;
-cious /shəs/ atrocious delicious;
-ciate /shē-āt/ associate

66. -que /k/ plaque opaque
-ique /ēk/ critique unique
-gue /g/ league tongue vague
-igue/ēg/ fatigue intrigue

65. table cradle rifle
bugle maple title needle
pickle apple battle dazzle
tumble handle jungle purple

72.French: -age /äzh/ garage corsage
é /ā/ café décor; ç /s/ façade;
ch /sh/ chef machine; **eau** /ō/ beau
plateau; **-et** /ā/ ballet buffet

71. -ate /āt/ [v] donate rotate
-ate /it/ [n] climate senate
-ace /ās/ [v & n] face place
-ace /is/ [n. only] palace

70. -less /lis/ **-let** /lit/ **-ness** /nis/
careless endless flawless timeless
anklet booklet bracelet leaflet
clearness deafness goodness

69. ar-r /air/ arrow carry marry
er-r /air/ berry cherry merry
ar-V /air/ care Carol Mary Paris
er-V (Not e) /air/ merit America

BIBLIOGRAPHY

*Other presentations of material and rules; [+]Contains workbook material.

Algeo, John and Pyles, Thomas. *The Origins and Development of the English Language.* New York, NY: Harcourt Brace Jovanovich College Publishers, 1993.

*[+]Anderson, Wilson C. *VAK Tasks for Vocabulary and Spelling.* Cambridge, MA: Educators Publishing Service, Inc., 1987.

Aronoff, Mark and Dobrovolsky, Michael and O'Grady, William. *Contemporary Linguistics, An Introduction.* New York, NY: St. Martin's Press, 1989.

Biehler, E. *Shona Dictionary.* Capetown, South Africa: Longmans, Green, & Co. LTD

*Bliss, Barbara A. *Understanding & Using the Orton-Gillingham Approach To Teaching Reading & Spelling.* Madison, WI: Barbara Bliss, 1993.

*Blumenfeld, Samuel L. *Alpha-Phonics (A Primer for Beginning Readers),* Boise, ID: The Paradigm Co., 1993.

Borror, Donald J. *Dictionary of Word Roots and Combining Forms.* Mountain View, CA: Mayfield Publishing Co., 1960.

*[+]Bowen, Carolyn C. *Angling For Words.* Novato, CA: Academic Therapy Publications, 1972.

Claiborne, Robert. *Our Marvelous Native Tongue.* New York, NY: Times Books, 1983.

Dandy, Evelyn B. *Black Communications: Breaking Down the Barriers.* Chicago, IL: African American Images, 1991.

Dillard. J. L. *Black English, Its History and Usage in the United States.* New York, NY: Vintage Books, 1973.

Dorland's Illustrated Medical Dictionary. Philadelphia: W. B. Saunders Co., 1988.

*[+]Engelmann, Siegfried. *Distar Language: An Instructional System.* Chicago, IL: Science Research Associates, 1976.

Finegan, Edward. *Language, Its Structure and Use.* New York, NY: Harcourt Brace & Co., 1994.

Fowler's Modern English Usage. R. W. Burchfield, ed. Oxford, England:: Clarendon Press.

*Fry, Edward B. and Fountoukidis, Dona Lee and Rolk, Jacqueline K. *The New Reading Teacher's Book, of Lists.* Englewood Cliffs, NJ: Prentice-Hall, Inc., 1985.

Funk & Wagnalls Standard College Dictionary. New York, NY: Funk & Wagnalls, 1973.

Galvin, Herman and Tamarkin, Stan. *The Yiddish Dictionary Sourcebook.* Hoboken, NJ: KTAV Publishing House, Inc. 1986.

*Gillingham, Anna and Stillman, Bessie W. *Remedial Training for Children with Specific Disability in Reading, Spelling, and Penmanship.* Cambridge, MA: Educators Publishing Service, Inc., 1987.

*[+]Green, Victoria E. and Enfield, Mary Lee. *Project Read Lesson Plans (Grades 1, 2, 3, 4); Phonology Guide.* Bloomington, MN: Language Circle Enterprise, 1990.

*[+]Hall, Nancy and Price, Rena. *Explode the Code.* Cambridge, MA: Educators Publishing Service, Inc. 1990.

*[+]Henry, Marcia K. *Words (Integrated Decoding and Spelling Instruction Based on Word Origin and Word Structure).* Los Gatos, CA: Lex Press, 1990.

*+Johnson, Kristin and Bayrd, Polly. *Megawords, Multisyllabic Words for Reading, Spelling, and Vocabulary.* Cambridge, MA: Educators Pub. Service, Inc. 1986.

Karnow, Stanley. *Vietnam, A History.* New York, NY: Penguin Books, 1983.

Kennedy, John. *A Stem Dictionary of the English Language.* Detroit, MI: Gale Research Co., 1971.

*+Kleiber, Margaret H. *Specific Language Training.* Bronx, NY: Decatur Enterprises, 1993.

Ladefoged, Peter. *A Course In Phonetics.* New York: Harcourt Brace Jovanovich, 1975.

Langenscheidt's New Pocket German Dictionary. Berlin, Ger.: Langenscheidt KG, 1970.

Levine, Harold. *Vocabulary for the College-Bound Student.* New York, NY: Amsco School Publications, Inc., 1965.

Liddell and Scott's Greek-English Lexicon (Abridged). Oxford, England: Oxford University Press, 1990.

Liles, Bruce L. *A Basic Grammar of Modern English.* Englewood Cliffs, NJ: Prentice-Hall Inc., 1987.

Machan, Tim William and Scott, Charles T., Editors. *English In Its Social Contexts, Essays in Historical Sociolinguistics.* New York: Oxford University Press, 1992.

Mansion's Shorter French and English Dictionary. Boston, MA: D. C. Heath and Co., 1965.

Marckwardt, Albert and Cassidy, Frederic. *Scribner Handbook of English.* New York, NY: Charles Scribner's Sons, 1967.

McCrum, Robert and Cran, William and MacNeil, Robert. *The Story of English.* New York, NY: Viking Penguin Inc., 1986.

Merriam-Webster's Collegiate Dictionary. Springfield, MA: Merriam-Webster, Inc., 1993.

Myers, Patricia I. and Hammill, Donald D. *Learning Disabilities (Basic Concepts, Assessment Practices, and Instructional Strategies).* Austin, TX: Pro-Ed, 1990.

New Dictionary of the Portuguese and English Languages. H. Michaelis, editor. New York, NY: Frederick Unger Pub., 1955.

Oxford English Dictionary. Oxford, England: Clarendon Press, 1989.

Oxford Latin Dictionary. P.G.W. Glare, editor. London: Oxford University Press, 1976.

*+Rak, Elsie T. *Spellbound (Phonic Reading and Spelling).* Cambridge, MA: Educators Publishing Service, Inc., 1977.

*Rome, Paula D. and Osman, Jean S. *Language Tool Kit.* Cambridge, MA: Educators Publishing Service, Inc., 1985.

Shipley, Joseph T. *Dictionary of Word Origins.* New York, NY: Philosophical Library, 1945.

Simpson, D. P. *Cassell's Latin Dictionary.* New York: MacMillan Publishing Co., 1968.

Smitherman, Geneva. *Talkin and Testifyin, The Language of Black America.* Detroit, MI: Wayne State University Press, 1985.

Velázquez Spanish and English Dictionary. Piscataway, NJ: New Century Pub., 1985.

Webster's Third New International Dictionary. Springfield, MA: G. & E. Merriam Co., 1968.

Wolfram, Walt and Johnson, Robert. *Phonological Analysis, Focus on American English.* Englewood Cliffs, NJ: Prentice Hall Regents, 1982.